Socioeconomics of Surgery

Socioeconomics of Surgery

Ira M. Rutkow, MD, MPH, DrPH

Clinical Associate Professor of Surgery
University of Medicine
and Dentistry of New Jersey
Newark, New Jersey

with **22** illustrations

The C. V. Mosby Company
ST. LOUIS • BALTIMORE • TORONTO   1989

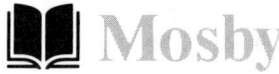

Editor: Terry Van Schaik
Assistant Editor: Patricia L. Gregory
Project Manager: Teri Merchant
Production Editor: Betty Hazelwood
Design: Liz Fett

Copyright © 1989 by The C.V. Mosby Company

All rights reserved. No part of this publication may be reproduced, stored in a retrieval system, or transmitted, in any form or by any means, electronic, mechanical, photocopying, recording, or otherwise, without prior written permission from the publisher.

Printed in the United States of America
The C.V. Mosby Company
11830 Westline Industrial Drive, St. Louis, Missouri 63146

Library of Congress Cataloging-in-Publication Data

Socioeconomics of surgery / [edited by] Ira M. Rutkow.
    p.   cm.
  Includes bibliographies and index.
  ISBN 0-8016-4306-6
  1. Surgery—economic aspects—United States. 2. Surgery—United States. I. Rutkow, Ira M.
  [DNLM: 1. Delivery of health care—United States. 2. Health policy—economics—United States. 3. Surgery—United States. WO 100 S678]
RD27.42.S63   1989
362.1'970973—dc19   88-13140
DNLM/DLC
TS/MV/MV 9 8 7 6 5 4 3 2 1

Contributors

Michael A. Ashworth, MB
Department of Surgery, Queens University,
Kingston, Ontario, Canada

Oliver H. Beahrs, MD
Professor of Surgery, Emeritus,
Department of Surgery, Mayo Clinic,
Rochester, Minnesota

Dorothy J. Buchanan-Davidson, PhD
University of Wisconsin-Madison, School of
Nursing,
Madison, Wisconsin

John P. Bunker, MD
Professor, Departments of Health Research and
Policy and Anesthesia,
Stanford University Medical School,
Stanford, California

Thomas C. Chalmers, MD
Technology Assessment Group,
Harvard School of Public Health,
Boston, Massachusetts

John R. Clarke, MD
Professor, Department of Surgery,
Medical College of Pennsylvania,
Philadelphia, Pennsylvania

Don E. Detmer, MD
Vice President Health Sciences,
University of Virginia School of Medicine,
Charlottesville, Virginia

William R. Drucker, MD
Professor, Department of Surgery, Uniformed
Services University of the Health Sciences,
Bethesda, Maryland

Paul A. Ebert, MD
Director, American College of Surgeons,
Chicago, Illinois

Sal Fiscina, MD, JD
George Washington University,
Law and Medical Schools,
Washington, D.C.

J. William Gavett, MME, PhD
Professor Emeritus, Department of
Preventive Medicine and Community Health,
University of Rochester Medical Center,
Rochester, New York

Brigid Goody, MBA, MPH
John F. Kennedy School of Government,
Harvard University,
Cambridge, Massachusetts

Darryl T. Gray, MD, MPH
Technology Assessment Group,
Harvard School of Public Health,
Boston, Massachusetts

Ward O. Griffen, Jr., MD, PhD
Executive Director/Secretary-Treasurer,
American Board of Surgery,
Philadelphia, Pennsylvania

Lynn R. Gruber, JD
InterStudy,
Excelsior, Minnesota

Susan Hartwell, MS
InterStudy,
Excelsior, Minnesota

Peg Hewitt, MS
Technology Assessment Group,
Harvard School of Public Health,
Boston, Massachusetts

Susan D. Horn, PhD
Professor, Department of Health Policy
and Management,
The Johns Hopkins School of Hygiene and
Public Health,
Baltimore, Maryland

Barry M. Manuel, MD
Associate Dean, Administration Department,
Boston University School of Medicine,
Boston, Massachusetts

Charles K. McSherry, MD
Professor, Department of Surgery,
Mount Sinai School of Medicine,
New York, New York

Francis D. Moore, MD
Moseley Professor of Surgery, Emeritus,
Department of Surgery, Harvard Medical School,
Boston, Massachusetts

Eric Munoz, MD, MBA
Dean's Office,
University of Medicine and Dentistry
of New Jersey,
Newark, New Jersey

Cynthia L. Polich, MA
InterStudy,
Excelsior, Minnesota

Leslie L. Roos, PhD
Professor, Departments of Business Administration
and Community Health Sciences,
University of Manitoba,
Winnipeg, Manitoba
Canada

Noralou P. Roos, PhD
Professor, Departments of Business Administration
and Community Health Sciences,
University of Manitoba,
Winnipeg, Manitoba
Canada

Ira M. Rutkow, MD, MPH, DrPH
Department of Surgery, University of Medicine and
Dentistry of New Jersey,
Newark, New Jersey

Ralph W. Schaffarzick, MD
Blue Shield of California,
San Francisco, California

Mark Schlesinger, PhD
John F. Kennedy School of Government,
Harvard University, Cambridge, Massachusetts

Steven Sieverts, MS
Blue Cross and Blue Shield of the National
Capital Area,
Washington, D.C.

John E. Wennberg, MD, MPH
Professor of Epidemiology, Department of
Community and Family Medicine,
Dartmouth Medical School,
Hanover, New Hampshire

IRA M. RUTKOW

Ira M. Rutkow was born in Newark and raised in Springfield, NJ. He received his undergraduate degree (1970) at Union College (New York). His medical degree was obtained at Saint Louis University School of Medicine (1975). Dr. Rutkow took the first two years of his general surgical training at Boston University—Boston City Hospital Medical Center. From 1977 through 1980 he served as a surgical resident and research fellow at the Johns Hopkins Medical Institutions. While there he was a Robert Wood Johnson Clinical Scholar and an Edwin L. Crosby Memorial Fellow of the Hospital Research and Educational Trust. In addition, he received the degrees of master of public health (1978) and doctor of public health (1981) from the Johns Hopkins School of Hygiene and Public Health. Dr. Rutkow completed his general surgical training at the University of Medicine and Dentistry of New Jersey (Newark) in 1982. Currently he is surgical director of The Hernia Centers of Manhattan and New Jersey. He also serves as clinical associate professor of surgery at the University of Medicine and Dentistry of New Jersey. Dr. Rutkow is a diplomate of the American Board of Surgery and a fellow of the American College of Surgeons. His other major research interests are the study of eighteenth, nineteenth, and early twentieth century American surgery and the editing of William Halsted's personal correspondence.

To my wife *Beth* and children *Lainie* and *Eric* I dedicate this volume. You have provided me with all the love, patience, and support that any husband and father could possibly ask for. Without your enthusiasm and sustenance I would accomplish little.

To my parents *Bea* and *Al Rutkow* this work stands as testimony to your conviction in my education. Your fostering of a love for intellectual endeavors and the sacrifices that you made will never be forgotten.

Preface

This volume is written for a wide spectrum of individuals, including surgeons, other physicians, medical students, nurses, health care delivery researchers and analysts, public health planners, hospital administrators, executives and other workers within the health care industry, politicians, and members of legislative staffs. Any person who daily confronts the many pressing issues in the delivery of surgical health care in the United States should be able to find material of interest in this book.

It is estimated that by the twenty-first century national health care expenditures will total almost 15% of our country's gross national product. Therefore economic reality dictates that efforts to promote cost effectiveness must continue. Because almost half of all adult nonmaternity hospital admissions involve diagnostic and/or therapeutic surgical procedures, it would be anticipated that many of these cost-controlling endeavors will be directed at the surgeon.

As Bosk points out in his 1979 book *Forgive and remember: managing medical failure:*

> The very features of surgery that make surgeons 'heroes' from one point of view at one point in time and that make them symbols of corruption, mendacity, and greed from another point of view at another time are the very features that make surgeons so well suited to serve as subjects. . . . These features are the precise and definitive nature of surgical intervention—its visibility, the expectation of success that surrounds this intervention, and the relatively short time frame in which outcomes are known. All of these make surgeons more accountable than their colleagues in other specialties.

Surgical therapy appears ideally suited for socioeconomic research because of its discretion, accomplishments, and costs. Now and in the future, the public and representatives from industry, labor, and the government will demand to know how their surgical health care dollars are spent. More important, they will want to be assured that the quality of their surgical care is "the best that money can buy."

In the past, the surgeon's primary interest revolved around the art and science of surgery, whereas the socioeconomic issues that affected medical and surgical health care were deemed of secondary importance. Consequently, little of the research concerning delivery of surgical health care has been conducted by surgeons. When I graduated from medical school in 1975, I wanted to combine a general surgical residency with some type of training in public health and policy formation. Unfortunately, there were no surgeons at my institution able to provide any guidance toward reaching my goal. One of the surgical faculty even went so far as to write in my letter of recommendation:

> He has a notion of finding his place in the world by combining surgery and public health. I have not been able to come to a good clear appraisal myself as to exactly how this will qualify him for a productive career in surgery despite several lengthy discussions.

Certainly, priorities have changed. As Vayda pointed out in his *New England Journal of Medicine* article (1973) comparing surgical rates in Canada and England and Wales:

> ... further socioeconomic research must be performed by investigators who do surgery and understand its many difficulties.

At present, no area of scientific investigation is more intricate, intriguing, and imperative than that involving our health care delivery system. Such research combines all the disparate elements of a mystery by Poe, a novel by Melville, and a poem by Whitman. It is my belief that surgeons must become actively involved in research on surgical health services and assume leadership roles in this growing and important field. Their continued passivity will only lead to ever greater restrictions on the practice of surgery.

Unfortunately, it is the rare surgeon in the United States who has additional formal education in areas such as business administration, economics, sociology, or health care policy formation. This lack of a critical mass of surgeons who share an interdisciplinary approach to surgical health care is among the surgical community's major research failures. Without such expertise, it becomes difficult to formulate pragmatic and efficacious public policy.

Because many of the investigations into the economic impact of surgical services are published in journals not read by the surgeon, it is difficult for the active practitioner to be aware of the dynamic areas of the discipline. There is also a distressing total lack of information in surgical textbooks on health care delivery. Finally, major surgical organizations have shown little real interest in providing national forums for discussion of socioeconomic issues.

To help alleviate some of these concerns, this volume brings together a large number of well-known researchers in the area of surgical health services. This is done with the hope of stimulating greater interest in research on the socioeconomics of United States surgical health care. More important, this text is meant to serve as an in-depth and collective source of information on all facets of surgical health care delivery. Perhaps surgeons will be stimulated to take a more active role in the formulation of future work in surgical health services research.

The book is divided into five sections. Each chapter is constructed to provide a substantial amount of information on a particular topic. They are meant to stand on their own and should be read accordingly.

The work is purposely intended to be comprehensive and encyclopedic in nature. The 1200 references are indicative of this goal. Accordingly, both a subject and author's indexes are provided. The material is current through late spring 1988. Because the socioeconomic conditions of health care in the United States change so rapidly, both the C.V. Mosby Company and I have made certain that the work has been published in an expeditious fashion.

The book encompasses a wide range of topics, each focusing on an important facet of the socioeconomics of surgery and surgeons. The book should provide a more comprehensive picture of the surgical delivery system and its providers than is available elsewhere in a single volume.

Certain caveats must be mentioned. It is not expected that any reader will agree with every author's opinions. In providing the authors with editorial guidelines, I suggested that a complete review of the literature must be included as well as a substantial list of references. The book is not intended to present pro and con arguments over each topic in surgical health care. To do so would have yielded an unwieldy tome. Instead, it is designed to stimulate the reader to appreciate the various areas that are currently being researched. Although individuals might totally disagree with the presentation of a chapter, they should be able to arrive at additional conclusions by reading some of the given references.

In order to assure a collective depth of research and clinical skills, I have deliberately included both surgeons and nonphysician authors.

In this way, the volume should appeal not only to the medical profession but also to other persons who must administer or formulate surgical policy.

Some discussions of the inefficiency and lack of quality of surgical care will seem familiar. They are encountered daily in the nation's newspapers and lay press. There are no easy solutions, and those who assume that all the ills can be corrected in a painless fashion do not understand the depth of the many problems. However, this work is an attempt to facilitate our economic and sociologic understanding of surgery and surgeons. It is designed to clarify our thinking about surgical health care. Whether any of its many proposals ever become accepted health care dogma is not important. Instead, its mission will be achieved by lifting the collective conscience of the surgical community, the medical profession, and the lay public to better understand the problems that surround surgical health care delivery.

In conclusion, the discussions in this book should create an atmosphere that provides a series of approaches that prove of continued value in reaching solutions for the betterment of the surgical health in our nation. It is evident that many chapters will soon be outmoded or in need of much revision. Such is the stage on which United States' health care is being conducted. In the end, it is hoped this volume will contribute in multiple ways to the design of future surgical health services research and to our understanding of socioeconomic issues as they relate to the surgeon.

Ira M. Rutkow
September 13, 1988

ACKNOWLEDGMENTS

I wish to express my sincerest appreciation to the staff of the C.V. Mosby Company for their farsightedness in allowing me to bring this book to fruition—to Jerry Freeland for his understanding of the importance of such a work, to Thomas Manning for providing it an existence, to Terry Van Schaik for her editorial guidance, and to Betty Hazelwood for her manuscript editing. In addition, a special personal thank you to all the individual contributors. Your expertise and excellence in health services research are what make this volume so valuable.

Contents

Part One Surgical Demographics

1. Surgical Operations and Manpower: Can Technical Proficiency be Maintained? 3
   IRA M. RUTKOW

2. Ambulatory Surgery, 30
   DON E. DETMER
   DOROTHY J. BUCHANAN-DAVIDSON

3. Socioeconomic and Practice Characteristics, 51
   IRA M. RUTKOW

4. Small Area Variations and the Practice Style Factor, 66
   JOHN E. WENNBERG

5. Determining the Rates of Surgical Operations, 93
   IRA M. RUTKOW

Part Two Delivery and Financing of Surgical Services

6. Impact of Diagnosis Related Groups and the Prospective Payment Assessment Commission, 108
   ERIC MUNOZ

7. Adjusting DRGs for Severity of Illness, 132
   SUSAN D. HORN
   MICHAEL A. ASHWORTH

8. Reimbursement in the Future: the Physician Payment Review Commission, 142
   OLIVER H. BEAHRS

9. Regionalized Surgical Health Care, 154
   RALPH W. SCHAFFARZICK
   JOHN P. BUNKER

10. The Impact of Managed Health Care Systems on Surgeons, 164
    LYNN R. GRUBER
    SUSAN HARTWELL
    CYNTHIA L. POLICH

11. For-profit Health Care and the Practice of Surgery, 182
    MARK SCHLESINGER
    BRIGID GOODY

12. Surgical Second Opinion Programs, 200
    IRA M. RUTKOW
    STEVEN SIEVERTS

Part Three Quality of Surgical Care

13. Quality Assurance and Utilization Review, 216
    CHARLES K. McSHERRY

14. The Evaluation of Surgical Therapies, 228
    DARRYL T. GRAY
    PEG HEWITT
    THOMAS C. CHALMERS

15. Large Databases and Research on Surgery, 258
    LESLIE L. ROOS
    NORALOU P. ROOS

16. The High-cost Surgical Patient, 276
    WILLIAM R. DRUCKER
    J. WILLIAM GAVETT

17. Commercial Constraints on Surgical Quality, 298
    FRANCIS D. MOORE

18. Implications of Federal Legislation for Surgical Practice, 306
    PAUL A. EBERT

Part Four Legal and Ethical Issues in Surgery

19 Clinical Surgical Decision Making, 314
    JOHN R. CLARKE

20 Unnecessary Surgery, 333
    IRA M. RUTKOW

21 Surgical Education and Certification Requirements, 352
    WARD O. GRIFFEN, JR.

22 The Malpractice Crisis and the Surgeon, 368
    BARRY M. MANUEL

23 The Surgeon in Court, 386
    SAL FISCINA

Part Five Summary

24 Recommendations: a Personal Perspective, 401
    IRA M. RUTKOW

PART ONE

Surgical Demographics

1. SURGICAL OPERATIONS AND MANPOWER: CAN TECHNICAL PROFICIENCY BE MAINTAINED?
   Ira M. Rutkow
2. AMBULATORY SURGERY
   Don E. Detmer
   Dorothy J. Buchanan-Davidson
3. SOCIOECONOMIC AND PRACTICE CHARACTERISTICS
   Ira M. Rutkow
4. SMALL AREA VARIATIONS AND THE PRACTICE STYLE FACTOR
   John E. Wennberg
5. DETERMINING THE RATES OF SURGICAL OPERATIONS
   Ira M. Rutkow

1

Surgical Operations and Manpower: Can Technical Proficiency Be Maintained?

IRA M. RUTKOW

During the past 20 years there have been extraordinary socioeconomic changes relative to the practice of medicine.[38] This has been especially true for all branches of surgery as reflected by vociferous debate about unnecessary surgery, quality assurance, surgical second opinion programs, and other consumer-related topics.* A dominant societal belief is that surgical operative rates in the United States show steady yearly increases, which suggests that an excessive number of surgical procedures are done. It is assumed that surgeons can create need for their services merely by moving into a given community.

These are difficult problems for the profession to address. The imprecision of indications for surgery usually is sufficient to prevent a clear determination of whether surgeons in this country operate too often. Whether too many surgeons are being trained and what constitutes an appropriate operative caseload for both an individual surgeon and a given society are vigorously debated. Within this discussion looms the overall questions of technical proficiency and quality of total surgical care. Will future surgeons in an extremely competitive environment be able to deliver efficient, competent, and skillful services?

To answer these questions, this chapter contains an analysis of operative rate data from 1970 to 1985, with particular attention to the years 1970 to 1974 and 1979 to 1985. In addition, attempts to quantify and determine appropriate manpower levels are reviewed. Last, scenarios regarding concerns about future technical proficiency and overall surgical health care delivery are proposed.

OPERATIVE RATE DATA

Since 1965 the National Center for Health Statistics (NCHS) through its National Hospital Discharge Survey (NHDS) compiled data on the number of operations performed annually in the United States. This information is from patients' medical records of an approximate 5% to 8% national sample of short-stay general and specialty noninstitutional hospitals, exclusive of military and Veterans Administration facilities.[33,34]

Before 1979 the International Classification of Diseases, 8th Revision, Adapted for use in the United States (ICDA-8) was used by short-stay hospitals in the country as the primary system for

---
*References 5, 12, 36, 40, 41.

coding diagnoses and procedures on their patients. Since 1979 the International Classification of Diseases, 9th Revision, Clinical Modification (ICD-9-CM) has been used. It allows for greater detail in a hospital's reporting of its surgical operative caseload. An extensive list of the types of operations listed in the NHDS can be found in several federal government publications.[33,34] In general, minor surgical operations and other procedures, such as termination of pregnancy, vasectomy, angioplasty, cystoscopy, and cardiac catheterization, are not included in the report.

Through a complex system of weighting measures, the sample NHDS data are expanded to produce national estimates by age and sex of the absolute number of operations performed in any given year. As in all surveys, results are subject to both nonsampling and sampling errors. Accordingly, approximate relative standard errors of estimated numbers of procedures are as follows: 10,000 operations, 18%; 100,000 operations, 11%; 1,000,000 operations, 7% and 10,000,000 operations, 5%.

To analyze surgical manpower, numbers of surgical operations were linked with numbers of physicians who perform those operations. To accomplish this, the American Medical Association's (AMA) annual publication Physician Characteristics and Distribution in the United States (PCD) was consulted. The PCD is derived from a physician masterfile that is started on each physician on admission into medical school or, in the case of foreign and Canadian graduates, on entry into the country. As a physician's training and career develop information is added to the file, including a self-designation of primary and secondary specialty. Participating in this self-labeling process are both board-certified and noncertified surgeons, and perhaps even general practitioners who consider themselves surgeons. What is not known is how many of the total numbers of surgeons are actually doing surgery and how many are, for instance, retired or in administrative roles or fellowships. However, if the same data source is used for all years in the study, there should be little distortion of the figures. The AMA also maintains yearly totals of individual surgical residents on duty.

The raw NHDS data were analyzed by studying more than 3000 ICDA-8 and ICD-9-CM procedure subheadings to distinguish actual operations from nonsurgical entries. Special emphasis was then placed on determining each specialty's most frequently performed surgical procedures. This was conducted for the years 1979, 1981, 1983, and 1985. The surgical specialties include (with ICD-9-CM rubrics in parentheses): neurosurgery (01-05); otolaryngology (18-22, 25-31); cardiothoracic (32-39); general surgery (06, 07, 38-54, 85, 86); urology (55-64); obstetrics and gynecology (65-71, 74); and orthopedics (77-84). Ophthalmology is not included, and plastic surgery could not be individually studied because it has no separate ICD-9-CM codes.

A few caveats must be introduced when 1980s' operative numbers are analyzed. A surgical operation counted in a particular specialty does not necessarily mean that all or nearly all of those operations were performed by members of that specialty. For example, there is considerable overlap between orthopedic surgery and neurosurgery regarding back surgery, and osteopathic surgeons are not included. Second, some procedures, although listed under a surgical specialty, are performed by nonsurgeons. Examples of this include family practitioners who practice general and obstetric-gynecologic surgery and podiatrists who perform orthopedic operations. However, the general practitioner who does surgery and the nonspecialty trained physician who considers himself a surgeon are having decreasing impact on surgical health care.

Beginning in 1983, I noticed trends for certain specialties that indicate an increasing impact resulting from the ambulatory surgical movement on validity of the NHDS and its ability to generate surgical rate data. In most instances, the NHDS includes inpatient procedures only. However, a gray area does appear in that some outpatient cases are being counted as inpatient cases. This occurs because the definitions of inpatient and outpatient vary among hospitals. For instance, a patient is admitted to a hospital in the morning, undergoes an inguinal herniorrhaphy, and is discharged later that afternoon. Is that an inpatient or an outpatient surgical operation? The patient occupied a hospital bed but did not stay overnight. At present, there is no way of determining how many actual hospital-based outpatient cases are included in the NHDS.

Another type of outpatient facility is the free-standing surgical unit. Before the 1980s there were few such surgical centers, and most operations were done on inpatients. Consequently, the ability of the NHDS to generate data that reflected "all" operative surgery in the nation's hospitals (excluding VA and military facilities) was possible. Unfortunately that is no longer the case. It is estimated that there are almost 800 free-standing surgical centers. In addition, there is a growing trend by surgeons to perform a range of operations such as dilation and curretage of the uterus and cosmetic repairs in their offices. If the NHDS is to maintain its overall validity it will need to extend its data base to include hospital-based outpatient as well as inpatient surgical operations and maintain distinction between the two. Provisions must be made also to incorporate surgical operations performed in free-standing units and physicians' offices.

On a practical level this inability to delineate outpatient surgical procedures is most obvious when numbers of certain operations are examined. For instance, in 1979, 579,000 inguinal hernia repairs were done. This level remained constant through 1984. In 1985, according to the NHDS, only 476,000 inguinal herniorrhaphies were done. The reason for the large decrease was that surgeons were beginning to perform more herniorrhaphies on outpatients, who are not included in the NHDS report.

For the specialties of otorhinolaryngology and ophthalmology this outpatient effect is substantial. According to the NHDS, the number of cataract extractions decreased from 630,000 in 1983 to 212,000 in 1985. For other specialties (general surgery, obstetric-gynecologic surgery, and urologic surgery) the decrease is moderate. Outpatient surgery has had little effect on thoracic and cardiovascular surgery, and neurosurgery. The use of arthroscopic procedures is the primary influence on the number of outpatient orthopedic procedures. I estimate that 10% to 15% of the country's total surgical operations, as defined for this book, are being done on an outpatient basis. Undoubtedly, this will increase substantially during the coming years.

It should be emphasized that even with the shift toward outpatient surgery, there is no reason to expect drastic changes in the number of surgical procedures done yearly in the United States. It merely suggests that the manner in which surgical health care is being delivered has been altered. In fact, if numbers of surgical procedures that can be performed only on an inpatient basis are analyzed, for example, cholecystectomy, appendectomy, mastectomy, colostomy, hysterectomy, cystocele-rectocele repair, and prostatectomy, it is noted that few of these operations have shown an increase during the past decade.

In 1970, 11,984,000 surgical operations were reported in the NHDS for seven surgical specialties (general surgery, obstetric and gynecologic surgery, orthopedic surgery, urologic surgery, ENT surgery, thoracic and cardiovascular surgery, and neurosurgery). In 1974 this had increased 25% to 14,948,000. During this 5-year period there was an 8% increase in the number of surgeons in six of these specialties (58,378 in 1970; 62,801 in 1974). Figures for thoracic and cardiovascular surgery were not available. In 1970 there was a total of 13,979 residents clinically active in the seven surgical specialties. In 1974 the number had increased by 16% to 16,164.

In 1979, 16,223,000 surgical procedures were reported by the NHDS for the seven surgical specialties. There was a decrease to 16,050,000 surgical procedures in 1985. This represents a change of less than 1%. It should be remembered that the effect of outpatient surgery was now present in the NHDS data base. During this 7-year period there was a 25% increase in the total number of surgeons (85,136 in 1979; 106,324 in 1985). In 1979 the seven specialties had 17,727 residents on duty. By 1985 this had increased by 5% to 18,657 residents. Although there was spectacular growth in numbers of surgical procedures during the 1960s and early 1970s, it is apparent that numbers of operations and cases per surgeon have significantly decreased during the past 5 to 10 years.

The first table of each appendix provides detailed information on each specialty's most frequently performed surgical procedures, and rankings of the 50 most common inpatient surgical procedures in the United States in 1985. In addition, the second table of each appendix shows the total operations, surgeons, and residents on duty for each specialty for the periods 1970 to 1974 and 1979 to 1985.

DATA RELIABILITY

Reliability of data must be ascertained in any report of the frequency of surgical operations. Currently there are numerous national data systems providing surgical discharge information, including the NCHS' NHDS, the American Hospital Association National Hospital Panel Survey, the Professional Activity Study of the Commission on Professional and Hospital Activities, and the Professional Review Organization Hospital Discharge Data System of the Health Care Financing Administration. Reports comparing the reliability of these systems have shown general agreement when the number of operative procedures is estimated.[21]

To assure reliability, the researcher's use of the same system consistently is as important as the data source itself. With the use of the same data source over an extended time the researcher can observe long-term trends and comparisons.

Accordingly, because I had previously used NHDS data, they were again surveyed.[37-52]

One of the major drawbacks of ICD-9-CM data is difficulty with the actual codes. For instance, in Table 1-1 the third most common general surgical operation is lysis of peritoneal adhesions. Primary operations for lysis of peritoneal adhesions without other diagnoses, for example, intestinal obstruction or cancer, have become extremely rare. A review of this code reveals that 50% of these operations were for exploratory laparotomies in women who had pelvic pain and in whom no specific pathologic condition could be found other than pelvic adhesions. Of these, 25% to 30% were for intestinal obstruction and 10% were for exploratory laparotomy in which no pathologic condition other than generalized peritoneal adhesions was noted. The remaining 10% were classified as unknown pathologic condition. Coding nuances such as this can be found throughout the ICD-9-CM codes. These can create confusion in distinguishing surgical procedures and in attempting to compare one specialty's patient numbers with another.

PREVIOUS MANPOWER STUDIES

Awareness of past and present numbers of surgical operations allows manpower prognostication to evolve in a rational and pragmatic manner. The all-important questions concerning the future maintenance of technical proficiency and overall surgical health care delivery can then be discussed on a more factual basis. Unfortunately, few surgical manpower studies have utilized such information. Before 1965 little was known about surgical caseloads in the United States. The earliest report on numbers of surgical procedures in this country was by Collins of the Public Health Service in 1938.[8,9] Investigating the frequency of surgical operations on 8758 white families in 18 states, he found that there were 6500 surgical operations per 100,000 population per year. Tonsillectomy accounted for almost one third of all procedures, with the setting of a fractured bone second, and appendectomies third. This report, although rudimentary in design, was the forerunner to all future data-collecting attempts by the federal government.

Throughout the subsequent decades, health care planners have offered projections of future need and supply of physicians in this nation. Among such prominent forecasts have been the 1933 report by Lee and Jones for the Committee on Cost of Medical Care of the American Medical Association, the Ewing Report (1948), the Mountin-Pennel-Berger forecast in 1949, the 1953 President's Commission on the Health Needs of the Nation, the Bayne-Jones Report of 1958, and the Bane Committee Report (1959). The latter appears to have furnished the foundation for the Health Professions Educational assistance Act of 1963 (PL 88-129). This legislation established the first federal program to provide substantive funds for medical education through grants for construction of medical schools and loans to medical students. It was amended in 1965 (PL 89-290) to provide further monetary assistance. Five years later the Carnegie Commission on Higher Education declared in a report[7]:

> The most serious shortages of professional personnel in any occupational group in the United States are in health services.

In 1970 Bunker compared rates of surgery between the United States and England and Wales.[4] He showed that overall rates of surgery in the United States were twice that of England and Wales. It was not unexpected that he also demonstrated per capita numbers of United States surgeons to be twice that of England and Wales. This finding was in striking agreement with Lewis' 1969 proposal of a surgical variation of Parkinson's Law[20]:

> Patient admissions for surgery expand to fill beds, operating suites and total surgical manpower.

These and other studies propagated the concept that surgeons coming to a community perform surgery according to their own financial requirements. However, if surgeons truly practiced their craft in a capricious manner, as numbers of surgeons increase, numbers of surgical operations should correspondingly change. Research has shown this not to be true, and the widely held societal belief that surgeons create their own distinctive supply and demand curve is a false and misleading statement.[38,49] Evidently there are professional, economic, and sociologic forces that do not allow a surgeon's scalpel to be wielded in an unbridled fashion.

Of all reports that provide surgeons a partial glimpse into these forces, the Study on Surgical Services for the United States (SOSSUS) remains most prominent.[54] It had its inception within the American Surgical Association (ASA) and the American College of Surgeons (ACS) in 1969 to 1970. It was a 5-year effort in which numerous issues were explored, including surgical manpower and individual surgeons' caseloads.

The SOSSUS was published as a multivolume work in 1975, and among its more interesting findings was the remarkably low number of operations performed per surgeon yearly. Approximately 15% of board-certified surgical specialists did fewer than 50 operations a year, 31% between 100 to 199 and slightly more than 33% did 200 or more surgical procedures. It was concluded that far too many physicians perform surgical operations and that workloads of surgeons were much more modest than originally thought. It was suggested that the total volume of operations performed in this country could be handled by a substantially smaller cadre of busier board-certified surgeons. In order to accomplish this, the following were specifically recommended:

1. The number of training programs should be reduced and identified more closely with university centers as "affiliated hospitals."
2. The total number of persons entering practice who have board certificates in general surgery and the surgical specialties should

be reduced over the next 10 years. The total number of persons in training needs to be reduced and tasks now performed by trainees would need to be assumed by other personnel.

The wholly unanticipated SOSSUS findings were being corroborated by other studies. Hughes et al. investigated workloads among general surgeons in a community practice and found them to be only 4.3 hernia equivalents per week. Additional reports by Hughes demonstrated similar conclusions.[15-17] This prompted his recommendation, closely paralleling the SOSSUS', that there appeared to be underutilization of costly and highly specialized surgical skills in the United States. It was suggested that a diminution in numbers of residents might result in increased efficiencies in the delivery of surgical health care.

After publication of the SOSSUS, suggestions to place constraints on surgical manpower became prominent. Moore et al. outlined four trial assumptions to determine future manpower goals.[32] They included (1) maintaining the current rate of increases in residency output, (2) maintaining a constant ratio of surgeons to population, (3) maintaining board-certification rates fixed and constant at the present average, and (4) maintaining a manpower goal to achieve growth of the surgeon/population ratio at the rate of 1% each 5 years. The latter plan was considered the most practical. To achieve this growth goal of 1% would have required a reduction in the number of physicians entering surgical residencies during the late 1970s and throughout most of the 1980s. After that, as the population grew, residency levels would be permitted to return to their present numbers. Many prominent surgeons were advocating the formation of some type of national agency to monitor surgical manpower rates.[31]

As proposals to place constraints on surgical manpower became more vociferous,[3] the SOSSUS' recommendations were soon being questioned by the ACS. Although the ACS was a parent of the SOSSUS, it directly challenged the accuracy of certain findings. Haug, director of the ACS Department of Surgical Practice, wrote[14]:

> Unreliable data such as those cited [SOSSUS] provide a poor basis for manpower estimates or for advanced planning.

It was not unexpected that without organized and academic surgery's support the SOSSUS would never achieve its hoped-for impact on surgery in the United States. Williams showed that the SOSSUS' recommendations were having no demonstrable effect and that surgical manpower continued to grow.[55] The SOSSUS had become an orphan in the world of surgical politics.

The generally expansionist policies for physician manpower, recommended by medical-manpower commissions and implemented by medical schools and State and Federal governments during the late 1960s and early 1970s, were beginning to have noticeable effects on the delivery and financing of United States' health care. In 1970 there were 152 nonfederal physicians for every 100,000 civilian population. A decade later there were almost 200 physicians per 100,000 civilians. It is projected by the Department of Health and Human Services that in 1990 the number of physicians per 100,000 population will be 235 and in the year 2000 will stand at 260.[13] From 1945 to 1965 there were 6000 to 7500 graduates of United States medical schools yearly. In 1970 the number rose to 8400, and by 1975 was 12,700. The total continued to rise and in 1980 was 15,135. In 1985, 16,347 physicians graduated from this country's schools of medicine.[11]

Clearly, government and society had managed to increase the physician population to such a point that there was a controversy about whether control of residency positions was an appropriate means of alleviating perceived specialty maldistribution. This debate was partially responsible for passage of the Health Professional Educational Assistance Act of 1976 (PL 94-484).

The law required medical schools to reserve training positions in internal medicine, family practice, and pediatrics in order to receive federal capitation grants.

Because of these and other concerns the Graduate Medical Education National Advisory Committee (GMENAC) was chartered in April, 1976, by Joseph Califano then Secretary, Department of Health, Education, and Welfare. Its goal was to review residency training from the points of view of geographic and specialty distribution, as well as finance, entry procedures, examination, and foreign medical graduates.[13]

Published in 1980, the GMENAC estimated a surplus of surgeons in 1990 of 38,600: specifically, general surgeons, 11,800; obstetrician-gynecologic surgeons, 10,450; orthopedic surgeons, 5000; Ophthalmologic surgeons, 4700; neurosurgeons, 2450; urologic surgeons, 1650; plastic surgeons, 1200; thoracic and cardiovascular surgeons, 850; and ENT surgeons, 500. To deal with this anticipated problem the following recommendations were made[13]:

1. All medical schools should reduce entering class size in the aggregate by a minimum of 10% by 1984 relative to the 1978 enrollment.
2. To correct surpluses in a manner not disruptive to the graduate medical education system, no specialty should increase or decrease the number of first-year trainees in residency more than 20% by 1986, compared with 1979.
3. Medical school graduates in the 1980s should be strongly encouraged to enter those specialties where a shortage of physicians is expected.

Much criticism was directed at GMENAC and its methodology.[24,35] However, the major findings could not be easily discounted, and it remains the standard work on which policy and health care planners rely when looking for information on future medical personnel needs. An important concern about GMENAC from a surgeon's standpoint is whether its estimations are accurate. Williams cited numerous deficiencies and recalculated the overall surplus of surgeons to be 56,000.[56]

Other warnings about surgeons surpluses were being heard. Most notable among them was Moore.[29] Instrumental in coordinating the manpower studies of the SOSSUS, he utilized the community size model for surgeon distribution and wrote[27]:

> By the year 2000, approximately two surgeons will be standing on the turf occupied by one surgeon in the years 1971 and 1972. The growth in the number of surgical specialists in this country is much faster than that of the population . . . and is rising quickly. . . .
>
> We believe that for surgery we will look and feel severely overcrowded. There is no escaping this fact.

With the SOSSUS and GMENAC part of medical political history, it should be possible to begin measuring their effects. The present review of numbers of surgical residents on duty for the years 1970 through 1985 showed that no specialty except urology had fewer residents in 1985 than in 1975.[11] It would be difficult to picture a more dismal response to the urgings of the SOSSUS and GMENAC reports.

As with SOSSUS, no major surgical organizations came forward to lend support to GMENAC's findings. A few months after publication of GMENAC, the Bulletin in the ACS carried a critique of the manpower projections.[2] In June, 1985, the ACS' Board of Regents stated[1]:

> The College does not endorse any of the GMENAC recommendations regarding manpower because each one lacks a data base sufficiently firm and convincing to warrant acceptance by the College.

In April, 1986, a study regarding surgical residents in the 1980s published by the ACS concluded[26]:

> This study has uncovered substantial evidence that the estimates of surgical residents in accred-

ited programs used as the surgical manpower bases in the GMENAC and DHHS studies are not as large as initially believed. This, in turn, has probably led to inflated projections of new, fully trained surgeons.

Although the ACS has not formally acknowledged the existence of a surgeon surplus, a recent study from their Executive Services Department investigating surgical workloads changes showed that the average number of operative procedures done by a general surgeon decreased 25% from 1982 to 1985.[25] Coincidentally, in the same report, more than 50% of surveyed surgeons thought that fewer surgeons were needed in their particular communities.

To further complicate the manpower equation, certain states, most notably New York and California, are contemplating legislative restrictions on the number of hours a resident may work on a given shift of duty and per week. This move is in response to a growing concern over errors made in the treatment of patients, believed related to resident fatigue and impairment of judgment. Limiting total work hours could conceivably lead to the need for more surgical residents or possibly more physician assistants. The end result could cause further decreases in operative cases available on a per surgeon basis.

Among other indirect effects on surgical manpower is recent growth in managed health care organizations. As the alphabet soup of United States health care delivery systems enlarges, for example, HMO, PPO, and IPA, there is the assumption that such entities will inevitably decrease utilization of surgical services. If this proves true, the need for surgeons would correspondingly decrease. As a result the growing surgeon surplus would be further aggravated.

IMPLICATIONS FOR PRESENT AND FUTURE SURGICAL CARE

With all the conflicting data on surgical manpower and future surgical health care delivery, where does reality lie? Certain facts stand out.

Numbers of surgical operations have shown virtually no increases since the mid-1970s. This is contrasted with an ever changing supply of surgeons, which has changed 25% from 1979 to 1985 alone. From 1970 to 1974, the increase in numbers of operations was far greater than the increase in numbers of surgeons. Now the equation is inversed.

Is a manpower crisis upon us? Some authorities think it does not exist; others believe it has been present since the early 1980s.[18] I consider it to be just beginning! For the average surgeon, there are 4 years of medical school, generally followed by 5 to 7 years of graduate training. Upon leaving residency, it usually takes 3 to 5 years to establish a practice and have an impact on the surgical health delivery system; this is 12 to 16 years. Therefore, in 1988 surgeons who are beginning to have major impact on numbers of operations would have graduated medical school in the period 1972 through 1976. If medical school enrollment did not reach its present peak levels until after 1975, it can be seen that these newer surgeons will not influence the delivery system until well after 1990. If there is the perception of a plethora of surgeons in 1988, the situation will only worsen during the remainder of this century and well into the 21st.

Critics of this scenario believe that recent federal legislation affecting foreign medical graduates will decrease the supply of physicians. However, this remains unclear because the United States-born foreign medical graduate is rapidly replacing the foreign-born foreign medical graduate.[53]

Within certain segments of surgery there has been a generally propagated concept that there are not too many surgeons, but too many "other" individuals, that is, non-board-certified and nonsurgically trained physicians, performing surgical operations. This position is tenuous at best and undoubtedly shortsighted, considering the rapid and spectacular decline in the number of non-board-certified surgeons in the United States.[30] Nevertheless, any truth that remains in this ostrichlike mentality should provide an even stronger stimulus to those who call for an elevation of surgical standards. As Moore writes[28]:

> We can hope that the voluntary national surgical organizations will see this surgical surplus as a realistic problem and face it squarely rather than adopting the juvenile view that surgeons are such wonderful people that one can never imagine a situation in which there are actually too many of them.

A surplus of surgeons will have a potentially far different effect on our society's ability to provide efficient and affordable health care than a surplus of nonsurgical physicians. The rationale for this concerns the value of cognitive versus noncognitive medical skills. Many cognitive functions can, if necessary, be taught and initially learned with a minimal of patient interaction. Although no one would condone such educational policy, the young physician initially learns to treat many pathologic processes, for instance, from textbooks or by observing other physicians. However, noncognitive skills, that is, technical surgical proficiency, cannot be similarly taught. They can be learned only with repetitive hands-on performance. For this reason, if the large number of young surgeons our medical education system is currently producing does not have adequately sized patient bases to procure these skills, their technical proficiency must become suspect.

The performance of a surgical operation can be a technically demanding feat. Accordingly, studies have begun to document the relationship between a surgeon's operative volume and surgical mortality.[6,22] They demonstrate that for many surgical operations surgeons, like most individuals, do best what they do most often. It is difficult to imagine that in the future, a surgeon who performs just two or three major operations a week will maintain technical competency. This is the very reason why regionalization of surgical health care and super-specialization, that is, a surgeon's performing only one type of operation in a high-volume practice, is beginning to appear.[10]

How will the problem of surgical manpower impact on patients' rights? If future caseloads are decreased to the level where clinical competence can be questioned, should surgeons be required to inform the public of their overall experience, including morbidity and mortality, with particular operations?

It is my opinion that the United States unknowingly and unwittingly faces a surgical manpower crisis of unprecedented proportions. The current direction of minimal increases in numbers of operations combined with extraordinary increases in the number of practicing surgeons, will create an exigency relative to technical surgical quality assurance. If 1988 seems bad, 1998 will prove worse, and 2008 an unmitigated disaster.

Accordingly, what situations may emerge from the current perplexities? As surgeons perform fewer operations, their technical skills might decline most notably for the more complex but less frequently completed procedures. This may lead to increased morbidity and mortality. Indications for surgical operations may become less stringent leading to unnecessary surgery. Because of their shrinking operative caseload, surgeons may be forced to practice nonsurgical, that is, primary care, medicine to maintain their livelihoods. This will further erode their technical skills and shift them into specialties for which they received little training. In the past the concern of the surgeon was that nonqualified physicians were practicing surgery. In the future the concern of the nonsurgical physician may be that nonqualified surgeons are practicing primary care. The cost of training a surgeon might become burdensome to society relative to what the surgeon returns to it in the way of surgical skills.

Invariably, the older, more established surgeon might experience a decrease in the size of his or her practice. Concurrently, the younger surgeon might not be able to secure a practice of sufficient size to provide adequate operative experience.

The current direction may produce two classes of surgeons: those who are splendid technicians and perform large numbers of surgical operations and a larger dispirited and deprived group who complete little in the way of operative surgery and have a strong sense of disenfranchisement. All this points to a potentially crippling and tragic effect on the future quality of our country's surgical health care.

The good news is that this chapter conveys a mixed message. There are reassuring data concerning unnecessary surgery because of supplier-induced demand for operations. It is evident, at least so far, that increasing numbers of surgeons do not necessarily drive up rates of surgical operations. Whether this remains true in the future is unknown. The worrisome part concerns surgical caseloads. The prospect of more surgeons performing fewer operations has become a major problem. Solutions are difficult at best, but a proper balance of surgeons and surgical operations must be achieved.[19]

APPROACHING THE MANPOWER SURPLUS

What can be done? It is a propitious time for a conclave of clear thinking and pragmatic surgeons to review the foundations on which United States surgery is built. The very fabric of our surgical education and training programs must be reevaluated to move us from the deadcenter position regarding socioeconomic changes that has been occupied for the last decade and a half.

1. Groups such as organized surgery, academic surgeons, and the various specialty boards must acknowledge that a surgical surplus, if not already present, will soon be upon us. They must accept the immensity of the problem and deal with it in a forthright and rational manner. Their unwillingness to confront the situation has created many of the current difficulties.
2. Numbers of surgical residency positions need to be reduced. This will create a substantial amount of turmoil but will add to the betterment of the profession. Nonuniversity-affiliated training centers should be brought under a university umbrella. Academic surgeons are the teachers of surgery. This position needs to be reemphasized and strengthened.
3. The study of socioeconomics must be recognized by the surgeon as a legitimate academic discipline. It is imperative that departments of surgery in major teaching institutions establish formalized sections that have as their principal function the responsibility for studying and carrying out research on the organization and delivery of surgical care. Forums for the discussion of socioeconomic problems must be provided at all national meetings. A cadre of young surgeons must be directed toward obtaining advanced degrees in such fields as economics, sociology, hospital administration, and business. The United States is in need of surgeons who have the ability not only to perform operations, but also to conduct economic and sociologic research into the delivery of surgical health care.
4. The federal government should continue to finance medical socioeconomic research groups, specifically the NCHS. The NHDS must be expanded to cover outpatient as well as inpatient surgical operations. The loss of such vital data would be immeasurable and make rational national surgical manpower planning both implausible and impossible.
5. The federal government in conjunction with organized and academic surgery should form a National Council on Surgical Manpower. This council should have decision making capabilities and be able to bring logic to the current chaos that exists in studying surgical manpower.

6. It is time for a new SOSSUS-like study to be conducted under the combined auspices of all surgical specialties. There have been massive socioeconomic changes that have occurred since 1970. These need to be documented in a well-coordinated effort to guide us into the twenty-first century of surgical health care. The surgical community and the nation must address these important questions in an expeditious manner. Continued passivity will surely lead to greater and perhaps unwanted restrictions on the practice of surgery and have possible dire consequences on our future national health care.

References

1. American College of Surgeons in an era of societal transformation, Chicago, 1985, American College of Surgeons.
2. Anonymous: A critique of the GMENAC physician manpower projections for 1990, Bull Am Coll Surg, Oct 1980.
3. Bloom BS, and Peterson OL: Changing the number of surgeons, N Engl J Med 303:1227, 1980.
4. Bunker JP: Surgical manpower: a comparison of operations and surgeons in the United States and in England and Wales, N Engl J Med 282:135, 1970.
5. Bunker JP, Barnes B, and Mosteller F, editors: Costs, risks, and benefits of surgery, New York, 1977, Oxford University Press, Inc.
6. Bunker JP, Luft HS, and Enthoven A: Should surgery be regionalized? Surg Clin North Am 62:657, 1982.
7. Carnegie Commission on Higher Education: Higher education and the nation's health: policies for medical and dental education, New York, 1970, McGraw-Hill, Inc.
8. Collins SD: Frequency of surgical procedures among 9,000 families, Public Health Rep 53:587, 1938.
9. Collins SD: Percentage of illnesses treated surgically among 9000 families, Public Health Rep 53:1593, 1938.
10. Crane M: Does a practice need a gimmick to survive today? Med Econ, p 52, March 1986.
11. 85th Annual Report on Medical Education in the United States, 1984-1985, JAMA 254:1567, 1985.
12. Finkel ML, McCarthy EG, and Ruchlin HS: The current status of surgical second opinion programs, Surg Clin North Am 62:705, 1982.
13. GMENAC Summary Report, vol 1, Report of the Graduate Medical Education National Advisory Committee to the Secretary, Department of Health and Human Services, United States Department of Health and Human Services, 1980, US Government Printing Office.
14. Haug JN: Misconceptions on surgical residency positions, Bull Am Coll Surg, Sept 1976.
15. Hughes EFX, et al: Surgical workloads in a community practice, Surgery 71:315, 1972.
16. Hughes EFX, et al: Utilization of surgical manpower in a prepaid group practice, N Engl J Med 291:759, 1974.
17. Hughes EFX, Lewit EM, and Lorenzo FV: Time utilization of a population of general surgeons in community practice, Surgery 77:371, 1975.
18. Iglehart JK: The future supply of physicians, N Engl J Med 314:860, 1986.
19. Levey GS: Organizing to begin physician manpower planning, N Engl J Med 315:1344, 1986.
20. Lewis CE: Variations in the incidence of surgery. N Engl J Med 281:880, 1969.
21. Lubitz J: Different data systems, different conclusions? Comparing hospital use data for the aged from four data systems, Health Care Finan Rev, p 41, 1981.
22. Luft HS, Bunker JP, and Enthoven AC: Should operations be regionalized? N Engl J Med 301:1364, 1979.
23. McCarthy EG, and Finkel M: Surgical utilization in the USA, Med Care 18:883, 1980.
24. McNutt DR: GMENAC: its manpower forecasting framework, Am J Public Health 71:1116, 1981.
25. Misek G: The surgical manpower survey: workload changes among general surgeons, Bull Am Coll Surg Feb 1987.
26. Misek G and Hynds-Karnell L: Surgical residents in the eighties, Bull Am Coll Surg April 1986.
27. Moore FD: A Community size model for physician distribution in the United States, J Clin Surg 1:162, 242, 1982.
28. Moore FD: Medical and surgical manpower and economic phenomena, Surgery 95:374, 1984.
29. Moore FD: Surgical manpower: past and present reality, estimates for 2000, Surg Clin North Am 62:579, 1982.
30. Moore FD and Lang SM: Board-certified physicians in the United States, specialty distribution and policy implications of trends during the past decade, N Engl J Med 304:1078, 1981.
31. Moore FD, Zuidema GD, and Ballinger WF: Surgical manpower and public policy, Surgery 83:116, 1978.
32. Moore FD, et al: National surgical patterns as a basis for residency training plans: the response of a panel of surgeons, Arch Surg 112:125, 1977.
33. National Center for Health Statistics: Development and maintenance of a national inventory of hospitals and institutions, Vital and Health Statistics. PHS Pub No 1000-series 1-No 3, Public Health Service, Washington, DC, Feb 1965, US Government Printing Office.
34. National Center for Health Statistics: Detailed diagnoses and surgical procedures for patients discharged from

short-stay hospitals, United States, 1979, DHHS Pub No (PHS) 82-1274-1, Washington, DC, Jan 1982, US Government Printing Office.
35. Reinhardt UE: The GMENAC forecast: an alternative view, Am J Public Health 71:1149, 1981.
36. Rutkow IM: "Unnecessary surgery": an update, Surgery 84:671, 1978.
37. Rutkow IM: Delivery of surgical health care in the United States, Arch Surg 116:963, 1981.
38. Rutkow IM: Surgical rates in the United States: 1966 to 1978, Surgery 89:151, 1981.
39. Rutkow IM: Rates of surgery in the United States: the decade of the 1970s, Surg Clin North Am 62:559, 1982.
40. Rutkow IM, editor: Surgical health care delivery, Philadelphia, 1982, W B Saunders Co.
41. Rutkow IM: Unnecessary surgery: what is it? Surg Clin North Am 62:613, 1982.
42. Rutkow IM: Ear, nose and throat operations in the United States, 1979 to 1984, Arch Otolaryngol Head Neck Surg 112:873, 1986.
43. Rutkow IM: General surgical operations in the United States, 1979 to 1984, Arch Surg 121:1145, 1986.
44. Rutkow IM: Obstetric and gynecologic operations in the United States, 1979 to 1984, Obstet Gynecol 67:755, 1986.
45. Rutkow IM: Orthopaedic operations in the United States, 1979 to 1983, J Bone Joint Surg 68-A:716, 1986.
46. Rutkow IM: Thoracic and cardiovascular operations in the United States, 1979 to 1984, J Thorac Cardiovasc Surg 92:181, 1986.
47. Rutkow IM: Urological operations in the United States, 1979 to 1984, J Urol 135:1206, 1986.
48. Rutkow IM: Surgical operations and manpower: an assessment of future quality, Health Aff 6:82, 1987.
49. Rutkow IM: Surgical operations in the United States, 1979 to 1984, Surgery 101:192, 1987.
50. Rutkow IM and Ernst CB: Vascular surgical manpower: too much? enough? too little? unknown? Arch Surg 117:1537, 1982.
51. Rutkow IM and Ernst CB: An analysis of vascular surgical manpower requirements and vascular surgical rates in the United States, J Vasc Surg 3:74, 1986.
52. Rutkow IM and Starfield BH: Surgical decision making and operative rates, Arch Surg 119:899, 1984.
53. Stimmel B: Medical students trained abroad and medical manpower, recent trends and predictions, N Engl J Med 310:230, 1984.
54. Surgery in the United States: a summary report of the Study On Surgical Services in the United States (SOSSUS), Chicago, 1975, American College of Surgeons, and the American Surgical Association.
55. Williams DC: Surgeons and surgery in Rhode Island, 1970 and 1977, N Engl J Med 305:1319, 1981.
56. Williams DC: Surgery and the GMENAC report: a reality test, Surgery 95:347, 1984.

CHAPTER ONE
Appendixes

APPENDIX 1-A

General Surgery

Table 1-1. General surgery: 20 most frequent operations

Procedure	1985 total*	1985 US rank	1983 total	1981 total	1979 total
1. Inguinal herniorrhaphy (53.0, 53.1)†	476	4	585	605	579
2. Cholecystectomy (51.2)	475	5	487	482	445
3. Lysis of peritoneal adhesions (54.5)	309	11	298	259	230
4. Appendectomy (47.0)	283	12	282	312	311
5. Debridement of wound, burn, or infection (86.22)	265	13	219	211	164
6. Partial excision of large intestine (45.7)	182	19	169	152	133
7. Biopsy or local excision of breast lesion (85.12, 85.21)	162	24	233	287	323
8. Excision of hemorrhoids (49.46)	120	28	129	170	164
9. Free skin graft (86.6)	118	29	120	130	126
10. Mastectomy (85.4)	116	30	116	112	112
11. Carotid endarterectomy (38.12)	107	34	95	73	54

*Yearly totals are tabulated in thousands.
†Figures in parentheses represent ICD-9-CM codes.

Continued.

Table 1-1. General surgery: 20 most frequent operations—cont'd

Procedure	1985 total*	1985 US rank	1983 total	1981 total	1979 total
12. Exploratory laparotomy (54.1)	104	36	82	107	111
13. Other hernia of anterior abdominal wall (53.5, 53.6)	97	39	97	106	104
14. Incision of bile ducts for relief of obstruction (51.4, 51.5)	88	42	79	92	75
15. Colostomy (46.1)	67	46	71	65	64
16. Local excision or destruction of lesion or tissue of large intestine (45.4)	63	48	75	59	43
17. Other excision of small intestine (45.6)	60	50	45	43	37
18. Temporary gastrostomy (43.1)	55		52	42	26
19. Repair of umbilical hernia (53.4)	52		63	69	65
20. Unilateral or partial thyroid lobectomy (6.2, 6.3)	46		50	55	63

Table 1-2. Number of general surgical operations, surgeons, and residents, 1970 to 1974 and 1979 to 1985

	1970 to 1974		1979 to 1985	
Operations	3,755,000	4,370,000	4,729,000	4,753,000
	16%*		1%	
Surgeons	22,619	23,750	32,059	38,169
	5%		19%	
Residents	6539	7354	7689	8070
	12%		5%	

*Percent increase from 1970 to 1974 and 1979 to 1985.

APPENDIX 1-B

Obstetric-Gynecologic Surgery

Table 1-3. Obstetrics-gynecology: 15 most frequent operations

Procedure	1985 total*	1985 US rank	1983 total	1981 total	1979 total
1. Cesarean section (74)†	879	1	809	704	601
2. Hysterectomy (68.3 - 68.6)	669	2	673	673	638
3. Unilateral or bilateral open destruction or occlusion of fallopian tubes (66.3 - 66.6)	531	3	568	595	547
4. Unilateral or bilateral salpingo-oophorectomy (65.4, 65.6)	472	6	457	420	400
5. Diagnostic dilation and curettage of uterus (69.09)	349	9	632	833	935
6. Diagnostic laparoscopy (54.21)	212	16	262	267	203
7. Repair of cystocele and rectocele (70.5)	165	23	150	175	175
8. Local excision or destruction of ovarian lesion or tissue (65.2)	106	35	107	114	92
9. Bilateral endoscopic destruction or occlusion of fallopian tubes (66.2)	52		105	177	196
10. Unilateral or bilateral oophorectomy (65.3, 65.5)	52		55	60	47

*Yearly totals are tabulated in thousands.
†Figures in parentheses represent ICD-9-CM codes.

Continued.

Table 1-3. Obstetrics-gynecology: 15 most frequent operations—cont'd

Procedure	1985 total*	1985 US rank	1983 total	1981 total	1979 total
11. Repair of fallopian tube (66.7)	38		33	28	15
12. Conization of cervix (67.2)	38		71	82	88
13. Other excision or destruction of lesion or tissue of cervix (67.3)	37		46	54	71
14. Excision or destruction of lesion or tissue of uterus (68.2)	36		37	36	28
15. Obliteration of vaginal vault (70.8)	32		23	24	20

Table 1-4. Number of obstetric-gynecologic operations, surgeons, and residents, 1970 to 1974 and 1979 to 1985

	1970 to 1974		1979 to 1985	
Operations	2,841,000	3,987,000	4,339,000	3,951,000
	40%*		−9%	
Surgeons	16,357	17,532	23,963	30,867
	7%		29%	
Residents	2655	3421	4496	4630
	29%		3%	

*Percent change from 1970 to 1974 and 1979 to 1985.

APPENDIX 1-C

Orthopedic Surgery

Table 1-5. Orthopedic surgery: 15 most frequent operations

Procedure	1985 total*	1985 US rank	1983 total	1981 total	1979 total
1. Open reduction of a fracture and internal fixation (79.3)†	393	7	331	293	274
2. Excision or destruction of an intervertebral disc (80.5)	228	15	188	129	132
3. Total hip replacement or arthroplasty of the hip (81.5, 81.6)	197	17	159	155	130
4. Arthroplasty of the knee or ankle (81.4)	178	20	161	148	123
5. Closed reduction of a fracture without internal fixation (79.0)	177	21	183	193	238
6. Arthroscopy (80.2)	176	22	260	228	130
7. Placement or removal of an internal fixation device without reduction of a fracture (78.5, 78.6)	160	25	173	202	160
8. Excision of a bunion or bunionette (77.5)	153	26	182	139	112

*Yearly totals are tabulated in thousands.
†Figures in parentheses represent ICD-9-CM codes.

Continued.

Table 1-5. Orthopedic surgery: 15 most frequent operations—cont'd

Procedure	1985 total*	1985 US rank	1983 total	1981 total	1979 total
9. Amputation of the lower limb (84.1)	115	31	118	90	80
Toe	43				
Foot	12				
Below the knee	29				
Above the knee	31				
10. Local excision of a lesion or tissue of bone (77.6)	109	33	136	120	95
11. Excision of semilunar cartilage of the knee (80.6)	97	40	147	155	155
12. Spinal fusion (81.0)	95	41	70	59	52
13. Partial ostectomy (77.8)	83	43	95	78	84
14. Division of bone (77.3)	65	47	116	85	56
15. Arthroplasty of the foot or toe (81.3)	61	49	103	71	43

Table 1-6. Number of orthopedic operations, surgeons, and residents, 1970 to 1974 and 1979 to 1985

	1970 to 1974		1979 to 1985	
Operations	2,005,000	2,576,000	2,858,000	3,312,000
		28%*		16%
Surgeons	7786	8950	12,657	17,166
		15%		36%
Residents	2015	2375	2572	2817
		18%		10%

*Percent increase from 1970 to 1974 and 1979 to 1985.

APPENDIX 1-D

Urologic Surgery

Table 1-7. Urology: 10 most frequent operations

Procedure	1985 total*	1985 US rank	1983 total	1981 total	1979 total
1. Prostatectomy (60.2 - 60.6)†	367	8	357	348	293
2. Transurethral excision or destruction of bladder tissue (57.4)	113	32	135	128	120
3. Transurethal removal of obstruction from ureter and renal pelvis (56.0)	68	45	52	48	46
4. Unilateral and bilateral orchiectomy (62.3, 62.4)	57		52	41	42
5. Circumcision (excludes newborn) (64.0)	52		91	104	102
6. Retropubic urethral suspension (59.5)	51		47	54	45
7. Ureterotomy (56.2)	48		53	40	41
8. Nephrotomy and nephrostomy (55.0)	43		23	14	16
9. Release of urethral stricture (58.5)	37		45	47	29
10. Partial or complete nephrectomy (55.4, 55.5)	33		38	34	32

*Yearly totals are tabulated in thousands.
†Figures in parentheses represent ICD-9-CM codes.

Table 1-8. Number of urologic operations, surgeons, and residents, 1970 to 1974 and 1979 to 1985

	1970 to 1974		1979 to 1985	
Operations	1,221,000	1,512,000	1,576,000	1,542,000
	24%*		−2%	
Surgeons	4963	5455	7242	8836
	10%		22%	
Residents	1011	1117	1077	1057
	10%		−2%	

*Percent change from 1970 to 1974 and 1979 to 1985.

APPENDIX 1-E

Otolaryngologic Surgery

Table 1-9. Otolaryngology: 10 most frequent operations

Procedure	1985 total*	1985 US rank	1983 total	1981 total	1979 total
1. Tonsillectomy (28.2, 28.3, 28.6)†	338	10	478	517	584
2. Repair and plastic surgery on nose (21.8)	193	18	263	255	242
3. Myringotomy (20.0)	104	37	187	191	225
4. Turbinectomy (21.6)	73	44	90	82	58
5. Temporary tracheostomy (31.1)	48		49	48	42
6. Excision and plastic repair of mouth and/or lip (27.4, 27.5)	46		57	56	56
7. Submucous resection of nasal septum (21.5)	38		49	52	59
8. Reduction of nasal fracture (21.7)	37		37	44	44
9. Excision or destruction of lesion of nose (21.3)	37		50	53	55
10. Frontal or other nasal sinusotomy and sinusectomy (22.4 - 22.6)	36		33	33	32

*Yearly totals are tabulated in thousands.
†Figures in parentheses represent ICD-9-CM codes.

Table 1-10. Number of otolaryngologic operations, surgeons, and residents, 1970 to 1974 and 1979 to 1985

	1970 to 1974		1979 to 1985	
Operations	1,687,000	1,838,000	1,816,000	1,340,000
	9%		−26%	
Surgeons	4595	4828	6117	7267
	5%		19%	
Residents	910	994	1038	1094
	9%		5%	

*Percent change from 1970 to 1974 and 1979 to 1985.

APPENDIX 1-F

Cardiothoracic Surgery

Table 1-11. Cardiothoracic surgery: 10 most frequent operations

Procedure	1985 total*	1985 US rank	1983 total	1981 total	1979 total
1. Coronary artery bypass (36.1)†	230	14	191	159	114
2. Insertion, replacement, revision, and removal of cardiac pacemaker system (37.7, 37.8, -37.72)	147	27	133	129	147
3. Incision of mediastinum, mediastinoscopy, medistinal biopsy, and excision or destruction of lesion or tissue of mediastinum (34.1, 34.2, 34.26, 34.3)	48		44	45	33
4. Lobectomy of lung (32.4)	33		28	24	22
5. Implantation or removal of heart assist system (37.6)	22		14	11	9
6. Replacement of aortic valve (35.22)	21		16	18	17
7. Excision or destruction of lesion or tissue of lung (32.2)	20		20	13	14
8. Replacement of mitral valve (35.24)	15		16	11	11
9. Repair of atrial and ventricular septa (35.7)	8		9	6	7
10. Scarification of pleura (34.6)	8		5	3	2

*Yearly totals are tabulated in thousands.
†Figures in parentheses represent ICD-9-CM codes.

Table 1-12. Number of cardiothoracic operations and residents, 1970 to 1974 and 1979 to 1985

	1970 to 1974		1979 to 1985	
Operations	258,000	349,000	452,000	651,000
		35%*		44%
Surgeons		not available		
Residents	271	296	276	285
		9%		3%

*Percent increase from 1970 to 1974 and 1979 to 1985.

APPENDIX 1-G

Neurosurgery

Table 1-13. Neurosurgery: 10 most frequent operations

Procedure	1985 total*	1985 US rank	1983 total	1981 total	1979 total
1. Exploration and decompression of spinal canal structure (3.0)†	100	38	98	82	70
2. Lysis of adhesions and decompression of peripheral and cranial nerves; including carpal and tarsal tunnel (4.4)	56		104	117	101
3. Incision and excision or destruction of brain and cerebral meninges (1.3, 1.5)	54		45	39	33
4. Incision, division and excision of peripheral and cranial nerves (4.0)	43		69	69	60
5. Extracranial ventricular shunt, including placement, revision and removal (2.3, 2.4)	36		36	28	21
6. Craniotomy and craniectomy (1.2)	34		36	35	43
7. Suture and neuroplasty of peripheral and cranial nerves (4.3, 4.7)	33		32	29	31
8. Cranioplasty (2.0)	12		12	17	13
9. Transposition of peripheral and cranial nerves (4.6)	12		13	13	7
10. Sympathectomy (5.2)	11		19	17	22

*Yearly totals are tabulated in thousands.
†Figures in parentheses represent ICD-9-CM codes.

Table 1-14. Number of neurosurgical operations, surgeons, and residents, 1970 to 1974 and 1979 to 1985

	1970 to 1974		1979 to 1985	
Operations	217,000	316,000	453,000	501,000
	46%*		11%	
Surgeons	2058	2286	3098	4019
	11%		30%	
Residents	578	607	579	704
	5%		22%	

*Percent increase from 1970 to 1974 and 1979 to 1985.

DON E. DETMER

Don E. Detmer is Vice President for Health Sciences and Professor in the Department of Surgery and in the Darden School of Business at the University of Virginia, Charlottesville, Virginia. He received his doctorate degree in medicine from the University of Kansas in 1965 and completed his surgical training at Duke University, Johns Hopkins University, and the National Institutes of Health. He received a health policy fellowship at the Institute of Medicine, National Academy of Sciences in 1972-73.

DOROTHY J. BUCHANAN-DAVIDSON

Dorothy J. Buchanan-Davidson was born in Monmouth, Illinois. She did her undergraduate work at Monmouth College and Washington State University and her graduate work in biochemistry at the University of Cincinnati College of Medicine and Childrens' Hospital Research Foundation. After receiving her PhD in 1950, she was on the staff of the Department of Biochemistry at Vanderbilt University School of Medicine. Subsequent to her postdoctoral training at the Lister Institute in London and the Pasteur Institute in Paris (1953 to 1956), she came to the University of Wisconsin where she has done biochemical research. Currently she serves as a medical writer and editor for the University of Wisconsin School of Nursing.

2

Ambulatory Surgery

DON E. DETMER
DOROTHY J. BUCHANAN-DAVIDSON

Ambulatory surgery is an accepted reality. Because of improved anesthetics, a healthier public, economic pressures, and good educational preparation, there has been a dramatic change, both in the number of patients who are receiving surgical treatment in an ambulatory setting and in the procedures performed in such settings.[84] It is estimated that by 1992, 40% to 50% of all surgical operations will be done as outpatient procedures. We do not know where this trend will peak. However, continued changes in technology and increases in procedures such as organ transplants will undoubtedly temper the number of procedures that can be done in such settings.

HISTORY AND GROWTH

The Edwin Smith Surgical Papyrus is evidence that ambulatory surgery dates to at least 3000 BC in ancient Egypt when 48 kinds of surgical procedures were described. Among these surgical operations were the treatment of flesh wounds, nasal and mandibular fractures, and simple long bone trauma.[67] In this century the earliest report on ambulatory surgery was in 1909 from the Royal Glasgow Hospital for Children. However, it was not until the mid-1950s, when early ambulation after surgery was popularized, that the concept of outpatient surgery was revived.[21]

UTILIZATION

Today's ambulatory surgery units in the United States developed from two prototypes—one located within the hospital and the other free-standing. In 1971, Davis and Detmer developed a successful hospital-based ambulatory surgery unit at the Watts Community Hospital in Durham, North Carolina.[18] They demonstrated that surgery could be done safely and economically in such a setting. As a result of various interacting demographic, market, technologic, attitudinal, and policy forces, a variety of ambulatory surgery services rapidly developed, so that within the next 10 years 18% of surgical procedures were being done in an outpatient setting.[59] Outpatient surgery increased 77% from 1979 to 1983 at hospitals, while inpatient surgery fell 7%.[3] In 1983 almost 5 million ambulatory surgery procedures were done in hospitals, constituting 24% of all hospital surgery, an increase from 14% in 1979.[28] By 1986, it was estimated that 38% of surgeries were being completed on an outpatient basis, a 277% increase from 1979.

Reports of the impact of ambulatory surgery on hospitals have varied. The overall movement of medical care to outside the traditional in-hospital setting has not yet abated. A 1985 survey by the National Research Corporation showed that 83% of hospitals reported increased use of outpatient services, compared with 70% in 1984, and that 13% planned to add free-standing ambulatory surgery in the coming year.[77] Federal reimbursement policies and tax laws may well become the major determinants for the near future. Midsized hospitals reported the largest increases: facilities with 100 to 199 beds showed a 20% gain; those with fewer than 100 beds, a 15% increase; and those with more than 300 beds remained the same. The greatest increases were in the Southeast (88%) and West (80%).[77]

In 1985 it was believed that more than 60% of American hospital managers planned to expand the hospitals' ambulatory surgery programs during the next 2 years. More independent hospitals (89%) showed an interest in expanding than multihospital corporations (50%). Fewer nonprofit hospitals (65%) or teaching hospitals (67%) than for-profit hospitals (80%) planned to expand, and more midwestern hospitals (more than 70%) planned expansions, compared with about 63% in other areas.[51,79]

Although free-standing surgical centers began in 1970 with the successful surgicenter unit of Reed and Ford in Arizona,[64] the number did not increase dramatically until 1975.[21] During the next 6 years, 12 to 18 centers opened each year. In the early 1980s the American College of Surgeons (ACS) issued this formal statement on ambulatory surgery: "The American College of Surgeons approves the concept that certain operative procedures may appropriately be performed in an ambulatory surgical facility, defined as a facility where the patient may have a procedure performed under general or regional anesthesia without overnight hospitalization."[39] That same year the number of new centers doubled the 1980 number. In 1985, 3.4% of 22.8 million surgical procedures in the United States were done in free-standing surgical centers compared with less than 2% of 22 million in 1984; also, 129 centers opened, representing a 39% increase in the number of existing centers. It is predicted that the number of free-standing facilities will increase to 817 in 1990 compared with 459 in 1985[36,37,52,82] (Table 2-1).

There are 12 corporate surgery center chains with approximately 125 free-standing centers open or being built. About 25% of all surgery centers' procedures are done at these free-standing centers. Medical Care International has a 34% corporate market share, Surgical Care Affiliates has 20%, and American Medical International and Alternacare each have a 16% share.[36,37] Independent facilities account for 70% of the market and perform 63% of the surgical procedures.[36]

The recent slowdown in the development of centers reflects difficulties of market entry and recent competitive marketing by hospitals. Facilities owned by hospitals had the highest utilization rates, and independently owned centers had the lowest because many were single-specialty centers with fewer doctors and operating rooms. Factors affecting use were geographic distribution, state legislation, certificate-of-need requirements, legal regulation, competitive pressures,

Table 2-1. Growth projections for free-standing surgery centers

Year	Number of Facilities*	Surgical Operation Projections, Total
1983	239	377,266
1984	330	517,851
1985	459	783,864
1986	592	1,033,604
1987†	652	1,259,664
1988†	693	1,433,124
1989†	748	1,661,308
1990†	817	1,919,133

Reprinted with permission from the June 5, 1987 issue of *Modern Healthcare Magazine*. Copyright Crain Communications, Inc., 740 N. Rush Street, Chicago, Il 60611.
*Open as of December 31, 1987.
†Projected figures.

and reimbursement policies. California and Florida have the most centers, followed by Louisiana, Arizona, Illinois, North Carolina, and Michigan. The 817 facilities anticipated to be in operation nationally by 1990 will generate almost 2 million outpatient procedures a year compared with about a million outpatient procedures in 1986[37,76] (Tables 2-2 and 2-3).

The American Hospital Association (AHA) estimates that 40% of hospital surgery could be done on an outpatient basis; others project as much as 50% to 60% when experimental technologies enter mainstream medicine.[28] At Methodist Medical Center, Peoria, Illinois, 51% of surgeries are now outpatient.[83] Mt. Sinai Medical Center in Miami Beach, which has a 75% Medicare-age patient population, does 53% of its surgery on an outpatient basis.[26] The University Hospital at the University of Utah is also at the 50% level.

Table 2-2. Free-standing facilities by type of ownership

Type	Facilities			% of Total			Under Development			% of Total		
	1984	1985	1986	1984	1985	1986	1984	1985	1986	1984	1985	1986
Corporate chain	150	125	115	33.2	23.6	18.1	57	15	10	46.7	21.4	23.2
Independent	274	367	461	60.6	69.3	72.5	61	52	30	50.0	74.3	69.8
Hospital owned	28	37	59	6.2	7.1	9.4	4	3	3	3.3	4.3	7.0
TOTAL	452	529	635	100.0	100.0	100.0	122	70	43	100.0	100.0	100.0

Reprinted with permission from the June 6, 1986 issue of *Modern Healthcare Magazine.* Copyright Crain Communications, Inc., 740 N. Rush Street, Chicago, IL 60611.

Table 2-3. Outpatient surgical procedures in the United States

Region	Outpatients, % of Total		
	1984	1985	1986
New England	35	42	46
East North Central	32	39	44
West North Central	29	37	42
Mountain	31	36	41
Pacific	29	36	41
South Atlantic	27	34	40
Middle Atlantic	25	31	37
West South Central	22	29	36
East South Central	23	27	36

Total number of hospitals in 1986: 6841

From AHA Annual Surveys of Hospitals, 1984-1986.

In a recent study by the Rand Corporation of 1132 patients hospitalized in six cities, about 17% of adult hospital admissions were for surgical procedures that were judged to have been acceptable for ambulatory care. The study concluded that 40% of hospital admissions were probably unnecessary.[55,73]

A health care survey by the Equitable Life Insurance Company of New York found in 1984 that at least half of lay people, physicians, hospital administrators, insurance executives, corporate benefits officers, and union leaders favored "a system that encourages people to have tests and minor surgery done in clinics and offices rather than hospitals."[35] Lagoe says that about 80% of people prefer ambulatory surgery.[46]

A National Research Corporation national survey showed that 82% of consumers 18 to 54 years of age were aware of outpatient services compared with 70% of those older than 55. Also, 80% of those 25 to 44 years versus 65% of those older than 44 years and 60% of Medicare patients prefer same-day surgery. Eighty percent of commercially insured people and 75% of HMO members preferred same-day surgery. Likewise, 74% of women and 83% of men preferred same-day surgery. Those patients who considered themselves to be in excellent or good health were more likely to prefer same-day surgery (81%) compared with 68% of those in fair or poor health. Patients who were more educated were more aware of alternative delivery methods and outpatient services—88% who had undergraduate and postgraduate degrees compared with 75% without college educations. Fifty-eight percent of those who had completed grade school preferred out-patient services, as did 74% of high school graduates, and 86% of college graduates. Acceptance varied with the geographic area: 82% in the Northeast, 81% in the North Central, 79% in the West, and 74% in the South.[42]

Pineault et al.[62] found that there was a limit beyond which one-day surgery became less acceptable to patients. It appears that we are beginning to push up against the limits if one judges on the basis of patient perceptions. They found that 54% of one-day surgery patients felt that the hospital stay was too short compared with 21% of inpatients. More one-day surgery patients expressed preference for hospitalization than did inpatients for one-day surgery. Clinical outcomes were as satisfactory with one-day surgery, but the recovery period was longer for those who had meniscectomies.[62]

Hospital-based ambulatory surgical units are preferred by 72% of American physicians for outpatient procedures, 7% prefer free-standing units, and 59% prefer their own offices. These percentages exceed 100% because physicians could respond to more than one category. More general and family practice doctors perform office-based surgeries (77%) than those with medical (34%) or surgical (24%) specialties. Fewer than 10% of physicians of any specialty use free-standing centers.[22] Perceived opportunities for better assessment and communication with patients and their families, more freedom to efficiently schedule their time, reduction in hospital red tape, and opportunity to train their own staff are mentioned as advantages for physicians who prefer free-standing units.[9,49]

In hospital outpatient units, physicians typically are perceived to have more and better equipment and backup equipment, a larger variety of supplies and instruments, better postoperative management of general anesthesia cases, no financial investment, and no management worries; however, they lack control over scheduling and management.[61]

> Over 90% of physicians are satisfied with ambulatory surgery because it eliminates the need for preoperative and postoperative in-hospital patient-physician contact, reduces the time between cases, facilitates block scheduling, and there are few cancellations. Those who do many quick, purely elective operations (eye, ear, nose, throat, and plastic surgery) are especially pleased. Acceptance of ambulatory surgery appears to be inversely proportional to the age of the surgeon.[12]

The development and maturation of ambulatory surgery appears to be progressing along a 20-year time frame. From 1971 until 1981, ambulatory surgery was in its infancy. From 1981 until 1986, it was in an adolescent stage. It is now in a stage of maturation and should reach a peak about 1991. By then the critical issues such as an adequate accreditation process, federal and private financing, a slowing of the rapid expansion of ambulatory surgery centers, and general acceptance of outpatient surgery will have occurred.

CLASSIFICATION

Today synonyms such as outpatient, ambulatory, day surgery, one-day surgery, short-stay surgery, same-day surgery, and out-of-hospital surgery are used interchangeably. They do not differentiate a 15-minute procedure done under local anesthesia from an hour procedure done under general anesthesia that requires a 2- to 3-hour recovery period before discharge. It is especially misleading when the term same-day surgery is applied to ambulatory surgery to denote surgical care delivered to a patient who is admitted that day and plans to remain in the hospital one night or longer.

In 1982 Detmer and Buchanan-Davidson[21] defined ambulatory surgery as

> the performance of surgical procedures that are more complex than office procedures that are usually done under local anesthesia but are less complex than major procedures that require prolonged postoperative monitoring and hospital care in order to guarantee the patient a safe recovery and a desirable outcome.

At least since the mid-19th century surgical procedures have been put into a binary classification of minor and major. As ambulatory surgery has gained widespread adoption in the United States, the inappropriateness of this classification system has become more apparent. We need to go beyond the concept of minor and major procedures that developed in the nineteenth century. In 1986 James E. Davis suggested the following three-part classification of minor ambulatory, major ambulatory, and inpatient care:

Level I Minor ambulatory (outpatient) surgery includes procedures performed on nonhospitalized patients followed by immediate discharge.

Level II Major ambulatory (outpatient) surgery is performed on nonhospitalized patients under any type of anesthesia, followed by a period of postoperative care and observation.

Level III Inpatient surgery is performed on hospitalized patients.[15,17]

Detmer and Buchanan-Davidson[21] previously defined classifications of surgical procedures and proposed three major and two minor categories. The three major categories were designated as primary, secondary, and tertiary surgical care. We used the terms primary, secondary, and tertiary surgical care as the major titles for the different categories, because primary care and tertiary care were already well-defined concepts in policy circles. What had been uniformly poorly defined was secondary care. Today we feel that to adequately describe all surgical procedures, a four-level classification is needed. Level IV adds a quaternary level generally associated with emerging highly technologic and very specialized care. Procedures may move between classification levels depending on advances in the procedures and changes in surgical indications. For the purposes of ambulatory surgery, levels I, II, and III are relevant (Fig. 2-1). In addition, between primary and secondary we felt that conceptually there should be a subclassification A to represent those cases that in a given patient or circumstance might be considered appropriate for either primary or secondary surgery. Also, between secondary and tertiary there should be a subclassification B to represent those procedures that may be either secondary or tertiary depending on the given patient or the circumstances. Finally, there also may well be need for a

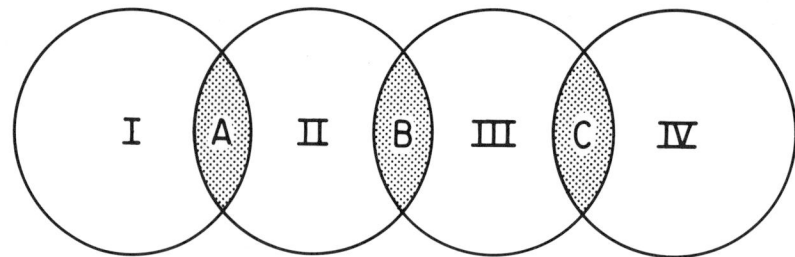

Figure 2-1. Proposed intensity classification for surgical procedures. Level I comprises primary surgery, that is, procedures appropriate for office settings. Subclass A includes procedures appropriate for either level I or level II, depending upon the particular case. Level II is secondary surgery, procedures appropriate for ambulatory surgery settings. Subclass B includes procedures appropriate for either level II or level III, depending upon the particular case. Level III consists of tertiary surgery, that is, procedures appropriate for in-hospital care. Subclass C includes procedures appropriate for either level III or level IV. Level IV consists of quaternary surgery, that is, procedures appropriate for highly technical, very specialized inpatient settings and typically intensive care for at least some period of time after surgery.

subclassification C between tertiary and the most complex procedures.

Primary surgical care (level I) incorporates those surgical procedures that are sufficiently simple that they may be performed in an office setting, typically using local anesthesia and not requiring any sophisticated care before and after the procedure. This does not imply that primary surgical procedures are simple in the sense that a physician who does not have adequate training and/or supervision may be able to perform these operations.

Secondary surgical procedures (level II) refer to those now primarily being called *ambulatory* surgical procedures. These procedures historically have been major procedures, but through advances in surgery and anesthesia are being managed increasingly on an ambulatory basis. The magnitude of these procedures is sufficiently more complex than primary procedures to warrant a different classification. These procedures are clearly in the domain of surgical specialists and, as reflected in Davis' classification, are not minor operations.

Tertiary surgical care (level III) refers to operative care involving surgical procedures that require the patient to be in an inpatient environment. These procedures uniformly involve major regional or general anesthesia and sufficient postoperative care to mandate in-hospital management. And level IV care is well beyond the reach of the ambulatory care setting.

This four-level major and three-level minor surgery categorization scheme should replace the previous three-level major and two-level minor surgery ones. The principle reasons for the surgical community to adopt a four-level system are both for planning and management purposes and especially to guide reimbursement and payment. Unless the surgical community helps define what can be quite routinely considered primary (level I), secondary (level II), tertiary (level III), or quaternary (level IV) procedures, there will be a great tendency for insurers who are without surgical knowledge to place far too many complex procedures into the secondary category and too many secondary procedures into the primary surgical category.

In addition, for the present at least, the boundary categories A, B, and C are desirable, because those procedures that are legitimately in boundary categories A, B, and C have not been well defined through either a consensus panel method or an analysis of actual clinical outcomes. Depending on the health and psychologic status of the individual patient, the response to anesthesia, the trauma caused by the surgical procedure, or complications that are found or that develop during the surgery and recovery, a procedure normally classified as primary might need to be cared for as a secondary procedure, a secondary procedure might require tertiary care, and a tertiary procedure might require quaternary care.

There is also the consideration that without the boundary categories (A, B, and C), surgeons may be legitimately underreimbursed for services they deliver or, worse, some patients may be inappropriately treated on an outpatient basis because of excessive concerns for reductionist fiscal policies out of step with achieving high-quality surgical results. Finally, universalizing the ambulatory surgery site as a norm for certain procedures may conflict with patients' rights to be assured protection against mishap.[53]

It would make sense for the American Colleges of Surgeons and Anesthesiologists to convene consensus panels to identify procedures as being, for example, primary or secondary, and, equally important, through a consensus approach and an analysis of contemporary practice patterns, that types A, B, and C procedures be identified.

Until or unless the surgical and anesthesiology community reaches consensus on what constitutes primary, secondary, tertiary, and quaternary surgical care and subclassifies groups A, B, and C, both will be buffeted by continuing struggles and debates from financing entities principally driven by a desire to contain costs. The drive for greater fiscal efficiency in the delivery of care is not a poor one, but it can produce poor results as well as a less than optimal image if not properly managed.

Who better than the specialists can study and define the proper current distribution of surgical procedures between these three major categories and the two intermediate subcategories? Until more precise information has been developed, consensus groups could go a long way toward giving us at least a start in the right direction.

Could we develop a classification system in the near future that would meet both national and international needs? Presently, no. There is sufficient variation in the level of development of surgery and anesthesia and/or pressing environmental conditions that would yield a uniform international categorization of this type inappropriate for the present. However, proceeding with a classification effort would represent a sufficient and important enough improvement over the old *minor* and *major* categorization to warrant development and implementation.

At present we are living with an anachronistic classification (minor and major) that serves neither the surgeon nor the policy maker well. And most important, if neither the surgeon nor the policy maker is served well, it is most likely that the patient is not being served well. Ultimately it is the benefit of the patient that will be positively affected by progress with a relevant contemporary classification.

PROCEDURES AND PATIENT SELECTION

To correctly determine which patients are suitable for outpatient surgery, consider the following: nature of the procedure, incidence of postoperative complications, probability for more extensive procedures than originally planned, reliability of the patient, psychological acceptance by patient of the same-day surgery procedure, health and cardiovascular stability of the patient, center's ability to handle possible complications, capability for self- or family care outside the hospital setting,[69] type of surgery planned, type of anesthesia used, and the skill of the surgeon.[2,4,19]

The decision rule that must be rigidly followed is to consider the patient's age and potential for immediate and delayed postoperative complications.[44] Sikes and Detmer[72] in 1979 found that, generally, patients younger than 75 years had normal operative risks, those older than 80 years had twice the risk, and those older than 90 years had 3 times the risk, regardless of the complexity of the procedure.

Hospital-based centers typically serve older patients. More than 25% of those seen in these centers are older than 65 years. In free-standing centers, 20% are younger than 10 years and only 10% are older than 60 years.

Before surgery a patient should be told how to actively prepare by (1) avoiding drinking, (2) practicing deep breathing and coughing, (3) communicating fully during preoperative evaluation, (4) reporting all medications taken, and (5) asking questions to alleviate fears and to develop a positive frame of mind. If the patient is to have general anesthesia, the anesthesiologist should be told about any crowns, bridges, or loose teeth.[81]

After the surgeon has scheduled a patient for surgery, the patient is contacted by phone, and the medical history carefully screened for significant medical, surgical, and anesthesia problems. As needed, proper and adequate laboratory, x-ray, and other diagnostic studies are done before surgery. Normally, hemoglobin and hematocrit levels and examination of urine by dipstick are the only tests done. This permits early detection of problems that need evaluation. Both verbal and written instructions are given to the patient before surgery.

At the Center for Ambulatory Surgery in Washington, D.C., a history and physical examination are taken within 2 weeks before surgery. For patients who will have general anesthesia, testing criteria for patients age 39 and younger include a complete blood count and urinalysis, but hemoglobin and hematocrit levels and dipstick urine testing are acceptable. For patients older than 40 years, an EKG and chest film are required also.

At the Ambulatory Surgical Facility in Hollywood, Florida, an anesthesiologist does a physical examination and takes a complete history. Basic laboratory requirements are a complete blood count and urinalysis, a chest film for patients older than 40 years, special test for sickle cell anemia in blacks, and most teenage patients and patients having nasal surgery have a coagulagram, including prothrombin time, partial thromboplastin time, and platelet count. At the Bailey Square Surgical Center in Austin, Texas, patients have a urinalysis and complete blood count done at preregistration. All patients older than 40 years have a chest film and electrocardiogram.

It is worth noting that the American College of Radiologists recommends chest films only for those exhibiting symptoms, those who have histories of pulmonary disease, or those from high-risk populations. According to these guidelines, far too many chest films are done routinely today. It is expected that fewer tests will become the routine in the future, and more attention will be given to the recording of the patient's history and the performance of the patient's physical examination.

At the Utah Center, a complete history and physical examination are taken by the anesthesiologist who "assumes all responsibility for patient problems when he initiates anesthesia." Wong, the anesthesiologist and director of the Center, emphasizes doctor-patient rapport. Only rarely is an adult given premedication, since most prefer to remain alert; this approach is foreign to many anesthesiologists. Wong prefers to give general anesthesia using inhalation agents. Also he feels that when bupivacaine is used to supplement general anesthesia, postanesthesia and postoperative recovery is smoother. Likewise, by minimizing use of parenteral medications, recovery is faster. There is a great psychologic benefit when patients can awaken with little pain, take fluids soon afterward, and return home in a few hours.[6,85]

The eight most common procedures done in outpatient settings are (1) diagnostic dilation and curretage, (2) diagnostic cystoscopy, (3) myringotomy, (4) biopsy of breast tissue, (5) local excision of a skin lesion, (6) diagnostic laparoscopy, (7) cataract extraction (laser), and (8) release of carpal tunnel. The Health Care Financing Association (HCFA) is currently expanding the list of outpatient procedures covered by Medicare from about 150 to 950.[21,25]

Gynecologists routinely perform outpatient culdoscopies, biopsies, cystoscopies, laparoscopies, hysteroscopies, vaginoplasties, minilaparotomies, and colpotomies. Aftereffects can be managed on an outpatient basis by using diuretics and uterine balloons to compress the interior of the uterus. Intraabdominal procedures that do not require abdominal incisions such as minilaparotomy, laser laparoscopies, removal of ovarian cysts through colpotomy incisions, vulvar procedures, vaginal procedures that can be managed with the use of local anesthesia, and cryotherapy can also be done.[32,65]

Cataract surgery has been especially common.[60] On the list of ambulatory procedures being developed by the HCFA, about 75% of eye procedures will be covered on an ambulatory basis.[33]

Between 40% to 60% of pediatric surgery is performed on an outpatient basis. It is less traumatic, children are healthier, they recover faster from surgery and anesthesia, anesthetics and other medications are less residual in children than in adults, and most surgical procedures are simple.[48]

After surgery, the recovery room staff monitors the patient for changes in vital signs and possible complications. Fortunately, many modern anesthetics act rapidly, and most produce only minimal drowsiness and nausea. If the patient has other than local anesthesia, it is essential that he or she be examined by a physician before discharge. When a patient's vital signs have been stable for an hour or longer, when there is no suggestion of complications, and when the patient appears alert and is not dizzy, a responsible adult may take him or her home. Someone must be at home to care for the patient. Short-acting analgesics can be used to control pain. Drugs are available to help manage vomiting or nausea that may develop. Patients are encouraged to move and become ambulatory. Specific directions are given about possible problems that might develop and where to obtain help if they do occur. Usually a nurse phones the next day to check on the patient's condition.[21]

COMPLICATIONS

In 1980, of more than 76,000 outpatient procedures, 10,700 complications occurred, or a 14% complication rate. Nausea and vomiting were most common. Only 0.4% required hospitalization because of bleeding, perforated uterus, hypotension, cardiac problems, unsuspected tubal pregnancy, appendectomy, and emotional problems. Eight patients (0.007%) had life-threatening complications.[78]

An Accreditation Association for Ambulatory Health Care (AAAHC) review of 42 of 59 freestanding facilities showed 263 complications of 103,341 procedures reported. These complications included 88 hemorrhages, 88 wound infections, and 29 anesthesia complications—a 0.25% incidence.[24]

The Freestanding Ambulatory Surgical Association (FASA) 1982 statistical survey of 23 of 31 centers reported 133 patients of 59,106 had major complications. Not surprisingly, there were fewer infections and errors in patient identification and drug dispensing.[7]

A study by FASA showed that 53 infections occurred in 700,000 procedures monitored. Natof in 1983 reported 10 infections in 1300 patients. Craig in 1983 showed an infection rate of less that 1%. A study by Garvey[29] in 1986 showed an insignificant difference between infection rates for gynecologic surgeries in hospitals and same-day basis in a separate operating room of the same hospital. In 1667 procedures there were 11 infections. Buch reported an infection rate of 1% to 5%. The rate tends to increase as the length of the procedure and the patient's hospital stay increase. Ambulatory surgery environment reduces likelihood of cross-infections—a patient is not in a room with two or three sick people for extended periods, and patients are more likely to be generally healthy.[38]

Of 105,000 outpatient eye surgeries, 40 cases of serious endophthalmitis were reported by ambulatory surgical centers.[60]

Analysis of almost 3000 tonsillectomy/adenoidectomy procedures showed that early discharge may be hazardous and economically unwarranted. It may have the risk of complications including hemorrhage, recurrent emesis, dehydration, aspiration, hypovolemia, and resulting complications such as pneumonia, anuria, and cardiovascular collapse, which would require emergency department visits. After surgery, 1.7% of the children bled. Persistent nausea and vomiting after discharge were the next most frequently occurring complications.[40] Variables not related to postoperative complications are patient gender, amount of blood loss during surgery, other procedures done at the same time, recovery room administration of physostigmine for delirium, an episode of emesis, or aggressive nursing care.[63] Care must be taken to avoid compromising the needs of the patients. The operation constitutes major pharyngeal trauma. In Massachusetts, New York, and Pennsylvania, a patient can be admitted if physician recommends, but in Alabama, Arizona, Idaho, Indiana, Kentucky, Michigan, Ohio, Oregon, Tennessee, and Washington, they must have prior approval from insurers to hospitalize, if third-party payment is to be assured.

At the Columbus, Ohio, Children's Hospital, 80% of participants who developed complications were likely to do so within the first 4 hours. Within the first 8 hours, without warning, patients may develop hemorrhage, emesis, and inability to take fluids. One physician concluded that patients should be kept at least 8 hours or overnight if they feel the patient is not doing well.[58] Admission can be justified on the basis of poor hydration, poor oral intake, or possibility of bleeding. The patient should be observed until the physican considers the patient fit for discharge. Any bleeding from the tonsil or adenoid bed should be stopped before discharge. Intravenous hydration should be administered as needed. The patient should demonstrate the ability to take fluids orally. Any symptoms of an obstructed airway should be treated and respiratory support given to patients who have difficulty breathing. Analgesics should be used as needed to make the patient comfortable.[58] Special care should be taken before sending a child home if the parents do not speak English, have no telephone, or live far away.

Reed has estimated that 1 to 2 patients of every 100,000 treated in ambulatory surgery centers will die. In a query of 135 centers, of 1,120,000 patients, 8 died at the surgery center and 9 died within 24 hours of surgery—a death rate of 1.4 per 100,000 patients.[5]

Complications are avoided best by preventive measures and careful screening before surgery—patients who are taking aspirin, who are menstruating, or who have hypertension should be treated cautiously and expectantly on an ambulatory basis. Complications occur most often after the patient has been discharged, so clear and concise postoperative instructions are vitally important. Complications may be attributed to surgery, anesthesia, preexisting disease, or a combination. Complications primarily related to surgery include hemorrhage, laceration of a major intraabdominal artery by the trocar during laparoscopy, or infection. Hemorrhage occurs most often after laparoscopy, tonsillectomy and adenoidectomy, nasal surgery, and augmentation mammaplasty. Other complications of laparoscopies include viscus perforation and bowel burn or bowel obstruction. Catastrophic complications may result from anesthesia, respiratory insufficiency, vomiting and aspiration, malignant hyperthermia, and sensitivity to or overdosage of local anesthetic drugs (because of rapid blood absorption). The staff should be aware of preexisting conditions such as heart disease, insulin-dependent diabetes, special drugs, or pregnancy. The drugs that patients take such as diuretics, tricyclic antidepressants, monamine oxidase inhibitors, and beta blockers must be evaluated. For some elderly patients, hospitalization may accelerate mental and/or physical deterioration to the point where long-term institutional care is needed.[7]

To avoid disasters in anesthesia, an adequate history and a physical examination must be taken, an advanced cardiac life support cart must be available, and the staff should not rush, should use a checklist, should understand every drug used, and should limit office-based procedures to low-risk patients who are ASA categories 1 and 11.[68] Successful outcomes often depend on having a relative or friend to escort the patient home and provide ongoing care. No patient should be allowed to drive himself or herself home after a secondary surgical procedure. And it can never be assumed that all surgery can be performed without inpatient admission.[46]

QUALITY CONTROL

What are the elements of quality control and recommendations for the next 5 years? To achieve real progress, we need (1) to have a good management information system and good management, (2) to refine procedure and patient selection, and (3) to begin outcome measurement as the Joint Commission for Accreditation of Health Care Organizations (JCAHCO) plans to do. All three elements of care need our attention: structure, process, and outcome.

With respect to structure, too many facilities called surgicenters are either glorified doctors' offices or poorly built or designed buildings. These should not be licensed or accredited. Process items also deserve attention. To maintain a quality assurance program, the most important issues are the proper credentialing of doctors, establishing reliable techniques of monitoring physicians' performance, and creating a system for looking at the outcomes of surgery over a period of time.[50]

A quality assurance program should begin with credentialing. Reviewing credentials in detail should take place every 2 years. To control staff credentials in isolated, separated environments, the qualified professionals in the area should initiate an area-wide credentialing system. The physical and mental condition of the doctor must be included. Reviews should include some determination of the justifiability of procedures. The results produced by the surgical procedures performed should also be examined periodically. Hospitals, clinics, and ambulatory surgery units have a concurrent and nondelegable duty to protect patients that includes stepping between the physician and the patient if it becomes necessary to assure the patient's safety.[70]

Both the JCAHCO and the AAAHC accredit free-standing and hospital-affiliated same-day surgery units, and their accreditations are recognized equally by third-party payers. Both use consultant surveyors, are in Illinois, charge similar rates, and have similar standards.

During a reorganization of the Joint Commission on Accreditation of Hospitals (JCAH) in 1979, AAAHC was created as a not-for-profit independent organization providing peer-based assessment, consultation, education, and accreditation. Six national organizations constitute AAAHC's membership—American College Health Association, FASA, American Group Practice Association, Medical Group Management Association, National Association of Community Health Centers, and the Outpatient Ophthalmic Surgical Association.

Members of the board of directors of AAAHC make accreditation decisions. Board members who are also the surveyors are practicing physicians, administrators, and other health care professionals from similar ambulatory care programs. The AAAHC is branching out into areas of ambulatory care, such as office-based surgery practices and urgent care centers. AAAHC's stated purpose is to help ambulatory health care organizations improve the quality of care their patients receive. For ambulatory surgical centers that seek accreditation, the association assesses the quality of care already provided, offers a professional consultation and educational exercises, and grants accreditation for those adhering to the prescribed standards.[1]

Accreditation decisions by the JCAHCO are not made in quite the same way as those of the AAAHC. The accreditation decisions work up through the accreditation committee of the board of the Joint Commission, which is made up of practicing physicians and administrators from the large health care organizations—AMA, AHA, ACS, American College of Physicians, and the American Dental Association. JCAHCO conducts a quality assurance workshop during the accreditation survey. It is focusing its efforts on policy issues such as creating medical staff standards.

Both try to make sure the standards are relevant, the procedures appropriate, and the program worthwhile. Both programs are voluntary. They follow federal protocols for research. Centers should not automatically grant privileges to physicians because they are on the staff of another facility. There must be quality assurance monitoring with special care to pinpoint problems.[41]

We have an issue today with process and outcome control, especially in free-standing units, since the current situation is a speculative market environment. Success or failure of units is not linked tightly enough to performance.

Many physicians are still deeply concerned about safety and possibility of complications during recuperation at home. As early as 1971 the AMA endorsed ambulatory surgery. In 1980 the ACS cautioned that quality control measures should be employed, that surgeons using surgery centers should have hospital privileges, that patients should be carefully selected to minimize risk, and that both free-standing surgery centers and hospital-sponsored facilities meet quality standards established by a nationally recognized accrediting body—JCAHCO for hospital-affiliated facilities or AAAHC for free-standing ambulatory surgery centers. The potential still exists for safety problems as more complex procedures (level II) are moved into the lower-cost office or primary care setting.

A prevalent argument against ambulatory surgery outside the hospital is that competitors are drawing off some of the simpler, more profitable cases from hospitals and leaving the more difficult, expensive ones. Hospitals are then forced to raise prices for more complex operations to cover their fixed costs. It is also possible that increasing one-day surgery could contribute to a long-run reduction in staff and hospital bed capacity—facilities that are expensive to maintain. Managing overall utilization is a thorny issue, and the total system level economics are not yet clear.[28,45]

The JCAHCO, AAAHC, and Medicare require staff to be trained in cardio-pulmonary resuscitation (CPR) and to be present when a patient is in the facility. A physician qualified in resuscitation should be present or immediately available until all patients have been discharged.[27]

In many respects, anesthesiologists are the watchdogs of ambulatory surgery. In an ambulatory setting, patients are not so much recovering from surgery as they are recovering from an anesthetic. Anesthesia safety standards should be comparable to those in a hospital, and no shortcuts can be tolerated. The medical director should be a physician able to assess both surgical and anesthesia risks, deal impartially with all surgical specialties, provide continuity of medical care until all patients have been discharged, and examine all patients before discharge who have received general anesthesia.

COSTS AND FINANCING

In their article in 1972 Davis and Detmer[18] reported a savings of 25% in hospital charges for each ambulatory patient. In 1985 Stephenson stated that ambulatory surgery could save 30% to 50%.[74] And a survey of Fortune 500 companies in 1986 showed that ambulatory surgery was ranked as the most important health care cost-containment strategy.[30] Indeed, ambulatory surgery is most frequently being pursued by American business.[46] At $325 a hospital day, Burns estimated that avoidance of 1 day of hospital stay for each surgical case transferred to an outpatient setting would save $2.5 billion in hospital charges in 1 year.[12]

Ambulatory surgery is one of the primary ways to reduce the cost of health care and the most dramatic cost-saving change initiated by the medical profession.[13] Ambulatory surgery should become more profitable because of escalating inpatient care costs and pressure from third-party payers to lower surgical expense. It is still an open question whether all services provided in the hospital setting are necessary or whether similar outcomes would be obtained if fewer services were provided.[7]

Two aspects of organizational arrangement that may affect cost of care and policy choices of interest to industry, third-party payers, and government are economies of scale and economies of scope—whether costs per unit of service decline as size of center increase and whether services are produced more inexpensively in combination with other hospital services or in separate physician offices.[12]

Hospital charges for surgery center procedures are only about one fifth of what the charges would be if the same procedure was done as an inpatient. As operations move to an outpatient setting, many hospitalized patients are staying longer, because they have had major surgery and are in critical condition. This is making the hospital more of an intensive care facility.[10,12]

Blue Cross/Blue Shield (BC/BS) of North Carolina found that ambulatory surgery for 18 various procedures saved more than $5 million in 1984. Individually, these procedures had savings ranging from 43% to 81% compared with inpatient charges.[28] The HCFA noted a 53% savings if the patient could be moved from an inpatient hospital setting to an ambulatory facility, a 63% savings if the patient were moved to a free-standing facility, and a 73% savings if moved to an office setting.[83] The hypothesis is that savings may result from a reduction of services provided to the ambulatory patient and/or from an incomplete evaluation of the services because the market value of relatives' support services are not included. Home care is less costly than hospital care if fewer services are provided or if cost assumed by relatives is not calculated. Nevertheless, the cost of preoperative workup for screening for ambulatory care does add to the cost.[7]

Group purchasing, heavy use of parttime staff, and highly refined computer services are consistently cited as cost-trimming methods used to improve bottom-line profits. Group purchasing of medical/surgical, laboratory, respiratory, pharmacy, and housekeeping equipment and supplies can result in cost savings of 15% to 40%, but there may be antitrust problems and caution must be taken to avoid illegal tie-ins.[31]

Rapid patient turnover, part-time hiring, and a limited partnership structure increased revenues at Surgical Care Affiliates of Nashville by $300,000 in 1986. They do 6000 procedures a year, get an average reimbursement of $425 per procedure, and incorporate physicians. At Lexington, Kentucky, block scheduling means lower costs to patients, more convenience, and fast turnover time.[14]

Until now, Medicare payment for outpatient surgery procedures has varied with the type of facility where the procedure is performed. If done in a hospital outpatient unit or hospital-affiliated surgical center, reimbursement for the facility component is made on a reasonable cost basis.

The 1987 Omnibus Budget Reconciliation Act signed into law October 27, 1986, provides a major boost for free-standing ambulatory surgical centers and will significantly alter the manner in which hospital outpatient department are reimbursed for providing surgical services because of the following:

1. It requires the HCFA to annually review and update ambulatory surgery center facility rates, beginning in 1987.
2. It requires that the HCFA review and update the list of covered procedures at least every 2 years. Expansion of the list is important because covered procedures are eligible for facility reimbursement ranging from $231 to $504 and because physicians who accept Medicare assignment with respect to those services receive 100% rather than 80% of their surgery fees. The new payment method will apply to about 100 procedures that are approved for Medicare reimbursement in free-standing ambulatory surgery centers.
3. It requires HCFA to implement a permanent prospective payment system for hospital outpatient surgical services by Oct. 1, 1989, and to develop a similar payment system for all hospital outpatient services by Jan. 1, 1991. It will essentially eliminate some of the disparity between payments made to hospitals and to free-standing facilities. Medicare will gradually implement prospective payment for ambulatory surgical services performed in hospital outpatient departments and eventually for all outpatient services. Payments for outpatient departments will be a blend of hospital costs and the ASC rates. Beginning Oct. 1, 1987, the blend will be 75% of hospital outpatient department costs and 25% of ambulatory surgery center rates. Beginning in Oct. 1, 1988, until prospective payment is implemented, the blend will be 50% of hospital outpatient department costs and 50% of ambulatory surgery center rates.
4. Peer review of ambulatory surgical procedures was instituted in June 30, 1987.
5. Facilities will be required to collect from the patient the 20% portion of the bill usually paid by coinsurance, regardless of whether their surgery is performed in a hospital outpatient department or at a surgical center. No coinsurance will be applied to physician charges. Physicians who accept assignment will be paid 100% for their allowable charges for ambulatory surgery procedures. Surgery centers, especially ophthalmic facilties, may no longer be able to offer no-cost surgery.
6. Congress did not approve a bundling provision, which would have required HCFA to include reimbursement for expenses such as for laboratory work and prosthetic devices within ambulatory surgery center facility payments.[8,47]

These changes will cause significant reduction in Medicare payments for outpatient surgery for most hospitals. The assumption is that the secretary of Health and Human Services is going to recommend reducing the physician payment by 30% to 40%.[31]

According to one policy observer, the ambulatory surgery provision is "an extremely large black box in which most of the questions aren't known, let alone answered." At this time it is difficult to predict exactly how hospitals will fare, but advocates for free-standing surgery centers are enthusiastic about the proposed changes.

Payment to designated ambulatory surgery centers for facility charges and ancillary services related to the procedures is based on prospectively determined rates for five procedure groups. All eligible procedures are in four groups except intraocular lens implants. If more than one procedure is done at the same time, the procedure classified in the highest payment group is paid at the full rate and the others at 50% of the applicable rate. The groups were developed by comparing a facility's charge for a procedure with the average charge for all procedures offered. The rates were set by selecting a group rate that would pay the center the average approximate cost for the procedure in the group.

About 100 procedures but more than 400 CPT-4 codes are covered by these rates. It is assumed that the expanded list of 900 to 1000 approved procedures will refer to the CPT-4 codes. The rates, which have not been updated since they were originally set in September 1982, range from $231 to $504. Each rate is adjusted for local wages. It is proposed that the rates be updated annually. With both the hospital cost reimbursement and the ambulatory surgery center prospective rate methods, the physician's fee is paid separately according to the customary locally prevailing rates. Ancillary costs such as for laboratory tests and durable medical equipment billed by physicians, hospitals, and laboratories, that are not related to the procedure are also billed separately.

One concern about the limitation that hospital payment cannot exceed the DRG rate is that a DRG does not correspond to the ICD-9-CM coded procedure but is assigned based on a combination of diagnosis, surgical procedure, and patient characteristics. Hospitals may have to use both codes on the same claim to determine the DRG to which the case would have been assigned in an inpatient setting.

The HCFA's Common Procedure Coding System, which uses CPT-4 codes plus additional codes for various medical supplies and services is unfamiliar to hospital medical records staffs. And it is hard to interchange ICD-9-CM codes and CPT-4 codes, since multiple ICD-9-CM codes may convert to a single CPT-4 code. The costs of complying will be imposed only on hospitals because free-standing centers already use CPT-4 codes, and unless the DRG limitation is placed on them, they will not be required to use ICD-9-CM codes.

A prospective pricing system (PPS) will probably be established for ambulatory surgery, but few hospitals have prepared for the transition. About 20% of hospitals price surgical services by a charge specific for a given procedure plus add-on expenses such as additional equipment and supplies, whereas 80% base prices on the length of time in surgery or a fixed rate per procedure basis. Free-standing centers already operate under an all-inclusive fixed payment rate established by the HCFA.

Hospitals will have to separate costs related to ambulatory surgery procedures from the cost of other outpatient service areas. They will have to identify direct costs of listed services as well as an appropriate allocation of overhead. A critical cost item will be capital payment.[54] It is regrettable that federal policy is indirectly forcing hospitals to consider moving their outpatient surgery procedures from the inpatient surgery suites to a totally separate area. Of course in some instances it is possible that this would make costing procedures easier and might introduce efficiencies that are not possible in an integrated system.[54] With generally an excess capacity in the system, it is more probable that aggregate system costs will be increased by these changes in federal policy.

The new Medicare plan to bring most outpatient surgical procedures under prospective pricing by October 1, 1989 brings the HCFA closer to a "prudent buyer approach" to Medicare services. It is hoped that this plan will reduce Medicare expenditures by $120 million in 3 years.

Unfortunately, the true costs of many hospital ambulatory surgery units are not known, since they are integrated with other outpatient service costs. Managers of these units will need to identify discrete costs. To adapt to changes of the times that emphasize cost-effectiveness, hospital managers should examine their information systems to determine physician capabilities, duration of surgical procedures, and utilization of resources.[66]

Procedures can be organized into six groups: (1) surgeon-administered local anesthesia, (2) anesthesiologist-administered anesthesia with a 2 to 6 hour postoperative stay, (3) procedures requiring a stay longer than 6 hours, (4) anesthesiologist-administered anesthesia after which the patient does not require stage-one post-anesthesia care, (5) minor procedures, and (6) nonsurgical procedures. Flat rates can include all facility fees required in the operating room, recovery room, and outpatient care unit, but not variable charges, such as laboratory, pathology, pharmacy, or x-ray services. Professional fees for services are separate. Many anticipate that such simplified pricing will assist those who function in price competitive environments.[60] Pressures to reduce costs by using the ambulatory setting remain strong.

One procedure commonly done on an ambulatory basis is cataract surgery. About 815,000 cataract extractions were done in 1985 at a cost to Medicare of $3.3 billion. By 1990 an estimated 2 million operations will be performed at costs of $6 billion. As networking ophthalmologists and optometrists build volume, there could be more surgery fees even though each fee may be less.[31] The average cost is $1200 per procedure or $780 million to the government. If the procedure is done on an outpatient basis, the cost could be reduced by about 50% and would save Medicare a projected $390 million. The savings could reach $1.5 to $3 billion per year if facilities were utilized to their maximum.[74] Whether this volume of cataract surgery could be done safely in such settings will deserve continued scrutiny. Some observers believe that the HCFA plans to limit reimbursement of physician fees for durable supplies and services in cataract surgery represent the beginning of national fee schedules and rationing of medical services.[34]

Savings of one half of the dollar cost of care for pediatric urology have been reported.[53,71] Also, switching many dental procedures to the ambulatory setting has saved more than an estimated $100,000 annually, according to a Hartford PSRO study.[80]

Rutkow and Robbins have an ambulatory care center devoted exclusively to hernia repair. The total fee is $1750 for anesthesiologist, surgeon, and facility charges compared with $3000 to $4000 for inpatient billing. The fees are kept low because of high patient volume.[56]

It has been stated that office-based podiatric surgical charges are about $1597 less per patient than that charged by major hospitals, although these charges may be low. However, the potential savings are about $2.8 million.[75]

As early as 1972 Davis and Detmer[18] reported that insurance companies welcomed ambulatory surgery because of savings of hospital charges, inpatient hospital utilization charges, and fewer tests and services, but liability was a major concern. After 3 months of operation, seven private carriers had accepted liability, and by 9 months, 19 companies were participating.

The Health Insurance Association of American regards ambulatory surgery as a cost-saving program. It recommends that insurance plans cover ambulatory surgical services provided by licensed physicians in a recognized establishment, whether hospital sponsored or not, just as they would reimburse other surgical services.[12]

According to a survey of 1000 large companies, ambulatory surgery was covered in 96% of company policies in 1984 compared with only 35% a decade before. Of the 39% providing incentives for outpatient surgery, 84% reimburse fully but typically reimburse only 80% for inpatient surgery.[83] Distribution of reimbursement is currently: BC/BS, 24%; other private third-party payers, 54%; Medicare and Medicaid, 2%; self-pay, 19%; and other, 1%.[12]

BC/BS reports savings to subscribers of $9.7 billion in 1985. BC/BS enrollees include 38% of all people in the United States who have health insurance—a total of about 76 million people. Benefits for outpatient services such as ambulatory surgery, home health care, preadmission diagnostic tests, and hospice care have been broadened.[11]

In Philadelphia, ambulatory surgery is performed in short procedure units (SPUs) within hospitals. A utilization review ensures efficient use of the SPU by minimizing simpler procedures that can be done in hospitals' outpatient departments or in physicians' offices.[28]

Blue Cross of Philadelphia has optional programs such as second surgical opinions and required advance approval for inpatient admissions for specific procedures to encourage ambulatory surgery.

A number of insurance companies will pay 75% to 80% of a surgeon's fee if the procedure is performed on an inpatient basis, as much as full fee if the patient is a hospital outpatient, and an additional incentive of 10% to 25% more than full surgical fee if care is given in an office. Blue Cross and Blue Shield of Michigan expect to save more than $70 million a year in group benefits at Ford and Chrysler alone. Physicians will be provided 125% of normal and customary charges if they shift to outpatient care and only 75% if the patient is admitted to the hospital, unless there is a medical reason for admission.

The major concern is whether such incentives will cause injudicious selection of office or ambulatory care sites for doing surgery.[83] More physicians are electing to do office-based surgery even though they may have to absorb cost of special equipment, supplies, and staff. Blue Cross statistics show that 37% of all surgery is done in physicians' offices. In North Carolina, surgeons doing one of 88 office-based procedures can be reimbursed a minimum tray fee of $15 to as much as $100 to cover cost of equipment and sterile supplies. In New York, surgeons can receive a 20% bonus reimbursement for any of 32 procedures done in their offices, with a minimum reimbursement of $15. Illinois BC/BS provides an additional allowance of $50 for cost of supplies for any of 14 procedures done in physicians' offices.[57] Medicare pays only 80% of physicians' fee if the procedure is done in the office but 100% if it is done in a hospital or free-standing facility.

Medicare cost figures have become the basis for hospital pricing decisions, so hospital-based ambulatory care services are often priced higher than comparable services in a free-standing setting. Three basic approaches that can be used to specify price levels within the framework of chosen pricing strategies are (1) cost-oriented, (2) demand-oriented, and (3) competition-oriented.

The cost-oriented approach is the simplest method of price setting, but it does not reflect the dynamics of the market place. The demand-oriented approach focuses on attributing a dollar amount to the perceived value of a given service. Competition-oriented pricing results in use of either the standard going rate of the marketplace or competitive bidding for a particular contract. To a degree, all three deserve consideration.

Although full-cost pricing may be used for setting inpatient service prices, it will not work effectively in a highly competitive market. Market-based pricing is more appropriate, since it takes into account all three price-setting approaches and incorporates factors critical to the health care marketplace. It is based on a combination of information sources and reflects awareness of prices of competing providers and their probable reactions to changes. Price sensitivity or elasticity of demand is considered.[43] Correct use of insurance codes may be key to prompt and correct reimbursement for procedures.[38]

Managers are bundling prices and tracking physician practices to survive under Medicare's prospective payment system for ambulatory care, which will be implemented over the next few years. Any program that has good cost accounting information will be in a better position to adjust. They can take a few steps now by getting medical directors of units together and going through preoperative orders for various classifications of patients relative to risk—both status of patient and type of operation. The prospective payment system will cover everything from medications administered during or after surgery to preoperative tests, so patterns of testing and variations in medications ordered by different physicians need to be identified. Physicians then need to agree that certain tests will be ordered only on an exception basis under extenuating circumstances.

CHANGE IN SURGICAL CARE

Changes will continue in surgical care, especially in ambulatory surgical care during the next 5 to 10 years.[16] The next 5 years will be a corporate phase and by the tenth year we will probably be in a consumer phase.

Corporations, the government, and the buyers will be contracting and competing with one another and with the practicing professionals on who delivers what care, when, and where. The consumer will control the system by 1995 or 2000 unless a major intervention occurs. Only if a national health insurance were implemented in the mid-1990s would physicians be likely to exert greater control over their work. Physician performance data will be playing a significant role in deciding who gets paid for delivering care, and who does not. Quality and cost will drive the system. There will be real time performance analysis, and public or corporate results will help the consumers decide where they choose to receive their health care.

Makers of surgical care policy have yet to determine exactly those circumstances in which ambulatory surgery is almost always as good as, usually as good as, or better than inpatient surgery or alternative forms of therapy. But methods will be selected to pay patients and physicians so they will use the ambulatory setting.[12] Among the good things these changes will produce are some challenges to medical education.

Quality control will not be driven so much by certificates on a doctor's wall, since credentialism will give way to quality of services delivered and the results achieved. The system will be driven by waiting times, available hours, quality of performance, and cost. Hospitals and ambulatory surgery centers "must evaluate, set new trends, develop appropriate strategies, and sharpen their survival skills."[20] This is an era of caring for patients instead of simply treating medical illnesses.[23] Educating professionals for these realities must be addressed, since these changes in the wind have received far too little attention to date.

Classifications will be periodically revised based on performance of regions, clinics, freestanding or hospital-based units, and inpatient data analyses. Instead of three or five circles (see Figure 2-1), computers will generate tens of tens, each representing defined market and procedure segments.

Feedback can and does change behavior. It is the major responsibility of surgeons to assure that we set and achieve high standards. Ambulatory surgery is the most profound change in surgical care in the United States in the last quarter of the twentieth century. We must attend to this change through its final phase of maturation.

References

1. Accreditation association adds three new members to its board, Same-Day Surgery 8:47, 1984.
2. Accurate preassessment ensures quality SDS patient care, Same-Day Surgery 8:105, 1984.
3. AHA data shows outpatient surgery rose 77% between 1979 and 1983, Same-Day Surgery 9:126, 1985.
4. Alexander MAJ: How to select suitable procedures for outpatient surgery: the Shouldice Hospital experience, ACS Bulletin 71:7, 1986.
5. Ambulatory patients die at rate of 1.4/100,000, informal survey shows, Same-Day Surgery 10:88, 1986.
6. American Society of Anesthesiologists: guidelines for ambulatory surgical facilities, 1983.
7. Ancona-Berk VA and Chalmers TC: An analysis of the costs of ambulatory and inpatient care, Am J Public Health 76:1102, 1986.
8. Baldwin MF: Hospitals wary of impact of reforms in Medicare outpatient surgery pay, Modern Healthcare, p 22, Dec 5, 1986.
9. Bartlett MK et al: The role of surgery on ambulatory patients in one teaching hospital, Arch Surg 114:319, 1979.
10. Berk AA and Chalmer TC: Cost and efficacy of the substitution of ambulatory for inpatient care, N Engl J Med 304:393, 1981.
11. Blue Cross reports major savings through ambulatory surgery, Same-Day Surgery 10:91, 1986.
12. Burns LA: Ambulatory surgery: developing and managing successful programs, Rockville, MD, 1984, Aspen Publishers, Inc.
13. Cannon WB: Insights on outpatient surgery, ACS Bulletin 71:9, 1986.

14. Corporate takeovers cut costs with group purchasing, part-time staffing, Same-Day Surgery 10:80, 1986.
15. Davis JE: Ambulatory and outpatient surgery are overdue for precise definition, Same-Day Surgery 10:89, 1986.
16. Davis JE: The future of major ambulatory surgery, Surg Clin North Am 67:893, 1987.
17. Davis JE: The major ambulatory surgical center and how it is developed, Surg Clin North Am 67:671, 1987.
18. Davis JE and Detmer DE: The ambulatory surgical unit, Ann Surg 175:856, 1972.
19. Davis JE and Sugioka K: Selecting the patient for major ambulatory surgery: surgical and anesthesiology evaluations, Surg Clin North Am 67:721, 1987.
20. Detmer DE: Ambulatory surgery, N Engl J Med 305:1406, 1981.
21. Detmer DE and Buchanan-Davidson DJ: Ambulatory surgery, Surg Clin North Am 62:685, 1982.
22. Doctors prefer hospital setting over freestanding surgery center, Same-Day Surgery 9:54, 1985.
23. Experts outline strategies for survival in new medical market, Same-Day Surgery 9:153, 1985.
24. FASA statistical review highlights complications, Medicare data, Same-Day Surgery 8:73, 1984.
25. Federal Register, 13176, April 21, 1987.
26. Flexible care plans, good physician support spell success, Same-Day Surgery 10:77, 1986.
27. Follow accreditation guidelines; be prepared for emergencies, Same-Day Surgery 8:25, 1984.
28. Fruen MA and Field MJ: Ambulatory surgery comes of age, Business and Health, 27, Sept 1985.
29. Garvey JM et al: Surveillance for postoperative infections in outpatient gynecologic surgery, Infect Control 7:54, 1986.
30. Goodspeed SW and Earnhart SW: Planning, developing, and implementing a freestanding ambulatory surgery center, Health Care Strategic Management, p18, Feb 1986.
31. Group purchasing arrangements cut costs for surgery centers, Same-Day Surgery 10:105, 1986.
32. Gynecologist offers guidelines for expanding office-based caseload, Same-Day Surgery 10:90, 1986.
33. HCFA's ambulatory procedures list will be released 'in a few months', Same-Day Surgery 10:138, 1986.
34. HCFA 'reasonable charge' limits may portend national fee schedules, Same-Day Surgery 10:61, 1986.
35. Health Care Survey respondents strongly favor outpatient surgery, Same-Day Surgery 8:62, 1984.
36. Henderson JA: Cost containment, hospital competition aren't limiting surgery center expansion, Modern Healthcare, p 148, June 5, 1987.
37. Henderson JA: Surgery center growth slows; more procedures done, Modern Healthcare, p 154, June 6, 1986.
38. Infection control can be a problem in ambulatory surgery facilities, Same-Day Surgery 10:58, 1986.
39. In 1981, six SDS procedures ranked among top 10 operative procedures, Same-Day Surgery 8:4, 1984.
40. Is tonsillectomy and adenoidectomy safe for ambulatory surgery patients? Same-Day Surgery 9:123, 1985.
41. JCAH, AAAHC authorities discuss accreditation for SDS, Same-Day Surgery 7:95, 1983.
42. Jensen J and Jackson B: Consumers prefer same-day surgery to inpatient care for minor procedures, Modern Healthcare, p 76, May 10, 1985.
43. Krentz SE and Jennings MC: Pricing strategies for hospital-based ambulatory care services: case study of an ambulatory surgery program, J Ambulatory Care Management 9:15, 1986.
44. Lagoe RJ, Bice SE, and Abulencia PB: Ambulatory surgery utilization by age level, Am J Public Health 77:33, 1987.
45. Lagoe RJ, Mankiewicz DA, and Milliren JW: The impact of outpatient surgery on hospitalization, Business and Health, p 38, April 1986.
46. Lagoe RJ and Milliren JW: A community-based analysis of ambulatory surgery utilization Am J Public Health 76:150, 1986.
47. Make immediate plans for onset of ambulatory prospective payment, Same-Day Surgery 10:157, 1986.
48. Market researchers examine nontraditional health care, Same-Day Surgery 7:148, 1983.
49. Marks SD et al: Ambulatory surgery in an HMO: a study of costs, quality of care, and satisfaction, Med Care 18:127, 1980.
50. Mitchell RT: Organization of a major ambulatory surgery program, Surg Clin North Am 67:693, 1987.
51. Most hospitals plan to expand ambulatory surgery facilities, Same-Day Surgery, 9:47, 1985.
52. Moxley JH and Roeder PC: New opportunities for out-of-hospital health services, N Engl J Med 310:193, 1984.
53. Muller C: Outpatient surgery: are we satisfied? Am J Public Health 76:1086, 1986.
54. Nathanson S and Riffer J: Hospitals not ready for outpatient surgery PPS, Hospitals, p 81, Nov 20, 1986.
55. Nearly a fifth of adult surgeries could have been on outpatient basis, Same-Day Surgery 11:13, 1987.
56. New Jersey doctors form center for outpatient hernia treatment, Same-Day Surgery 10:15, 1986.
57. Office-based surgery is target of some insurer incentive plans, Same-Day Surgery 10:159, 1986.

58. Otolaryngologists take firm stand on T&A surgery payment restrictions, Same-Day Surgery 10:136, 1986.
59. Patterson JF, Bechtoldt AA, and Levin KJ: Ambulatory surgery in a university setting JAMA 235:266, 1976.
60. Physician urges eye surgery centers to keep edophthalmitis statistics Same-Day Surgery 10:125, 1986.
61. Physicians debate advantages of different outpatient settings Same-Day-Surgery 8:152, 1984.
62. Pineault R et al: Randomized clinical trial of one-day surgery: patient satisfaction, clinical outcomes, and costs, Med Care 23:171, 1985.
63. Raymond CA: Study questions safety, economic benefits of outpatient tonsil/adenoid surgery JAMA 256:311, 1986.
64. Reed WA and Ford JL: Outpatient clinic for surgery Med World News 12:58, 1971.
65. Rhu HS and Rust JA: Economics of ambulatory surgical gynecology, Clin Obstet Gynecol 17:291, 1974.
66. Rins WH and Rufener BL: Management of the freestanding surgicenter and the allocation of costs, J Ambulatory Care Manage 10:22, 1987.
67. Schneck LH: Ambulatory surgery, AORNJ 40:248, 1984.
68. SDS units can learn from major complications, Same-Day Surgery 7:25, 1983.
69. Should 'ambulatory' be taken literally? Same-Day Surgery 7:115, 1983.
70. Should complicated surgery cases be performed in the SDS unit? Same-Day Surgery 7:142, 1983.
71. Siegel Al: Outpatient pediatric urological surgery: techniques for a successful and cost-effective practice, J Urol 136:879, 1986.
72. Sikes ED Jr and Detmer DE: Aging and surgical risk in older citizens in Wisconsin, Wis Med J 78:27, 1979.
73. Siu Al: Inappropriate use of hospitals in a randomized trial of health insurance plans, N Engl J Med 315:1259, 1986.
74. Stephenson SV: Ambulatory surgical centers, JAMA 253:342, 1985.
75. Study shows office foot surgery costs less than hospital procedures, Same-Day Surgery 9:149, 1985.
76. Surgery center growth slowing, but more procedures being done, Same-Day Surgery 10:114, 1986.
77. Survey reports greater outpatient surgery use at 83% of hospitals, Same-Day Surgery 10:11, 1986.
78. Tang J: Ambulatory surgery, Tex Med 80:39, 1984.
79. Taylor J: Outpatient surgery: an institutional and community impact analysis, J Ambulatory Care Manage 9:38, 1986.
80. Tooth extraction criteria, PSRO combine to lower dental admissions, Same-Day Surgery 8:51, 1984.
81. Urge SDS patients to become fit before surgery begins, Same-Day Surgery 7:122, 1983.
82. Westman J: Same-day surgery: management issues and future growth, Int J Health Plann Manage 1:213, 1986.
83. Wetchler BV: Ambulatory surgery: the future is now, JANA 54:121, 1986.
84. Wolcott MW, editor: Ambulatory surgery and the basics of emergency surgical care, Philadelphia, 1981, JB Lippincott Co.
85. Wong HD: General anesthesia for ambulatory surgery, Int Anesthesiol Clin 20:37, 1982.

3

Socioeconomic and Practice Characteristics

IRA M. RUTKOW

Before 1960 the practice of medicine in the United States was essentially a laissez-faire system. Although there were always some grumblings about governmental interference, most physicians practiced in an unencumbered fashion with little in the way of external controls. It was not until the mid-1960s and President Lyndon Johnson's Great Society with the introduction of Medicare that governmental regulation became a reality. This was further augmented by the funding of medical education via the government's Health Professions Educational Assistance Act. These two laws permanently altered the way in which health care would be delivered.

THE ERA OF INVESTIGATIONS

As surgeons began to practice in this increasingly controlled environment, it was only natural that questions about the efficacy and efficiency of surgical health care delivery would be raised. As such, it was during the late 1960s and early 1970s that initial investigations into the socioeconomic and practice characteristics of surgeons were first carried out.[63,66]

The Study on Surgical Services for the United States

Among the earliest and certainly most comprehensive of these reports was the Study On Surgical Services for the United States (SOSSUS).[4,77,78] This was a vast undertaking by the surgical community to study itself and its role in the future care of patients. It was unlike any previous investigation, and because of its immense scope, it stimulated smaller but similar studies by other medical and surgical specialties.

The roots of SOSSUS can be traced back to January 1969 when Owen Wangensteen, as president of the American Surgical Association, appointed a committee chaired by Jonathan Rhoads to study the future course of that organization. This committee delivered its report in April 1970 and recommended a broad approach to the major issues facing surgery in the United States. This led to the formation of another committee on issues, under the chairmanship of George Zuidema. Concurrently, the American College of Surgeons' Board of Regents had appointed a steering committee on distribution and adequacy of surgical care under the chairmanship of Francis Moore. As these two studies began, it became obvious to both organizations that the entire effort could be pursued in a more efficacious manner by combining the resources of the two associations. In July 1970 the merger was accomplished, and SOSSUS came into being. George Zuidema accepted the chairmanship of the executive committee and directed the overall study.

The first 24 months of its existence were spent in organizing the effort and finding funds for its operation. Ultimately, almost $1.5 million was raised, and the actual gathering of information took place during the early 1970s. Numerous subcommittees were appointed including academic surgical manpower; surgical manpower; allied surgical manpower; organization, delivery, and financing of surgical services; legal and ethical issues in surgery; community-physician relations; interprofessional relations; surgical research; quality of surgical care; and government relations.

Throughout the first 4 years of SOSSUS' existance, preliminary results from its investigations were published in various medical journals.[49,55] The final version was presented in Fall 1975 as a soft-cover 207-page report that outlined the 10 subcommittees' investigations. A formal three-volume, hardbound, 2782-page edition was offered for sale in the spring of 1976.

Data collection. The SOSSUS utilized two methods to obtain data. One was a questionnaire to obtain information and opinions from a representative sample of surgeons about their practice organization, workloads, work time, and other relevant data. The second was a comprehensive examination of surgeons' work loads in four diverse geographic areas of the United States (the Southeast, the Pacific coast, the Atlantic coast, and New England). In the first method 6201 usable questionnaires were returned of a national sample of 10,000 physicians identified as performing surgery. In the second method, all surgical operations done by 2700 physicians who performed any surgery during the study year were obtained in the four areas.

Data findings. The results were surprising for a number of reasons. The mean professional workweek for a surgeon was found to be 46 hours. This varied from 57 hours for a board-certified thoracic surgeon to 38 hours for a board-certified ophthalmologist. The average workweek was noted to vary greatly by type of practice arrangement. An academic board-certified surgeon averaged 52 hours while a hospital-based board-certified surgeon worked 42 hours. Much of professional time was devoted to direct patient care. Differences between the specialties ranged from 37 hours for a board-certified general surgeon to a low of 31 hours for a board-certified ophthalmologist. Approximately 35% of all respondents were members of incorporated practices. This was most frequent among the board-certified surgeons. Almost 40% of all surgeons were in group or partnership arrangements.

The manner by which patients came to a surgeon for consultation showed 50% of both office and hospital visits were self-referred. One third came via other physicians. Physician referral, however, varied greatly by specialty. Slightly fewer than 50% of all office or other ambulatory patients were evaluated for nonsurgical illnesses. This also varied by specialty. Thirty-three percent of board-certified surgeons stated their patients in need of routine elective surgery had to wait more than 6 days for a hospital bed to be available. A similar percentage noted their patients had to wait at least 1 week for a nonemergency office appointment.

The most controversial aspect of SOSSUS concerned data on workloads and manpower. The total number of individuals carrying out surgical operations, approximately 30% of all active practitioners, was felt to be excessive. Of the physicians performing surgery in the United States, approximately 20% to 25% did not have the established credentials of the specialty boards. This fact was tempered by the fact that 75% to 95% of all major surgical cases were performed by only board-certified practitioners. For some specialties such as neurosurgery and thoracic surgery the figure approached the 95% mark, while for the general surgeon and gynecologist it was from 60% to 75%. Surgical specialists with certification were noted to have workloads 46% to 89% higher than those without such credentials.

A relative abundance of surgeons was demonstrated in the Northeast, Middle Atlantic, Northwest, and Pacific regions of this country. The central portion occupied a middle range as did the Mountain states, which had an even distribution of all specialties. The South Atlantic, East South Central, and West South Central regions had fewer surgeons as well as all other specialists and had fewer hospital beds. Despite these differences, the distributional discrepancies for surgeons were not large compared with those for other medical specialists and total medical facilities.

The SOSSUS failed to identify large or small areas of this country that were significantly undersupplied with personnel suitably qualified to carry out surgery. Rural counties averaged fewer surgical specialists than did large cities. This concentration of surgical personnel in urban areas often reflected the secondary, tertiary, or highly specialized nature of some specialties. This was particularly noticeable for neurosurgery. By contrast, general surgeons, gynecologists, urologists, and orthopedic surgeons could be found in most nonurban areas.

The most startling finding of the SOSSUS was the remarkably low number of operations performed per surgeon on a yearly basis. Approximately 15% of the board-certified surgical specialists carried out fewer than 50 operations a year, and 31% between 100 to 199. Slightly more than 33% performed 200 or more procedures. These figures ranged from a high of 300 procedures for a board-certified plastic surgeon, 215 for a board-certified general surgeon, to a low of 90 procedures for the board-certified ophthalmologist. Operative workloads were highest among the board-certified surgeons in single specialty or multispecialty groups and partnerships. Operative workloads rose sharply for board-certified surgeons who were between the ages of 40 to 50 years and then declined rapidly.

The study concluded that far too many physicians perform surgical operations and that the workloads of surgical specialists were much more modest than originally expected. Further, the study suggested that the total volume of operations performed in the United States could be handled by a substantially smaller cadre of busier board-certified surgeons.

Responses to SOSSUS' findings. After the presentation of SOSSUS' findings, numerous spinoff articles containing data from SOSSUS appeared in various journals.* All these reports brought SOSSUS into more public view, which allowed its recommendations to be heard at various levels of society in the United States. Partially as a result, SOSSUS was embroiled in controversy from its outset.[10,16,34] Most prominent was its recommendation for controls or constraints on residency output. Accusations of artificially induced doctor shortages were made, and a Congressional committee hurled the shibboleth "unnecessary surgery" at the surgical community.

To make matters worse, the American College of Surgeons began to question many of the recommendations from SOSSUS. This was most evident in a number of articles from the College's Department of Surgical Practice. Williams repeated the 1970 SOSSUS analysis of Rhode Island, using 1977 data from that state. Comparisons of the results for 1970 and 1977 indicated that, at least in Rhode Island, surgical manpower had continued to grow. As of 1977, the SOSSUS recommendations were having no demonstrable impact in Rhode Island. The number of surgeons continued to increase without apparent change in their operative workloads.

Corroborating studies. The major findings from the SOSSUS were corroborated by other studies. Hughes et al. investigated workloads in a general surgical practice.[35] They introduced the term hernia equivalents as a ratio of the relative

---

*References 11-14, 18, 27-30, 52, 53, 55, 56, 58, 59.

value of a procedure to the relative value of an inguinal herniorrhaphy. This then affords a measure of the relative amount of surgical work entailed in an operation. Thus, a vagotomy and pyloroplasty with a relative value of 70, twice that of an inguinal herniorrhaphy at 35, may be said to equal two hernia equivalents of surgical work.

Utilizing this type of weighting scale, Hughes et al. demonstrated a large variation in the workloads among 19 general surgeons in a community practice.[32] The busiest surgeon performed 13 hernia equivalents per week, but the mean weekly workload was only 4 hernia equivalents, and the median was 3. Thus, half of this population of general surgeons performed less operative work per week than the equivalent of three inguinal herniorrhaphies.

Applying this quantification technique to the operative workloads of surgeons in training, Hughes et al. observed operative workloads of 0.7 to 3.0 hernia equivalents per week and mean operative complexities of 1.0 to 1.6 during the first 4 years of training.[33] Chief residents, however, were found to perform 8.2 hernia equivalents per week. In the aggregate, residents performed surgery 21% more complex than the previously cited population of general surgeons in a neighboring community practice.

In a final comparison, the utilization of surgeons in a prepaid group setting were contrasted with the community practice fee-for-service general surgeons.[36,71] The median weekly workload of 9.9 hernia equivalents for the prepaid cohort was more than 3 times that of the fee-for-service surgeons. There was also a higher percentage of operations performed in an ambulatory setting by the prepaid practitioners, which accounted for a higher median complexity of inpatient procedures for that group. Hughes' et al. overall conclusion closely paralleled the SOSSUS' finding that there appeared to be an underutilization of costly and highly specialized surgical skills in a fee-for-service community practice setting. Accordingly, a diminution in the number of residents might result in increased efficiencies in the delivery of surgical health care.

A study of practice patterns in a nonmetropolitan area revealed that general surgeons spent an average of 22 hours seeing approximately 74 patients in one week.[22] Twenty-six percent of the presenting problems and 32% of the major diagnoses were defined as primary care problems. Approximately 22% of the general surgeons' patients required referral to other surgical specialists.

A 1968 analysis of a rural general surgical practice revealed that only 43% of the total cases would come under the category of general surgery.[64] Gynecology, orthopedics, and urology accounted for more than 40% of the procedures. Most subsequent urban/rural comparisons reveal the patterns of surgery to be strikingly similar.[45]

A 1973 report from California investigated the qualifications of practitioners who performed surgery and found a large percentage of operations were carried out by "unqualified" personnel.[65] Specific examples included: the repair of complex lacerations by nonsurgical physicians more than 75% of the time; appendectomy, 40%; tonsillectomy, 50%; and hysterectomy, 30%.

Comparisons between metropolitan and nonmetroplitan areas have shown that in some rural districts the non-board-certified general surgeon performed more surgical procedures on a weekly basis than did the board-certified practitioners. Kane et al. demonstrated in Utah that only 60% of those identifying themselves as general surgeons had specialty certification.[37] General practitioners performed one fourth of all procedures although there was an overall suggestion that the board-certified surgeons carried out a relatively larger proportion of the potentially more complicated surgery. Urban general practitioners performed proportionately more surgery than their rural counterparts. For most procedures, at least one third of the rural patients had surgery in urban hospitals.

Report of the Graduate Medical Education National Advisory Committee

For surgeons, the other major socioeconomic study of the 1970s was the Report of the Graduate Medical Education National Advisory Committee (GMENAC) chartered in April 1976 by Joseph Califano, then Secretary, Department of Health, Education, and Welfare.[26] Its goal was to review residency training from the points of view of geographic and specialty distribution. Submitted to the Secretary of Health and Human Services in September 1980, its seven volumes are a massive compendium of facts.

The GMENAC forecasted surpluses of surgeons in 1990 to be 28,600. Specific numbers were: general surgeons, 11,800; obstetrician-gynecologists, 10,450; orthopedic surgeons, 5000; ophthalmologists, 4700; neurosurgeons, 2450; urologists, 1650; plastic surgeons, 1200; thoracic and cardiovascular surgeons, 850; and otorhinolaryngologists, 500.

GMENAC also defined medical service areas to help assess the adequacy of medical services. Within such areas, standards could be established for the minimum number of surgeons per 100,000 population and the maximum travel time required to receive their service. It was thought that an area is medically underserved if the physician-to-population ratio is less than half that recommended for the nation as a whole or if the maximum travel time required is not feasible for 95% of the population. The standards for general surgery were 4.8 physicians per 100,000 total population and 90 minutes travel time. As with the SOSSUS, among GMENAC's numerous other recommendations were those that called for a reduction in the number of practicing surgeons and the number of entering medical students.

Controversy plagued GMENAC from the minute it was created. Its methodology has been severely criticized, but it remains the standard work on which health care planners rely when searching for information on future medical personnel needs.[51,69] Interestingly, Williams, who had shown the lack of support for SOSSUS' findings, demonstrated that GMENAC's calculations for a surgeon surplus should really have been 56,000.[75]

Conclusions

The presentation of GMENAC's recommendations symbolically brought the many research projects started in the 1970s to a close. It would be safe to say that many of the findings from the previously cited papers are no longer applicable to United States surgeons. The socioeconomic conditions under which surgery in the United States is practiced have undergone dramatic alterations in a relatively short time. However, it is important to be cognizant of these investigations from an historical perspective and to utilize them as a guide for future projects.

CHANGES IN THE 1980s

The decade of the 1980s has seen fundamental changes in the delivery of health care in this country. In fact, there has been so much that research projects are often out of date before their conclusions can be presented. Unfortunately, this is one of the major difficulties in attempting to understand current socioeconomic and practice characteristics of surgeons. During the past few years there has been a relative dearth of such studies. There are various reasons for this, but in the final analysis our knowledge of the socioeconomic and practice characteristics of surgeons today is less than in the 1970s.

Increase in Specialization

One of the most important changes of the past two decades is the overwhelming motivation for graduate education and specialty certification. By the end of the 1960s it had become evident that postgraduate training and eventual board certification were to be the sine qua non of the total medical education experience. Previous studies had suggested that a sizable portion of surgery in this country was being performed by individuals who were not trained as surgeons and did not have credentials of their respective boards.[46] Levitt et al. demonstrated that more than 90% of graduates of medical schools in the United States in 1960 and 1964 sought residency training, and three fourths of them had achieved specialty certification.[42] The authors concluded that by the late 1970s this process would go on to completion and that virtually every graduate of a medical school in the United States would undergo formal training beyond the internship with a view to specialty certification.

This finding was supported by Moore and Lang's 1981 study that found the total number of board-certified physicians in medicine, surgery, and the clinical services to have increased from 106,300 in 1971 to 158,900 in 1978.[54] As a result the percentage of board-certified physicians in these specialty fields grew from 65% to 78%. It was concluded that board certification was becoming a virtually universal criterion that carried the implication of de facto licensing.

As such, Schwartz et al. studied the changing geographic distribution of board-certified physicians.[68,70] They showed that for the first time between 1960 and 1977, diplomates of specialty boards began to appear in many small nonmetropolitan communities. The percentage increase in numbers of specialists in small towns significantly exceeded that in cities, but the absolute increase in specialists per 100,000 persons was greater in metropolitan areas. For example, in 1960, 19% of towns with a population of 5000 to 10,000 had board-certified general surgeons. By 1977 the figure had increased to 38%. In urology, for towns of 10,000 to 20,000 population, the percentages changed from 9% to 26%. The findings suggested that the increased supply of specialists activated market forces that caused the observed changes in distribution.

Increased Delivery of Primary Care by Specialists

Interestingly, along with this dramatic surge in the number of specialists, there was a parallel increase in their delivery of primary care.[1] It seemed as though a continued shortage of primary care physicians was being compensated for by the specialist. Whether specialists' participation in primary care was the most appropriate or cost-effective way to improve access to such care remains unresolved.

Payment Arrangements and Numbers of Surgeons

One of the most effective ways in which to determine if the practice of surgery has truly changed is to query the practicing surgeon. Three such questionnaires, which span the 1970s and 1980s, document the evolving situation.[8,12,50] In 1971 a poll of fellows of the American College of Surgeons showed the following results: of the respondents, 77% thought a fee-for-service practice arrangement was most preferable; only 19% favored collection of fees by a group with payment to the surgeon via a negotiated formula. From the same questionnaire, surgeons were asked to estimate the number of surgeons who were active as compared with the number necessary to provide for best service in their specialty. Thirty percent stated there were too many, and 54% said there was an appropriate number.

In a report from 1977, similar questions yielded the following opinions. Forty-seven percent of general surgeons felt there was an excess of other general surgeons, and 46% thought the number was about right. A full decade later, 52% of general surgeons thought there were too many other surgeons, and only 39% felt there were just enough. Clearly, the general surgeons' image of overcrowding in their own field was increasingly evident.

Surgical Physician Assistants

One of the most ballyhooed aspects of surgical care in the late 1970s and early 1980s was utilization of surgical physician assistants. There were enormous policy implications for the future represented in this concept. Initially developed at Duke University and the University of Washington in the mid-1960s, it stimulated a surprising amount of interest and research. As the surplus of surgeons grew in the United States, it was anticipated that appropriately trained and supervised surgical physician assistants would play an increasingly important role in improving the care of surgical patients and, by functioning as junior housestaff, make it possible to reduce the number of surgeons being trained. Certainly, this scenario never developed.*

Some specialties use a large number of surgical physician assistants. However, this level of usage has not occurred across all surgical specialties. The surgeon surplus has brought forth enormous changes in health care delivery. Among these changes is a decrease in the individual surgeon's caseload. It would be unlikely to expect surgeons to further decrease their operative time by allowing physician assistants into the operating room to supplant fully trained surgeons. As Lewit et al. pointed out, it is difficult to advocate the modification of organizational and financial barriers that exist with the introduction of paraprofessionals as surgical assistants when there already exists an excess of surgeons.

As early as 1971 surgeons were indicating there would be some opposition to utilizing surgical assistants. Although from a policy standpoint, the concept of paraprofessionals assisting in the operating room would seem an enviable goal, in this era of surgeon surplus it can no longer be considered realistic. As would be expected, there has been little more formal research into the cost efficacy of surgical assistants, and the nationwide clamor for their presence is no longer strongly noted.

Specialty-specific Studies

During the last decade, each surgical specialty has realized that its specific needs and desires are not necessarily met by studies that consider surgery and surgeons as a whole.† Administrative bodies within each separate surgical specialty have presented or are preparing studies that look at practice characteristics of specialty surgeons. Unfortunately, in most cases these separate studies deal with little more than questions of manpower. Indepth analyses of how surgeons practice, current socioeconomic indicators, environmental trends likely to affect the practice setting, organization of practice, types and numbers of services provided, and mechanisms of payment for service need to be fully explored.

A recent study on elective foot surgery and the relative roles of podiatrists and orthopedic surgeons points out the importance of specialty-specific reports. Weiner et al. have demonstrated that more than 60% of all elective insured foot surgery for federal employees was completed by doctors of podiatric medicine.[73] Although they were not able to adjust for the severity of the patient's underlying condition or the appropriateness and outcome of surgery, the average per procedure charge submitted by an orthopedic surgeon was 17% higher than that of a podiatrist. More important, orthopedic surgeons were 5 times more likely to perform a surgical operation on an inpatient basis, and their admitted patients had longer hospital stays. The practical impact of such findings on the reimbursement mechanisms for elective foot surgery is enormous.

In another specialty-oriented report, the utilization of otolaryngologic surgical procedures performed in Syracuse during 1983 and 1984 was evaluated.[41] This citywide analysis demonstrated that 63% of otolaryngologic operations carried out during the study were performed in outpatient settings. Total utilization was highest for myringotomies, tonsillectomies, and adenoidectomies, more than 80% of which were performed on an ambulatory basis. The greatest number of these operations were performed in free-standing ambulatory surgical centers. Examples such as the preceeding two papers point out the necessity for each surgical speciality to complete its own report similar to SOSSUS.

---

*References 5, 19, 20, 31, 39, 40, 43, 47, 48, 61, 62.
†References 2, 3, 9, 15, 17, 21, 23, 25, 44, 57, 60, 67, 72, 76.

Comprehensive Studies

After the large number of investigations from the 1970s and early 1980s on socioeconomic and practice characteristics of surgeons, the present paucity of new studies is disappointing. Most data that are available come from sources such as the American Medical Association, American Hospital Association, or the American College of Surgeons.

AMA data on workload. Freiman and Marder studied changes in the hours worked by physicians from 1970 to 1980.[24] Utilizing the information from the AMA's Sixth Periodic Survey of Physicians, they noted a statistically significant decline in hours of approximately 3%, or 1½ hours per week. For surgeons, however, they found that the number of hours worked per week had dropped by about 2%. However, because the percentage of total weekly work hours spent in patient care had increased from 88.5% to 90.3%, the actual number of hours spent in patient care remained roughly equivalent. Unfortunately, most of the information in this study relates to a time that preceeds the enormous socioeconomic changes of the 1980s. For this reason the findings and conclusions appear somewhat outdated.

ACS data on workload. The American College of Surgeons through its annual Surgical Manpower Survey has noted definite workload changes among general surgeons.[50, 51] There have been sizeable declines in both time spent in direct patient care activities (approximately 6%) and in the number of operative procedures performed by an average general surgeon (25%) from 1982 to 1985. In 1985 an average of 19 hours per week was spent in the operating room, 14 hours in the office, and 11 hours making hospital rounds. Most important, there has been a decrease from 60% to 48% of general surgeons who felt their practice workload was satisfactory. Conversely, there has been an increase from 17% to 29% of general surgeons who consider their workload too light. These results suggest an overall drop in output of the average general surgeon and increasing dissatisfaction with daily activities. This study points out the futility of utilizing data from reports more than 5 years old to understand current practice characteristics.

Another study from the American College of Surgeons shows that it is still not known exactly what operations currently constitute the typical surgical workload of a board-certified general surgeon.[38] The delivery of surgical health care is undergoing such rapid change that the style of practice this year can be dramatically different from what it was only 3 or 4 years ago.

AMA data on physician characteristics and distribution. The American Medical Association, through its annual survey on physician characteristics and distribution, provides historical and current data on this country's physician population. The following data (based on the 1987 AMA survey) furnish a basis for comparison essential for health services research, program planning, and policy development.[6] As of January 1, 1987, there were 569,160 physicians in the United States. In absolute numbers, the total physician population grew by 119% between 1960 and 1987 (approximately 260,000 to 569,000). The country's total population increased by 35% (183,000,000 to 247,000,000) in the same period. These data indicate physician growth was 240% greater than that of the total population. In 1986 there were 60% more physicians per 100,000 population than a quarter of a century earlier. Fifteen percent of physicians in the United States are women. Foreign medical graduates constitute 22% of the total, Canadian graduates slightly more than 1%, and United States graduates 77%. Eighty-one percent of physicians are involved in patient care. Proportionate percentages of physicians in residency training or fellowship since 1965 showed virtually no fluctuation. However, the total number of residents and fellows since 1965 grew by 45,234 or 104% (Tables 3-1 and 3-2).

Socioeconomic and Practice Characteristics

Table 3-1. Physicians in the United States

	1963	1970	1983	1986
Total physicians	276,475	334,028	519,546	569,160
Men	257,818 (93%)	308,627 (92%)	449,958 (87%)	482,490 (85%)
Women	17,322 (7%)	25,401 (8%)	69,588 (13%)	86,670 (15%)
United States graduates	238,571 (86%)	270,637 (81%)	398,142 (77%)	436,556 (77%)
Foreign medical graduates	30,925 (11%)	57,217 (17%)	112,005 (22%)	123,090 (22%)
Canadian graduates	5644 (3%)	6174 (2%)	7863 (1%)	8148 (1%)
Patient care	NA	278,535 (83%)	423,361 (82%)	462,126 (81%)
Residents and fellows	43,506 (15%)	51,228 (15%)	73,171 (14%)	88,650 (15%)

Table 3-2. Total physicians per 100,000 total population

Year	1965	1970	1975	1980	1985
Ratio	150	161	180	200	222

Among the 569,160 physicians in the United States, 129,234 (23%) designate themselves as surgeons. Of these a total of 22,412 (18%) are foreign medical graduates. There are 10,221 (8%) women surgeons (Table 3-3).

Of the 118,687 male physicians who consider themselves surgeons 26,694 (22%) are younger than the age of 35; 33,597 (28%) from 35 to 44 years of age; 28,694 (24%) age 45 to 54 years; 19,291 (16%) from 55 to 64 years of age; and 10,412 (9%) are 65 years of age and older (Table 3-4).

Of the 10,547 female physicians who designate themselves surgeons, 5797 (55%) are younger than the age of 35; 3079 (29%) from 35 to 44 years of age; 962 (9%) age 45 to 54 years; 450 (4%) from 55 to 64 years of age; and 259 (2%) are 65 years of age and older.

The importance of board certification as a measure of postgraduate training and overall medical education is well established. Of the 569,160 total physicians, 254,637 (45%) are not board certified. Among the 129,234 physicians self-designated as surgeons, 46,977 (36%) do not have board certification (Table 3-5). The majority of the non-board-certified group fall into two categories. Either they are the older surgeons, who began practice when board certification was not as important as it is today, or the younger surgeons who are in the middle of or just completing training and have not had the opportunity to take the board examination. At present, approximately 3500 to 4000 new certificates are issued yearly by the ten surgical specialty boards (Table 3-6). In the future, it will be the rare surgeon who does not have the full credentials of his specialty board.

AMA data on characteristics of medical practice. The American Medical Association

Table 3-3. Total surgeons by specialty

	1965	1975	1986
General surgery	27,693	31,562	37,214
Foreign medical graduates	NA	6786 (22%)	7701 (21%)
Women	NA	567 (2%)	2009 (5%)
Obstetrics/gynecology	16,833	21,731	31,364
Foreign medical graduates	NA	4209 (19%)	6579 (21%)
Women	NA	1777 (8%)	6136 (20%)
Orthopedic surgery	7549	11,379	17,659
Foreign medical graduates	NA	1095 (10%)	1757 (10%)
Women	NA	60 (1%)	326 (2%)
Ophthalmology	8397	11,129	15,180
Foreign medical graduates	NA	950 (9%)	1362 (9%)
Women	NA	395 (4%)	1248 (8%)
Urology	5045	6667	8980
Foreign medical graduates	NA	1050 (16%)	1776 (20%)
Women	NA	16 (<1%)	110 (1%)
Otolaryngology	5325	5745	7577
Foreign medical graduates	NA	777 (14%)	1130 (15%)
Women	NA	69 (1%)	326 (4%)
Plastic surgery	1133	2236	4185
Foreign medical graduates	NA	319 (14%)	715 (17%)
Women	NA	62 (3%)	243 (6%)
Neurologic surgery	2045	2926	4126
Foreign medical graduates	NA	477 (16%)	664 (16%)
Women	NA	18 (1%)	104 (3%)
Thoracic surgery	1477	1979	2114
Foreign medical graduates	NA	442 (22%)	527 (25%)
Women	NA	4 (<1%)	23 (1%)
Colon rectal surgery	650	661	835
Foreign medical graduates	NA	89 (13%)	201 (24%)
Women	NA	5 (1%)	22 (3%)

Table 3-4. Surgeons by age

	<35	35-44	45-54	55-64	65 >
General surgery	11,161 (30%)	8891 (24%)	7339 (20%)	6181 (17%)	3642 (10%)
Obstetrics/gynecology	7943 (25%)	9283 (30%)	6782 (22%)	4951 (16%)	2405 (7%)
Orthopedic surgery	4635 (26%)	5357 (30%)	4279 (25%)	2330 (13%)	1058 (6%)
Ophthalmology	3500 (23%)	4526 (30%)	3645 (24%)	2093 (14%)	1416 (9%)
Urology	1697 (19%)	2693 (30%)	2469 (27%)	1450 (16%)	671 (8%)
Otolaryngology	1723 (23%)	2240 (30%)	2055 (27%)	907 (12%)	652 (9%)
Plastic surgery	646 (15%)	1664 (40%)	1164 (28%)	507 (12%)	204 (5%)
Neurologic surgery	932 (23%)	1149 (28%)	1114 (27%)	644 (16%)	287 (7%)
Thoracic surgery	172 (8%)	580 (27%)	638 (30%)	520 (25%)	204 (10%)
Colon/rectal surgery	82 (10%)	293 (35%)	170 (20%)	158 (19%)	132 (16%)

Table 3-5. Board certification status of surgeons

	Board-certified	Not board-certified
General surgery	20,614 (55%)	16,600 (45%)
Obstetrics/gynecology	19,041 (61%)	12,323 (39%)
Orthopedic surgery	11,714 (66%)	5945 (34%)
Ophthalmology	11,000 (72%)	4180 (28%)
Urology	6447 (72%)	2533 (28%)
Otolaryngology	5267 (70%)	2310 (30%)
Plastic surgery	3109 (74%)	1076 (26%)
Neurologic surgery	2538 (62%)	1588 (38%)
Thoracic surgery	1860 (88%)	254 (12%)
Colon/rectal surgery	667 (80%)	168 (20%)

Table 3-6. Annual certificates issued by surgical specialty boards

	1971	1974	1977	1980	1983	1986
General surgery	873	806	954	1,081	911	912
Obstetrics/gynecology	620	734	829	780	927	596
Orthopedic surgery	504	657	719	570	299	629
Ophthalmology	383	426	567	496	481	480
Urology	206	215	402	332	273	237
Otolaryngology	332	275	284	121	255	251
Plastic surgery	89	144	157	155	163	176
Neurologic surgery	92	66	104	138	108	83
Thoracic surgery	160	158	146	110	136	147
Colon/rectal surgery	23	20	31	38	31	45
TOTALS	3282	3501	4193	3821	3584	3556

also conducts a socioeconomic monitoring system. The following data are from the 1987 edition of its publication on socioeconomic characteristics of medical practice.[7] The average surgeon works 47 weeks of the year and performs 49 hours per week of direct patient care. Twenty-one hours are for office visits; 9 are for hospital rounds; 15 are spent in the operating room; and 5 hours for other visits. However, when other professional responsibilities are included, the mean number of hours worked per week increases to 58.

For surgeons the mean number of hours of direct patient care activities per week has increased from 47.6 in 1982 to the 1986 figure of 49.2. The obstetrician/gynecologist has noticed an even larger increase from 49.2 hours in 1982 to 54.4 in 1986.

In 1986 surgeons were discharging on average 5.3 patients from the hospital per week. For obstetrician/gynecologists the number was 7.4. For all surgical specialties the amount of hospital discharges has shown steady declines since the beginning of the 1980s. Currently the average length of stay for a surgical patient is 4 days. The obstetric/gynecologic patient has an average stay of only 3½ days. As expected, the mean number of days for hospital stays per patient has shown a progressive decline over the last 5 years.

CONCLUSIONS

Unfortunately, there are few other current studies that investigate the demographics and practice characteristics of surgeons in the United States. For this reason, our understanding of the mechanics of surgical practice is less in the 1980s than it was in the 1970s. Unless there are concerted efforts on the part of both organized surgery and the federal government to institute new SOSSUS-like studies, it can be anticipated that policy implementation, which depends on the presence of up-to-date socioeconomic data, will be haphazard and perhaps misguided.

References

1. Aiken LH et al: The contribution of specialists to the delivery of primary care: a new perspective, N Engl J Med 300:1363, 1979.
2. Alford BR: Manpower needs in otorhinolaryngology, Arch Otolaryngol 104:725, 1978.
3. American Academy of Orthopaedic Surgery: 1982 manpower survey, document 270-82, Chicago: The Academy, 1982.
4. American College of Surgeons–American Surgical Association: Surgery in the United States: a summary report of the study on surgical services for the United States (SOSSUS), Chicago: American College of Surgeons & American Surgical Association, 1975.
5. American College of Surgeons Subcommittee on Allied Health Personnel: Essentials of an approved educational program for the surgeon's assistant, Bull Am Coll Surg 58:58, 1973.
6. American Medical Association: Physician characteristics and distribution in the United States, 1987, Chicago: American Medical Association, 1987.
7. American Medical Association: Socioeconomic characteristics of medical practice, 1987, Chicago: American Medical Association, 1987.
8. Anonymous: Results of the fellowship questionnaire, Bull Am Coll Surg Dec 1971.
9. Ansell JS: Trends in urological manpower in the United States in 1986, J Urol 138:473, 1987.
10. Blackstone EA: The condition of surgery: an analysis of the American College of Surgeons' and the American Surgical Association's report on the status of surgery, Milbank Mem Fund Quart 55:429, 1977.
11. Bloom BS and Peterson OL: Changing the number of surgeons, N Engl J Med 303:1227, 1980.
12. Bloom BS et al: Surgeons in the United States: opinions on current issues related to surgical practice, Surgery 82:635, 1977.
13. Bloom BS et al: Surgeons in the United States: practice characteristics. Arch Surg 113:188, 1978.
14. Bloom BS et al: Thoracic surgeons and their surgical practice, J Thorac Cardiovasc Surg 78:167, 1979.
15. Cleveland RJ, Orthner HG, and Bahnson HT: Thoracic surgery manpower: the third manpower study, J Thorac Cardiovasc 84:921, 1982.
16. Colton T: Quality of care and unnecessary operations: a comment on the condition of surgery, Milbank Mem Fund Quart 55:461, 1977.
17. Council on long range planning and development with the cooperation of the American College of Obstetricians and Gynecologists, JAMA 258:3547, 1987.
18. DeJong RH: Too many surgeons? JAMA 237:267, 1976.
19. Detmer DE and Perry HB: The utilization of surgical physician assistants: policy implications for the future, Surg Clin North Am 62:669, 1982.
20. Detmer DE et al: Surgical trainees in the Duke physician's associate program, Surgery 72:142, 1972.
21. Ernst CB et al: Vascular surgery in the United States: report of the joint SVS-ISCVS committee on vascular surgical manpower, J Vasc Surg 6:611, 1987.
22. Folse R et al: Surgical manpower and practice patterns in a nonmetropolitan area, Surgery 87:95, 1980.
23. Fraley EE and Watkins E: Surgical and urologic manpower in the United States, 1969 to 1978, J Urol 127:218, 1982.
24. Freiman MP and Marder WD: Changes in the hours worked by physicians, 1970-80, Am J Public Health 74:1348, 1984.
25. Glenn JF: Urologic manpower and training program survey, J Urol 117:137, 1977.
26. Graduate Medical Education National Advisory Committee: Report of the Graduate Medical Education National Advisory Committee to the Secretary, Department of Health and Human Services, Vol 1, Summary Report. USDHSS, HRS, Office of Graduate Medical Education, Washington, DC, 1980, US Government Printing Office.
27. Hauck WW et al: Osteopathic surgeons in the United States, The DO 119:125, 1976.
28. Hauck WW et al: Surgeons in the United States, JAMA 236:1864, 1976.
29. Hauck WW et al: Urologists and their surgical practice, Urology 12:557, 1978.
30. Hauck WW et al: General surgeons and their surgical practice, Surgery 85:303, 1979.
31. Heinrich JJ et al: The physician's assistant as resident on surgical service, Arch Surg 115:310, 1980.
32. Hughes EFX, Lewit EM, and Lorenzo FV: Time utilization of a population of general surgeons in community practice, Surgery 77:371, 1975.
33. Hughes EFX, Lewit EM, and Rand E: Operative workloads in one hospital's general surgical residency program, N Engl J Med 289:660, 1973.
34. Hughes EFX, Lewit EM, and Pauly MV: The study on surgical services for the United States: a valid prescription for American surgery? Milbank Mem Fund Quart 55:465, 1977.
35. Hughes EFX et al: Surgical workloads in a community practice, Surgery 71:315, 1972.

36. Hughes EFX et al: Utilization of surgical manpower in a prepaid group practice, N Engl J Med 291:759, 1974.
37. Kane RL et al: Giving and getting surgery in Utah: an urban-rural comparison, Surgery 83:375, 1978.
38. Karnell LH: The surgical manpower survey: selected operative procedures performed by board-certified general surgeons, 1982-1985, Bull Am Coll Surg 72:9, 1987.
39. Laws HE and Elliott RL: Experience with a surgeon's assistant in a community practice, Am Surg 38:214, 1972.
40. Laws HL et al: Training and use of surgeon's assistants, Surgery 83:445, 1978.
41. Leopold DA and Lagoe RJ: Patterns of otolaryngologic surgery utilization in Syracuse, NY. Arch Otolaryngol Head Neck Surg 112:623, 1986.
42. Levit EJ, Sabshin M, and Barber-Mueller C: Trends in graduate medical education and specialty certification, N Engl J Med 290:545, 1974.
43. Lewit EM et al: A comparison of surgical assisting in a prepaid group practice and a community hospital, Med Care 18:916, 1980.
44. Loop FD et al: The fourth manpower study of thoracic surgery, Ann Thor Surg 44:450, 1987.
45. Majure JA and Abernathy CM: Rural surgeons of Colorado: the scope of their practice, Bull Am Coll Surg 66:251, 1981.
46. Mason HR: Manpower needs by specialty, JAMA 219:1621, 1972.
47. Miller JI, Craver JM and Hatcher CR: Use of physicians' assistants in thoracic and cardiovascular surgery in the community hospital, Am Surg 44:162, 1978.
48. Miller JI and Hatcher CR: Physicians' assistants on a university cardiothoracic surgical service: a five year update, J Thorac Cardiovasc Surg 76:639, 1978.
49. Miller LD et al: The training of surgeons: how many, in what, and by whom? Surgery 76:170, 1974.
50. Misek G: The surgical manpower survey: workload changes among general surgeons, Bull Am Coll Surg 72:13, 1987.
51. Misek G and Hynds-Karnell L: The surgical resident pipeline, Health Affairs 6:119, 1987.
52. Moore FD: Contemporary American surgery: hard data at last, N Engl J Med 295:953, 1976.
53. Moore FD: Manpower goals in American surgery, Ann Surg 184:125, 1976.
54. Moore FD and Lang SM: Board-certified physicians in the United States: specialty distribution and policy implications of trends during the past decade, N Engl J Med 304:1078, 1981.
55. Moore FD et al: The production, attrition and biologic life time of surgeons in relation to the population of the United States, Ann Surg 176:457, 1972.
56. Moore FD et al: National surgical work patterns as a basis for residency training plans, Arch Surg 112:125, 1977.
57. O'Neil JA: Update on the analysis of the need for pediatric surgeons in the United States, J Pediatr Surg 15:918, 1980.
58. Nickerson RJ et al: Doctors who perform operations: a study on in-hospital surgery in four diverse geographic areas, N Engl J Med 295:921, 982, 1976.
59. Nickerson RJ et al: Otolaryngologists and their surgical practice, Arch Otolaryngol 104:718, 1978.
60. Pearse WH et al: Manpower for obstetrics-gynecology: III. Contributions to total female medical care, Am J Obstet Gynecol 144:332, 1982.
61. Perry HB: Physician assistants: an overview of an emerging health profession, Med Care 15:982, 1977.
62. Perry HB, Detmer DE, and Redmond EL: The current and future role of surgical physician assistants, Ann Surg 193:132, 1981.
63. Peterson OL: Practice characteristics of surgeons in the United States, Surg Clin North Am 62:641, 1982.
64. Phillips RB: Analysis of a rural general surgical practice, Am J Surg 115:795, 1968.
65. Roemer MI and Gartside F: Effect of peer review in medical foundations on qualifications of surgeons, Health Serv Rep 88:808, 1973.
66. Rutkow IM: Delivery of surgical health care in the United States, Arch Surg 116:963, 1981.
67. Rutkow IM and Ernst CB: An analysis of vascular surgical manpower requirements and vascular surgical rates in the United States, J Vasc Surg 3:74, 1986.
68. Schwartz WB et al: The changing geographic distribution of board-certified physicians, N Engl J Med 303:1032, 1980.
69. Steinwachs DM, Weiner JP, and Shapiro S: A comparison of the requirements for primary care physicians in HMOs with projections made by the GMENAC, N Engl J Med 314:217, 1986.
70. Tarlov AR: The increasing dispersion of specialists, N Engl J Med 303:1058, 1980.
71. Watkins RN et al: Time utilization of a population of general surgeons in a prepaid group practice, Med Care 14:824, 1976.
72. Watts C: Neurosurgical manpower requirements for 1990, Neurosurgery 8:277, 1981.
73. Weiner JP et al: Elective foot surgery: relative roles of doctors of podiatric medicine and orthopedic surgeons, Am J Public Health 77:987, 1987.

74. Williams DC: Surgeons and surgery in Rhode Island, 1970 and 1977, N Engl J Med 305:1319, 1981.
75. Williams DC: Surgery and the GMENAC report: a reality test, Surgery 95:347, 1984.
76. Worthen DM, Luxemberg MN, and Gutman FH: Ophthalmology manpower studies for the United States. Part III: a survey of ophthalmologists: viewpoints and practice characteristics, Ophthalmology 88:45A, 1981.
77. Zuidema GD: SOSSUS and the outlook for American surgery. Ann Surg 184:125, 1976.
78. Zuidema GD: The study on surgical services for the United States (SOSSUS) and its impact on American surgery, Surg Clin North Am 62:603, 1982.

JOHN E. WENNBERG

John E. Wennberg is a professor in the Department of Community and Family Medicine at Dartmouth Medical School, Hanover, New Hampshire. He received his MD degree from McGill Medical School (1961) and his MPH from Johns Hopkins University (1967).

4

Small Area Variations and the Practice Style Factor

JOHN E. WENNBERG

In the 1930s school children living in Oxford, England, were about 10 times more likely to have a tonsillectomy than their counterparts living in Cambridge.[15] In the 1960s the chances that a child would have the operation by age 20 if he or she lived in Morrisville, Vermont, was about 60% and for Middlebury children the chances were less than 10%. In the 1970s the probability of having a hysterectomy in Rockville, Maine, was about 25% by age 75, whereas it reached 70% for the women of Lewiston.[38] In 1982 the rate for carotid endarterectomy among people living in Boston was more than twice that of New Haven, but the rate for coronary bypass surgery was the reverse. Hysterectomies were substantially more common among New Haven women, but hip and knee replacements were performed at a higher rate among Bostonians.[36]

These statistics are examples of small area analysis (SAA), a technique that uses large administrative databases to obtain population-based measures of rates of treatment or resource use. SAA is part of a broader strategy for improving clinical decision making by increasing understanding of the respective roles patients and physicians play in determining the utilization of services and by decreasing uncertainty about the outcomes of care through use of the evaluative sciences. The evidence from SAA indicates a dominating influence of physician practice style in the decision to use surgery and its importance in influencing utilization among defined populations including those living in academically and medically sophisticated communities such as Oxford, Cambridge, Boston, and New Haven.

There is a direct connection between small area variations, practice style, and the professional uncertainty that results when clinical decisions must be based on unevaluated medical theory. The influence of practice has its origins in defects in the scientific basis of medicine, in failure to give priority to the evaluation of the outcomes of alternative treatment theories, and in failure to structure clinical decision making to assure that clinical evidence is correctly interpreted and that patient preferences dominate the value judgments that must be made in choosing treatments. Indeed, I use the term practice style to encompass the idiosyncratic clinical decision-making behavior of physicians that inevitably arises when outcome-based standards of care, based on well-tested clinical hypotheses concerning the outcomes of alternative treatments or on an accurate assessment of the utility or value of care to patients, are not available to guide everyday practice. The challenge to physicians is to improve the scientific basis of medicine by an organized program of research to reduce uncertainties about the basic probabilities for outcome after alternative treatments and to learn how to structure medical decision making to assure that patient preferences for outcomes and attitudes toward risk determine the choice of treatment.

In this chapter I will review the evidence for the importance of practice style as a causal influence in small area variations and discuss briefly the role of the evaluative sciences in improving the scientific basis of medicine. I frame the case with a review of the history of medical care epidemiology's contribution to an understanding of the determinants of variation in the utilization of tonsillectomy and then turn to a more general review of the epidemiology of common surgical practices to emphasize the pattern of variation itself as a major clue to the importance of practice style for a particular operation. Particular attention is focused on the pattern of variation of hospitalization of common orthopedic conditions and then of inguinal hernia repair, appendectomy, cholecystectomy, hysterectomy, and prostatectomy. In a final section of the chapter, policy options for reducing professional uncertainty about correct practice, which in turn can lead to a reduction in unwanted variations in surgical utilization, will be presented.

PRACTICE STYLE THEORY AND THE CASE OF TONSILLECTOMY
The Contribution of J. Alison Glover

The history of the contribution of medical care epidemiology to practice style theory is in many ways a footnote to J. Alison Glover.[15,16] In his classic 1938 study of tonsillectomy among British school children living in different communities, Glover uncovers the small area variation phenomenon for the first time:

> Comparisons of the rates in different areas . . . revealed striking differences in areas apparently similarly circumstanced. . . . the operation rate in Margate was eight times that in Ramsgate; that of Enfield was six times that of Greenwood and four times that of Finchley; that of Bath five times that of Bristol; that of Guildford four times that of Reigate; that of Salisbury three times that of Winchester.

Glover's studies lead him to the importance of what he called "medical opinion" in determining geographic variation:

> Great variations in local incidence appear to depend almost entirely upon medical opinion in the individual area.

Glover uses the term medical opinion to mean clinical attitudes toward diagnosis and treatment that are the products of different learned traditions, rules of thumb, and untested practice theories concerning the nature of disease and outcomes of treatments. His usage is thus very close to the meaning I give to practice style. His main argument is based on "the strange bare facts of incidence," a res ipsa loquitur argument made credible by the sheer magnitude of the variations and the strength of the circumstantial evidence associating physician decision making with the variations. But his argument for the contribution of medical opinion is by no means limited to descriptive epidemiology. In retrospect I can find many uses in epidemiology in his papers that foreshadow the approach of the latter day small area analysts in terms of methodology as well as strategies for establishing causality. There is also a lesson for today in the tone of his approach and his aspirations that the unresolved controversies be settled by appeal to evidence about outcomes.

The Method and the Geographic Unit of Analysis

Glover was an opportunist in his uses of epidemiology to study surgical practice: he found out the available sources of data and put them to use. The post–World War I period in the United Kingdom was a felicitous time for the investigator interested in the epidemiology of tonsillectomy. Beginning in 1919 a tonsillectomy became a subsidized benefit for British school children under the School Medical Service. Throughout the 1920s and 1930s statistics on the number of tonsillectomies performed and the number of children in attendance in each school district were kept and published in the Reports of the Chief Medical Officer. Glover used these reports to estimate the cumulative probability of having a tonsillectomy by place of residence, a technique later formalized by Fairbairn and Acheson,[10] and Gittelsohn and Wennberg.[14] School records also enumerated episodes of otitis media and the results of tests conducted to evaluate hearing loss, and Glover turned this data to advantage to examine the relationship between tonsillectomy and medical care outcomes. In this use of routine data, Glover foreshadows the work of Lembcke,[17] Lewis,[18] Wennberg,[37] Gittelsohn,[13] Roos,[28] Roos,[25] McPherson,[20] Vayda,[32] Barnes,[2] and others[7] who would rely on routine hospital discharge reporting systems and health insurance claims for studies of small area variations or medical care outcomes.

Glover also was the first to demonstrate the principal advantages of organizing epidemiologic studies that concentrate on the impact of physician decision making on utilization. It is the size of the population and the specificity of the relationship between the population and the physicians who are responsible for the decisions to do tonsillectomies that are key to Glover's ability to detect variations. When large regional populations were compared, for example, the rate for London, for county boroughs and for urban districts, he noted the rates were about the same. It was only when these regions were broken down to the level of the individual school district that the great variations were exposed with the "extremes often being in adjacent areas." By achieving a close relationship between the decision-maker physician and the population served, Glover's epidemiology captures the effect of clinical policies on utilization, namely the effect on rates of the school medical officer responsible for the diagnosis and referral of patients for evaluation by the surgeon for tonsillectomy. Differences in policies among school medical officers, which are "averaged out" at the regional level, became a major source of variation when rates among school districts are compared.

Modern day SAA of physician practice styles emulates as closely as possible this specificity between populations and physicians achieved by Glover. In the United States and other countries, where no natural relations exist between administrative boundaries and the providers of care, SAA techniques involve patient origin studies at the postal code or minor civil division level of aggregation to create hospital market areas. In these markets the demographic situation is often such that the clinical decisions of only a few physicians contribute to the overall rate for a specific treatment. For example, in Lewiston five gynecologists were responsible for the hysterectomies, and in the Rockland area there were two.

Examination of the Pattern of Variation

Glover's use of statistics for describing medical practice set the tone of his analysis. "The strange bare facts of incidence" carried most of the weight of his argument as he painted a picture of variability that seemed incredible in terms of the conventional wisdom that medical services were prescribed on the basis of need. In addition to statistics describing cross-sectional variations, Glover made use of the decades-long monitoring of tonsillectomies available from the School Medical Service to show the contrasting consistency of the rates in an area compared with the variation that exists between areas. More recent investigations by the Roos team in Canada[27] and Wennberg and Gittelsohn[38] have noted this broad stability in the rates for a variety of surgical procedures within a particular community and labeled this the surgical signature phenomenon.

Glover paid little attention to the quantitative measure of variation: the actual amount of variation. In the case of tonsillectomy, a frequently performed operation with order of magnitude differences in rates at the extremes, this mattered little. But the systematic application of small area analysis required the development of adequate statistical tools for assessing the variation if the important differences in the pattern of variation between common services was to be appreciated and evaluated. Much of the progress in small area studies have been possible because of the work of McPherson and Clifford,[20] who developed a method for isolating the systematic component of variation, thus allowing the comparison of the degree of variation for the same operation between different sets of small areas as well as the comparison of the degree of variation associated with different operations. Shephard and Cooper have recently suggested a similar approach.[31]

As it turns out, the variation associated with tonsillectomy is about the same, whether the studies are undertaken in the United Kingdom, the United States, or Scandinavia. It also turns out that specific operations appear to have characteristic patterns of variation, and tonsillectomy is among the most variable of operations.

Documentation of Professional Uncertainty and Critique of the Theory Underlying Surgical Practice

Glover's conclusion on the role of medical opinion in small area variations is made plausible by his analysis of the controversies and the disagreements about treatment philosophies that he uncovers through his review of the literature and his discussions with colleagues and consultants. A common theme is the lack of understanding about the natural history of the untreated condition and the important but unsubstantiated future benefits of the operation in preventing bad outcomes. His review suggests that prophylactic removal of the tonsil to prevent the subsequent incidence of sore throat, otitis media, or hearing loss is an unsubstantiated extension of surgical theory based on reasoning by analogy: the theory (evidently correct to Glover) that the operation is effective in properly selected cases with demonstrated morbidity, such as those with "frequently repeated attacks of acute tonsillitis that cannot be explained by extraneous infections," led some physicians to advocate a role for the operation in preventing future impairment in the mildly symptomatic patients. In addition to faulty logic, action based on the preventive theory denies the "probability that the tonsil serves some useful purpose, its tendency for spontaneous involution, and the success of nonoperative methods of treatment that are often likely overlooked . . ." It also is risky, a point Glover makes by showing that 424 British school children died after tonsillectomy between 1931 and 1935.

Glover as a pediatrician may be less neutral about which rate is right than other students of practice variations, but he nonetheless builds his case for the importance of medical opinion by exposing controversy and citing inadequately tested theory concerning outcomes. In this way he sets a tone for subsequent investigations.

Causal Arguments Based on Changes in Practice Style or Physician

Glover's case for the importance of practice style does not rest entirely on circumstantial evidence. He sought out direct evidence, and the most convincing he found is the changes in the rates of tonsillectomy that occurred when the school medical officer changed:

> In 1929, [in] his first year as school medical officer, [Dr Garrow] reduced the number of operations from 186 (2.9% of all children in average attendance) in 1928 to 12 in 1929.

He notes the persistence of the changes: in Dr. Garrow's district the average rate in the 7 years preceding 1929 was 2.6%; in the 8 years after Garrow's employment the rate was more than 10 times less—0.2%. These and similar changes in other school districts were attributed by Glover to the change in medical opinion associated with the change in personnel. Taking advantage of this natural experiment, Glover went on to investigate the association between changes in practice style and health status:

> Judging by the returns for otitis media (which is now very low) and from other conditions, nothing harmful, but rather the reverse, has happened from the substitution, in all but a most carefully selected fraction of cases, of conservative methods for operation, a substitution that has been carried out for 10 years.

Since Glover's time, small area analysts have emphasized the example of the association between changes in personnel and rates of service as an important link in the causal argument for the importance of practice style.

But rapid changes in practice patterns have also been shown to occur in the absence of changes in physician personnel as a result of changes in clinical policies among local physi-

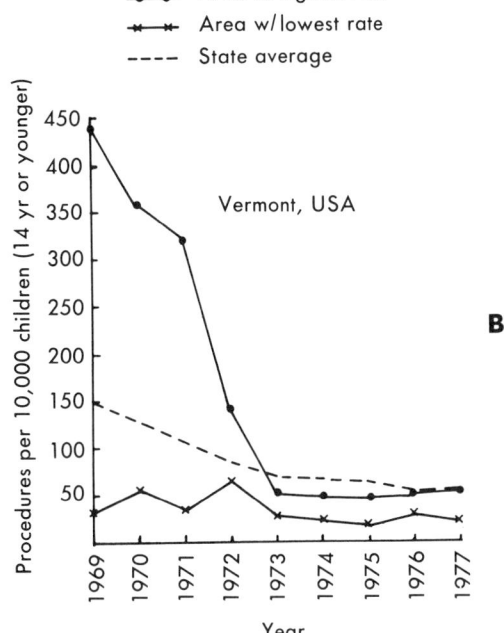

Figure 4-1. Changes in tonsillectomy rates in Hornsey Borough (UK) and Morrisville, Vermont. The figure shows the change in tonsillectomy rates associated with changes in physician practice style. **A,** Variations in tonsillectomy rates among British school children living in Hornsey Borough school district. In pre–World War II Britain, tonsillectomies were prescribed as part of the School Health Service. After 1929, when Dr. Garrow succeeded to the position of school health officer, the rates dropped precipitously. The school health officer was responsible for the initial clinical evaluation. Dr. Garrow's opinion about the value of tonsillectomy differed from his predecessor's. The figure also shows the rate for otitis media, which Glover used as evidence against the theory that tonsillectomy was effective in preventing this condition. **B,** Effect of feedback of information on utilization rates to practicing physicians. The rates compare Morrisville, Vermont, with Middlebury, Vermont, and with the state average. In late 1972, after learning about the rates in their own and in other areas, Drs. Blower and Parker of Morrisville took steps to reduce the rates in their area. The reductions in rates from 1969 to 1970 are explained by the departure from the area of one active surgeon.

cians after the feedback of information to educate physicians about the extent of variation and the rates of surgery in their own areas. This evidence is important not only because the causal relationship between professional decision rules and the level of utilization is directly demonstrated but also because the constructive responses to feedback holds significant promise for reforms that could substantially improve clinical decision making. My colleagues and I learned this in the early 1970s when we became aware of the large variations in tonsillectomy rates among Vermont communities and took the information to the Vermont Medical Society. Without formal program support and principally through the efforts of its past president, Roy Buttles, the society circulated the information on tonsillectomy rates to Vermont hospitals. The rate in the Morrisville area was such that the preadult probability of having a tonsillectomy was 65%; within 2 years the risk dropped to less than 10% because of changes in local practice styles. On learning of the high rate in their area, two physicians, Lewis Blowers, a general surgeon, and Robert Parker, a pediatrician, undertook an active review process that led to the rapid decline[40] (Figure 4-1). They described their experience as follows:

> Awareness of the differences among the areas led us to review the literature on indications for tonsillectomy and we subsequently accepted Haggerty's viewpoint on the indications for tonsillectomy and adenoidectomy. We also agreed between us to review each candidate for tonsillectomy, whether seen on referral or in our own practices. By the end of 1972, we reviewed most of the tonsillectomies performed at our local hospital. We believe this process of obtaining a second opinion helped us standardize the decision process.

Patient Demand as a Cause of Small Area Variation

Glover examined the possibility that illness rates were responsible for the large variations and could find little relationship with "any impersonal factor" such as overcrowding, poverty, bad housing, or climate. Because the services were subsidized and provided as part of attending school, economic factors and access to care were not issues in Glover's situation. In the main, Glover relied on the "strange bare facts of incidence" to make his case, banking more on the epidemiologic common sense of his readers than on systematic, direct demonstration of his thesis:

> In each of these categories there are extreme variations in the operation rate, the extremes often in adjacent areas. . . . Possible factors such as the efficiency of school dental service, rainfall, climate, [overcrowding, unemployment] and nutrition returns have been considered, but with one extremely doubtful exception—urbanization—not the slightest suggestion of correlation has been obtained. . . . But if urbanization be a factor there are inexplicable anomalies. . . . the highest rates of all are in certain agricultural counties and the [urban areas] with the higher rates include residential towns and health resorts famed for their beauty, climate and spaciousness.

Although Glover gave a plausible account of the lack of importance of illness differences, his approach is nonetheless indirect, an argument of exclusion. Because he can find nothing that correlates with utilization, the differences must rest on the supply side where a good case for the rate of medical opinion has been built. Direct evidence would require some form of trial in which the same patients were examined by different physicians with different results.

Unbeknownst to Glover, the "experiment" that was needed to demonstrate directly the lack of importance of variations in patient characteristics or illness rates in the recommendation for tonsillectomy had already been performed. In 1934 the American Child Health Association wanted to make certain that no New York City school child who needed a tonsillectomy went without.[1] They needed, therefore, to know how much "unmet need" there really was. To find out, they undertook a sophisticated study that, ironically, not only provided direct "experimental" evidence for the extraordinary variability in professional judgment, but also led to considerable doubt about the very notion of unmet need.

The research design required the sampling at random of 1000 school children. The examiners found that 60% had already had tonsillectomies. The remaining 40% were examined by the school physicians who selected 45% as needing operations. The investigators wanted to make sure no one in need of a tonsillectomy was left out, so the children who were not selected were then reexamined by another group of physicians. Perhaps to everyone's surprise, the physician recommended that 40% of these have the operation. The third examination of the twice-rejected children by yet another group of physicians produced recommendations for the operation in 44%; only 65 children of the original 1000 survived the screening examination without recommendation for tonsillectomy.

In the discussion of Glover's paper before the Royal Society of Physicians, a discussant raised an additional consumer-based theory of causality of small area variations in tonsillectomy that I have personally encountered on several occasions—that parents learn to expect tonsillectomies and demand them for their children. This theory was the basis for some concern to the physicians in Morrisville who feared that their patients might seek tonsillectomy from physicians in adjacent areas when they became relatively unavailable locally. The dramatic drop in rates and the direct evidence of no increase in use of out-of-area facilities for tonsillectomies after the significant decrease in tonsillectomy rates in Morrisville demonstrates that this is probably not an important factor.

A Missing Link in the Glover Thesis

The evidentiary support of practice style theory would also be strengthened by direct observation of the practice styles of physicians as they interact with their patients, in order to document the differences and to show the relationship between practice style and rates in the area. Bloor, Venters, and Samphier provide this missing link.[4,5,6] Compelled by the logic of Glover's explanation, these workers set out to document the role of medical opinion or practice style theory directly.

They took as their laboratory two health districts in Scotland with substantially different tonsillectomy rates. The high rate district, they showed, had higher rates of referral from general practitioners to surgeons as well as acceptance rates, but with considerable differences among individual physicians within each area. They then observed and characterized practice styles to show how the surgical decision rules of the surgeons varied and how they correlated with propensity to operate. Their work thus provides direct evidence in support of the practice style theory: the differences in rates between the regions, to use Bloor's words,

> can be attributed to differences between specialists in their assessment practices: local differences in the nature of specialist practice "create" local differences in surgical incidence. . . . [The findings] amount to a detailed vindication of Glover's conviction that variations in the incidence of surgery are largely the product of medical opinion rather than the product of the differential distribution of morbidity.

Bloor's examples of practice style are worth reviewing in some detail. The researchers obtained their information by sitting in on the clinical sessions of the surgeons to describe the history taking and physical examination and to develop profiles of the decision rules each surgeon used. They then met individually with each surgeon to review and modify the profiles to make certain that they accurately reflected the surgeon's practice pattern. Variations were found in many of the routines used by the surgeons for assessing the need for tonsillectomy. Differences were noted in the specific clinical features that the surgeons thought were important to take into account in making their decision. Bloor illustrates these differences by direct quotes from three surgeons who had opposite attitudes concerning the importance of clinical evidence for chronic infection, as measured by inflammation in the area near the tonsil (the anterior pillars) or in the lymph nodes or glands:

> Anterior pillars being injected [infected] is a fairly constant [ie reliable] sign: in the healthy they don't seem to be, whereas in the unhealthy there seems to be a sort of injected . . . [appearance].

> All the anterior pillars will tell you [is] if there's been a recent infection—they'll be a bit reddened. It's not of very great importance. The [cervical] glands are important—persistent glands are a sign of persistent infection.

> I don't worry about large cervical glands . . . some people say if they're visible it's significant: if a child comes with visible cervical glands I get their blood examined—one child had leukemia. . . . If they're not visible but palpable it doesn't worry me in the slightest.

Bloor found that physicians with less restrictive definitions of abnormal were "likely to consider a higher proportion of any given child population suitable candidates for operative treatment than colleagues employing more restrictive definitions."

The physicians' practice styles also differed on the basis of the relative importance they gave to the history versus the physical examination. Surgeons with a high proclivity to operate tend to stress the importance of the physical examination. For example, one surgeon felt that three physical signs, that is, purulent material in the tonsil, reddened anterior pillars, and palpable cervical nodes, were decisive, and his rule of thumb was to operate on any child with two or more of these signs. Among low operators, the reverse was the case: much more stress was put on the history. The views of one surgeon represented an extreme of this position:

> I think in almost every instance it's the history rather than the examination. Somebody is supposed to have said once that the only point in looking at the child's throat is to make sure the tonsils are still there, that no one else was there before you! That is an exaggeration but it puts the point over.

Practice style differences were also found in the details elicited from the history and the interpretation of the meaning of referral. One high-operator doctor felt that the mere fact of referral implied an extensive history of morbidity, and in most cases his decision-making strategy combined an examination of the child with a simple check on his assumption of morbidity by asking the parent if the child "suffered lot of trouble." In direct contrast, a second physician (Dr. 1), a low operator, acted as an independent assessor, seeking to reconstruct the clinical history in highly specific terms.

Bloor found that such differences among specialists in the specificity and extensiveness of their history taking linked naturally to similar differences in the decision rules they use in recommending operations. Dr. 1's decision rules could be characterized as a set of conditional probabilities that Dr. 1 estimates from the information he gathers through the history and physical. "Thus, Dr. 1's decision rules constitute a series of linked qualifying clauses on the lines of the following: if a child is, of A age, and if the child suffers sore throats of recurrence rate B, and if the attacks are of severity C, and if the examination findings are of D nature, then the child will receive E disposal." Bloor found that the more specific and extensive the decision rules, the more symptomatically differentiated were the patients receiving surgery and the more restrictive the criteria for surgical admission. In other words, the less likely surgeons were to use crude rules of thumb and the more likely they were to use ad hoc decision analytic techniques, the more conservative were their estimates of the benefits of operation.

Another difference in practice style documented by Bloor is the tendency to temporize, to let nature take its course before making a final decision on the surgery. Low operators were characterized as having a high tendency to wait and see, to arrive at the decision that an operation was not an immediate ethical necessity, and that some intermediate approach such as antibiotic treatment could be used:

What we're really doing is playing for time. I don't know whether the [sulfonamide] really helps or not—it certainly helps in the sense that the parents are pleased that she's getting some treatment—but the important thing is that we gain time to allow the trouble to resolve itself.

Differences in opinion on the outcomes of watchful waiting versus immediate operation, that is, differences in belief in the value of the preventive theory of surgery, are an important source of variation in clinical decision making for a number of common operations.

EPIDEMIOLOGY OF COMMON SURGICAL PRACTICES
A Simple Model of the Determinants of Variation

So far we have discussed only one operation, tonsillectomy, as the epitome of a "high variation" operation. I will show that there are systematic differences in the degree of intrinsic variation in the rates of hospitalization or the use of surgery: the amount of variation is different, depending on the cause of admission or type of surgery. I also will show that the degree of variation serves as an indicator of the relative importance of practice style in influencing utilization rates.

I have found a simple model of the determinants of utilization particularly helpful in organizing my own thinking about variation, and it may be helpful to the reader. Consider first the possible sources of variation in utilization rates. The rate of use of a specific service in a population group, for instance, the rate of tonsillectomy in Morrisville, Vermont, can be viewed as the result of the interaction of four factors. Factor one is the illness rate: the number of individuals per capita who have the illness or condition that makes them eligible for a treatment. Factor two is the rate that those who have the illness or condition actually decide to seek care. Factor two is under the influence of a variety of socioeconomic and personal factors such as income, health insurance, or beliefs in medical care. In the language of the economist, factors one and two are typically demand factors. Factors three and four result from the decisions made by medical professionals, primarily physicians. Factor three covers the diagnostic decisions—the proportion of patients with a given illness who end up with a particular diagnosis. Factor four is the treatment decision of the physician when the diagnosis is made: the proportion of patients who receive tonsillectomy (rather than some alternative treatment such as an antibiotic or watchful waiting). The relationship between rates and behavior is mathematically presented in the box on page 76.

When physicians make consistent diagnoses and when they select the same treatment, factor three and factor four will be constant from area to area and will play no role in the variations. Indeed, a few "anchor" or "low variation" conditions have been found for which the contribution of physician decision making to the rates of hospitalization or surgery is minimal, constrained by a demonstrable professional consensus on correct practice.[34] The classic example is hospitalization for fracture of the hip: all physicians agree on the criteria for diagnosis and the implementation of these criteria is objective and reproducible by virtually all physicians. Physicians also agree on the need for hospitalization. Factors three and four do not vary from physician to physician and any systematic variation in the admission rates to hospital must relate to illness rates (factor one), differences in access (factor two), and/or errors in the data (a source of variation not summarized in the model in the box on page 76).

Practice Style and the Rates of Hospitalization for Orthopedic Conditions

By comparing the pattern of variation in incidence of hospitalization for low variation causes of admission with other causes of hospitalization where professional behavior is less constrained, one can obtain an indication of the impact on total variation that likely derives from practice

---

A Simple Model of the Impact of Illness Rates, Decisions by Patients to Access Care, and Physician Decisions Concerning Diagnosis and Treatment on the Surgery Rate

Variations in the incidence of surgery may occur because of four sets of factors that are intrinsic to the patients or to the physician. Illness rates may vary (factor one); patients may vary in their proclivity to seek care and from whom they seek it from (factor two). Once patients seek the care of a physician, physicians may vary in their diagnosis (factor three) and/or in the treatment they prescribe (factor four). The probability for operation S_k for a particular disease g can be expressed as a function of the conditional probabilities of these four factors:

Factor one (illness rates)

P_{gh} = Probability of disease (g) in individual (h)

Factor two (physician contact rate, given illness)

$\Omega_i|g, h$ = Probability of care from physician (i) given (g) and (h).

Factor three (a physician's diagnosis, given contact and illness)

$R_j|g, h, i$ = Probability of condition label (j) given g,h, and i.

Factor four (a physician's decision on need for a specific procedure, given the diagnosis, contact and illness)

$S_k|g, h, i, j$ = Probability of operation (k), given g,h,i and j.

The expected number of operations (k) may be represented as the sum over all disease states (g) of individuals (h), condition label (;) and physicians (i):

$$E\ S_k = \text{Expected number of operations k in population}$$
$$= \Sigma_{g, h, i}\ (P_{g, h})\ (\Omega_i|g, h)(R_j|g, h, i)(H_k|g, h, i, j).$$

Finally, the overall rate of surgery (SR) in a population of size (N) is a function of the expected number of procedures for each constituent operation that is part of current practice of medicine:

$$E\ S_t = \text{Total expected number of operations in population.}$$
$$= \Sigma\ ES_k$$
$$SR = Es_r \times \frac{1}{N}$$

---

style. As an example, consider the variation in hospitalization rates for orthopedic conditions (Figure 4-2). Ankle and forearm fractures are clearly more variable than hip fractures. Surely the reason for increased variation is not failure of injured people in low rate areas to seek care for their broken bones. It can be said with confidence that virtually all people with fractures will seek medical attention. Factor two is not an important factor, nor is factor three. Except in rare circumstances, fractures are easily diagnosed by physical or x-ray examination, and diagnosis is no more difficult for ankle or forearm than for hip fractures. The factors likely to contribute to the variations are differences in the incidence of fractures (factor one) and differences among physicians concerning the need to treat patients with these fractures in the hospital rather than in the ambulatory setting (factor four).

Although it is logically possible that the incidence of ankle and forearm fractures is much more variable from community to community than hip fracture, there is no sound theoretical reason or any epidemiologic data suggesting the existence of such differences. The most likely source of the increase in variation for ankle and forearm fractures alone and beyond that seen for hip fracture, I argue, is factor four. In the case of hip fracture, the decision to hospitalize is nar-

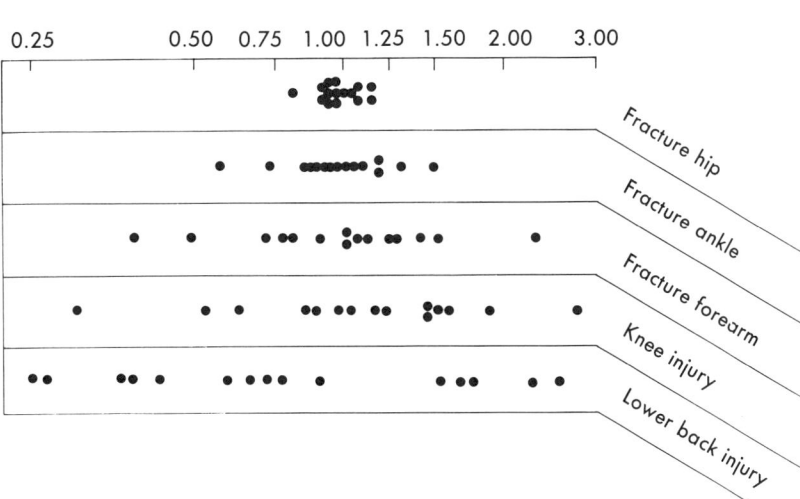

Figure 4-2. Variations in hospitalization rates for common orthopedic conditions. The data are age adjusted and expressed as the ratio to the state average. Each dot is the rate in one of the 15 most populated hospital markets in Maine, 1980 to 1982. The person-years of experience in these areas range from 55,019 in Houlton, Maine to 581,543 in Portland. The expected number of hospitalizations for the least frequent injury in Houlton is 26.7.

rowly constrained because fractures of the hip are very serious injuries with high death rates. The professional standard of practice is firm in its requirement that all patients be hospitalized. By contrast, for the other fractures the implicit standards of care do not tightly constrain the decision to hospitalize.

The same line of reasoning is helpful for understanding the increasing variation seen in Figure 4-2 for back and knee injuries. These conditions offer many alternative treatments ranging from hospitalization with or without surgery to medication and preventive exercises. Orthopedic surgeons are familiar with the controversies concerning the preferred treatment of back and knee injuries and recognize there is little professional consensus on these matters.

Figure 4-2 gives a qualitative feeling for the relative variation of hospitalization rates for the five injuries, but it is often useful to use the more quantitative summary measure of variability made possible because of the McPherson-Clifford statistic, which has become known as the systematic component of variation, or SCV.[20] Under the assumption that variations in the incidence rates for common orthopedic injures are about the same among small areas, the SCV measure for the magnitude of variation in the hospitalization rates for hip fractures can be used to estimate the proportion of variation in hospitalization rates attributable to illness (and errors in the data). For the reasons given above, it is reasonable to assume that patients with fractures virtually always contact the medical care system and that the fractures are virtually always diagnosed correctly. Accordingly, the proportion of variation because of the four factors in the model of utilization can be estimated (Table 4-1). Under

Table 4-1. Proportionate influence of the factors of variation

Injury	Total variation (SCV × 1000)	Estimated Proportion of Variation (%) Because of			
		Factor One (Illness)	Factor Two (Access)	Factor Three (Pt diagnosis)	Factor Four (Pt treatment decision)
Fracture of the hip	7	100%	0%	0%	0%
Fracture of the ankle	47	15%	0%	0%	85%
Fracture of the forearm	138	5%	0%	0%	95%
Back injury	296	2%	?%	(<====?95%===>)	

the assumption that variations because of illness and errors in the data are similar for each of the four injuries, only a small proportion of the variation in hospitalization for ankle and forearm fractures can be attributed to factor one; I estimate that practice style concerning the decision to hospitalize accounts for 85% and 95%, respectively. For back injuries, only 2% of variation is attributable to illness rates; for this condition, differences in diagnostic styles may well play an important role in this injury, and I have indicated this uncertainty in the table. A small amount of variation for this condition may be because of factor two, but the discussion that follows shows that factors affecting patient decisions to seek care are not important causes of small area variation.

Pattern of Variation of Common Operations

Consider now "the strange bare facts of incidence" as they apply to inguinal hernia repair, appendectomy, cholecystectomy, hysterectomy, and prostatectomy and how they compare with tonsillectomy. Figure 4-3 shows the distribution of rates for these operations among the larger communities of Maine, Vermont, and Rhode Island as they were in 1974 and 1976.[20,38] I have deliberately chosen these older data to avoid the possible contribution of outpatient surgery to the pattern of variation. At the time of these studies, all of these operations were performed in hospitals. In each state, inguinal hernia repair is the least variable operation. In none of the areas was the rate statistic significantly different from the state average. The SCV was 8—about the same as hip fracture. The dispersion of rates for appendectomy and cholecystectomy looks more variable than inguinal hernia repair and, indeed, the quantitative measures of variation bear this out: the SCV for cholecystectomy is 17 and that of appendectomy is 17, a ratio to that of hernia of 2.1. These differences are significant.

Next on the scale of variation are prostatectomy and hysterectomy, each significantly more variable than cholecystectomy or appendectomy. For hysterectomy, the SCV is about the same as for fracture of the ankle and about 6 times more variable than inguinal hernia. Eleven or 33% of areas were significantly different from the state average. Prostatectomy is approximately as variable as hysterectomy, showing an SCV of 50. Seven of the areas are significantly different from the state average. Finally, there is the "very high variation" operation, tonsillectomy, with an SCV of 208—some 26 and 4 times more variable than inguinal hernia repair and hysterectomy, respectively. Tonsillectomy is substantially more variable than fracture of the forearm but less than hospitalization for back injury. The ratio

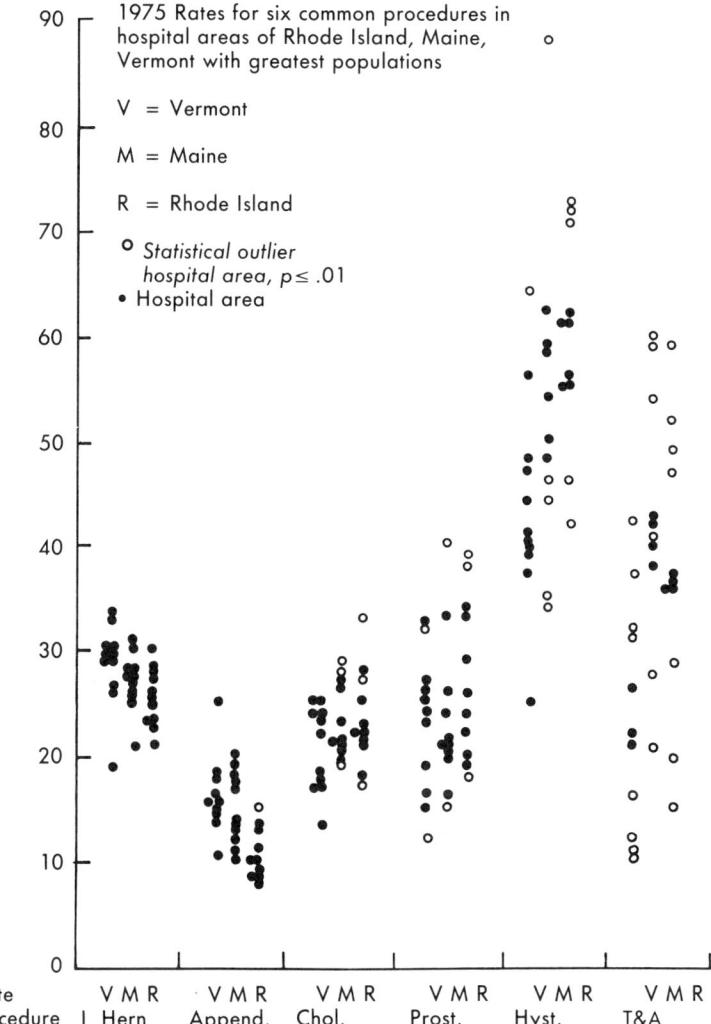

Figure 4-3. The distribution of rates for surgery in the 11 most populous communities in Rhode Island, Maine, and Vermont. The open circles are areas that are statistically different from the average for the state (one degree of freedom, chi-square test, $p<.01$). Note the consistency in the pattern of variation from one state to another for a given operation. The greater the variation, the greater the contribution of physician practice style to the utilization rate.

from high to low in each state is 6 or more and 22 of the 33 areas (66%) are significantly different from the state average.

The reader, in considering the data in Figure 4-3, may be struck by the consistency of the pattern of variation from state to state. This may seem surprising, since the populations have quite different ethnic backgrounds. For example, the populations in many of the hospital markets of Rhode Island are strongly influenced by the Portuguese immigrations that occurred in the late 19th century whereas many hospital markets in Maine and Vermont are predominantly settled by immigrants from French Canada. But despite these differences, the patterns are quite similar, suggesting that for the low variation conditions the incidence of illness is about the same and that for the high variation operations, the practice style factor plays a similar role in each state.

Since the completion of the three-state comparison in the late 1970s, my colleagues and I have replicated these studies in as many different regions as we could to test the hypothesis that the pattern of variation is a function of the procedure rather than of the population or of the way medical care is organized or paid for. Our reasoning went as follows: if professional practice styles are the dominant component of variations, the pattern of variation should tend to be more or less similar from one part of the country to another and, unless explicit differences in professional opinions exist between countries, they should also be similar from one nation to another. Clinicians in different parts of the world tend to have similar clinical options, and they certainly share a common world medical literature; difficulties in interpreting physical signs and symptoms respect neither state nor international boundaries. Given the small area approach, which isolates the decision patterns of a few local surgeons, the population-based analyses would show similar levels of variation on a procedure-specific basis, even though there may well be differences in illness rates and certainly differences in ethnic background, methods of payment, and organization of services.

The common operation study has been replicated in Massachusetts, Iowa, and California.[33] The pattern of variation for these six operations is quite similar, even though population characteristics are obviously different.[29] The most severe test of our hypothesis that the pattern of variation was intrinsic to the procedure came when Klim McPherson, Oli Hovind, and I compared the patterns of variation among three New England states, Norwegian counties, and British health districts, which correspond roughly to our hospital market areas.[20] Altogether we studied nine operations: the six shown in Figure 4-3 plus lens extraction, hemorrhoidectomy, and varicose vein stripping. Despite the known national differences in (1) the organization of medical practices, (2) the numbers of surgeons, and (3) the ethnic and social characteristics of Norwegians, Americans, and the British, the variation in each of the countries was essentially the same, except that for inguinal hernia operations it was (as we shall see, understandably) higher in England, while hysterectomies were less variable in Norway. Our conclusion from the international study was:

> The degree of variation generally appeared to be more characteristic of the procedure than of the country in which it was performed. Thus, differences among countries in the methods of organizing and financing care appear to have little relation to the intrinsic variability in the incidence of common surgical procedures among hospital areas in these countries.

Despite the differences in average rates of use, the rates in England were often much lower than in the United States.

> The degrees of controversy and uncertainty seemed to be similar among clinicians in all three countries.

Professional Uncertainty and the Pattern of Variation of Common Operations

There are controversies and disagreements concerning the diagnosis and/or treatment of the conditions for which these operations are used, and these controversies can be linked in the fashion of Glover to the propensity toward variation.[35]

Inguinal herniorrhaphy. This procedure is recommended by virtually every physician in the United States for patients with hernias, excluding only premature infants and patients with associated diseases that substantially increase the risk of morbid or mortal complications. Authors of medical texts and journals do not view this as a controversial operation. The uniformity in rates reflects the absence of alternatives. This is not so, however, in the United Kingdom where the opinion among US physicians is not shared by their British compatriots. In England there is a long tradition of treating some hernia patients with trusses; the greater variations observed among English health districts suggest that this option is chosen more commonly in some districts than in others.

Since 1982 we have seen a gradual increase in the SCV measure for inguinal hernia repair in the United States, reflecting the differential adoption of the new philosophy of ambulatory surgery in some areas.

Appendectomy. There is little controversy concerning the theoretical reasons for undertaking appendectomy because virtually all physicians recommend this operation for patients with evidence of the classic progression of appendicitis. The controversies concern the diagnosis (factor three): other causes of abdominal pain and nausea and vomiting are commonly confused with appendicitis, leading to appendectomy in patients who do not have appendicitis. The percentage of cases that are shown by pathologic examination to be false positive varies among hospitals, but I have not found any studies to show that the percentage of false positive operations correlates with the appendectomy rate in an area. deDombal and his associates have shown that computer-assisted diagnoses can improve clinical judgment in this area and help physicians reduce the number of false-positive cases.[9]

The SCV for appendectomy is typically 2 or 3 times higher than that for hip fracture or inguinal hernia repair. The curious exception is in West Germany where Lichtner and Pflanz[19] have shown much greater variations interpreted as a response by German surgeons to a specific incentive that, ironically, was designed to assure surgical proficiency.[22] In that country board certification in general surgery requires that a resident complete 1000 appendectomies! Pflanz felt that this incentive clouds clinical judgment. It is curious how a rule that in one context seems so rational may have pernicious effects on utilization.

Cholecystectomy. Agreement exists within the profession that cholecystectomy can provide substantial symptomatic relief and is sometimes lifesaving when done for obstructive jaundice and/or biliary colic secondary to cholelithiasis, for a severe attack of acute cholecystitis, or for cancer of the gallbladder. The disagreements that are easily documented in the literature and through conversations with physicians are about the treatment of asymptomatic "silent" or minimally symptomatic gallstones. Some physicians advocate the prophylactic or preventive removal of such stones while others believe the benefits are not worth the risks.

The situation is similar to the controversies Glover reported in his review of the theoretical reasons for the routine use of tonsillectomy and similar also to arguments we found concerning the theory for intervening operatively in the natural history of prostatism. The argument concerns future probabilities, in this case life expectancy. Some believe life expectancy is improved by early operation because it removes the possibility of a complication in the future when the patient is older and sicker and therefore more at risk for the surgery that would then be needed. Others believe that the risk of developing a complication and the associated probability of death is sufficiently low and that the initial loss in life expectancy caused by the prophylactic surgery will never be regained.

A clinical trial to compare watchful waiting with prophylactic surgery would be very costly. It would require large numbers of patients and would need to be continued for many years. But controversies concerning the preventive use of surgery can be tested using decision analysis, a newer method for testing medical care outcomes that is conceptually similar to a clinical trial but that uses estimates for the probabilities for outcomes derived from synthesizing various reports in the literature. Fitzpatrick and his colleagues evaluated international literature to obtain a set of estimates of the probabilities (1) for operative death rates by age and comorbid conditions, (2) for the incidence of complications, given a silent stone, and (3) for competing causes of death.[11] They then integrated these probabilities in a decision analysis to estimate life expectancy given the two treatment choices. Their results showed little effect on life expectancy, and they concluded that the decision must be based on other issues, namely the patients peace of mind and attitudes toward risk. More recently, Ransohoff and his colleagues conducted a similar analysis but used newer data that included a retrospective cohort study they conducted on the natural history of the unoperated patient that was organized to improve on the estimates found in the literature.[23] The Ransohoff decision analysis showed a slight decrease in life expectancy for those who chose prophylactic surgery. When they included discounting or monitory costs in their model, surgery was further disfavored.

Hysterectomy. This operation is highly variable with an SCV that is typically about 60. When undertaken for cancer of the uterus, the operation shows the low pattern of variation typical for that of hip fracture or inguinal hernia repair, but fewer than 10% of the hysterectomies performed in the United States are for cancer. Most reasons for hysterectomy show extensive small area variations. The most common therapeutic goal for hysterectomy is probably treatment of pain and bleeding, with sterilization and cancer prophylaxis as important secondary objectives. Exactly how often hysterectomy is performed for sterilization or cancer prevention as a primary objective is difficult to say because of controversies concerning the use of hysterectomy for these objectives and because in situations when reimbursement does not cover these objectives, other diagnoses such as stress incontinence or pelvic relaxation may be listed as the reason for hysterectomy.

In contrast to cholecystectomy for silent stones, prophylactic hysterectomy does appear to increase life expectancy. A recent decision analysis by Sandberg and colleagues indicates that prophylactic hysterectomy in a good-risk 40-year-old woman probably does increase life expectancy by slightly longer than 4 months.[30] It is not clear, of course, that the individual patient, if fully informed about the costs, risks, and benefits, would choose the operation for this purpose. For most women there is no gain at all because the increase in life expectancy applies only to the 1.3% of women otherwise destined to die of cancer of the endometrium of cervix. The risk of anesthetic or surgical death, although relatively small compared with some other operations, is not zero. Sandberg estimates the death rate is about 1 in 700 for a 40-year-old woman. There is little information on functional status changes postoperatively, but the available information suggests mixed results. One study suggests the postoperative recovery period is typically longer for this operation than for cholecystectomy and appendectomy. Forty days after hysterectomy, 5% of women reported they felt "worse" than they did before surgery.[24] The Roos team reports that although the number of women making visits to their physicians for uterine-related diagnoses decreases after hysterectomy, the number of visits for urinary tract infections, menopausal symptoms, skin infections, and back problems increases. There is an apparent increase in emotional disturbances among women with hysterectomy compared with those who have had cholecystectomy or appendectomy, as evidenced by the percentage of postoperative patients seeking psychiatric care.[26]

Prostatectomy. This procedure for treatment of benign hypertrophy of the prostate is a highly variable operation with a small area study SCV usually of about 60, and poses many of the same issues. A careful review of the literature and consultations with practicing urologists reveal many gaps in the scientific basis for clinical decision making. There are two schools of thought. One group of physicians are early interventionists who believe that prostatic resection should be carried out when there is clinical and anatomical evidence of benign prostatic hypertrophy, particularly if the patient is relatively young and in reasonably good physical health. These clinicians subscribe to the preventive theory: operate now to avoid greater risks to patients later. Members of the conservative school hold the contrasting belief. Their view is that the natural history of the disease is such that the underlying prostatic hypertrophy will not progress to threaten life expectancy for most patients. If everyone who has evidence of benign hypertrophy were operated on, overall life expectancy would be reduced. For such clinicians the operation in patients without upper urinary tract obstruction is done to reduce symptoms and to improve the quality of life. In this view—the quality of life theory for surgical intervention—rational decision making depends on the prefer-

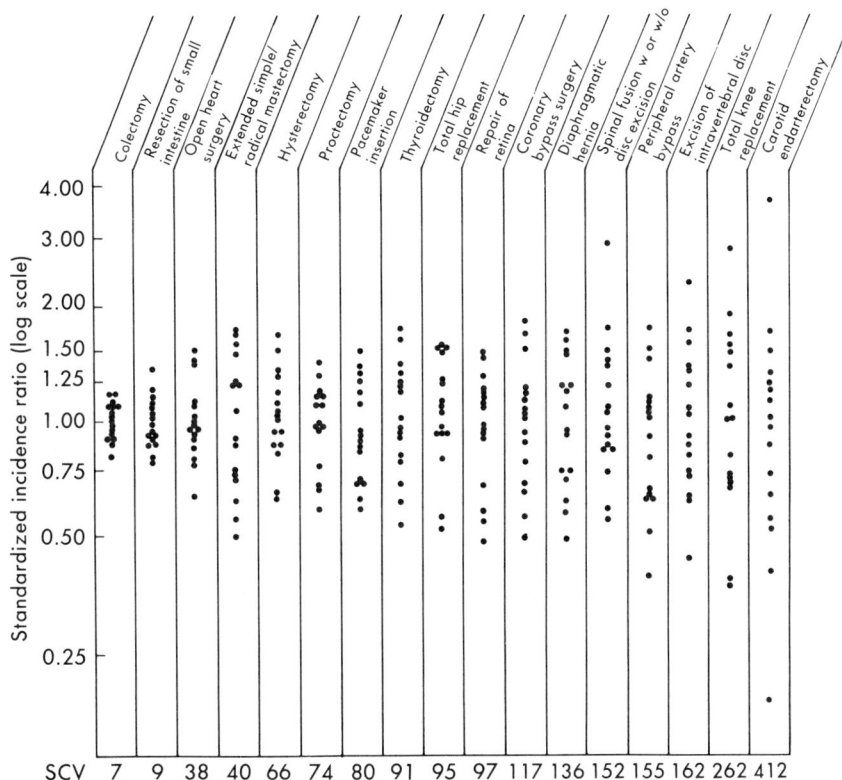

Figure 4-4. Variations in surgery rates for 17 common operations among selected communities in California, Connecticut, Iowa, Massachusetts, and New York. Each dot represents the age and sex standardized rate in one of 16 communities located within the five states. Several of these communities contain well-known academic medical centers (see text). The pattern of variation seen among academic areas (where most services are provided by physicians affiliated with medical schools) is similar to that seen among other areas. The SCV index can be used to point to operations that need assessment because of underlying differences in professional opinion on correct practice. Most of the operations exhibit a variation profile that has greater intrinsic variation than hysterectomy.

ences of the patient for either the various outcomes associated with surgery or its alternative, watchful waiting.

Note the similarity of this controversy to the situation for cholecystectomy. Surgery will entail lower risks if carried out electively today than later as an emergency. On the other hand, elective surgery does carry significant risks and, if deferred, may never become necessary. The question of the impact of the choice of treatment on life expectancy and quality of life, such as that of cholecystectomy and hysterectomy, requires the integration of various conditional probabilities including the probability for operative death and complications, for death and complications from the untreated condition, and for death (and morbidity) from all other cases. It also requires the evaluation by the patient of his attitudes toward these outcomes.[3,12,41]

On the Extent of Variation in Hospital Practice

Using the SCV, we have extended the analysis of variation to evaluate each discrete medical and surgical cause of admission. We used hysterectomy as a reference operation, regarding each operation or cause of admission that was more variable than this operation as "high variation," suggesting that utilization is substantially influenced by practice style. We used the diagnostic related group (DRG) classification system, but in designing the study we were concerned that variations might be caused by minor differences in coding practices.[40] To reduce variation from this source, we grouped similar DRGs to provide a total of 111 modified DRGS (M-DRGs). Among medical causes of admission, only three M-DRGs were less variable than hysterectomy: myocardial infarction, gastro-intestinal hemorrhage, and stroke. As a group, medical admissions were more variable than were surgical admissions. But discretionary professional decision making is apparently playing a role in the decision to use most major surgery. In addition to inguinal hernia repair, appendectomy, and cholecystectomy, only major small bowel surgery and large bowel surgery were less variable than hysterectomy.

Similar studies have now been repeated in several states, and the relative ranking of specific M-DRGs is quite consistent. Recently we compared the rates of surgery in 16 larger communities in California, Iowa, New York, and Massachusetts. Several of these communities contain well-known academic medical centers, including Stanford, the University of Iowa, the University of Rochester, the University of Massachusetts (Worcester), the University of California (Sacramento-Davis), Yale, and the three medical schools in Boston. Figure 4-4 shows the distribution in rates among these areas for the common operations, excluding those represented in Figure 4-3 with the exception of hysterectomy, which stands as a marker for "high variation" operations. Colectomy, small bowel surgery, open heart surgery, and extended simple or raical mastectomy are less variable than hysterectomy. Proctectomy, pacemaker insertion, thyroidectomy, total hip replacement, repair of retina, coronary bypass surgery, diaphragmatic herniorrhaphy spinal fusion, peripheral artery bypass, excision of intravertebral disc, total knee replacement, and carotid endarterectomy each rank as high variation operations.*

---

*Small area studies among communities where most residents receive their treatments in university hospitals demonstrate some of the consequences of the failure of contemporary medical science to provide a workable basis for rationing medical treatments. For example, the per capita costs of hospitalization among residents of Boston are about twice that of the residents of New Haven, even though the populations of these two cities are quite similar demographically. Most of the differences in costs is related to the greater numbers of hospital beds per capita used to treat Bostonians. It should be of interest to surgeons that small area studies show that most of the variation in total per capita costs for hospitalization between communities relates to differences in the use of hospitals for medical admissions rather than surgical procedures. For example, the total rate for surgery among Bostonians and New Havenites is about the same.[36]

The Practice Style Factor and the Supply of Surgeons

The supply of surgeons is of considerable importance to the per capita rate of surgery as shown by the correlations between surgeons and the overall rate for surgery.[18,21,37] However, the correlations between the number of surgeons and the rates for individual procedures are not always strong. This is well illustrated by surgical signature phenomenon, which has been reported by our research team[38] and by the Roos team in Manitoba.[27] In Figure 4-5 taken from studies in Maine, the numbers of gynecologists in low and high hysterectomy rates were approximately equal, but the relative proportions of various gynecologic procedures performed were quite different. Left undisturbed by feedback or by migration of physicians in or out of area, the surgical signature of a community tends to remain constant from year to year.

Boston and New Haven comparisons are interesting in that although the rate for total surgery is quite similar in both communities, the rates for individual procedures vary substantially and in a fashion inconsistent with the theory that surgical care is rationally allocated between competing clinical priorities. For example, carotid endarterectomies are more than 2 times as

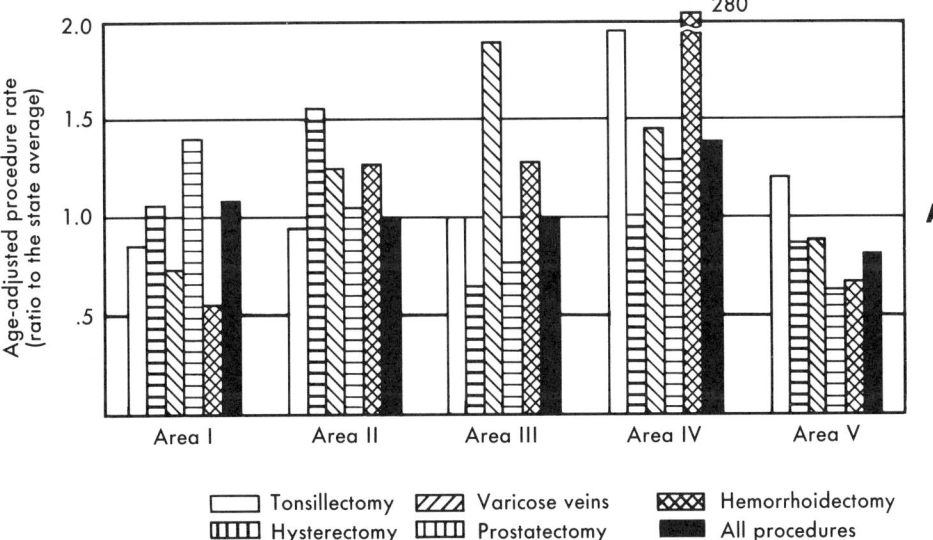

Figure 4-5. The surgical signature. **A,** The numbers on the vertical axis are the ratio of the state average rate to the area rate. The figure gives data for the five most populous hospital areas in Maine. It shows that the rates at which specific procedures are performed within an area vary markedly and to a large degree are independent of the total operation rate. Area II and area III have the same total operation rate, but area II exceeds in hysterectomies doing 56% more than the state average whereas area III exceeds in varicose veins. In each of the five areas a different procedure is performed most often; in four of the five areas, the least performed procedure is different. The number of surgeons and their specialty distribution do not vary to the same degree. It appears that variations in physician supply represent a less important contribution to small area variations in rates of high variation surgical procedures than differences in the opinions about the proper indications for surgery.

Continued.

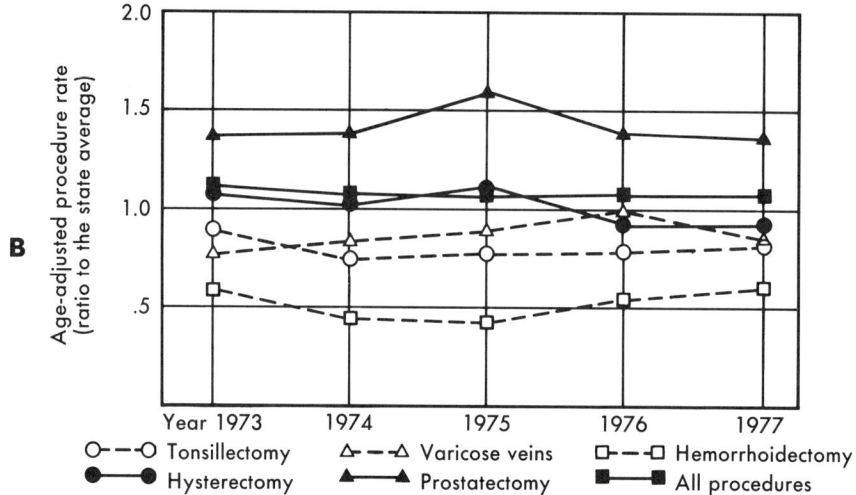

Figure 4-5.—cont'd. B, The surgical signature tends to remain constant over time. The trend lines give the rates of area I for a 5-year period.

common for Bostonians, but coronary bypass operations are twice as common among New Havenities. Hysterectomies are more common in New Haven, but knee and hip replacements are more common in Boston.[36]

When the use of surgery is not governed by a professional consensus on correct medical practice, the rates of surgery reflect the practice styles they adopt, which are in turn the result of a complex interaction between the available supply of surgeons and acceptable (but untested) theory about appropriate practice. This is illustrated by the effect on utilization associated with physician migration. As an example, consider the rapid increase in surgery associated with the arrival of two surgeons in one Maine area who subsequently invested much of their time in back surgery (Figure 4-6). The exhibit also illustrates the counter influence on rates of the Maine Assessment Program's effort to establish implicit regional standards for laminectomy. This effort subsequently led to an assessment of the outcomes comparing medical with surgical management of herniated discs.

BEYOND PRACTICE STYLE: THE ROLE OF THE EVALUATIVE CLINICAL SCIENCES
The Promise of the Evaluative Clinical Sciences

It is possible to go beyond the "incredible bare facts of incidence". The chain of circumstances that now connects small area variations, practice style, and professional uncertainty can be broken. The need is to evaluate untested medical theory, and this is feasible. The past 20 years or so have seen remarkable progress in statistical and epidemiologic techniques and in methods for measuring patient symptoms and evaluating the quality of life. They have also brought equally remarkable progress in computer and information science, in new approaches for evaluating patient preferences, and in the adaptation of clinical decision theory to medical decision making. It is now possible to speak of a new set of disciplines that together constitute the evaluative clinical sciences. They offer the promise of a scientific program that can greatly improve clinical decision making by decreasing uncertainty about

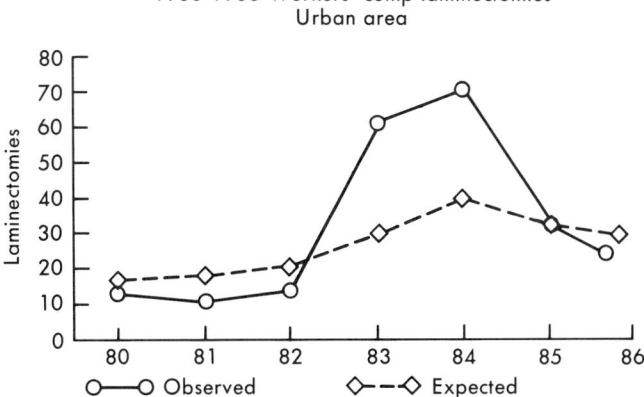

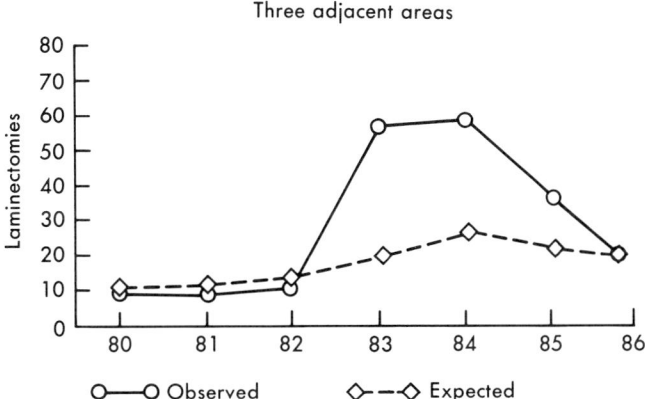

Figure 4-6. The effect on surgery rates of physician migration. Area II in Maine had a low rate for laminectomy in the early 1980s. In early 1983, two new physicians entered this market, and the rate for the operation increased dramatically. The figure shows the number of laminectomies performed on local residents and on residents of three adjacent areas in relation to this change in manpower. The dotted line in the figure gives the expected number of cases based on the state average rate. The increase in expected numbers of cases after 1982 is caused almost entirely by the increases brought about by the two surgeons. Although the population served by the hospitals in area II is less than 20% of the state population (including the three adjacent referral areas), the numbers of laminectomies performed by these two new surgeons resulted in nearly a doubling of the state rate. In late 1984 the Maine Medical Assessment program met with the surgeons to discuss the indications for laminectomy. The rates dropped precipitously and have continued to fall in 1986.

the probabilities and the value to patients of the outcomes of care. They also offer new ways of communicating information to physicians and patients that can greatly increase understanding about the consequences of medical choices and thus help patients make the decisions they truly want.

We recently undertook an assessment of prostatectomy that takes advantage of some of the progress in the evaluative sciences.[3,12,41,42] The assessment was made possible because of the Maine Medical Assessment Program, a program of the Maine Medical Association organized to inform practicing physicians about small area variations and to help them evaluate the role and significance of practice style in these variations.[8] The evaluation began with a detailed review of the surgical literature and with consultations with urologists practicing in high rate and low rate areas to achieve a detailed understanding of the theoretical reasons for using prostatectomy and to obtain the best available estimates for the probabilities for the various outcomes associated with the watchful waiting and the surgical strategies for treating benign prostatic hypertrophy. We then sought to improve on the estimates for outcomes we found in the literature by using claims data to measure the postoperative death rates and the incidence of complications after surgery. Because of the long period of patient follow-up and the size and representative nature of the patient population in the claims database (virtually all patients 65 years and older treated in Maine and Manitoba), the estimates based on this data source were more accurate than those available in the published literature (Figure 4-7). These estimates were integrated into a decision analysis to show that life expectancy is actually a little longer for those who do not undergo early operation.*

---

*The initial loss of life because of the operation is not regained by avoiding the risks for surgery among those who may need the operation in the future to treat significant chronic obstruction.

The failure to demonstrate an extension in life expectancy when prostatectomy is prescribed under the preventive theory means that for patients without chronic obstruction the operation is justified only under the quality-of-life theory for surgery. Therefore patient preferences provide the rationale for the choice between surgery and watchful waiting in the individual situation. Information on the probabilities for symptom relief, improvements in the quality of life, and the importance of symptoms to the patients is thus of critical importance for rational decision making. Our literature review revealed a virtual absence of information about the probabilities for these "soft" outcomes after prostatectomy. To obtain this critical information we developed a patient questionnaire incorporating many of the methodologic advantages for measuring symptoms, functional status, and quality of life and interviewed patients before their surgery and at 3, 6, and 12 months after prostatectomy. We were therefore able to fill in many of the missing gaps in the estimates of the probabilities for symptom reduction and improvement in the quality of life and were able to obtain estimates for incontinence, impotence, and other complications not easily documented by claims data.

The patient interview results emphasize the complexity of clinical decision making when the objective is to improve the quality of life and shows the importance of establishing which of the treatment options the patients truly want. Although we found a rough correlation between the level of symptoms and the degree to which patients were bothered by their symptoms, we found no data that permitted us to predict accurately how a particular patient would feel about his symptoms. For example, some severely symptomatic patients were not much bothered by their symptoms. Presumably, some of these patients, if informed that they truly have an option and if told about the risks and benefits of surgery as well as those of watchful waiting, might have a different attitude toward surgery

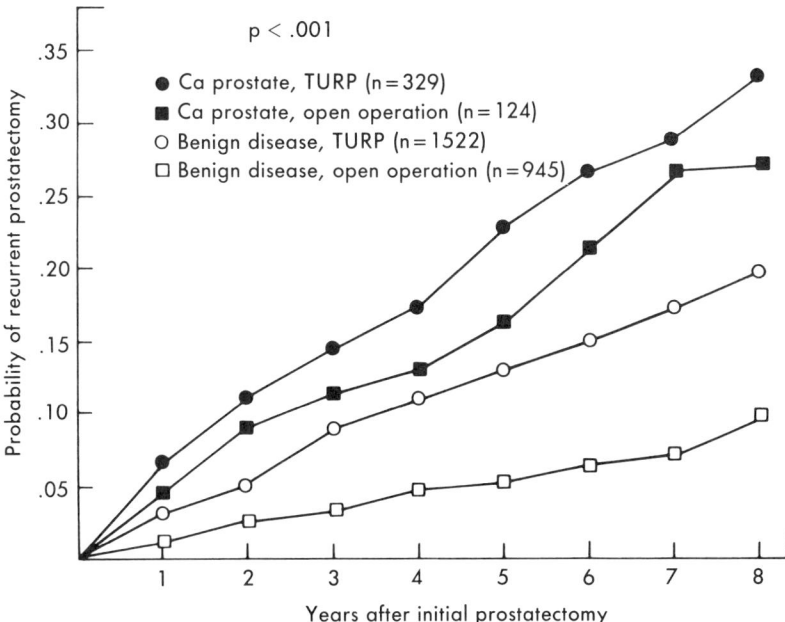

Figure 4-7. Cumulative probability for recurrent prostatectomy by type of prostatectomy. This figure gives the 8-year cumulative probability for one or more secondary prostatectomies by diagnosis and type of primary prostatectomy. Patients who received an open operation had a lower probability for receiving a second operation. For those with no evidence of malignancy during the first operation, the relative risk of recurrence was 2.0. In the Cox regression model, the only significant covariable was cancer of the prostate. Age, size of hospital, teaching status of hospital, and all patient illness covariables were not significantly associated with the probability of undergoing a secondary operation.

than those who are bothered a lot by their symptoms. Such findings emphasize the need for an active role of the patient in the decision to undergo this operation.

The prostatectomy assessment also offers a more specific diagnosis of the practice style–related causes of small area variation for prostatectomy than previously possible. For this operation, we concluded, the origins of the practice style factor were an unjustified belief in the preventive theory as well as failure, under the quality of life theory, to base patient decision making on the patient's own preferences for outcome. By providing more accurate estimates for the probabilities for outcomes as well as formal tests of the underlying surgical theory, such assessments should be broadly useful for improving the scientific basis of surgical practice. Although not intended to replace randomized clinical trials (RCT) when the latter is clearly indicated, the nonexperimental study designs we used should be helpful in determining whether an RCT is scientifically and ethically justified and helpful in designing an optimum clinical trial. In situations where the outcome events are rare or so far in the future that RCTs are difficult or impossible, or where sham surgery is needed as a control for the placebo effect of surgery, they may offer the only reasonable means for testing surgical theory.

The Professional Uncertainty Hypothesis as Null Hypothesis

Failures to test clinical theory adequately vitally affects the interests of patients and physicians. For patients the implications are starkly evident in that the everyday practice routinely involves the use of treatments that have not been established as scientifically correct. The problem is not that such experiments exist—they are an essential part of innovation in medicine, and progress is impossible without them. The problem is that often the experiments are unevaluated and therefore contribute nothing to the orderly development of the scientific basis of medicine.

It must be understood that the current situation is not the fault of clinicians. More than anyone, clinicians want to know the truth of what they do. They are forced to act: their patients expect action and their biomedical training gives them a large number of reasonable theories on which to base their actions. The problem is not that they theorize and act but that the framework necessary for evaluating actions and theories does not ordinarily exist. As a result, in the academic as well as in the nonacademic setting, the theories often go untested, and the knowledge base of clinical medicine remains stuck.

There are important implications for physicians who have counted on their education and the scientific literature as the guarantor of their special status. More and more, the profession finds itself under attack for "unscientific" variations in the costs and quantity of medical care. With the increasing concern about rising costs, policy makers, employers, and third party carriers are increasingly asking the profession to explain the variations. But the weak nature of the scientific knowledge means in many instances the variations cannot be explained on the basis of known differences in need or outcome. There seems to be a growing realization that the profession can no longer combat threats to professional status and interferences in the organization and economics of medical practice by raising a general alarm that these disturb the doctor-patient relationship or lead to the rationing of care.

I close by suggesting that the effective response of the profession to the small area variation phenomenon is to reaffirm its commitment to the medical model—that allocation should be based on the efficacy of treatments and the preferences of patients for outcomes—and to accept the responsibility for the systematic evolution of the theories that are behind the costly differences in practice style. An assessment program should be organized to evaluate the costly differences in practice style, to eliminate those theories that are wrong, and to establish the scientific basis for those that are right. An orderly agenda is needed to bring under protocol the common medical and surgical practices that have escaped evaluation. Surgeons must play a leadership role. The number of assessments that could be done is potentially quite large so priorities must be set. I have suggested that the profession concentrate first on those clinical practices and conditions where the uncertainty involves the greatest measurable risk to the largest numbers of patients and on those that involve the greatest significance for costs. For surgeons this would mean concentrating on those highly variable major operations that involve the use of the hospital or outpatient departments such as those illustrated in Figure 4-5.

References

1. American Child Health Association: Physical defects: the pathway to correction, New York, 1934, Res. Div. American Child Health Association.
2. Barnes BA et al: Report on variation in rates of utilization of surgical services in the Commonwealth of Massachusetts, JAMA 254:371, 1985.
3. Barry MJ et al: Watchful waiting versus immediate transurethral resection for symptomatic prostatism: the importance of patients' preferences, JAMA 259:3010, 1988.
4. Bloor M: Bishop Berkeley and the adenotonsillectomy enigma: an exploration of variation in the social construction of medical disposals, Sociology 10:43, 1976.
5. Bloor MJ, Venters GA, and Samphier ML: Geographical variation in the incidence of operations on the tonsils and adenoids: an epidemiological and sociological investigation. 1. J Laryngol Otol 92:791, 1978.

6. Bloor MJ, Venters GA, and Samphier ML: Geographical variation in the incidence of operations on the tonsils and adenoids: an epidemiological and sociological investigation. 11. J Laryngol Otol 92:883, 1978.
7. Copenhagen Collaborating Center for the Study of Regional Variations in Health Care (Sponsored by WHO): CCC Bibliography on Regional Variations in Health Care, Copenhagen, Denmark, 1985, Institute of Social Medicine.
8. deDombal FT et al: Human and computer-aided diagnosis of abdominal pain: further report with emphasis on performance of clinicians, Br Med J 1:376, 1974.
9. Department of Health Care Review, Division of Health Policy and Program Evaluation: Confronting regional variations: the Maine approach, Chicago, 1986, American Medical Association.
10. Fairbairn AS and Acheson ED: The extent of organ removal in the Oxford area, J Chronic Dis 22:111, 1969.
11. Fitzpatrick G, Neutra R, and Gilbert JP: Cost-effectiveness of cholecystectomy for silent gallstones. In Bunker JP, Barnes BA, and Mosteller F, editors: Costs, risks, and benefits of Surgery, New York, 1977, Oxford University Press.
12. Fowler FJ, et al: Symptom status and quality of life following prostatectomy, JAMA 259:3018, 1988.
13. Gittelsohn AM, and Wennberg JE: On the incidence of tonsillectomy and other common surgical procedures. In Bunker JP, Barnes BA, and Mosteller F, editors: Costs, risks, and benefits of Surgery, New York, 1977, Oxford University Press.
14. Gittelsohn AM, and Wennberg JE: On the risk of organ loss, J Chronic Dis 29:527, 1976.
15. Glover JA: The incidence of tonsillectomy in school children: proceedings of the Royal Society of Medicine 31:1219, 1938.
16. Glover JA. The Paediatric approach to tonsillectomy. Arch Dis Child 23:1, 1948.
17. Lembcke PA: A scientific method for medical auditing, Hospitals 33:65, 1959.
18. Lewis CE: Variations incidence of surgery, N Engl J Med 218:880, 1969.
19. Lichtner S, and Pflanz M: Appendectomy in the Federal Republic of Germany, Med Care 9:311, 1971.
20. McPherson K, et al: Small area variations in the use of common surgical procedures: an international comparison of New England, England, and Norway, N Engl J Med 307:1310, 1982.
21. Mitchell JB, and Cromwell J: Variations in surgery rates and the supply of surgeons. In Rothberg DL, editor: Regional variations in hospital use, Lexington, Ma., 1982, DC Health and Co.
22. Personal communication, 1975.
23. Ransohoff DF, et al: Prophylactic cholecystectomy or expectant management for silent gallstones, Ann Intern Med 99:199, 1983.
24. Richards DH: A posthysterectomy syndrome, Lancet 2:983, 1974.
25. Roos LL, and Roos NP, Assessing existing technologies: the Manitoba study of common surgical procedures, Med Care 21:454, 1983.
26. Roos NP. Hysterectomy: variations in rates across small areas and across physicians' practices. Am J Pub Health 1984; 74:327-335.
27. Roos NP and Roos L: High and low surgical rates: risk factors for area residents, Am J Public Health 71:591, 1981.
28. Roos NP, Roos L, and Henteleff PD: Elective surgical rates—do high rates mean lower standards? Tonsillectomy and adenoidectomy in Manitoba. N Engl J Med 297:360, 1977.
29. Roos NP, Wennberg JE, and McPherson K: Using DRGs for studying variations in hospital admission patterns, Health Care Fin (in press).
30. Sandberg SI et al: Elective hysterectomy: benefits, risks, and costs. Med Care 23:1067, 1985.
31. Shepard DS, and Cooper GS: Small area variations in rates of hospitalization and surgery within Rhode Island, AM J Prev Med 3:101, 1987.
32. Vayda E et al: Five-year study of surgical rates in Ontario's counties, Can Med Assoc J 131:111, 1984.
33. Wennberg JE: Small area variations in hospitalized case mix for DRGs in Maine, Massachusetts, and Iowa: final report to the National Center for Health Services Research and Technology Assessment, US DHHS, Grant No. HS-04932.
34. Wennberg JE, Barnes B, and Zubkoff M: Professional uncertainty and the problem of supplier-induced demand, Soc Sci Med 16:811, 1982.
35. Wennberg JE, Bunker JP, and Barnes B: The need for assessing the outcome of common medical practices, Annu Rev Public Health 1:277, 1980.
36. Wennberg JE, Freeman JL, and Culp WJ: Are hospital services rationed in New Haven or over-utilized in Boston? Lancet 8543:1185, 1987.
37. Wennberg JE, and Gittelsohn A: Small area variations in health care delivery, Science 182:1102, 1973.
38. Wennberg JE, and Gittelsohn AM: Variations in medical care among small areas, Sci Am 246:120, 1982.
39. Wennberg JE, McPherson K, and Caper P: Will payment based on diagnosis-related groups control hospital costs? N Engl J Med 311:295, 1984.
40. Wennberg JE et al: Changes in tonsillectomy rates associated with feedback and review, Pediatrics 59:821, 1977.
41. Wennberg JE et al: An assessment of prostatectomy for benign urinary tract obstruction: geographic variations and the evaluation of medical care outcomes (in press).
42. Wennberg JE et al: Use of claims data systems to evaluate health care outcomes, JAMA 257:933, 1987

5

Determining the Rates of Surgical Operations

IRA M. RUTKOW

Among the most difficult questions to be answered by health care research is that of determining the appropriate rate of surgical operations for a given society.* Paralleling this query is an important secondary issue. What determinants go into the establishment of surgical operative rates.

Unfortunately, it is a commonly accepted belief that a physician-induced demand for surgery exists. Fuchs has argued that surgeons shift the need for operations.[19] With all things being equal, a 10% increase in the surgeon/population ratio results in an approximate 3% increase in per capita utilization. Cromwell and Mitchell, in a follow-up to Fuchs' report, found definite support for the concept of competitive market failure; that is, the supply of surgeons, numbers of operations, and surgical fees do not follow normally expected supply/demand curves.[14]

These and other papers use sophisticated economic models to provide estimates and arrive at conclusions.[59,64] However, research that employs actual numbers of practicing surgeons and operations fails to support the concept that surgeons perform operations in a capricious manner and possibly according to their own financial requirements.[52,56,58] Numerous investigations have demonstrated that recent large increases in the number of practicing surgeons in this country have failed to generate any evidence of parallel increases in the number of surgical operations. The belief that surgeons are able to create need for their services in 1988, as opposed to before 1970, by merely moving into a given community has proven to be fallacious and adversely fuels the entire question of unnecessary surgery.[57] In an attempt to answer some of these questions, this chapter presents a detailed look at the numerous factors that impact on the surgical decision-making process. This process, in turn, becomes the ultimate determinant of rates of surgical operations.

DIFFERENCES AMONG COUNTRIES

It is well known that different countries tolerate substantial differences in their frequencies of surgery without consistent unfavorable outcomes. Vayda and Rutkow showed that from 1966 to 1976 overall surgical rates in Canada remained relatively unchanged and consistently 60% higher than those in England and Wales.[68] United States' rates were the highest of the three countries and increased 25% during the study period. The authors demonstrated that mortalities for selected surgical conditions were unrelated to rates of surgery. For instance, the United States

---
*References 30, 47, 50, 52, 55, 69.

and England and Wales had comparable death rates for gallbladder diseases despite the fact that their cholecystectomy rates varied by almost 300%. Interestingly, Canada's death rates for gallbladder diseases and its cholecystectomy rates were both highest. England and Wales had the lowest prostatectomy rates and the lowest mortality for prostatic carcinoma and hyperplasia. On the other hand, its mortality for malignant disease of the breast is highest with the lowest breast surgery rates.

One of the most telling statistics concerning a country's attitudes toward surgical health care is the percentage of gross domestic product utilized for health expenditures.[60] According to Vayda and Rutkow, a society's overall health care expenditures appear to better reflect national priorities and values and thus be more important than other factors in explaining cross-national differences in rates of surgery.

Among industrialized countries, the United States has always had one of the highest figures, which currently is more than 11% (Table 5-1). For our country at least, this amount seems to correlate with its high surgical operative rate. The basic difficulty, which persists in interpreting these data with regard to surgical policy formulation, is a lack of health outcome measures and clinically defined standards of surgical appropriateness.[9]

THE SURGICAL DECISION-MAKING PROCESS

Although the periodical literature is rich in studies attempting to elucidate factors that influence rates of surgery, concrete conclusions are not at hand. Before variations in surgical rates can be fully appreciated, it is important to completely understand the manner in which surgeons make an operative decision and the factors that can influence this choice. Accordingly, this chapter will present a model of the surgical decision-making process and discuss its various determinants.

The importance of having such a model is apparent because if rates of surgery are largely a function of societal philosophies, ethics, and health expectations, the cost-containment approaches targeted to individuals, such as surgical second opinion programs and prospective payment mechanisms incorporating physician fees, may not have much impact.[51,54] If there were a

Table 5-1. Total health expenditures as a percentage of gross domestic product

Country	1965	1975	1985*
Australia	5.2	7.4	7.6 ($904)
Canada	6.1	7.3	8.6 ($1282)
France	5.3	7.6	9.4 ($1072)
West Germany	5.1	7.8	8.1 ($983)
Italy	4.6	6.7	7.4 ($678)
Japan	4.5	5.6	6.6 ($783)
Spain	2.7	5.1	6.0 ($456)
Sweden	5.6	8.0	9.3 ($1172)
Switzerland	3.8	7.1	7.9 ($1144)
United Kingdom	4.1	5.5	5.7 ($627)
United States	6.0	8.4	10.8 ($1776)

*Dollar amount in parentheses represents per capita total health expenditure in 1985.

relationship between particular types of professional organizations and inclination to operate, approaches targeted to institutions or their patterns of staffing would be indicated.

The overriding theme of the model is the postulate that multiple determinants impact on the determination of surgical operative rates (Figure 5-1). These determinants are found on three levels and include: (1) social, political, and economic forces (society-community level), (2) characteristics of organizations in which surgeons work (professional organization level), and (3) characteristics of individual clinicians (individual surgeon level). It is expected that factors at one level may affect those at another level. Consequently, it is often difficult to isolate and examine specific influences. In most instances a higher level will have a dominating force over lesser ones.

Care Implications of Differing Rates

What remains most uncertain with this model and numbers of surgical operations in general is the importance of high rates versus low rates. Do high rates mean lower standards or vice versa? This issue is most clearly stated in the numerous papers that examine the question of variations in rates of surgery among different countries and specific localities. These differences have been documented for almost a quarter of a century. Logan and Eimerl demonstrated wide variations in surgical rates for removal of hemorrhoids, tonsils, and the uterus between the United States and Canada, which were twice those of Great Britain and Sweden.[29] Conversely, the Swedish rates for removal of the gallbladder, prostate, and varicose veins were double those of the other two countries. Pearson et al. showed that the rate of tonsillectomy and/or adenoidectomy, inguinal herniorrhaphy, and cholecystectomy performed in New England were 2 to 4 times higher than in Liverpool, England.[39] Liverpool and Uppsala, Sweden, were found to have similar surgical rates except for gallbladder and gynecologic operations.

It was a study by Bunker in 1970 that brought the existence of variations to the level of intense public scrutiny.[10] He compared operations and surgeons in the United States with those in England and Wales and noted that per capita, the United States had twice as many surgeons as England and Wales and twice the number of operations performed per population. Vayda in a 1-year comparison of Canada with England and Wales found that the overall Canadian operative rates was 1.7 times greater than that in England and Wales, and sex-specific age/standardized rates for common, primarily discretionary operations were 2 to 7 times greater in Canada.[65] The

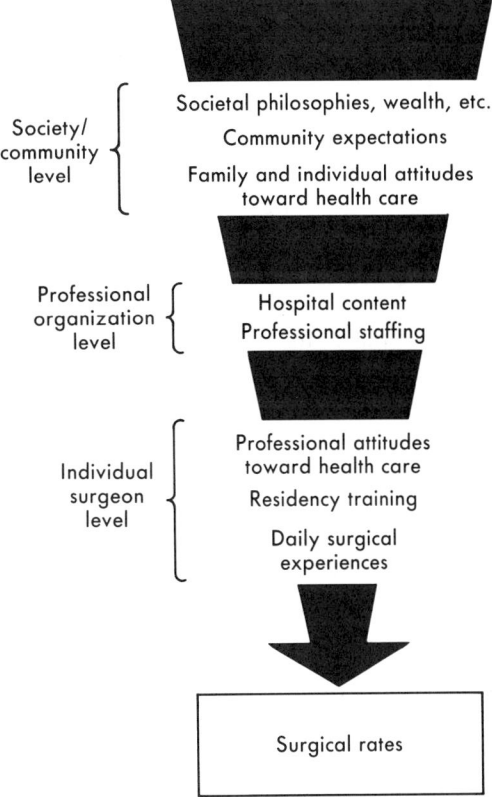

Figure 5-1. The surgical decision-making process: determinants of surgical rates. (Redrawn from Rutkow IM: Health Serv Res 17:380, 1982.)

appendectomy rates in both West Germany and Japan have been demonstrated to be 2 to 3 times greater than in other industrialized countries.[28,78] McPherson et al. have documented wide variations in the use of common surgical procedures within and between England and Wales, Canada, and the United States.[35,36]

Variations at the regional and local levels have also been well studied. In the earliest such report, Glover demonstrated persistent variations in the incidence of tonsillectomy in school children.[22] This was followed by Lembcke's 1952 paper that analyzed appendectomies in 23 hospital services areas in and around Rochester.[26] He noted a range from 250 to 690 operations per 100,000 population. No correlation between low appendectomy rates and high mortality from appendicitis could be demonstrated. In a now classic report, Lewis studied the Kansas Blue Cross Association record and showed a threefold to fourfold variation in state regional rates for the performance of six common elective procedures.[27] In Massachusetts a fourfold variation in the tonsillectomy rate from one community to the next was noted.[2] Wennberg and Gittelsohn have reported extreme variations, as much as 1000% in the patterns of use of nine common surgical procedures in Vermont and Maine.[74,75] Gornick showed large variation in surgical utilization by Medicare patients.[23] Detmer and Tyson analyzed population-based surgical rates for primary appendectomy, cholecystectomy, herniorrhaphy, and tonsillectomy in Wisconsin.[16] They noted variations of as much as 800% in the rates of the procedures, even within large health-planning districts. Barnes et al. reported twofold and threefold variations across geographic areas for 14 common operative procedures in Massachusetts.[3] Wennberg et al. recently showed that a Bostonian is about twice as likely to undergo a carotid endarterectomy as an individual living in New Haven; for coronary bypass operations the risk is the reverse.[73] Those in New Haven experience a substantially higher operative rate for hysterectomies and back surgery, whereas the rates for knee and hip replacements are much greater in Boston.

Small area variation studies are not limited to the United States. Numerous studies have documented similar findings in other countries for a host of surgical operations including adenotonsillectomy, cataract extraction, appendectomy, and hysterectomy.*

The studies that have examined variations in surgical rates across geographic areas suggest that the differences are a function of numerous factors including physician attitudes toward indications for surgery, the prevalence of third-party insurance, availability of hospital beds, physician age, place of training, and, most important, the supply of surgical manpower. Lewis even went so far as to state almost 20 years ago that a surgical variation of Parkinson's law, "patient admissions for surgery expand to fill beds, operating suites, and total surgical manpower," might be present.[27]

It is probably not unreasonable to assume that all of these factors contribute to geographic variations in surgical rates. Such differences in themselves, however, cannot be taken to mean that unnecessary surgery is being performed in those areas with higher rates. Because there are no guidelines for determining which of the surgical rates are the most appropriate, could not, in fact, the higher rates represent the meeting of previously unmet needs for surgery? Conversely, it can be argued that because the areas with lower rates do not appear to have significantly higher mortality statistics than the high rate areas, the higher rates represent unneeded surgery. However, the mortality-data argument can be countered, since so few of the operations are a matter of life or death.[30,33]

Perhaps the essence of geographic variations can be explained by inappropriateness. Is it possible that in areas with high surgical rates surgeons are performing less appropriate or more

---

*References 7, 37, 44, 46, 49, 63, 66, 67, 76.

inappropriate procedures and vice versa for low use areas? The findings from a recent article that examined appropriateness of use of carotid endarterectomy, coronary angiography, and upper gastrointestinal tract endoscopy appear to refute this hypothesis.[13] Chassin et al. selected geographic areas of high, average, and low use of these procedures and randomly sampled Medicare beneficiaries who had undergone one of the procedures. Differences among sites in levels of appropriateness were small. For example, in the high-use site for carotid endarterectomy, 37% of the procedures were appropriate, compared with 42% in the low-use site. Carotid endarterectomy was performed 5.3 times as frequently in the high-use site compared with the low-use site. The authors concluded that differences in appropriateness cannot explain geographic variations. Interestingly, significant levels of inappropriate use (29% to 40%) were found at all the sites for carotid endarterectomy. In a similar study Chassin found the same findings in a population of Medicare-age patients.[12]

Society—Community Level

Having noted the large variation in operative rates that any given society may have, we must return to the model of the surgical decision-making process and describe the various levels and factors that constitute it.[5,6] Of the three levels, the most broad-based and significant is the society-community level. Within this category are broad external forces that shape a society's and a community's delivery of surgical health care. It is here that such socioeconomic conditions as the amount of industrialization, the degree of affluence, and general attitudes toward health care come into focus. Community expectations regarding their health needs constitute an important contribution.

The most fitting example within this society-community level is the paucity of surgical operations performed in third world nations. It must be assumed that the need for surgical intervention exists there. For instance, there is no reason to believe that the prevalence of inguinal hernias would be any different from that in the industrialized world, yet inguinal herniorrhaphy is not performed in the underdeveloped countries to the extent that it is in developed countries. Recent articles point out the shortage of surgeons and consequent low operative rates in Pakistan and Africa.[6] In 1983 Gil and coworkers demonstrated a distressing underutilization of health care personnel and facilities and low productivity of surgeons in Colombia.[21] The less affluent a society is the less likely will be its need for surgical health care. Public health problems such as sanitation, hygiene, and vaccination will command greater importance than an elective surgical schedule.

According to the model, factors at the society-community level can influence the other two levels, and factors at the professional organization level can influence the individual surgeon level. The reverse effects are unlikely. Any one or a combination of all three alternatives should account for the final rates of surgery, and their relative impact can vary across national boundaries. In addition, the levels will often overlap, and it may be difficult to distinguish among them.

Professional Organization Level

The professional organization level is made up mostly of the characteristics of professional organizations by which surgeons organize themselves. At this level such organizational criteria as staffing, type of practice, and remuneration are operative. Within this category the most prominent example of professional organization is hospital physician staffing. The ability to selectively close or open a hospital staff to new physicians could have a substantive impact in determining a hospital's operative rate. In addition, the manner in which surgeons organize themselves, such as American College of Surgeons, American Medical Association, and specialty societies, would be expected to have an impact on rates of surgery.

Individual Surgeon Level

At the individual surgeon level, for example, the characteristics of the individual practitioner, such factors as professional attitudes toward health care, residency training, and daily surgical experiences shape the category. Such characteristics can be measured either individually or as an aggregate. For a surgeon, professional attitudes on health care would be noted in a predisposition toward surgical intervention. The factor of a surgeon's skills and technical knowledge is composed of two components: (1) training and education, that is, residency, and (2) daily medical experiences.

Socioeconomic Influences on Physician Performance

Roemer and Friedman have demonstrated the presence of broad social controls on physician performance at the society-community and professional organization interphases.[43] These socioeconomic forces form the types of services provided by a hospital and hence the patterns of professional staff organization required to provide those services effectively. In the middle of this structuring process is the surgical practitioner, who is molded in patterns of practice that conform to the norms of the organization. A growing example in the United States is the providing of surgical care within the confines of a health maintenance organization (HMO), preferred provider organization (PPO), independent practice association (IPA), or a strictly private practice. In addition, the norms of the community regarding health care will also affect the surgeon's decision making. If, for example, a surgeon practices in a relatively affluent and educated community, some research has shown that the surgical rate can be expected to be higher than in a less educated region.[11,47]

Family and individual attitudes. In addition to societal and community expectations, family and individual attitudes about health care are important. Predisposing factors such as family composition, social structure, and health beliefs, and enabling factors including family resources and individual needs regarding illness and its prevention, coexist with the societal and community influences.

Professional organization. Flood et al. developed measures for evaluating the professional organization.[18] Included within their scheme were: the entire organization—the hospital; the responsible organizational unit—the professional staff; and the relevant performance unit—the individual surgeon. It would be logical to expect all these units to have an impact on the surgical decision-making process. At the professional organization level, Flood et al. showed that hospital features, including capital expenditures, and hospital staff professional organizational features, including proportion of contract or salaried physicians and number of surgical specialties represented at a hospital, have greater impact on surgical outcomes than do individual surgeon characteristics.[17] For instance, the establishment of an ambulatory surgical unit under the auspices of a hospital would have a major influence on the number of outpatient operations being performed. Similarly, Nobrega et al. demonstrated that the organization of medical care plays an influential role on surgical usage and even overrides such considerations as fee-for-service versus prepaid delivery systems.[38]

Socioeconomic status. Socioeconomic status is an important variable that affects surgical care at the society-community level. It is accepted that poor people often carry a burden of ill health far greater than those living in better circumstances. However, there is no reason to suppose that certain surgical abnormalities such as inguinal hernia, cataract formation, and prostatic hypertrophy should have a predilection for a particular socioeconomic level.

Educational level. Bunker and Brown assessed the question of overuse of surgical services in the United States, which is often attributed to lack of consumer education.[11] Assuming that physicians are the most educated group about medical problems, Bunker and Brown examined the use of surgical services by physicians and their families and compared it with lawyers, ministers, and businessmen. They found surgical rates for physicians and their families to be as high or higher than for the other groups. Overall, surgical rates for the four groups were estimated to be 30% higher than those for the country as a whole. It was concluded that as the public became better informed about surgical services, the demand for surgery would increase. What was not measured concerned the availability of surgical services. It might be that the better educated groups in society have greater access to surgical care. If less-educated individuals had better access to surgeons, their rates of surgery might also be proportionately higher.

Roos and Roos also found that high surgical rate areas contained a more educated populace.[47] This was in contrast to Bombardier et al. who showed the opposite correlation with education.[8] In addition, they noted a large increase in surgical use among economically disadvantaged groups, the aged, the less educated, and nonwhites. Scott and Mackie, in a similar report, found many frequently performed surgical procedures to have the same rate of occurrence for all socioeconomic levels.[62]

Health care delivery systems. At the professional organization level, variations in rates of surgery have been noted between different health care delivery systems. Most notable in this regard are the fee-for-service versus prepaid plans. Why is it that research has demonstrated a difference in surgical rates between similar populations when they receive surgical care under varied payment schemes?

One of the earliest reports to investigate this issue was Densen's et al. study of surgical care in a dual choice situation.[15] They analyzed two populations: one was enrolled in the Group Health Insurance Plan, which had its medical care provided through fee-for-service solo practice; the other cohort was enrolled in the Health Insurance Plan of Greater New York, which received its surgical care on a prepaid basis. When the data were classified into admissions involving surgery and those without surgery, the biggest difference between the two plans occurred among female surgical patients. The prepaid group's admission rates were lower at all age groups.

Six years later, Perott also demonstrated that prepaid health plans had lower surgical rates than did the fee-for-service mode.[42] He considered the hospital experience of federal employees covered under different insurance plans. In comparing the rates of hospitalization for surgery, the data showed a tonsillectomy and/or adenoidectomy rate for the government Blue Shield plan more than 2.5 times that of the prepaid group practice plan; for various types of gynecologic surgery it was 1.5 times that of the group practice; and an appendectomy rate was twice that of the prepaid group practice enrollees. For all surgical procedures, the Blue Shield–insured employees had a rate of 7000 per 100,000 covered persons, while the prepaid practice had a rate of 3900 per 100,000.

A 1968 study of surgical rates between comprehensive, family-oriented pediatric care (experimental cohort) and conventional hospital-based care (control group) demonstrated the experimental group to have operative rates 50% to 70% lower than the controls after the study was 6 months old.[1] The precise method of payment was apparently not a subject of special consideration in this report. However, prepayment was in effect provided by the experimental cohort. Certainly, a change in delivery system was affecting surgical rates.

Kisch et al. outlined an approach for studying the environment of surgical procedures by epidemiologic analysis.[25] Significant differences in incidence rates between prepaid practice hospitals and proprietary institutions were invariably noted. Differences between the prepaid hospitals and voluntary hospitals were less striking.

Bellin and Geiger studied the rates of surgical admissions among a geographically isolated low-income group in Boston, both before and after the installation of a comprehensive health care clinic.[4] Within 1 year of operation of the center, the annual surgical admissions and total number of surgical hospital days had greatly decreased. Within 2 years, surgical admissions were only 24% of prestudy levels. The study demonstrated the potential effectiveness of an ambulatory health care center in reducing the demand for surgical beds in a low-income community.

A 1973 report studied a 1-year utilization of medical and hospital services by more than 3000 Canadian steelworkers and their families who belonged to a prepaid group practice plan.[23a] This was contrasted with utilization by families of fellow workers whose care was provided by independently practicing surgeons. For rates of tonsillectomy and/or adenoidectomy among children, the prepaid members had a figure of 8800 per 100,000 population while the fee-for-service rates was 27,000 per 100,000. Additionally, there was a 20% to 40% lower secondary surgical procedure rate for the prepaid group.

Hughes et al. studied the utilization of surgical manpower in a prepaid group practice versus that of general surgeons in a fee-for-service community practice.[24,70] The prepaid group practice achieved economies in the delivery of surgical services through the utilizaton of an ambulatory modality for the performance of almost 25% of all operations.

Gaus compared various aspects of HMO's performance in 10 plans with that of the fee-for-service system for a Medicaid population.[20] As was hypothesized, hospital use was significantly lower by 250% in group practice plans than in the fee-for-service systems. Specifically, the prepaid group practice had a surgical admission rate of 24,000 per 100,000 population, while the fee-for-service rate was 82,000 per 100,000.

Wilson and Longmire found the method of surgeon payment to influence several important aspects of surgical care.[77] The preoperative processes of laboratory tests and radiographic procedures were ordered more frequently and less selectively by salaried surgeons without any corresponding improvement in outcome. In appendicitis, there was a trend for fee-for-service physicians to undertake earlier exploration, resulting in fewer secondary complications. Operative workloads were highest for surgeons receiving salary plus percentage in fee-for-service group practice.

LoGerfo et al. assessed the care received by persons enrolled in either a large prepaid group practice or in a prepaid independent practice setting in which surgeons were reimbursed on a fee-for-service basis.[31,32] They found that for quite similar low-income enrollee groups with full prepaid benefits, the frequency of appendectomy, tonsillectomy and/or adenoidectomy, cholecystectomy, and hysterectomy were much higher under the plan in which physicians were reimbursed on a fee-for-service basis.

Although most studies appear to support the hypothesis that enrollees in prepaid insurance plans have lower surgical utilization rates than do members in fee-for-service systems, there are some additional investigations that refute these findings. Perkoff et al. found the lack of effect of an experimental prepaid group practice on utilization of surgical care in a university medical center.[40,41] The study investigated surgical rates over a 3-year period, and contrary to what was expected, the prepaid enrollees used the same or more surgical care than did fee-for-service members. Both male and female ambulatory enrollees also had fewer surgical procedures. Scitovsky and McCall also demonstrated that surgical admission rates were higher for a fee-for-service group plan when contrasted to a prepaid Kaiser plan.[61] However, when surgical procedures performed in the hospital on a nonadmission basis are added to surgical admissions, the surgical rates under the two plans became almost identical.

LoGerfo et al. studied the care of patients undergoing cholecystectomy, hysterectomy, appendectomy, and tonsillectomy with or without adenoidectomy in the Seattle Model Cities Health Care Program.[31] Patients in the prepaid group plan were more likely to have met criteria for appropriate or necessary surgery than were those in the independent practice association. In the independent practice association, 79% of hysterectomies and 32% of tonsillectomies were judged appropriate. The groups were similar in the proportion of patients having elements of good care documented in their records. In addition, they studied possible underprovision of care in an indirect manner. The study suggested that there were more enrollees in the prepaid group plan who would have met criteria for having a hysterectomy and tonsillectomy but who did not have surgery. Whether this represents underprovision of surgical care is an unresolved issue.

Even with the marked differences in the rates of surgical procedures, there is little in the way of data that proves outcomes of essential care are different under various types of HMO arrangements as opposed to traditional fee-for-service settings. For instance, Francis and Polissar studied patients with colorectal cancer and found similar 4-year survival and recurrence rates in a prepaid group plan form of HMO as compared with patients in other settings.[31]

Although one possible explanation for the lower surgical rates observed in prepaid group practice is that the absence of a financial incentive for the surgeon to overutilize reduces the amount of unnecessary surgery performed, a counterexplanation can be offered: the prepaid system might be denying some patients surgery that is appropriate. As stated previously, the problem with all studies of variation in rates of surgery between competing health care delivery systems is the absence of a definition of what the appropriate or correct rate of surgery is or should be.

Because there had been much debate over consumer satisfaction with one delivery system compared with the next, Gaus asked a number of questions regarding general satisfaction with regard to accessibility and physician care of enrollees in both groups.[20] When the responses were analyzed, more than 90% of both prepaid and fee-for-service groups were satisfied or very satisfied. Wilson and Longmire specifically studied satisfaction with surgical care in six different organizations.[77] Although satisfaction with care was generally high, only 86% of patients in the sample from a prepaid group plan responded favorably compared with 99% in a community hospital. In an interesting corollary finding, they found that fewer patients in the prepaid group plan could recall the name of their surgeon than in the other situations. In a third study, Marks et al. studied costs, quality of care, and satisfaction regarding ambulatory surgery in an HMO.[34] They noted no differences in quality of care for inpatients and ambulatory patients, and both providers and patients were very satisfied with the type of surgical service they received. It would appear that patients who undergo surgical procedures are generally happy irrespective of the manner in which the surgical health care is delivered.

Differences in Individual Surgical Practices

Much research attention is now being focused on the bottom rung of the decision-making process model, the individual surgeon level. Unfortunately, findings are inconclusive regarding the importance of the individual surgeon to the overall surgical decision-making process and its endpoint: rates of surgical operations. Wennberg et al. have discussed this puzzling problem in a number of papers.[71-73] Their evidence supports the hypothesis that variations in rates of surgery occur to a large extent because of differences among physicians regarding their evaluation of patients, that is, diagnostic studies, or their belief in the value of a surgical operations for meeting patient needs, that is, therapeutic initiatives. They have termed this the "professional uncertainty hypothesis" and consider it germane to current controversies regarding the nature and extent of the surgical decision-making process and its effect on rates of operations.

According to Wennberg, the very uncertainty of surgical decision making explains why physicians can influence utilization. He feels that the wide range of professionally acceptable alternate diagnoses and therapies is a major factor in the wide variation in rates of surgical operations. A lack of professional consensus on the role of surgery in a given community will contribute to the varying rates of appropriate surgical usage. For instance, the rate of appropriate surgery will be higher when larger proportions of patients with appropriate indications seek the advice of physicians preferring surgical therapy. Thus the importance of the practice style for the rates of utilization for specific treatments will depend on the mix of primary physicians, medical specialists, and surgeons. Therefore, those favoring either medical or surgical therapy will vary from one community to the next as will the proportion of patients with appropriate indications for treatment who end up with either surgery or medical management.

In an interesting investigation, Rutkow and Starfield studied the process of surgical decision making at the individual surgeon level.[55] To accomplish this, they factored out influences from the two higher levels (society/community and professional organizations) by posing two questions: (1) are there differences in the way surgeons from Canada, England, and the United States would treat a patient if various external influences such as those from the society-community and professional organization levels were not present? and (2) do such simple technical decisions regarding need for surgery have a major impact in determining a country's known surgical rate?

In order to study these questions, 4687 surgeons from these three countries were asked to assess the need for surgical intervention for patients presented as fictional case vignettes. Known operative rates in these countries were then obtained and compared with the surgeons' responses to judgment of need for surgery in the fictional cases. These comparisons provided answers to the two queries.

The most interesting finding was the enormous amount of international differences in surgical decision making. There was no evidence of any similarity in the way surgeons from one country answered the clinical vignettes compared with those of another country. This variation in surgical decision making was also evident in comparing surgeons from the same country with one another. More important, no correlations could be demonstrated in the way surgeons responded to the clinical situations and their own country's surgical operative rate. For instance, in breast surgery, English surgeons had the highest percentage of affirmative responses (indicating a more aggressive surgical attitude toward the vignettes than Canadian or United States surgeons), yet England has the lowest known breast surgical rate of the three countries. Similarly, for cholecystectomy, Canadian surgeons had the lowest affirmative response rates, yet in actuality Canada has a known cholecystectomy rate that is almost 50% greater than that in the United States and 300% greater than in England. An ancillary finding showed no correlations between the surgeons' responses and select socioeconomic and educational factors such as method of financial reimbursement, type of hospital at which they operate, structure of their practice, country of graduation from medical school, decade in which practice of surgery began, board certification, and type of hospital where clinical training took place.

The findings of this study indicated there are differences in the way surgeons from three industrialized countries would treat a patient if various external influences, that is, socioeconomic, organizational, and demographic factors, were not present. However, these simple technical decisions regarding need for surgery were not found to have a major impact in determining a country's or a region's known surgical rates. It would seem that differences in the socioeconomics and organizational frameworks of health care systems, rather than individual technical decisions of need for surgery, play a more influential role in determining a country's surgical rate.

CONCLUSIONS

As has been shown, the surgical decision-making process is a very complex and involved mechanism. The better it is understood the more realistic and pragmatic health care policy can be promulgated. Certainly, if rates of surgical operations are largely a function of political, economic, or social forces at the society-community and/or professional organizational levels, policy changes targeted at the individual practitioner will be relatively ineffective in the overall effort to control health care costs. For example, second-opinion programs, which take an individual approach to dealing with the problem of increasing amounts of surgery, may be nothing more than a short-lived solution to a long-term problem.

Exactly what management strategies will need to be implemented to modify or improve surgical outcomes remains unclear. However, a fuller understanding of the entire surgical decision-making process and its multiple determinants will need to be in place before effective changes can occur.

References

1. Alpert JJ, Heagarty MC, and Robertson L: Effective use of comprehensive pediatric care: utilization of health resources, Am J Dis Child 116:529, 1968.
2. Baldwin AD: Tonsillectomy and adenoidectomy in Massachusetts, N Engl J Med 285:1537, 1971.
3. Barnes BA et al: Report on variation in rates of utilization of surgical services in the commonwealth of Massachusetts, JAMA 254:371, 1985.
4. Bellin SS, Geiger HJ, and Gipson CD: Impact of ambulatory health care services on the demand for hospital beds, N Engl J Med 280:808, 1969.
5. Bernth-Petersen P and Bach E: Epidemiological aspects of cataract surgery: regional variations in frequency, Acta Ophthalmol 61:397, 1983.
6. Blanchard RJW et al: The epidemiology and spectrum of surgical care in district hospitals of Pakistan, Am J Public Health 77:1439, 1987.
7. Bloor MJ, Venters GA, and Samphier ML: Geographical variation in the incidence of operations on the tonsils and adenoids, J Laryngol Otol 92:791 and 883, 1978.
8. Bombardier C et al: Socioeconomic factors affecting the utilization of surgical operations, N Engl J Med 297:699, 1977.
9. Brook RH et al: Geographic variations in the use of services: do they have any clinical significance? Health Aff 3:63, 1984.
10. Bunker JP: Surgical manpower: a comparison of operations and surgeons in the United States, and in England and Wales, N Engl J Med 282:135, 1970.
11. Bunker JP and Brown BW: The physician-patient as an informed consumer of surgical services, N Engl J Med 290:1051, 1974.
12. Chassin MR et al: Variations in the use of medical and surgical services by the medicare population, N Engl J Med 314:285, 1986.
13. Chassin MR et al: Does inappropriate use explain geographic variations in the use of health care services? A study of three procedures, JAMA 258:2533, 1987.
14. Cromwell J and Mitchell JB: Physician-induced demand for surgery, J Health Econ 5:293, 1986.
15. Densen PM et al: Prepaid medical care and hospital utilization in a dual choice situation, Am J Public Health 50:170, 1960.
16. Detmer DE and Tyson TJ: Regional differences in surgical care based upon uniform physician and hospital discharge abstract data, Ann Surg 187:166, 1978.
17. Flood AB and Scott WR: Professional power and professional effectiveness: the power of the surgical staff and the quality of surgical care in hospitals, J Health Soc Behav 19:240, 1978.
18. Flood AB et al: Effectiveness in professional organizations: the impact of surgeons and surgical staff organizations on the quality of care in hospitals, Health Serv Res 17:320, 1982.
19. Fuchs VR: The supply of surgeons and the demand for operations, J Human Resources 13s:36, 1978.
20. Gaus CR, Cooper BS, and Hirschman C: Contrasts in HMO and fee-for-service performance, Soc Secur Bull, May 1975.
21. Gil AV et al: Surgeons and operating rooms: underutilized resources, Am J Public Health 73:1361, 1983.
22. Glover JA: The incidence of tonsillectomy in school children, Proc R Soc Med 31:1219, 1938.
23. Gornick M: Medicare patients: regional differences in length of hospital stays, 1969-1971. Soc Secur Bull, July 1975.
23a. Hastings JEF et al: Prepaid group practice in Sault Ste Marie, Ontario: analysis of utilization records, Med Care 11:91, 1973.
24. Hughes EFX et al: Utilization of surgical manpower in a prepaid group practice, N Engl J Med 291:759, 1974.

25. Kisch AI et al: An epidemiologic approach to the study of the incidence of surgical procedures, Med Care 7:471, 1969.
26. Lembcke PA: Measuring the quality of medical care through vital statistics based on hospital service areas: comparative study of appendectomy rates, Am J Public Health 42:276, 1952.
27. Lewis CE: Variations in the incidence of surgery, N Engl J Med 281:880, 1969.
28. Lichtner S and Pflanz M: Appendectomy in the Federal Republic of Germany: epidemiology and medical care patterns, Med Care 9:311, 1971.
29. Logan RFL and Eimerl T: Case loads in hospital and general practice in several countries, Milbank Mem Fund 43:302, 1965.
30. LoGerfo P: Variations in surgical rates: fact vs. fancy, N Engl J Med 297:387, 1977.
31. LoGerfo JP: Organizational and financial influences on patterns of surgical care, Surg Clin North Am 62:677, 1982.
32. LoGerfo JP et al: Rates of surgical care in prepaid group practices and the independent setting: what are the reasons for the differences? Med Care 17:1, 1979.
33. Marcus AC: Underprovision of elective surgery in a prepaid group practice: a difference of opinion, Med Care 19:774, 1981.
34. Marks SD et al: Ambulatory surgery in an HMO: a study of costs, quality of care and satisfaction. Med Care 18:127, 1980.
35. McPherson K et al: Regional variations in the use of common surgical procedures: within and between England and Wales, Canada and the United States. Soc Sci Med 15a:273, 1981.
36. McPherson K et al: Small-area variations in the use of common surgical procedures: an international comparison of New England, England, and Norway, N Engl J Med 307:1310, 1982.
37. Nilsen ST et al: A comparison of cesarean section frequencies in two Norwegian hospitals, Acta Obstet Gynecol Scand 62:555, 1983.
38. Nobrega FT et al: Hospital use in a fee-for-service system, JAMA 247:806, 1982.
39. Pearson RJC et al: Hospital caseloads in Liverpool, New England, and Uppsala: an international comparison. Lancet 2:559, 1968.
40. Perkoff GT, Kahn L, and Mackie A: Medical care utilization in an experimental prepaid group practice model in a university medical center, Med Care 12:471, 1974.
41. Perkoff GT et al: Lack of effect of an experimental prepaid group practice on utilization of surgical care, Surgery 77:619, 1975.
42. Perott GS: Federal employees health benefits program: utilization of hospital services. Am J Public Health 56:57, 1966.
43. Roemer MI and Friedman JW: Doctors in hospitals: medical staff organization and hospital performance, Baltimore, 1971, The Johns Hopkins University Press.
44. Roos L: Supply, workload and utilization: a population-based analysis of surgery in rural Manitoba, Am J Public Health 73:414, 1983.
45. Roos NP, Roos LL, and Henteleff PD: Elective surgical rates: do high rates mean lower standards? N Engl J Med 297:360, 1977.
46. Roos NP: Who should do the surgery? tonsillectomy-adenoidectomy in one Canadian province, Inquiry 16:73, 1979.
47. Roos NP and Roos L: High and low surgical rates: risk factors for area residents, Am J Public Health 71:591, 1981.
48. Roos NP and Roos L: Surgical rate variations: do they reflect the health or socioeconomic characteristics of the population? Med Care 20:945, 1982.
49. Roos NP: Hysterectomy: variations in rates across small areas and across physician's practices, Am J Public Health 74:327, 1984.
50. Rutkow IM: Delivery of surgical health care in the United States, Arch Surg 116:963, 1981.
51. Rutkow IM: Surgical decision making and operative rates, doctoral dissertation, Baltimore, 1981, The Johns Hopkins School of Public Health.
52. Rutkow IM: Rates of surgery in the United States: the decade of the 1970s, Surg Clin North Am 62:559, 1982.
53. Rutkow IM, editor: Surgical health care delivery, Philadelphia, 1982, WB Saunders Co.
54. Rutkow IM: The surgical decision-making process: determinants of surgical rates, Health Serv Res 17:380, 1982.
55. Rutkow IM and Starfield BH: Surgical decision making and operative rates, Arch Surg 119:899, 1984.
56. Rutkow IM: Surgical operations in the United States: 1979 to 1984, Surgery 101:192, 1987.
57. Rutkow IM: Quality of surgical operations and supply, Health Aff 6:82, 1987.
58. Rutkow IM and Zuidema GD: Surgical rates in the United States: 1966 to 1978, Surgery 89:151, 1981.
59. Sauter VL and Hughes EF: Surgical utilization statistics: some methodologic considerations, Med Care 21:370, 1983.
60. Schieber GJ and Poullier JP: Recent trends in international health care spending, Health Aff 6:105, 1987.
61. Scitovsky AA and McCall N: Use of hospital services under two prepaid plans, Med Care 18:30, 1980.
62. Scott HD and Mackie A: Decisions to hospitalize and operate: a socioeconomic perspective in an urban state, Surgery 77:311, 1975.
63. Simpson A: Variations in operation rates in New Zealand, NZ Med J 99:798, 1986.

64. Sloan FA, Valvona J, and Perrin JM: Diffusion of surgical technology: an exploratory study, J Health Econ 5:31, 1986.
65. Vayda E: A comparison of surgical rates in Canada and in England and Wales, N Engl J Med 289:1224, 1973.
66. Vayda E and Anderson GD: Comparison of provincial surgical rates in 1968, Can J Surg 18:18, 1975.
67. Vayda E, Morison M, and Anderson GD: Surgical rates in the Canadian provinces: 1968 to 1972. Can J Surg 19:235, 1976.
68. Vayda E and Rutkow IM: A decade of surgery in Canada, England and Wales, and the United States, Arch Surg 117:846, 1982.
69. Vayda E and Mindell WR: Variations in operative rates: what do they mean? Surg Clin North Am 62:627, 1982.
70. Watkins RN et al: Time utilization of a population of general surgeons in a prepaid group practice, Med Care 14:824, 1976.
71. Wennberg JE: The paradox of appropriate care, JAMA 258:2568, 1987.
72. Wennberg JE, Barnes BA, and Zubokk M: Professional uncertainty and the problem of supplier-induced demand, Soc Sci Med 16:811, 1982.
73. Wennberg JE, Freeman JL, and Culp WJ: Are hospital services rationed in New Haven or over-utilised in Boston? Lancet 1:1185, 1987.
74. Wennberg J and Gittelsohn AM: Small area variations in health care delivery, Science 182:1102, 1973.
75. Wennberg J and Gittelsohn AM: Health care delivery in Maine: patterns of use of common surgical procedures, J Maine Med Assoc 66:123, 1975.
76. West RR and Carey MJ: Variation in rates of hospital admission for appendicitis in Wales, Br Med J 1:1662, 1978.
77. Wilson SE and Longmire WP: Does method of payment affect surgical care? J Surg Res 24:457, 1978.
78. Yoshida Y and Yoshida K: The high rates of appendectomy in Japan, Med Care 14:950, 1976.

PART TWO

Delivery and Financing of Surgical Services

6. IMPACT OF DIAGNOSIS RELATED GROUPS AND THE PROSPECTIVE PAYMENT ASSESSMENT COMMISSION
   Eric Munoz
7. ADJUSTING DRGs FOR SEVERITY OF ILLNESS
   Susan D. Horn
   Michael A. Ashworth
8. REIMBURSEMENT IN THE FUTURE: THE PHYSICIAN PAYMENT REVIEW COMMISSION
   Oliver H. Beahrs
9. REGIONALIZED SURGICAL HEALTH CARE
   Ralph W. Schaffarzick
   John P. Bunker
10. THE IMPACT OF MANAGED HEALTH CARE SYSTEMS ON SURGEONS
    Lynn R. Gruber
    Susan Hartwell
    Cynthia L. Polich
11. FOR-PROFIT HEALTH CARE AND THE PRACTICE OF SURGERY
    Mark Schlesinger
    Brigid Goody
12. SURGICAL SECOND OPINION PROGRAMS
    Ira M. Rutkow
    Steven Sieverts

ERIC MUNOZ

Eric Munoz, born in the Bronx, New York, and raised in New Jersey, received a BA in psychology from the University of Virginia (1969), an MD from the Albert Einstein College of Medicine (1974), and an MBA in finance and economics from Columbia University (1983). He trained in general and vascular surgery at Yale University. He is the medical director for the University of Medicine and Dentistry of New Jersey University Hospital (Newark). He was recently appointed to the Prospective Payment Assessment Commission.

6

Impact of Diagnosis Related Groups and the Prospective Payment Assessment Commission

ERIC MUNOZ

This chapter will analyze national surgical health policy issues as they affect the surgeon, particularly regarding the inhospital payment of services, and will summarize recent research done in surgical economics and finance. Parts of this chapter contain a substantial discussion on the workings of national surgical health policy in America via fiscal incentives offered by the new Medicare diagnosis related groups (DRG) hospital payment system. The DRG payment system will ultimately affect all surgeons and their patients. In 1983 Congress passed a law that significantly altered Medicare's method of payment for inpatient hospital services. The Social Security Amendments of 1983 (PL 98-21) terminated hospital cost-based reimbursement by Medicare and began a 3-year transition to a prospective payment system (PPS) for inpatient hospital services. The system mandated by this law is based on fixed per-case payment rates for patients in 473 DRGs (see appendixes for all surgical DRGs).

The ultimate objective of Medicare's PPS was to reduce Medicare's expenditures for inpatient surgical hospital care while maintaining an acceptable level of quality and access for patients. This goal was to be accomplished through a fundamental alteration of the financial incentives facing hospitals, that is, the introduction of economic risk into hospital payment. Medicare's PPS is a marked change from the previous hospital payment system, that is, whereby all costs were reimbursed, yielding an entirely original set of new incentives.

One incentive under PPS is for hospitals to decrease the cost of treatments provided to surgical patients, most commonly by decreasing the hospital length of stay. PPS reduces the financial incentives for hospital managers and surgeons to provide added technologies (except where they may decrease costs to the hospital), and it encourages surgeons to assess the costs versus benefits of services. Because payment is per case, hospitals may have the incentive to increase the number of surgical admissions, particularly those that may be profitable, or to prevent those surgical admissions that may be unprofitable. PPS may also provide incentives for hospitals to find new sources of revenue by developing services not under DRG payment restrictions.[29]

Although the hospital incentives under PPS and some of their impacts were predicted by the designers of the DRG system, it was not known whether they would happen. This lack of data has not discouraged many from predicting serious undesirable results of PPS on the surgical patient's access to and quality of health care, on the introduction of new technologies into the practice of surgery, and on the level of clinical surgical research in the United States.* The concern that Medicare's PPS could result in a threat to the surgical health delivery system has made it a very important and controversial issue (Figure 6-1). Congressional awareness of problems with PPS was evident as the system was drafted; some of the problems were addressed in the Social Security amendments of 1983. The DRG law mandated that the Secretary of the Department of Health and Human Services (DHHS) prepare annual reports on the impact of PPS through 1987.[21] With PPS the Congress established an independent advisory body to analyze and recommend changes regarding DRG hospital payment. This advisory body, the Prospective Payment Assessment Commission (ProPAC), advises both the Congress and the Secretary of Health and Human Services regarding DRGs. ProPAC consists of 17 individuals who meet regularly; in addition, it has a professional staff of 25 analysts and an annual budget of just less than $4 million.

COMPONENTS OF DIAGNOSIS RELATED GROUPS

The DRG system was developed at Yale University during the 1970s as a way to group patients with similar resource consumption. This grouping was done to develop a standard grouping system to quantify patient care requirements. The system was later transformed into a payment scheme by several large pilot projects, most notably in New Jersey. It is a product classification system. Although there are differences across a given DRG population, on average the system describes for each DRG similar patients, similar diseases or operations, and similar outcomes.

These DRGs were created by aggregating 10,000 diseases or procedures by International Classification of Diseases, Ninth Revision, Clinical Modification (ICD-9-CM) code into 23 major diagnostic categories (MDCs) and then disaggregating them into 468 DRGs. DRGs describe patients with similar resource consumption in a way that is medically meaningful to physicians. The key components of the system are principal diagnosis, primary operative procedure, comorbidities or complications, age, and discharge status. Each DRG is characterized by a particular procedure (operation) or several related procedures, age (younger than or older than 70 years), the presence or absence of complicating conditions, for example, wound infection or pulmonary embolism, or comorbidities such as hypertension or diabetes mellitus, and at times whether the patient is discharged alive or dead.

Each DRG has its own weight intensity. The weight index is a figure that describes the average consumption of resources in the United States around a weight index of 1.0000, which is the degree of resources consumed by the average inpatient. Each patient's chart is evaluated at discharge and grouped into the most intense (highest weight index) DRG. Thus a patient entering the hospital (admission) with shortness of breath (chronic obstructive pulmonary disease, DRG No. 88, weight index 1.0412) who has an upper gastrointestinal bleed and undergoes a gastric operation (hemigastrectomy, DRG No. 154, weight index 2.6901), will be coded at discharge and reimbursed for DRG No. 154 because this DRG yields the highest reimbursement.

This system allows a hospital, surgeon, or health care system to assess its products (DRGs). Because products (DRGs) can now be assessed more accurately, input (dollars, tests, hospital days) in relation to output (morbidity, mortality,

---
*References 1, 3, 5, 7, 32, 34, 35.

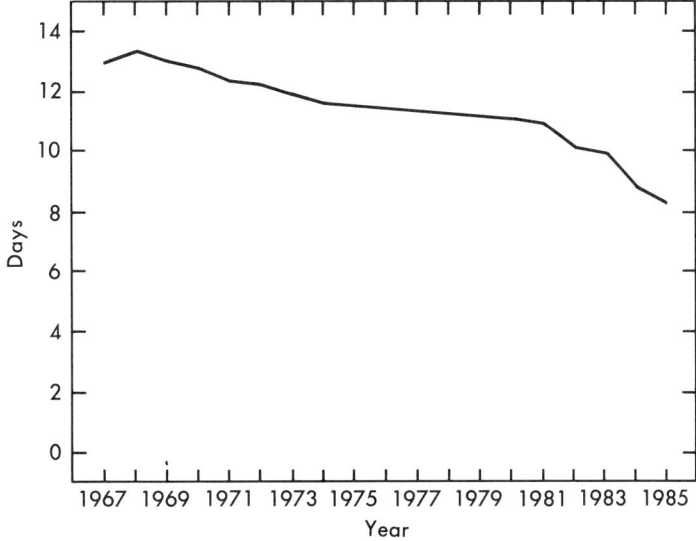

Figure 6-1. Average length of stay for Medicare patients, 1967-1985.

cure) can be better evaluated. This product classification system has strengths and weaknesses. It may change the traditional approaches to some types of surgical practice and may tend to reward treatments that are not more profitable to the hospital. The system will also cause a relatively rapid expansion of administrative changes needed at the institutional level to deal with the payment scheme. The new payment system makes accurate medical record keeping and coding a much more vital area for each hospital, since the economic well-being of each institution is now directly related to this department.

THE PROSPECTIVE PAYMENT ASSESSMENT COMMISSION: ITS ROLE, RESPONSIBILITIES, AND PROCESSES

The Congress established ProPAC as a permanent independent commission with responsibilities to maintain and update the new DRG payment system. In 1986 the Congress expanded the Commission from 15 to 17 members. The Commission members are appointed by the director of the Office of Technology Assessment (OTA), within the Congress of the United States. Members of ProPAC are chosen to provide independent expertise in health care delivery, financing, and research.

ProPAC's Priorities

Maintaining access to high-quality health care. ProPAC's first priority is maintaining access to high-quality surgical health care for citizens of the United States covered by Medicare (about 31 million people, primarily the elderly, certain groups of permanently disabled patients, and those with end stage renal disease). With the changing financial incentives for hospitals, PPS may affect the maintenance of quality surgical health care while restraining health care costs. Hospitals that are paid under DRGs by Medicare and other payers must be sensitive to the costs for patient care because they now face some economic risk. PPS may encourage a decrease of hospital tests, procedures, supplies, equipment, personnel, and hospital days. As the increase in hospital expenditures slows, and cost savings are realized, methods to detect adverse effects on quality and access of surgical care will be needed (Figure 6-2). ProPAC is interested in the issues related to quality of care. The DRG classifications and weights also must be modified appropriately to reflect changes in surgical practice. In addition, the DRG update factor must be used to allow hospitals to maintain an adequate delivery of surgical services.[29]

Encouraging hospital productivity and long-term cost effectiveness. Another priority of ProPAC is encouraging productivity and long-term cost effectiveness in surgical health care delivery. PPS uses DRGs to categorize patients and define the various hospital surgical products, that is, patients. Hospital care is only one of many "inputs" that contribute to a surgical patient's overall health status. Other types of care outside of the hospital also contribute to an individual's health status. PPS may provide incentives to move surgical services to other settings. If these services can be delivered at a lower cost and equal quality in these settings, efficiency will be improved. The emphasis on reducing costs, however, may retard the adoption of new services that may at first increase costs, although in the long term could improve patient surgical care, productivity, and/or cost effectiveness.

Facilitating innovation and appropriate surgical technologic change. Concerns regarding changes in technology are highly relevant to the surgeon. It is hoped that Medicare's DRG prospective payment system will have an unbiased effect on surgical technologic advancement. A third priority of ProPAC is that of encouraging innovation and the appropriate surgical technologic change. PPS payment levels should be neutral concerning the development, diffusion, or adoption of new surgical technologies and practices. Concerning the potential effects of PPS on the adoption of new technologies and practices, ProPAC is interested in payment policies and amounts that are adequate to enable hospitals to adopt new technologies. One approach ProPAC has chosen to ensure adequate surgical technologic innovation under PPS is to modify current DRG classifications and weights to reflect changes in technology and surgical practice.[29]

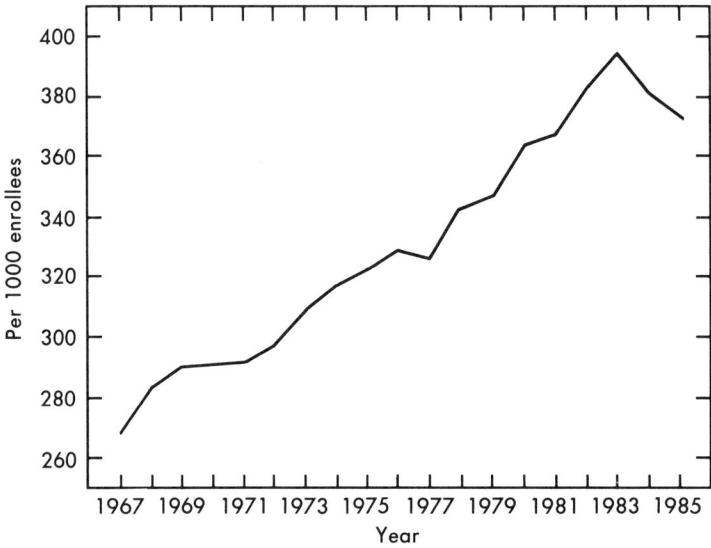

Figure 6-2. Medicare hospital admissions, 1967-1985.

Maintaining stability for providers, consumers, and other payers. A fourth priority of ProPAC is the maintenance of a stable environment for surgeons, hospitals, patients, and other payers. ProPAC feels that in a rapidly changing surgical health care delivery and financing era, its recommendations should provide as much predictability and stability as possible.[29]

Decision making based on reliable, timely data and information. ProPAC's fifth priority is to base its deliberations on reliable, timely data and information. ProPAC's major contribution to DRGs are recommendations based on accurate analytic study.[29] ProPAC presented recommendations on ways to change and improve surgical DRGs for fiscal year 1988 (outlined in this chapter). The 28 ProPAC recommendations reflected the collective judgment of ProPAC's 17 commissioners regarding issues of importance to surgical patients, surgeons, hospitals, and the Medicare program. The following major areas were addressed: updating DRG payments (the update factor); earlier availability of DRG cost data; incorporating capital payments into DRGs, improving hospital labor areas; concerns regarding beneficiaries (surgical patients); issues related to rural hospitals (those that tended to be in sparsely populated areas of the United States), improvements to surgical DRGs, and the study of DRG surgical case mix change.[29]

Updating PPS Payments (the Update Factor)

The amount of increase of DRG hospital payments each year is a major issue to both surgeons and hospitals. The update factor together with cost increases at the hospital level will generate the financial risk facing surgeons, surgical departments, and hospitals. For fiscal 1988 ProPAC recommended an increase in the level of PPS prices of 2.2% of urban hospitals and 3% for rural hospitals. These update factors were derived by combining a number of components, the analyses of which are quite complex and quantitative to the clinical surgeon. One component was a 5.4% average reduction, to be phased in over 3 years to reflect recent differences between projected and actual costs during the first year of PPS, because it was widely felt that the DRG rates were at first too generous. This reduction resulted in a decrease of 1.9% for urban hospitals and 1.1% for rural hospitals for fiscal year 1988.[29] The other components of the update factor were: an increase of 4.9% for inflation in the hospital market basket (increases in hospital goods and services), a 0.5% increase for scientific and technologic advances (improved technologies), and a 1.3% increase for real case mix changes (a more complex patient); and a decrease of 1% for improvements in hospital productivity (input relative to output), a .3% decrease for shifts in the site of service (usually out of the hospital), and a 1.3% decrease for expected changes in the DRG case mix index.[29]

Improvements to the DRGs

A significant debate has risen over improving the accuracy of surgical DRGs. The health policy problem involves whether to attempt small improvements in DRG prediction using the data currently captured by hospitals, that is, UHDDS hospital discharge data, or whether to attempt large improvements in DRGs by requiring hospitals to collect new data, which would be administratively costly and which would require further medical record analysis.[12] ProPAC believed that the current DRG system is the most appropriate at this time for hospital DRG case mix payment. ProPAC recommended several specific refinements to the DRG system that could be done using currently available hospital discharge data. ProPAC also advocated the development of longer term improvements in surgical DRGs by incorporating new data not currently collected in the patient's discharge abstract. ProPAC also believed that current outlier payment policy, that is, very costly surgical cases should be further refined to improve resource accuracy and to reduce the financial risk associated with caring for extremely costly surgical cases.[29]

Study of Case Mix Change

A number of issues related to medical record coding and abstracting may impact on the dynamics of surgical DRGs. ProPAC urged the development of more complete data and methods to analyze changes in surgical DRGs over time. Previously, ProPAC noted there has been difficulty in distinguishing between changes in real DRG case mix (a more complex surgical patient) and coding improvements ("DRG creep") when developing the DRG update factors. This problem requires a very complex health policy analysis confounded by many variables. ProPAC is working with the Health Care Financing Administration (HCFA) in analyzing the reabstraction of medical records to test and refine methods to measure DRG surgical case mix change.[30]

Propac Recommendations for Fiscal Year 1988

Updating PPS payments.

(Detailed analysis of these recommendations are contained in the ProPAC Technical Report.)[31]

Recommendation 1	Update factor
Recommendation 2	Adjustment to the level of standardized amounts
Recommendation 3	Allowance for scientific and technological advancement, productivity goals, and site-of-care substitution
Recommendation 4	Adjustments for case mix change
Recommendation 5	Update factor for excluded hospitals and distinct-part units
Recommendation 6	Timely availability of Medicare cost report data
Recommendation 7	All-inclusive rate
Recommendation 8	Level of federal capital payment
Recommendation 9	Capital payment transition
Recommendation 10	Institutional neutrality
Recommendation 11	Capital exceptions process
Recommendation 12	Improving the definition of hospital labor market areas
Recommendation 13	Improving the area wage index
Recommendation 14	Extension of volume protection to all isolated, rural hospitals
Recommendation 15	Clarification of sole community hospital volume exception criteria
Recommendation 16	Evaluation of current PPS payment policies for rural hospitals
Recommendation 17	Improvements in outlier payment policy

Beneficiary concerns

Recommendation 18	Inpatient hospital cost-sharing requirements
Recommendation 19	Evaluating the results of PRO Quality of Care Review
Recommendation 20	Improving the measurement of hospital case mix
Recommendation 21	The use of patient age in defining DRGs
Recommendation 22	Improving the use of complications and comorbidities in defining DRGs

Recommendation 23	Updating the surgical hierarchies and the list of operating room procedures
Recommendation 24	Improving grouper logic and ICD-9-CM coding
Recommendation 25	Temporary DRG for the implantable defibrillator
Recommendation 26	Temporary DRG for the cochlear implant
Recommendation 27	Additional payment for magnetic resonance imaging scans
Recommendation 28	Record reabstraction study

The Future

Surgical health policy in the future will be increasingly driven by fiscal incentives provided to surgeons and hospitals. Surgical practice involves a complex interaction between economic forces affecting the surgeon and those facing the hospital, in addition to medical and surgical indications for diagnoses and treatments. Many surgeons provide a substantial amount of their surgical care (and both surgeon and hospital revenue) at the inpatient hospital setting. It is likely that some conflicts may develop in the future between financial incentives offered to hospitals and those offered to surgeons. Although the new Medicare DRG hospital payment system covers a substantial number of patients (the elderly), other payers still retain a cost-based reimbursement system. Currently 13 states, however, have adopted some form of DRG prospective pricing system for surgical patients based on the Medicare DRG method. It is likely that for the foreseeable future, DRG prospective pricing will become the dominant payment scheme for the majority of hospitalized surgical patients. Thus the DRG system is likely to be a significant driving force for national surgical health policy for the next decade.[33] It is also likely that surgery in the United States will begin to experience "future economic shocks" in the next decade, as national and international forces interact with our discipline.

The rapidly changing reimbursement system in the United States will affect the hospital care of all surgical patients whether or not they are under DRG reimbursement. Unfortunately, surgeons have not been trained in the science of surgical economics; this will change. It is probable that the fiscal flows affecting health care delivery in the next decade will have a far greater incremental effect on the average surgical patient in the average hospital in the United States compared with the incremental effect of any other medical discipline during this same period. In addition, there are going to be inequities and weaknesses within large aggregate grouping schemes such as DRGs.[36,37] This is a distressing point when most surgeons understand little of the science of economics or surgical health policy. The limited resource problem that is now upon us in surgical care will never abate. Surgical services (as with all health care services) on the margin provide decreasing returns to scale. Surgeons face an exciting challenge for the future to improve efficiency, that is, input relative to output. In addition, the United States is providing more expensive surgical care to increasingly fewer of its citizens. The number of uninsured and underinsured in this country is growing and becoming increasingly visible to those in national public policy. These issues will require study and analysis by surgeons.

SURGICAL ECONOMICS AND FINANCE

The surgical world is changing because of a variety of forces impinging on both surgeons and hospitals. During the 1970s research appeared on surgical manpower issues, rates of surgical procedures and factors affecting same, various quantitative analyses related to the marginal utility of various treatments or types of operations (either using cost effectiveness or cost-benefit analysis), factors that influenced surgical practice patterns, and some historical data on surgical expenditures.[2-4,10,17] As recently as 1981 Rutkow reviewed the existing literature on surgical health care delivery and showed that much of the analyses along these lines had appeared primarily in nonsurgical journals.[31] The remaining portion of this chapter will analyze more recent research on surgical health delivery data including analysis of: (1) surgical expenditures, (2) the DRG system and findings related to surgeons, (3) refining surgical DRGs, (4) effects of DRGs on the surgeon, (5) future policy issues related to DRGs, and (6) data on the costs of treatment for selected surgical disorders. This analysis will deal mainly with issues related to the hospital-based treatments of surgical disorders. Although there has been an increase of these types of analyses in the surgical literature, a substantial number of these studies still appear in journals not read routinely by surgeons.

Aggregate Surgical Health Expenditures

Moore has previously analyzed the dollar flow for United States surgical care in terms of a six-level model.[7] Of the $310 billion expended for health care in 1981, it was estimated that $85 to $95 billion was the "surgical stream," that is, that amount expended to take care of surgical patients at a variety of institution types including ambulatory care and surgeons' fees (Table 6-1). Some of the determinants of surgical flows were reviewed in Moore's study, as well as potentially controllable costs and case mix pressures. Surgical complications, when severe, increased routine operative costs by a factor of 8 to 20. The maintenance of high quality in the United States, despite new manpower pressures, was felt to be the single most important factor in cost containment. By voluntary or imposed controls on fees, malpractice premiums, case mix selection, and hospital utilization, a saving of $2 to $4 billion was believed by this researcher to be attainable and practical. This would be 5% of the surgical stream; the realistic "achievable" savings of total surgical flow was estimated by Moore to thus be about $5 billion.[17]

The economic costs of trauma in the United States were analyzed by Munoz by utilizing available data from United States Vital Statistics and using models to convert to dollar costs for trauma fatalities and nonfatalities.[18] Trauma cost the nation approximately $61.025 billion in fiscal 1982 (1977 figures indexed to 1982 dollars) or 6.9% of total US health care expenditures and 2.3% of the total US gross national product (GNP).[19] This included $19.278 billion for direct costs (treatment related) and $41.746 billion in indirect costs (forgone earnings). The largest sin-

Table 6-1. An estimate of surgical streams in total dollar flow (1981)

	Totals (billion)	Surgical estimates (billion)
Acute care hospitals budgets	$122	$73.2 (60%)
Nursing home budgets	$ 24	$ 0.72 (3%)
Practice charges of physicians and dentists	$ 72	$14.4 (20%)
Brokers and bureau costs	$ 11	$ 1 (10%)
All other provider budgets	$ 81	$ 5 (6%)
TOTAL SURGICAL	$310	$94.3 (30%)

From Moore FD: Ann Surg 201; 132, 1985.

gle category by group was indirect costs (forgone earnings) for male fatalities ($26.635 billion) followed by direct costs (treatment related) for male nonfatalities ($12.145 billion).

The DRG System and the Surgeon

The DRG hospital payment system has begun to dramatically alter financial incentives provided to surgeons and hospitals.[24] Rhodes compared the length of hospitalization of 329 patients undergoing femoropopliteal bypass during 1982 with that allowed under Medicare's DRGs for major reconstructive vascular surgery (DRG Nos. 110 and 111).[30] The mean length of stay in this study was found to be related to the patient's age, increasing at a rate of about 1% per year. The site of distal anastomosis, a factor not considered in establishing the criteria for these DRGs, was also important. The lengths of stay for above-the-knee popliteal, below-the-knee popliteal, and tibioperoneal anastomoses were significantly different, with lengths of stay increasing for more distal anastomoses. Rhodes found that more distal anastamoses were also associated with increased rates of postoperative morbidity, reoperation, and mortality. It was concluded (1) that the DRG system did not take account of certain important variables for this surgical DRG influencing the length of hospitalization for femoropopliteal bypass, (2) that it could favor younger patients undergoing proximal bypass, and (3) that it is biased against distal bypass for limb salvage.[30]

Munoz analyzed hospital charges (excluding physician fees) for all patients who underwent cholecystectomy without common bile duct exploration (DRG Nos. 197 and 198) to quantify mean hospital charges, variances, and components of hospital charges.[19] The mean total hospital charge for elective cholecystectomy was $4763 ± $1656; the mean length of stay (LOS) was 8 days ± 3.2 days. Low and high trim points were $3211 to $10,639 and 5 to 19 days LOS. Analysis of services showed that laboratory work (urinalysis, hematology, coagulation, microbiology, and biochemistry) averaged $451 (9.5% of total), room and board $2635 ± $1044 (55.3% of total), operating and recovery room $924 ± $167 (19.4% of total), and central supply/pharmacy $350 ± $158 (7.4% of total). The mean total hospital charge for patients undergoing emergency cholecystectomy was $11,436 ± $4185; mean LOS was 17.8 days ± 6.5 days. Low and high trim points were $6353 to $19,734; LOS was 9 to 30 days. Services as percent of total were laboratory, 15.8%; room and board, 53.7%; operating and recovery room, 9.4%; central supply/pharmacy, 7.4%; and other, 13.8%. Munoz concluded that: (1) for a given surgical disease or DRG there was marked variance of hospital charges; (2) mean charges of emergency patients were 240% that of elective patients; and (3) consumption of services varies significantly within each group and between groups.[19] This was one of the earliest health services studies to suggest that route of admission (emergency versus nonemergency) might be an important determinant of hospital resource consumption.

Another report by Munoz demonstrated that a majority of surgical DRGs would be unprofitable under the proposed DRG reimbursement scheme.[22] A method was developed for allowing the hospital to group patients within each DRG to show differences in hospital charges and be clinically meaningful to surgeons. Munoz tested the hypothesis that entities called identifiers, arbitrarily chosen as mode of admission (emergency [+ER] versus nonemergency [-ER]) and the presence (+T) or absence (-T) of blood transfusion, would show differences in charges (mean hospital charge exclusive of physician fees) within a surgical DRG. In nine DRGs encompassing general surgery, thoracic surgery, cardiac surgery, neurosurgery, orthopedics, urology, and head and neck surgery, 905 patients were studied. For the ER identifier, eight of nine DRGs were found to be positive (greater than 20% difference in charges between positive and negative identifier); for T identifier, all nine DRGs were positive. It was evident that clinical variables could be used to stratify differences in cost within surgical DRGs.[22]

Craniotomy without trauma (DRG No. 1) has been characterized as to the cost dynamics of its DRG.[25] The findings from this study showed that: (1) each hospital service category had wide charge variances around the mean; (2) emergency (ER) admissions were 200% more expensive than nonemergency (non-ER) admissions; (3) ER admissions seemed to have no greater severity of illness than non-ER admissions but had a significantly different referral pattern, that is, admission from the ER to a nonneurosurgical service with a subsequent neurosurgical referral; and (4) this DRG when grouped into clinical "subproducts", such as craniotomy for tumor, hematoma, hydrocephalus, aneurysm, and benign cyst, showed marked differences. Among the most important findings were that "referral dynamics" (change in clinical service) may provide some explanation of cost variance within a DRG and that surgical DRGs could be grouped by cost by the reason or diagnosis for a particular procedure (clinical subproducts).[25] This can have the most potential impact in understanding DRGs.

The implementation of prospective payment systems for hospitals, most notably the Medicare DRG mechanism, will encourage surgeons and hospitals to characterize populations that create financial risk.[13] A previous study has demonstrated that certain factors (called identifiers), such as emergency admission or necessity for blood transfusion, predicted higher-cost patients per DRG.[22] It has also been shown that surgical complications and deaths can generate financial risk under DRG payment and that the degree of risk would vary by the dynamics of the complications and death.[26] Munoz et al. examined all surgical admissions (n = 5596) to a large voluntary hospital and determined general and vascular surgical complications and deaths (170 patients: complication rate, 3.1%) for 1983 and 1984. Total charges exclusive of physicians fees for these patients were $4,683,670 (mean per patient, $27,551) resulting in a DRG loss of $2,304,967 (mean per patient, $13,558). Charges and financial risk generated by the origin of the surgical morbidity and death differed as follows: (1) iatrogenic origin only (n = 41)—mean charge per patient, $15,321 (19.5% of whom had unusually long hospital stays or unusually high costs [outliers]); (2) origin intrinsic to the patient's disease only (n = 75)—mean charge per patient $28,391 (38.7% outliers); and (3) combined iatrogenic origin and patient's disease (n = 54)—mean charge per patient, $35,669 (48% outliers). This study demonstrated that general and vascular surgical morbidity and deaths generated significant financial risk under DRG reimbursement. The degree of financial risk was greatest for patients who had combined iatrogenic and intrinsic complications, followed by patients with intrinsic complications only, then by patients with only iatrogenic complications.[26]

Refining Surgical DRGs

The current patient classification schemes used in DRG case mix reimbursement appear not fully sensitive to variations in resource consumption that are associated with differential disease severity. Severity of illness describes the range of illness for a given disease — from a simple uncomplicated case to a very complex case ending in death. A number of methods such as the Horn Severity of Illness Index and the Acute Physiologic and Chronic Health Evaluation (APACHE) are currently being evaluated by HCFA and ProPAC as potential modifiers within the DRG payment scheme.[29] Patient management categories (PMCs) are a clinically based measure of severity of illness that uses objective medical criteria to assess the stage of disease progression.[6] Its availability in automated form increases its ease of implementation in hospital reimbursement and management. Results of recent studies by Young have demonstrated that PMCs are useful DRG case mix tools that explain significant variation in cost per discharge within current diagnosis related groups. Patient management categories appear to be clinically relevant, to describe variances in severity, and to identify comorbidities.[37]

The Horn Severity of Illness Index has been suggested as a refinement to DRGs.[11] It consists of a seven-tier model that appears to stratify severity of illness. Comparative analyses of the DRG case mix groups within hospitals and an application of severity-adjusted diagnosis related groups case mix definitions appear enhanced by the Horn index. The index also describes the contribution of the variation in physician practice patterns to the variation in resource use per patient within a hospital in addition to cross-hospital comparisons.[11]

Another severity modifier of DRGs is the acute physiology score (APS) of the Acute Physiologic and Chronic Health Evaluation (APACHE) II.[34] The APS is defined by a relative value scale applied to 12 objective physiologic variables routinely measured on most hospitalized patients shortly after hospital admission. In a study by Knaus for intensive care patients, APS at admission appeared strongly related to subsequent resource costs of intensive care for 5790 consecutive admissions to 13 large hospitals, both across and within diagnoses. Knaus suggests that the APS could also be used to evaluate quality of care, medical technology, and the response to changing financial incentives.[15]

The health policy problem of adjusting DRGs for severity of illness involves the "incremental" utility of the various severity of illness modifiers. Some forms of severity modifiers such as PMCs use data already captured and coded with routine discharge data (called UHDDS discharge data). These types of UHDDS severity modifiers appear very modest at improving DRG resource prediction; however, a system based on currently available data would be relatively inexpensive to implement. Other forms of DRG severity modifiers, such as the Horn index and the APACHE II system, require substantial additional data collection by hospitals. Although these non-UHDDS based systems might increase DRG accuracy more substantially, they would do so at a significant cost to the hospital. At this time it appears that the current DRG system will undergo no modification regarding severity of illness.

Although DRGs were originally devised as a research instrument for the evaluation of medical resource allocation, a study by Delguercio et al. compared the actual physiologic status of patients within the DRG classification.[7] One hundred consecutive high-risk elective surgical patients entered a preoperative intensive care unit for prospective analyses of physiologic assessment, resource utilization, DRG classification, and outcome. Swan-Ganz catheters inserted 1 or 2 days before surgery were used to compute physiologic profiles and stage according to previously published criteria. This paper suggested that although the DRG system as set up by HCFA correctly predicted that age and comorbidity factors led to increased utilization of resources, the extent to which they underestimated the increased needs for these patients could lead to significant financial risk. Delguercio concluded that high-risk, referred surgical patients were much sicker than they appeared to the DRG system, and in all 100 cases financial compensation was grossly inadequate.[7]

Effects of DRGs on Surgical Care

No one knows what the DRG hospital payment system will do to the quality and access of patients' surgical care. Some data suggest that the new DRG system may create problems for hospitals, surgeons, and their patients. A study by Munoz assessed the financial impact (revenues versus expenses) as measured by hospital charges and costs versus DRG revenues of prospective payment systems on emergency department generated admissions for a large teaching hospital under two payment systems: Medicare and an all-payer system.[21] All emergency department admissions were analyzed for the years 1983 and 1984 under both systems by clinical specialty, using standard DRG methodology. Findings suggested that: (1) with charges as a measure of expense under both payment schemes, all clinical departments had large groups of unprofitable patients: Medicare, $12,895,038; all-payer system, $15,553,893; (2) when costs were computed as the expense measure (using our hospital's cost-to-charge ratio), Medicare patients produced a deficit ($2,363,163); however, under an all-payer system, there was a small net profit ($4,267,859); and (3) the implementation of federalized DRG reimbursement rates increased losses for this population from 1983 to 1984. Reductions in outliers reimbursement (10%) and teaching costs (25%) caused revenues to drop substantially, potentiating losses. Munoz et al. suggested that hospitals with large emergency department admission populations, particularly Medicare patients, may be at a significant financial disadvantage under prospective payment systems. In effect, they were suggesting that DRG prospective pricing schemes could limit the "access of hospital care for some Americans."

In another study Munoz et al. tested the hypothesis that financial risk would be generated by surgical patients transferred to tertiary care hospitals from other acute care hospitals under DRG reimbursement.[28] Hospital costs (exclusive of physician fees) were analyzed for 97 adult general surgical patients transferred between January 1, 1985, and December 31, 1986. Transferred patients had significantly higher resource utilization (hospital costs) than nontransferred patients within the same surgical DRGs as follows: total mean costs per patients, $17,348 versus $9460; mean length of stay, 21.4 days versus 10.9 days; mean laboratory cost per patient, $1849 versus $975; and mean radiologic cost per patient, $794 versus $397. Transferred patients generated a yearly deficit of $238,717 ($4922 loss per patient) for the hospital, whereas other patients within the same surgical DRGs generated a profit of $727,632 ($489 profit per patient). Munoz et al. suggested that DRG reimbursement may provide a financial disincentive for teaching hospitals to accept surgical transfer patients from other acute care hospitals, thus potentially decreasing the access of care for these complexly ill surgical patients.[28]

One study by Fitzgerald et al. suggested that Medicare DRG payment may have actually caused a decrease in the quality of surgical care for a group of elderly hip fracture patients. Demographic and clinical data were reviewed for a group of orthopedic surgical patients treated at a municipal hospital both before and after the implementation of DRG payment. It was found that after DRG payment implementation, the mean length of hospitalization fell from 16.6 to 10.3 days, and the mean number of physical therapy sessions decreased from 9.7 to 4.9. The proportion of patients discharged to nursing homes increased (from 21% to 48%), as did the number receiving nursing home care at six months after discharge.[8]

Previous studies by Munoz showed that certain clinical variables (identifiers) would differentiate hospital expenses within surgical DRGs. Another study by this group demonstrated that the clinical variables of admission (emergency versus non-emergency, blood transfusion, and surgical intensive care unit admission) could stratify both differences in severity of illness and hospital charges for patients in general surgical DRGs.[27] It was suggested that these three identifiers might be useful to surgeons and hospital administrators in evaluating surgical patients for differences in resource consumption during their hospitalization, and for better management of hospital-based inpatient costs. Cholecystectomy (DRG No. 197) as analyzed by Munoz et al. demonstrated the practical application of this concept. Emergency admissions in this DRG had total charges that were more than double those of nonemergency admissions; this was caused in part by long preoperative lengths of stay (about 8 days). Because emergency DRG No. 197 patients were financial losers, there was an economic incentive for the hospital to improve efficiency in this group. The utilization review coordinator and the administrative staff believed that the preoperative workup for these patients, who were usually admitted with the diagnosis of acute cholecystitis, could be done more quickly without changing the quality of care or outcome for the patient. The effort involved decreasing the lag time for the diagnostic testing (usually Tc-labeled immunodiacetic acid (HIDA) scans, ultrasound, or both) and facilitating operative scheduling for these patients.[21]

Another study by Munoz et al. found that certain "identifiers" may assist hospital management in reversing physician-related referral behavior that could result in higher hospital costs per DRG.[25] An analysis of patients undergoing craniotomy (DRG No. 1) showed that emergency admissions had a pattern of referral dynamics that tended to expand costs per DRG. Emergency admissions in the craniotomy study were twice as expensive as nonemergency admissions but not more severely ill. However, they had significantly different referral patterns. Many of these patients were admitted to the neurology service with subsequent referral to the neurosurgery service, after which craniotomy was performed. This study suggested that hospital administration could promote savings by encouraging admission directly to the neurosurgical service for certain patients with admitting emergency diagnoses fitting the craniotomy DRG profile, that is, likely to need a craniotomy, and thus potentially shorten the preoperative length of stay for these patients. Munoz et al. have demonstrated in a number of studies that route of admission may be a powerful predictor of cost variances caused by a variety of factors, some of which may be reversible without altering the quality of surgical care.[25]

In another study, the financial components of a common surgical DRG (No. 62, inguinal and femoral hernias) that was unprofitable under DRGs, the appropriateness of hospital expenditures, and proposed strategies for cost containment without sacrificing the quality of care were all examined.[20] Hospital charges were examined by hospital service category and aggregated by total dollars per category, patient mean dollars plus or minus standard error of mean per category, and patient totals. Total hospital charges for this DRG were $493,432, DRG reimbursement (1983 Federal Register) would have been $447,799, resulting in a net loss (deficit) to the hospital of $47,434 or $212 per patient. Hospital services (room and board, laboratory and ancillaries) appeared overused in the treatment of this DRG. Munoz et al. suggested that strategies involving quite modest decreases in the hospital length of stay and use of ancillary services (laboratory, x-ray, electrocardiogram) would have saved at least $60,000 and have made this a profitable surgical DRG.[20]

The value of routine pathologic study of specimens taken at herniorrhapy was assessed by Munoz et al.[14] Although there may be some justification for routine tissue testing for medical and legal reasons and quality assurance purposes or for specimens that appeared abnormal at operation, it was suggested that for patients who undergo herniorrhapy, little positive effect on the outcome is gained from routine pathologic examination of specimens that appeared normal at operation.

Costs of Different Forms of Treatment

To date there have been few data to compare surgical treatments for the same disease (such as different operations), and to compare various types of treatments (for example, medical or surgical) for a particular disease. However, two recent studies demonstrate representative investigations along these lines.

Current data on the surgical management of breast carcinoma supports the selective use of conservative surgery, that is, lumpectomy, axillary sampling, and irradiation, rather than modified radical mastectomy. Munoz et al. conducted an economic comparison of these two forms of surgical therapy. Total charges for treatment (hospital and physician) of 79 patients with stage I or II breast cancer during 1983 and 1984, utilizing either therapy, demonstrated that mean total charges per patient for lumpectomy (n = 49) were $14,176 ± $4262, and for mastectomy (n = 30) were $10,345 ± $3134. Although hospital inpatient fees were significantly less for lumpectomy ($5741) than for mastectomy ($7328), mean total physician fees were significantly higher for lumpectomy ($4505) in this study. Radiotherapist fees and the substantial radiation therapy hospital outpatient charge for lumpectomy ($5015) made the mean total charges for lumpectomy significantly higher than for mastectomy. The authors suggested that incentives offered by DRGs may provide the hospital incentives to encourage one form of surgical therapy or the other.[23]

Cello et al. studied bleeding esophageal varices and compared a medical treatment (sclerotherapy) with a surgical treatment (portacaval shunt).[5] This study randomized Child's class C patients to either sclerotherapy or portacaval shunt. Forty-six percent of sclerotherapy patients survived compared with 42% of portacaval shunt patients; sclerotherapy patients had significantly more rehospitalizations after discharge for bleeding. There was no differences in long-term survival between either group, however. The total cost of treatment was much greater for the portacaval shunt group ($23,957) compared with the sclerotherapy group ($15,364). This study is important because it suggests that efficiency might be improved for the treatment of bleeding esophageal varices, that is, the same output with lesser input by the use of a nonsurgical therapy. This type of analysis will become very important as health care resources become more limited.

DRGs and the Future of Surgical Practice

The technical construction of DRGs may also provide physicians and hospitals with incentives to encourage certain types of treatments as suggested by Smits.[33] Both HCFA and ProPAC are studying DRG coding practices. The assignment of codes may affect surgical practice. Hospital bills submitted to Medicare for payment must be coded according to the International Classification of Diseases, Ninth Revision, Clinical Modification (ICD-9-CM). ICD-9-CM is an inclusive code; it accommodates all events in surgical practice without the addition of new codes to the system. A new operation is either coded in the same way as a similar operation or placed in one of the general or "grab bag" codes described in terms such as "other operations on the vagina." However, a new surgical procedure is handled, existing rules require that it continue to be coded in the same way until the next revision of the entire coding system; ICD-9-CM will be revised no earlier than 1991.

Coding and pricing may also have effects on the surgeon. The grouping of a number of diverse surgical procedures in a single grab bag code leads to the assignment of a single DRG and a single price for all the procedures in the group. An innovative vascular procedure assigned to code 39.99 would be given a weight of 2.35 and would be paid at a relatively high price. An innovative urologic procedure assigned to code 64.49 would, by contrast, be given a weight of 0.8330 and paid at a much lower price. DRG payments make coding an issue of national health policy in which each decision can have a multimillion dollar effect. The resolution of questions about the coding of new surgical procedures should now become the responsibility of a publicly accountable group established by the government. Smits suggests that a national coding committee composed of federal staff members and outside experts could resolve coding disputes and develop guidelines for the appropriate coding of new procedures.

CONCLUSIONS

This chapter has attempted to review the more important recent analyses in the field of national health policy, DRGs, surgical health care delivery, economics, and finance. Given the economic drives of the U.S. economy, it appears that surgical health care financial policy is at the core of surgical health care public policy. Transplantation surgery provides a good example. Although there are certain constraints affecting surgical transplantation, such as organ availability and rejection phenomenon, the most major factor affecting the "availability" of "transplant services" in this country during the remainder of the century will likely be its ability to pay for same. As it becomes clear to the United States' surgical community that it faces real constraints in the delivery of surgical care, issues of cost containment and surgical economics will be studied in earnest. Surgeons must come to understand the concept of marginal, that is, incremental or relative, value or utility of an action. Omitting those actions that provide little marginal value on the patient's outcome should provide additional dollars for other surgical therapies. Surgeons will need to do much further study of surgical expenditures and costs, access, and the quality of surgical care.

References

1. Avorn J: Benefit and cost analysis in geriatric care: turning age discrimination into health policy, N Engl J Med 310:1294, 1984.
2. Barnes BA: Cost benefit analysis of surgery: current accomplishments and limitations, Am J Surg 133:438, 1977.
3. Bloom BS et al: Surgeons in the United States: practice characteristics, Arch Surg 113:188, 1978.
4. Bombardier C et al: Socioeconomic factors affecting the utilization of surgical operations, N Engl J Med 297:699, 1977.
5. Cello IP et al: Endoscopic sclerotherapy versus portacaval shunt in patients with severe cirrhosis and variceal hemorrhage, N Engl J Med 311:1589, 1984.
6. Conklin JE et al: Disease staging: implication for hospital reimbursement and management, Health Care Finan Rev, 1984 Ann Suppl, p.1.
7. DelGuercio LRM, Savino JA, and Morgan JC: Physiologic assessment of surgical diagnostic related groups, Ann Surg 202:519, 1985.
8. Fitzgerald JF et al: Changing patterns of hip fracture care before and after implementation of the prospective payment system, JAMA 258:218, 1987.
9. Ginzberg E: Sounding board: a hard look at cost containment, N Engl J Med 316:1151, 1987.
10. Hauck WW et al: Surgeons in the United States: activities, output and income, JAMA 236:1864, 1976.
11. Horn SD, Horn RA and Sharkey PD: The severity of illness index as a severity adjustment to diagnosis related groups, Health Care Finan Rev, 1984 Ann Suppl, p. 33.
12. Jencks SF et al: Evaluating and improving the measurement of hospital case mix, Health Care Finan Rev, 1984 Ann Suppl, p. 1.
13. Jencks SF and Kay T: Do frail, disabled, poor and very old Medicare beneficiaries have higher hospital charges? JAMA 257:198, 1987.
14. Kassan M et al: Value of routine pathology in herniorraphy performed upon adults. Surg Gynecol Obstet 163:518, 1986.
15. Knaus WA et al: APACHE II: severity of disease classification system. Crit Care Med 13:818, 1985.
16. Moore FD: Contemporary American surgery: hard data at last, N Engl J Med 295:953, 1976.
17. Moore FD: Surgical streams in the flow of health care financing: the roles of surgery in national expenditures: what costs are controllable? Ann Surg 201:132, 1985.
18. Munoz E: Economic costs of trauma, United States, 1982, Trauma 24:237, 1984.
19. Munoz E et al: Surgonomics: the cost of cholecystectomy, Surgery 96:642-646, 1984.
20. Munoz E, Margolis IB, and Wise L: Surgonomics and cost containment, Surg Gynecol Obstet 162:137, 1986.
21. Munoz E et al: The financial effects of emergency department generated admissions under prospective payment system, JAMA 254:1763, 1985.
22. Munoz E et al: Surgonomics: the identifier concept: hospital charges in general surgery and surgical specialties under prospective payment systems. Ann Surg 202:119, 1985.
23. Munoz E et al: Lumpectomy versus mastectomy: the costs of breast preservation for cancer, Arch Surg 121:1297, 1986.
24. Munoz E et al: Source of admission and cost: public hospitals face financial risk, Am J Public Health 76:696, 1986.
25. Munoz E et al: Surgonomics: the cost dynamics of craniotomy, Neurosurgery 18:321, 1986.
26. Munoz E et al: The costs and dynamics of surgical morbidity and mortality, Surgery 100:905, 1986.
27. Munoz E et al: The identifier concept: clinical variables to manage costs for surgical patients, Hosp Health Serv Admin 32:85, 1987.
28. Munoz E et al: The transfer of surgical patients between hospitals, Arch Surg 123:68, 1988.

29. Prospective Payment Assessment Commission: report and recommendations to the Secretary, US Department of Health and Human Services, April, 1987.
30. Rhodes RS, Krasmiak CL, and Jones PK: Factors affecting length of stay for femoropopliteal bypass: implications of the DRGs, N Engl J Med 314:153, 1986.
31. Rutkow IM: Delivery of surgical health care in the United States, Arch Surg 116:963, 1981.
32. Schwartz WB: The inevitable failure of current cost containment strategies, JAMA 257:220, 1985.
33. Smits H and Watson R: DRGs and the future of surgical practice, N Engl J Med 311:1612, 1984.
34. Wagner DP and Draper EA: Acute physiology and chronic health evaluation (APACHE II) and Medicare reimbursement, Health Care Finan Rev, 1984 Ann Suppl, p. 91.
35. Waldo DR, Levit KF, and Lazenby H: National health expenditures, 1985, Health Care Finan Rev, 1986, 8, p. 1.
36. Wennberg JE, McPherson K, and Caper P: Will payment based on diagnostic related groups control hospital costs? N Engl J Med 311:295, 1984.
37. Young W: Incorporating severity of illness and comorbidity in case-mix measurement, Health Care Finan Rev, 1984 Ann Suppl, p. 23.

APPENDIX 6

Surgical DRGs by Specialties

DRG	Description	1988 Relative Weights
Cardiothoracic		
075	Major chest proc	3.0258
076	OR proc on resp system except major chest with CC	2.0885
077	OR proc on resp system except major chest w/o CC	1.0970
083	Major chest trauma age > 69 and/or CC	0.9698
084	Major chest trauma age < 70 w/o CC	0.5372
103	Heart transplant (not applicable for hospital)	11.9225
104	Cardiac valve proc with pump and with cardiac cath	7.3424
105	Cardiac valve proc with pump and w/o cardiac cath	5.7811
106	Coronary bypass with cardiac cath	5.5415
107	Coronary bypass w/o cardiac cath	4.2858
108	Cardiothoracic proc, exc valve and bypass with pump	5.3703
109	Cardiothoracic proc w/o pump	3.9142
115	Permanent cardiac pacemaker implant with AMI or CHF	4.0516
116	Permanent pacemaker implant w/o AMI or CHF	2.7694
117	Cardiac pacemaker replace and revise pulse gen; repl only	1.2261
118	Cardiac pacemaker pulse generator repl only	1.7563
General Surgery		
049	Major head and neck proc	2.8923
146	Rectal resection age > 69 and/or CC	3.4379
147	Rectal resection age < 70 w/o CC	2.1344
148	Major small and large bowel proc age > 69 and/or CC	3.2376
149	Major small and large bowel proc age < 70 w/o CC	1.8341
150	Peritoneal adhesiolysis age > 69 and/or CC	2.6797
151	Peritoneal adhesiolysis age < 70 w/o CC	1.4885
152	Minor small and large bowel proc age > 69 and/or CC	1.5988
153	Minor small and large bowel proc age < 70 w/o CC	1.0566
154	Stomach, esophageal, and duodenal proc age > 69 and/or CC	3.7961
155	Stomach, esophageal, and duodenal proc age 10-69 w/o CC	1.8195
156	Stomach, esophageal, and duodenal proc age <17	0.8382

Continued.

Surgical DRGs by Specialties—cont'd

DRG	Description	1988 Relative Weights
General Surgery		
157	Anal proc age > 69 and/or CC	0.9324
158	Anal proc age < 70 w/o CC	0.5449
159	Hernia proc except inguinal and femoral age > 69 and/or CC	1.1454
160	Hernia proc exc inguinal and femoral age 18-69 w/o CC	0.6810
161	Inguinal and femoral hernia proc age > 69 and/or CC	0.7541
162	Inguinal and femoral hernia proc age < 70 w/o CC	0.5004
163	Hernia proc age <17	0.7717
164	Appendectomy with complicated prin diag age > 69 and/or CC	2.4014
165	Appendectomy with complicated prin diag age < 70 w/o CC	1.4675
166	Appendectomy w/o complicated prin diag age > 69 and/or CC	1.4954
167	Appendectomy w/o complicated prin diag age < 70 w/o CC	0.8651
170	Other digestive system proc age > 69 and/or CC	2.7316
171	Other digestive system proc age < 70 w/o CC	1.4018
191	Major pancreas, liver, and shunt proc	4.6881
192	Minor pancreas, liver, and shunt proc	3.8625
193	Biliary tract proc exc tot cholecystectomy age > 69 and/or CC	3.0252
194	Biliary tract proc exc cholecystectomy age < 70 w/o CC	1.8505
195	Total cholecystectomy with CDE age > 69 and/or CC	2.3854
196	Total cholecystectomy with CDE age < 70 w/o CC	1.6898
197	Total cholecystectomy w/o CDE age > 69 and/or CC	1.8768
198	Total cholecystectomy w/o CDE age < 70 w/o CC	1.1152
199	Hepatobiliary diagnostic proc for malignancy	2.2693
200	Hepatobiliary diagnostic proc for nonmalignancy	2.4731
201	Other hepatobiliary or pancreas OR proc	2.3933
257	Total mastectomy for malignancy age > 69 and/or CC	1.0448
258	Total mastectomy for malignancy age < 70 w/o CC	0.8462
259	Subtotal mastectomy for malignancy age > 69 and/or CC	1.0046
260	Subtotal mastectomy for malignancy age < 70 w/o CC	0.6010
261	Breast proc for nonmalignancy Exc Biopsy and Loc Exc	0.6204
262	Breast biopsy and local excision for nonmalignancy	0.4312
267	Perianal and pilonidal proc	0.6248
269	Other skin, subcut tiss and breast OR proc age > 69 and/or CC	1.5177
270	Other skin, subcut tiss and breast OR proc age < 70 w/o CC	0.6834
276	Nonmalignant breast disorders	0.5245
277	Cellulitis age > 69 and/or CC	0.9695
278	Cellulitis age < 70 w/o CC	0.7063
280	Trauma to skin, subcut tiss, and breast age > 69 and/or CC	0.6197
281	Trauma to skin, subcut tiss, and breast age 18-69 w/o CC	0.4306
282	Trauma to skin, subcut tiss, and breast age < 17	0.3424

Surgical DRGs by Specialties

DRG	Description	1988 Relative Weights
General Surgery		
286	Adrenal and pituitary proc	2.7063
287	Skin grafts and wound debride for endoc, nutr, and metabolic disease	2.2274
288	OR proc for obesity	2.0018
289	Parathyroid proc	1.1470
290	Thyroid proc	0.8424
291	Thyroglossal proc	0.4991
292	Other endo, nutr and metabolic OR proc age > 69 and/or CC	2.6027
293	Other endo, nutr and metabolic OR proc age < 70 w/o CC	1.1698
392	Splenectomy age > 17	3.5252
393	Splenectomy age < 17	1.5206
394	Other OR proc of the blood and blood forming organs	1.2250
400	Lymphoma or leukemia with major OR proc	2.6900
401	Lymphoma or leukemia with minor OR proc age > 69 and/or CC	2.0871
402	Lymphoma or leukemia with minor OR proc age < 70 w/o CC	0.9252
406	Myeloprolif disord or poorly diff neoplasm with maj OR proc	2.7146
407	Myeloprolif disord or poorly diff neoplasm with maj OR proc W	1.4499
408	Myeloprolif disord or poorly diff neoplasm with min OR proc	0.8955
415	OR proc for infectious and parasitic diseases	3.5067
439	Skin grafts for injuries	1.7523
442	Other OR proc for injuries age > 69 and/or CC	1.9218
443	Other OR proc for injuries age < 70 w/o CC	1.2169
444	Multiple trauma age > 69 and/or CC	0.8207
445	Multiple trauma age 18-69 w/o CC	0.5183
446	Multiple trauma age < 17	0.4796
461	OR proc with diag of other contact with health service	0.7198
GYNECOLOGY		
353	Pelvic evisceration radical hysterectomy and vulvectomy	2.2997
354	Nonradical hysterectomy age > 69 and/or CC	1.5482
355	Nonradical hysterectomy age < 70 w/o CC	0.9929
356	Female reproductive system reconstructive proc	0.7983
357	Uterus and adnexa proc for malignancy	2.1591
358	Uterus and adnexa proc for nonmalignancy exc tubal interr	1.2941
359	Tubal interr for nonmalignancy	0.9025

Continued.

Surgical DRGs by Specialties—cont'd

DRG	Description	1988 Relative Weights
GYNECOLOGY		
360	Vagina, cervix and vulva proc	0.6957
361	Laparoscopy and endoscopy (female) except tubal interr	0.6442
362	Laparoscopic Tubal Interruption	0.4095
363	D&C, Conization, and Radioimplant for malignancy	0.6597
364	D&C, Conization except for malignancy	0.4262
365	Other female reproductive system OR proc	1.9060
380	Abortion w/o D&C	0.3124
381	Abortion with D&C	0.3694
NEUROSURGERY		
001	Craniotomy age > 17 except for trauma	3.4434
002	Craniotomy for trauma age > 17	3.8160
003	Craniotomy age < 18	2.9183
004	Spinal proc	2.5904
005	Extracranial vascular proc	1.5685
006	Carpal tunnel release	0.4393
007	Periph and cranial nerve and other nerv sys proc age > 69	2.5269
008	Periph and cranial nerve and other sys proc age < 70 w/o	0.7367
214	Back and neck proc > 69 and/or CC	2.1385
215	Back and neck proc < 70 w/o CC	1.3768
OPHTHALMOLOGY		
036	Retinal proc	0.6820
037	Orbital proc	0.7104
038	Primary iris proc	0.3779
039	Lens proc	0.5167
040	Extraocular proc except orbit age > 17	0.4675
041	Extraocular proc except orbit age < 17	0.3657
042	Intraocular proc except retina, iris, lens	0.6600
ORTHOPEDICS		
209	Major joint proc	2.4145
210	Hip and femur proc exc major joint age>69 and/or CC	2.1776
211	Hip and femur proc exc major joint age 18-69 w/o CC	1.6104

Surgical DRGs by Specialties

DRG	Description	1988 Relative Weights
ORTHOPEDICS		
212	Hip and femur proc exc major joint age 0-17	1.3764
213	Amputations for musculoskeletal sys and conn tissue disord	1.8460
214	Back and neck proc age>69 and/or CC	2.1385
215	Back and neck proc age<70 w/o CC	1.3768
216	Biopsies of musculoskeletal system and conn tissue	1.5973
218	Lower extr and humer proc exc hip, foot, femur age>17 with CC	1.6224
219	Lower extr and humer proc exc hip, foot, femur age 18-69 w/o CC	1.0186
220	Lower extr and humer proc exc hip, foot, femur age <17	0.9242
221	Knee proc age > 69 and/or CC	1.4523
222	Knee proc age < 70 w/o CC	0.7995
223	Upper extr proc exc humerus and hand age>69 and/or CC	1.1202
224	Upper extr proc exc humerus and hand age<70 w/o CC	0.6588
225	Foot proc	0.6775
230	Local excision and removal of int fix device of hip and femur	0.8868
231	Local excision and removal of int fix device exc hip	0.8346
232	Arthroscopy	0.8603
OTOLARYNGOLOGY—HEAD AND NECK SURGERY		
049	Major head and neck proc	2.8923
050	Sialoadenectomy	0.6681
051	Salivary gland proc except sialoadenectomy	0.5424
052	Cleft lip and palate repair	0.7033
053	Sinus and mastoid proc age > 17	0.6159
054	Sinus and mastoid proc age <17	0.6889
055	Misc ear, nose, and throat proc	0.4598
057	T and A Proc exc tonsillectomy and/or adenoidectomy age >17	0.7907
058	T and A Proc exc tonsillectomy and/or adenoidectomy age <17	0.3097
059	Tonsillectomy and/or adenoidectomy only age > 17	0.3845
060	Tonsillectomy and/or adenoidectomy only age <17	0.2616
061	Myringotomy age > 17	0.5401
062	Myringotomy age < 17	0.3089
063	Other ear, nose, and throat OR proc	1.1538

Continued.

Surgical DRGs by Specialties—cont'd

DRG	Description	1988 Relative Weights
PERIPHERAL VASCULAR SURGERY		
110	Major reconstructive vascular proc age > 69 and/or CC	3.6718
111	Major reconstructive vascular proc age < 70 w/o CC	2.2639
112	Vascular proc exc major reconstruction	1.8911
113	Amputation for circ system disorders exc upper limb	2.4590
114	Upper limb and toe amputation for circ sys disorders	1.7040
119	Vein ligation and stripping	0.8692
120	Other OR proc on the circulatory system	2.4776
128	Deep vein thrombophlebitis	0.8513
285	Amputations for endocrine, nutritional, and metabolic dis	2.9919
PLASTIC SURGERY		
049	Major head and neck proc	2.8923
051	Salivary gland proc except sialoadenectomy	0.5424
052	Cleft lip and palate repair	0.7033
056	Rhinoplasty	0.4471
216	Biopsies of musculoskeletal system and conn tissue	1.5973
217	Wnd debric and skin graft ex hand for musculoskeletal and conn tissue dis	2.8155
226	Soft tissue proc age > 69 and/or CC	1.3570
227	Soft tissue proc age < 70 w/o CC	0.6878
228	Ganglion (hand) proc	0.8201
229	Hand proc except ganglion	0.5202
233	Other musculoskeletal sys and conn tissue OR proc age>69 w/o CC	1.7267
234	Other musculoskeletal sys and conn tissue OR proc age<70 w/o	0.9057
261	Breast proc for nonmalig except biopsy and local exc	0.6204
263	Skin grafts for skin ulcer or cellulitis age>69 and/or CC	2.5967
264	Skin grafts for skin ulcer or cellulitis age<70 w/o CC	1.6179
265	Skin grafts exc for skin ulcer or cellulitis with CC	1.3909
266	Skin grafts exc skin ulcer or cellulitis w/o CC	0.6865
268	Skin, subcutaneous tissue, and breast plastic proc	0.5934
269	Other skin, subcut tissue, and breast OR proc age>69 w/o CC	1.5177
270	Other skin, subcut tissue, and breast OR proc age<70 w/o CC	0.6834
287	Skin grafts and wound debridement for endocrin nutr, metabolic	2.2274
291	Thyroglossal proc	0.4991
439	Skin grafts for injuries	1.7523
440	Wound debridements for injuries	2.2498
441	Hand proc for injuries	0.7185
458	Nonextensive burns with skin grafts	3.7113
459	Nonextensive burns with wound debridements and other proc	1.7964

Surgical DRGs by Specialties

DRG	Description	1988 Relative Weights
UROLOGIC SURGERY		
302	Kidney transplant	3.8463
303	Kidney, ureter, and major bladder proc for neoplas	2.7747
304	Kidney, ureter, and major bladder proc for nonmalig age > 69	2.3651
305	Kidney, ureter, and major bladder proc for non malig age < 70 w/o	1.3665
306	Prostatectomy age > 69 and/or CC	1.4376
307	Prostatectomy age < 70 w/o CC	0.9121
308	Minor bladder proc age > 69 and/or CC	1.5354
309	Minor bladder proc age < 70 w/o CC	0.8620
310	Transurethral proc age < 69 and/or CC	0.9026
311	Transurethral proc age < 70 w/o CC	0.5681
312	Urethral proc age > 69 and/or CC	0.8246
313	Urethral proc age 18-69 w/o CC	0.5286
314	Urethral proc age 0-17	0.4323
315	Other kidney and urinary tract OR proc	2.3635
334	Major male pelvic proc with CC	1.9237
335	Major male pelvic proc w/o CC	1.4080
336	Transurethral prostatectomy age > 69 and/or CC	1.0774
337	Transurethral prostatectomy age < 70 w/o CC	0.7505
338	Testes proc for malignancy	0.7865
339	Testes proc nonmalignancy age > 17	0.5930
340	Testes proc nonmalignancy age 0-17	0.4335
341	Penis proc	1.0294
342	Circumcision age > 17	0.4494
343	Circumcision age < 17	0.3788
344	Other male reproductive system OR proc for malignancy	1.1302
345	Other male reproductive system OR proc exc for malignancy	0.8284

SUSAN D. HORN

Susan D. Horn holds a PhD in statistics from Stanford University (1968). She is Professor, Department of Health Policy and Management, Johns Hopkins School of Hygiene and Public Health, and Associate Director, Center for Hospital Finance and Management, The Johns Hopkins Medical Institutions.

MICHAEL A. ASHWORTH

Michael A. Ashworth, an associate professor of surgery and of community health and epidemiology at Queen's University, Kingston, Canada, received his MDCM degree from McGill University (1961) and his MBA from Queen's University (1985). After basic surgical training in Montreal, he studied orthopedic surgery first in the Harvard residency program and then as a Fellow at Children's Hospital and the Peter Bent Brigham Hospital in Boston. He currently specializes in clinical pediatric orthopedic surgery and trauma.

7

Adjusting DRGs for Severity of Illness

SUSAN D. HORN
MICHAEL A. ASHWORTH

Historically, the science of patient classification has focused on the epidemiology of disease. The International Classification of Diseases (ICD) was developed because of public health officials' need to determine disease-specific mortality and morbidity. Although revised repeatedly to obtain greater specificity of disease, ICD was neither designed originally nor modified later to represent severity of illness.

As early as 1973, prospective reimbursement per case was proposed as an alternative to traditional fee-for-service payments as a means of controlling hospital costs.[19] In such a system, it is important that the patient groups that define the payment categories are homogeneous with respect to resource requirements, within the bounds of medical meaningfulness. The Diagnosis Related Groups (DRGs) system was the first widely recognized classification system to deal with this problem. Developed by researchers at Yale University, it attempted to create patient groups that were homogeneous with respect to length of stay, using a reduction in variance grouping algorithm. The DRG system was first tested in 1978 as a basis for prospective payment in the state of New Jersey. In that experiment and in other studies, patients within most DRGs were found to exhibit high variability of resource use, as measured by charge, cost, and length of stay.[12] Many researchers have suggested that much of this variability might be caused by differences in patient severity of illness.

The DRGs were subsequently revised in 1982, and Department of Health and Human Services' Secretary Schweiker stated in his Report to Congress in December 1982 that severity of illness, "defined as the risk of immediate death or permanent loss of function due to the patient's disease," was no longer a problem.[21] In particular, the report declared that the "DRGs account for the major differences in the cost of treatment among patients, due to severity of illness, in three ways": (1) if a patient is sicker and requires a certain type of operation, (2) if a patient is sicker because of complicating or comorbid conditions, or being older or younger, or (3) if a patient has certain diseases that indicate he/she is sicker, then DRGs take all these factors into account. However, many studies have shown that these three sets of labels are very limited in their ability to differentiate severity of illness.[15,20,22]

If a classification system is to function successfully as the basis for prospective payment, it must adequately differentiate resource requirements. Because different physicians tend to respond similarly to the same stimuli,[7] it is likely that resource use will follow severity of illness.

It is also desirable if a classification system can evaluate the quality of output. Quality assurance programs that look only at inputs of care, such as drug error rates, are of limited value. Success or failure in attaining short-term therapeutic goals should be an integral part of program analysis. A patient classification system that provides information on quality of care as well as homogeneous resource use groups can form a vital link between quality and productivity.

SEVERITY OF ILLNESS

One attempt to quantify severity of illness is the Disease Staging System.[8] "Staging defines the progressive levels of severity for disease in terms of the events and pathophysiological observations that characterize each stage. Within a given body system, higher degrees of involvement or greater degrees of disruption are identified as more severe."[6] The Disease Staging System was originally designed for manual data collection using the whole chart, but in its computerized form it uses only routine discharge abstract data. The Staging System was originally intended for education; its conception is similar to the staging of malignant disease. "It scans principal and secondary diagnosis codes and uses the relationships among codes to identify the underlying condition of highest severity."[6] However, many studies have found that whether used alone or as a refinement to DRGs, the Disease Staging System explains little more variation in resource use than do DRGs.[4,18] This lack of difference may be the result of either the limited severity information available from discharge abstract data and/or of insufficient consideration of the interactions of multiple diseases manifested by the patient.

The Patient Management Categories system (PMC) also uses standard discharge abstract data and attempts to account for levels of severity in the design and definitions of its approximately 840 categories.[23] However, the developers of PMCs state that "the objective . . . was not to capture severity distinctions among individual patients . . . rather, it was to identify and incorporate clinical and severity distinctions among patient types, where those distinctions reflect expected differences in patient management and, consequently, hospital resource requirements."[23] PMCs recognize comorbidity by categorizing patients into more than one PMC. However, the number of possible different patient groupings is very large. For example, considering at most one comorbidity, there could be 704,760 different PMC groups (840 × 839).

Numerous studies have found that the DRGs and other case mix systems based only on discharge abstract data, such as computerized Disease Staging and Patient Management Categories, provide a limited explanation (about 30%) of variation in resource use.[4,5] They deal in only a limited way with the severity issue and, as a consequence, may lead to inequitable prospective payment as well as to difficulties for physicians and hospital managers.*

Quantifying Severity of Illness

The quantification of severity of illness presents a complex and challenging problem. Because resource requirements, medical meaningfulness, and quality of output are all important, any proposed solution necessarily entails compromise. For example, ideally it would be desirable to employ only data that could not be affected by actions taken by patient care personnel, thus avoiding the influence of practice patterns and available technology. On the other hand, the exclusion of elements such as complications would ignore factors critical to the determination of the patient's total burden of illness. Most systems of patient classification, even when employed as a basis for prospective payment, accept this compromise to some degree to avoid the loss

---

*References 1,5,13,14,16.

of important information. For example, DRGs split initially on the basis of surgery/no surgery and include complications, such as urinary tract infections, that can be influenced by the care giver. However, current discharge abstract data appear insufficient to describe severity of illness, let alone the quality of output. Two approaches to quantifying severity of illness that use inputs beyond ordinary discharge abstract data are: MEDISGROUPS and the Computerized Severity Index (CSI), developed at Johns Hopkins University.

MEDISGROUPS. MEDISGROUPS uses about 260 "key clinical findings" to classify patients in the admission period into one of five severity groups.[3] This grouping is based largely on the highest key clinical finding present but also uses decision rules that incorporate combinations of findings. An additional severity measurement may be taken later in the hospitalization. The key clinical findings are determined by physical signs, the results of laboratory tests, radiologic and pathologic examinations, and the performance of certain diagnostic and life support procedures such as transfusion, bronchoscopy, and endotracheal intubation. The precise rules that specify what key clinical findings fall into what severity levels are proprietary, and they have been unavailable for study. A detailed review of the validity of the MEDISGROUPS system for possible use in adjusting DRGs for severity of illness has been performed by researchers at Boston University.[18] These researchers show that MEDISGROUPS-adjusted DRGs (RIV^{16} = 25.6%) explain only about 3% more of the variation in resource use than DRG's alone (RIV = 22.6%). Also, they question the medical validity of some of the classification decisions and the extensive use of procedures to define severity levels.

Computerized Severity Index. The manual Severity of Illness Index, the predecessor to the CSI, attempted to capture the patient's total burden or severity of illness by quantifying seven individual dimensions.[11]

- The stage of the principal diagnosis at admission
- Complications that develop during the hospital stay
- Preexisting comorbidities
- The degree to which the patient requires more than the minimal level of direct care expected for the principal diagnosis
- Diagnostic and therapeutic procedures performed outside of the operating room
- The patient's response to treatment
- The extent to which a patient shows residual evidence of the acute injury or illness at the time of discharge

The seven dimensions were not designed to be independent of each other but rather to reflect the burden of illness from different points of view; taken together, they were intended to describe accurately the patient's overall severity of illness.

Although it predicted resource use much better than DRGs,[14,16] (in one study, DRGs alone predicted 28% of the variation in cost per case, while severity-adjusted DRGs predicted 61% of this variation) the manual Severity of Illness Index has been subject to several criticisms. Specific concerns included subjectivity of judgments, possible circularity of some dimensions, and potential difficulty in administration on a national scale. The CSI deals with these issues and was developed to facilitate widespread collection of severity of illness data. A detailed discussion of the conceptualization of the CSI system, its comparison with other case mix systems, and its applications is presented elsewhere.[9]

Like the manual Severity of Illness Index, the CSI is based on how ill the individual patient is within each disease condition, not just that the patient has the disease condition. Our physician research team believed that to assess severity of illness accurately, one must know the extent of each disease and the interaction of the diseases present. With this information, we can relate a patient's resource needs, as described by the CSI levels, to the resources used and thereby create a measure of efficiency of care. We can also examine changes in CSI levels during the hospital stay to evaluate and measure the quality of patient care (effectiveness). And, finally, such a system can help to standardize and improve the collection of clinical information.

The CSI system was developed as an extension to the ICD-9-CM coding system.[17] Explicit severity criteria exist for each ICD-9-CM code. Severity criteria result in a severity rating of 0 to 4 for each diagnosis. If no data can be found in a patient's chart to substantiate any severity criteria associated with a diagnosis, that diagnosis receives a severity rating of zero, and it is natural to inquire whether the diagnosis is correct or if the medical record is properly documented. In addition, the CSI system produces an overall patient severity level on a scale of 1 to 5, with 5 reserved to indicate death.

The severity criteria used in the CSI system are based on patient characteristics and not treatment characteristics, so performance of treatments does not affect the severity level of the patient. The CSI criteria are objective clinical findings such as maximum temperature, maximum blood pressure, laboratory values and radiologic and physical findings. They are the same data items needed to establish the existence of a diagnosis, so they are easy to collect while performing abstract coding, quality assurance review, risk management, or utilization review of the record.

An example of a set of CSI criteria for the disease cholelithiasis is presented in Table 7-1. The signs and symptoms for cholelithiasis involve the cardiovascular and digestive systems and include fever, weight loss, pain, and abnormal laboratory findings. These are all included in the cholelithiasis criteria set, and the extent of abnormality of each is listed in columns under levels 1 through 4. Level 1 indicates normal to mild symptoms, level 2 indicates moderate symptoms, level 3 indicates serious symptoms, and level 4 indicates catastrophic or life-threatening symptoms. All criteria in a column are considered of equal severity. Thus, not all criteria appear in all four columns.

To determine the severity of a diagnosis, the two most severe criteria are used. If both criteria fall into level 4, then the CSI level for the disease is 4. If the two most severe criteria are in level 3, or one criterion is in 3 and one is in 4, then the CSI level for the disease is a 3, and so on. We require documentation of two criteria at (or above) a given severity level to rate a disease at that level so that a single extreme value of a patient characteristic cannot by itself determine the severity of a disease. Our research has shown that one extreme value is not a good indication of severity.

The severity criteria for all diseases are publicly available in a CSI code book entitled "Computerized Severity Index: ICD-9-CM Severity Modification, Adult Criteria," published by Health Systems International, New Haven, Conn. The CSI code book is organized as a fourth volume companion to the three-volume ICD-9-CM code book; it is arranged in the same order as the current ICD-9-CM code book so that severity criteria can be found easily. Public evaluation and comments on our CSI criteria are encouraged in order to refine the criteria over time.

To compute the overall CSI level for a patient, several steps are followed: First, the CSI software eliminates secondary diagnoses directly associated either with the principal diagnosis or with other secondary diagnoses, so that multiple coding of a single disease process (which may be appropriate under the rules for discharge abstract coding) will not influence the overall CSI level. Second, the CSI level of each disease is calculated using each patient characteristic only once. This prevents a single patient characteristic from having a disproportionate impact on the overall CSI level. Finally, the overall CSI level is produced using the severity of each diagnosis and disease-specific weighting rules that reflect the interaction of the diagnoses.

Because one of the development goals of the CSI system was to exploit the ability of a disease-

Table 7-1. Cholelithiasis; other disorders of gall bladder; of biliary tract

Category	Level 1	Level 2	Level 3	Level 4
Cardiovascular		Pulse rate 100-129	Pulse rate 130 or more	Life-threatening arrhythmias and/or hypotension
Digestive	Nausea 5 or fewer stools/day	Vomiting 6-10 stools/day Diffuse abdominal distention	Persistent vomiting 11-20 stools/day Absent bowel sounds	21 or more stools/day
Fever	Temperature 100.4F or less and/or chills	Temperature 100.5-102F	Temperature 102.1-103.9F and/or rigors	Temperature 104F or higher
General	Weight loss of 1%-5.9% of body weight	Weight loss of 6%-15.9% of body weight	Weight loss of 16% to 20.9% of body weight	Weight loss of 21% or more of body weight
Laboratory values				
Chemistry	Amylase $\leq 1.5 \times$ norm Bilirubin ≤ 2.0 mg/dl	Amylase $1.6-4.0 \times$ norm Bilirubin 2.1-5.0mg/dl	Amylase $4.1-5.9 \times$ norm Bilirubin 5.1-11.0mg/dl	Amylase $\geq 6.0 \times$ norm Bilirubin ≥ 11.1 mg/dl
Hematology	Hct (M) 41.4-30.0% (F) 35.0-30.0% Hb (M) 13.7-10.0 gm/dl (F) 11.9-10.0gm/dl WBC × 1000 4.5-11.0/cu mm Bands <10%	Hct 29.9-20.1% Hb 9.9-6.6gm/dl WBC × 1000 11.1-20.0/cu mm Bands 10-20%	Hct 20.0-15.1% Hb 6.5-5.1gm/dl WBC × 1000 20.1-30.0/cu mm Bands 21-40%	Hct ≤ 15.0% Hb ≤ 5.0gm/dl WBC × 1000 ≥ 30.1/cu mm Bands >40%
Pain			Abdominal guarding and/or + rebound; colicky pain	Abdominal rigidity

specific system to minimize required data entry, we were interested to see how many CSI questions would actually be presented to the CSI data collectors in practice. Using a representative data base of 150,000 patient records, we found that the median number of CSI questions presented per case was 28. The 25th percentile was 17 questions, and the 95th percentile was 68 questions.

Severity of illness, either for an individual diagnosis or for the patient as a whole, can be measured by using the CSI at any time from admission through discharge. Although the maximal severity level throughout the hospitalization may be the best determinant of resource requirements, admission versus discharge severity level comparisons (as well as the monitoring of diagnoses acquired while in the hospital) are useful for quality assurance purposes. With the CSI, the patient's progress through each disease, as well as the overall severity level, is open to serial evaluation.

Severity can be assessed with the present CSI software system up to five times for a patient's stay. If more times are needed, another record can be created for the patient. The most common ways to collect severity data now are: based on admission characteristics, based on discharge characteristics, and based on maximum characteristics throughout the hospital stay. Concurrent CSI determinations are also possible. The various disease-specific CSI levels representing severity at various times during the hospital stay can be added as additional digits at the end of the patient's five-digit ICD-9-CM codes, and the corresponding overall CSI levels can be stored in optional fields in the patient's record, as depicted in Table 7-2. In this case the patient came in for an elective gallbladder surgery. He had normal to mild signs and symptoms on admission. Although the severity of his cholelithiasis did not change, he developed signs and symptoms of ischemic heart disease and hypertension requiring the patient to stay in the hospital a total of 10 days. His overall maximum CSI level was 2, and

Table 7-2. Severity assessments during patient stay

	A	M	D
PDX (cholelithiasis) 574.0	1	1	1
IHD (ischemic heart disease) 411.1	1	2	1
HTN (hypertension) 401.0	1	2	1
OVERALL	1	2	1

A, admission; *M*, maximum throughout stay; *D*, last 48 hours; *PDX*, principal diagnosis.

everything resolved by discharge. This severity detail by diagnosis can be stored in an expanded discharge abstract data set that can be very useful in assessing efficiency and effectiveness of hospital care.

CSI information has many uses. Potential quality of care problems may be indicated by cases that go from a low admission CSI level to a higher maximum CSI level. These cases can be reviewed by physicians to determine if the CSI level increased from natural or iatrogenic causes. The CSI system can be used to develop institutional norms for patterns of change from admission to maximum CSI level for all patients, by department, by major diagnostic category (MDC), by DRG, or by diagnosis, and to identify deviations from the standard pattern that may indicate either extraordinarily good practice or possible quality of care problems. These uses are described in more detail elsewhere.[2]

The CSI system is an aid in utilization review because one can study resource use controlling for CSI level. There are well-known problems in using a heterogeneous classification system such as DRGs to indicate over utilization or underutilization: a physician who appears to be high-cost in a DRG-based analysis often responds, "my patients are sicker," within each DRG. Using CSI-adjusted DRGs for analysis eliminates this problem. Accurate and useful physician practice profiles produced with CSI-adjusted DRGs are described in detail elsewhere.[10]

The CSI system can also create a patient discharge summary based on the demographic information and detailed clinical information on each of a patient's diagnoses at multiple time points that is stored by the CSI system. Hence, the CSI software helps to minimize physician paperwork. In addition, a study is underway to determine if the discharge CSI level, possibly along with the maximum CSI level, can be used for accurate prediction of resource needs after hospitalization such as nursing home care or home health care.

The CSI can be used to create a whole new system of severity-adjusted DRGs. Age, complications, and comorbidities now form the final splits that carve out DRGs from MDCs, but they can be replaced by severity splits. For some DRGs, severity may not be an important predictor of variability in hospital resource use, for example, in the elective surgical procedure of carpal tunnel release. For most DRGs, however, severity will be an important predictor of variability in hospital resource use. It may not be necessary to divide every DRG into five severity levels; within a DRG, it may be possible to collapse two or more severity levels, based on medical meaningfulness and empirical data on resource use by severity level. When enough CSI data are available from hospitals, we will study the best way to use CSI to divide DRGs into homogeneous resource use groups. Also, since CSI is based on ICD-9-CM codes and can be added to DRGs easily, it can be used to adjust prospective payment levels based on the severity of the patient. PPO and HMO arrangements can be made using CSI-adjusted DRGs.

Because CSI information is disease specific and publicly available, physicians and nurses writing in the medical record can know in advance what information must be included so that the severity of the patient can be assessed accurately. Improved accuracy of the medical record and improved accuracy of discharge abstract coding should then be observed. Any diagnosis for which insufficient criteria are recorded in the medical record is scored as CSI level zero, and the system asks if the diagnosis is correct. Medical records personnel can then take such queries back to the physician with a request for more information. In the future, when there is a completely computerized medical record, answers to disease-specific CSI questions, such as these relating to laboratory data, radiology data, vital signs data, and physical findings data, can all be obtained directly from the hospital's central computerized data bank by the CSI software, which can then compute the severity of each of the diagnoses and the overall CSI without any additional data input.

In summary, the CSI is based solely on clinical characteristics that are available in the chart. Weighting rules are used to take into account the interactions of diseases that are found in hospitalized patients. The complete CSI criteria sets are published as a companion volume to the current three-volume ICD-9-CM coding system, and hence are available for study, evaluation, and refinement. A software package has been developed to facilitate collection of the CSI criteria and determination of an overall severity level according to specific weighting rules.

Surgical examples. The CSI is based on the severity of each recorded diagnosis, a concept that corresponds to the first three dimensions in the manual Severity of Illness system (Stage of principal diagnosis, Complications, and Interactions). Hence, the CSI is based on the same principles of disease interaction as its manual predecessor. Considerable data are available from use of the manual system that demonstrate the power of the system to define highly homogeneous groups, specifically within DRGs.[16] In Table 7-3 are combined data from 15 hospitals from DRG 110 (major reconstructive vascular procedures, age $\geq$ 70 and/or complication/comorbidity). The costs of these patients range from $926 to $107,362. Adjusting for Severity of Illness demonstrates improved homogeneity, quantified by both a 41.2% reduction in variance and a decrease in coefficient of variation from 100.1% to 46.0%

Another example is given by data from DRG 148 in Table 7-4 (major small and large bowel procedures, age ≥ 70 and/or complication/comorbidity). The costs of these patients range from $1183 to $153,708. Adjusting for Severity of Illness again demonstrates improved homogeneity, quantified by both a 30.6% reduction in variance and a decrease in coefficient of variation from 146.8% to 62.5%. The data on DRG 148 in Table 7-5 are drawn from one hospital. The improvement in homogeneity from Table 7-4 (RIV = 55.4% and coefficient of variation of 40%) may be because of elimination of the effects of interhospital accounting differences. Note that the average cost increases monotonically as the severity level increases in all these examples.

SUMMARY AND CONCLUSIONS

The economic environment in which the surgeon works has undergone considerable change since prospective payment was introduced in October 1983. No longer is the surgeon the object of indiscriminate hospital marketing in an environment of cost-plus pricing where more treatment implies greater profits. Beyond the expectations of the patient and the constant threat of litigation, the surgeon is now under scrutiny from both third party payers and hospital managers. He/she is now expected to function as the physician/manager. Efficient, quality treatment is the watchword.

Table 7-3. DRG 110: major reconstructive vascular procedures, age ≥ 70 and/or CC: cost data from 15 hospitals

Severity Level*	N	Average Cost	CV
	274	$10,659	100.1
1	46	$5118	39.1
2	170	$8131	41.3
3	38	$17,968	56.7
4	20	$31,004	82.2
	RIV = 41.2%		WTCV = 46.0

CV, coefficient of variation; RIV, reduction in variance; WTCV, weighted coefficient of variation.
*Manual Severity of Illness level.

Table 7-4. DRG 148: major small and large bowel procedures, age ≥ 70 and/or CC: cost data from 15 hospitals

Severity Level*	N	Average Cost	CV
	322	$12,094	146.8
1	49	$4042	41.6
2	180	7276	51.0
3	51	18,098	88.5
4	42	34,843	105.0
	RIV = 30.6%		WTCV = 62.5

CV, coefficient of variation; RIV, reduction in variance; WTCV, weighted coefficient of variation.
*Manual Severity of Illness level.

Table 7-5. DRG 148: major small and large bowel procedures, age ≥ 70 and/or CC: cost data from a single hospital

Severity Level*	N	Average cost	CV
	103	$8023	70.3
1	17	$4741	23.8
2	65	6959	38.6
3	17	10,986	37.3
4	4	26,690	57.2
	RIV = 55.4%		WTCV = 40.0

CV, coefficient of variation; RIV, reduction in variance; WTCV, weighted coefficient of variation.
*Manual Severity of Illness level

But how can one tell if one surgeon is more efficient than another? Because of factors such as geographic situation, experience, and the technology available to them, some practitioners consistently manage a more severely ill population of patients than do others. If efficiency or quality of care are to be evaluated and compared, severity differences among different surgeons' caseloads must be adequately recognized. Since each practitioner will treat his/her own particular mix of severity, it is only appropriate to compare individual efficiency and effectiveness with others with a similar patient mix.

Current economic and regulatory conditions have raised questions about the validity of past approaches to patient classification. Not only must disease mortality and morbidity be described; efficiency and effectiveness of care must also be scrutable. Traditional discharge abstract data are insufficient for this purpose. Not only does disease severity need to be quantified, but it also must be compared over time. This requires entering the body of the chart itself to use clinical findings that are not now part of the discharge abstract. The CSI provides the opportunity to perform sequential severity comparisons of both individual diseases and overall severity of illness using an expanded discharge abstract data base.

References

1. Ament RP et al: Three case type classifications: suitability for use in reimbursing hospitals, Med Care 20: 460, 1982.
2. Backofen J, Ashworth A, and Horn SD: The computerized severity index: a new sophisticated tool to measure hospital quality of care, Healthcare Forum, March/April: 35, 1987.
3. Brewster AC, Bradbury RC, and Jacobs CM: Measuring the effect of illness severity on revenue under DRGs, Healthcare Finan Manage, July, 52, 1985.
4. Calore KA and Iezzoni L: Disease staging and PMCs: can they improve DRGs? Med Care 25: 724, 1987.
5. Coffey R and Goldfarb M: DRGs and disease staging for reimbursing Medicare patients, Hospital Studies Program Working Paper No. 1, Rockville, Md, Oct 1984, National Center for Health Services Research.
6. Conklin JE et al: Disease staging: implications for hospital reimbursement and management, Health Care Finan Rev Ann Suppl Nov. 1984, p. 13.
7. Cullen DJ et al: Therapeutic intervention scoring system: a method for quantitative comparison of patient care, Critical Care Med 2: 57, 1974.
8. Gonnella JS, Hornbrook MC and Louis DZ: Staging of disease: a case-mix measurement, JAMA 251: 637, 1984.
9. Horn SD: Measuring severity: how sick is sick? how well is well? Healthcare Finan Manage, Oct: 21, 1986.
10. Horn SD: Physician profiling: how it can be misleading and what to do, Consultant, 27: 86, 1987.
11. Horn SD and Horn RA: Reliability and validity of the Severity of Illness Index. Med Care 24: 159, 1986.
12. Horn SD and Sharkey PD: Measuring severity of illness to predict patient resource use within DRGs, Inquiry 20: 314, 1983.
13. Horn SD et al: Inter-hospital differences in patient severity: problems for prospective payment based on diagnosis-related groups. N Engl J Med 313:20, 1985.
14. Horn SD et al: Severity of Illness within DRGs: impact on prospective payment, Am J Public Health 75: 1195, 1985.
15. Horn SD et al: Misclassification problems in diagnosis-related groups: N Engl J Med 314: 484, 1986.
16. Horn SD et al: Severity of Illness within DRGs: homogeneity study, Med Care 24: 225, 1986.
17. ICD-9-CM International Classification of Diseases 9th Revision Clinical Modification, Ann Arbor, Mich., 1978, Commission on Professional and Hospital Activities.
18. Iezzoni LI, Ash AS, and Moskowitz MA: MEDIS-GROUPS: a clinical and analytic assessment, Health Policy Research Consortium, Brandeis Univ., Waltham, Mass., July 1987.
19. Lave JR, Lave LB, and Silverman LP: A proposal for incentive reimbursement for hospitals, Med Care 11: 79, 1973.
20. Mullin RS: Diagnosis-related groups and severity: ICD-9-CM, the real problem, JAMA 254: 1208, 1985.
21. Schweiker R, Secretary DHHS: Report to Congress—Hospital prospective payment for Medicare, Dec. 1982.
22. Smits HL and Watson RE: DRGs and the future of surgical practice, N Engl J Med 312: 1612, 1984.
23. Young WW: Incorporating severity of illness and comorbidity in case mix measurement, Health Care Finan Rev. Ann Suppl 1984, p. 23.

OLIVER H. BEAHRS

Oliver H. Beahrs, an Alabama native, received his MD degree from Northwestern University in 1941. After 4 years in the US Navy, he trained in surgery at the Mayo Graduate School and then joined the Mayo Clinic staff in 1950. During a 29-year career there, his main areas of surgical interest included surgery of the head and neck and the gastrointestinal tract. He retired in 1979 and holds the position of emeritus professor of surgery, Mayo Medical School. He is immediate past chairman of the Board of Regents and now president-elect of the American College of Surgeons and an immediate past member of the Physician Payment Review Committee.

8

Reimbursement in the Future: the Physician Payment Review Commission

OLIVER H. BEAHRS

Medicare was adopted in 1965. Part A was established to cover hospital care of those people who were eligible for Medicare benefits, and part B was developed to provide for physician reimbursement. Physician reimbursement would be according to the customary, prevailing, and reasonable fee methodology, commonly known as the CPR approach. As long as the charge did not exceed, to a certain limit, physicians' fees in the previous year, it did not appear that there would be a financial problem. At first, payment for Medicare services was not a fiduciary concern because, in general, the amounts were relatively low. However, by the late 1970s and the early 1980s, serious questions regarding funding were becoming evident.

FLAWS IN CPR METHODOLOGY

Numerous criticisms of the CPR methodology have been voiced. Most prominent are those that relate to its apparent cost ineffectiveness because it: (1) increases charges and volume of the services, (2) contains inappropriate incentives for use of medical services, and (3) is administratively complex.

Increased Changes and Volume of Services

As the number of Medicare enrollees enlarged and as extremely expensive technology was introduced into American health care, inflation became rampant within the system. Consequently, costs of both parts A and B significantly increased. The methodology for payment for part A was altered in 1984 when reimbursement to hospitals was based on diagnostic related groups (DRGs). This change was thought to help control the costs of part A. Partially this would occur by moving some inpatient services to outpatient facilities and also by encouraging the discharge of patients at an earlier stage in their hospitalizations.

Although changes in the reimbursement for part A were being addressed and controlled to some extent, significant increases continued to occur in the costs of part B services. During the same period, the overall federal deficit increased significantly, putting pressure on attempts to control costs of all federal services. In 1982 the funding of part B Medicare services was $15 billion. By 1987 these costs had doubled to $30 billion. From 1975 to 1985, part B costs increased 16% per year. Two percent of the increase was because of increasing numbers of enrollees, 7% because of higher prices of health care services, and 7% because of an increase in the number of services provided to the beneficiaries.

From the beginning of Medicare, an attempt has been made to protect the beneficiary from significant costs of the program. In 1966 the monthly premium to the beneficiary was $3 per month. By 1975 it had increased to $6.70 and by 1985 to $15.50. Suddenly in 1988 the cost to the beneficiary was increased to $24.80 or 38% more than it had been the year before. Since the cost had not increased during the previous 2-year period, it has to be recognized that, in part, the 38% increase was a catch-up for the prior 2 years. Other reasons given for the need for the 38% increase include (1) new or improved capabilities of the health care delivery system, (2) meeting needs not previously provided to the Medicare population, (3) improved access to care for the beneficiaries of the program, (4) provision of services of little or no value to the patients and (5) physycan incentive (financial) to provide more services.

Inappropriate Incentives

Likewise, it was recognized that some physicians were abusing the system in order to maximize their financial return. Historically, many services (primarily surgical) for which a charge was applied were for a bundle of tasks related to the primary health care program. These bundled services for which a global fee had previously applied are now, in some instances, being unbundled. Consequently, charges are applied for each individual portion of the service. As an example, if a cholecystectomy is performed, separate charges are applied for the preoperative care, for the abdominal exploration carried out at the time of the operation, for freeing up the adhesions if they were present, for doing a related procedure that might be indicated such as an appendectomy, and then for the cholecystectomy itself. This, in part, is caused by the extensive coding system that is used to encourage recording of all aspects of the services provided. This is essential for record-keeping purposes but does not always seem appropriate for charge purposes. Unfortunately, in some instances the carriers encouraged this. There are even traveling seminars advertised to educate physicians and their personnel on how to maximize reimbursement by unbundling services. The magnitude of this abuse has been variously estimated to be as much as 50%, but more realistically is probably between 10% and 20% of claims.

Another abuse of the coding system is to upgrade services from a lesser one that carries a lower fee to a more complicated service that has a higher fee. The movement of some health care services from an inpatient environment to the outpatient mode has shifted costs of these services from part A to part B. Some of these shifts in costs were justified but not always so because on an outpatient basis, the service(s) could be provided at a lesser cost, but the charge applied to the service(s) did not always reflect this.

ESTABLISHING THE PHYSICIAN PAYMENT REVIEW COMMISSION

Other factors that made it very difficult to evaluate part A reimbursement were the variance in carrier performance and the lack of uniform instructions from the Health Care Financing Administration (HCFA) to the carriers. Because of the financial difficulties Congress was having with the budget and the increasing costs of the Medicare program, in 1985 it authorized a commission to consider physician payment issues. This task was accomplished under the auspices of the Office of Technology Assessment, which was to appoint a Physician Payment Review Commission (PPRC) to consider methods of controlling and reducing part B costs of Medicare.

The Commission was appointed early in 1986 but was not activated until November 1986 because of lack of funding. The authorizing legislation requested that the first report from the Commission be sent to Congress in March 1987 and then annually in March. The instructions to the Commission were to consider the methodology of physician reimbursement based on specialty, geographic location, service rendered, and other factors.

Roles of the PPRC

The roles of the PPRC are several: (1) to serve as an independent source of expert advice to Congress and the Secretary of the Department of Health and Human Services, (2) to provide an opportunity for beneficiaries of the Medicare program, physicians, and other parties to present views to be considered in policy deliberations on payment issues, (3) to conduct objective analyses of data as a basis for policy decisions regarding payment for health care services, and (4) to perform design work necessary to implement major changes in the method of physician payment.

Goals of the PPRC

The goals of the PPRC are numerous: (1) there should be financial protection of the beneficiary; (2) any system of physician reimbursement should not interfere with what should improve access to care; (3) quality of care should be maintained; (4) there should be equity among physicians (similar pay for similar services); (5) there should be a reduction in the growth of supplemental medical insurance (SMI)—the taxpayer paying approximately 75% of the costs, the beneficiary no more than 25%; (6) the method of physician reimbursement should be understandable; (7) there should be orderly change; and (8) there should be pluralism in the methods of reimbursement. In other words, there should be a place for fee-for-service as well as capitation, reimbursement, and perhaps other methods. Naturally, to reach these goals, trade-offs will be inevitable. In reaching the goals, the PPRC should address the current inequities in payment to physicians. However, it must be remembered that medicine is an art and science, and the program should incorporate society's concerns regarding limited resources but also maintain physicians' freedom to use clinical judgment.

Initial Suggestions

The PPRC made its first report to Congress on May 1, 1987. The report contained several suggestions and identified various areas that required further study and consideration before any final recommendations could be made. After consideration of several forms of physician reimbursement, the Commission made the following recommendation:

> The Commission endorses the concept of the fee schedule for paying for physician services to Medicare beneficiaries. The relative payments for services, location settings, and perhaps specialties would differ from the patterns of allowed charges under the current system. A recommendation that Medicare adopt a fee schedule or specific characteristics of a specific development process will require decisions on issues of design and development.

This recommendation continues the methodology of physician reimbursement through a fee schedule. A fee schedule based on other than charge factors, as is true of the CPR methodology, would then be simpler to administer and many of the disadvantages of the present system could be eliminated. Any fee schedule that might be recommended and subsequently put into effect likely would be based on a relative value scale (RVS). The RVS has been developed either on the basis of resource costs or of other factors in the provision of services. A fee schedule would then be established by developing and utilizing a multiplier against the RVS, which in turn would establish the actual fees to be paid for the services. The multiplier would take into account numerous factors such as geographic location, urban or rural locations, and specialty costs including professional liability and overhead expenses of providing the services.

As noted in the Commission's report, the single largest component of costs of production for physician services is the value of the physician's own input. Determination of value or cost of the physician's time and effort is difficult. For surgical procedures, time can be identified from the operating room records, but for other types of medical services, this is not true. Efforts to estimate the relative values of physician services have been based on surveys of physicians or on less formal judgment of physician panels. This has been investigated by Egdahl and Manuel, Hadley and Berrenson, and Hsiao and Staison (see suggested readings).

A national fee schedule would certainly simplify the administration of the Medicare reimbursement program over and above what it is today utilizing the CPR methodology. Undoubtedly, any fee schedule that might be utilized would have to undergo a political process of negotiation so that in the end, the actual fee schedule would be acceptable to both the physician community as well as to the payer or the government. Likewise, the beneficiaries or the Medicare patients would have to be participants with their views represented in the overall negotiating process. Even though the Commission currently recommends a fee-for-service method for physician reimbursement, this does not totally exclude other reimbursement methodologies that might subsequently evolve or that might take place concurrently. For instance, a comprehensive prepayment to medical entities for the provision of health care services (capitation) to groups of Medicare beneficiaries is another payment scheme under study.

Any program must have a mechanism for continuous updating, such as a fee schedule, because of the inflationary factors that might be present, changes in the costs of providing the services, or changes in technology that occur over time. A strong argument for a system of reimbursement that is satisfactory to the medical community is to make health care services accessible and available to the beneficiaries. If such a method of payment is not acceptable, there is the possibility of withdrawal of services or lack of participation by physicians in the program. Therefore, the Committees' actions will all have both direct and indirect effects on the quality of health care available to the Medicare patient.

For a variety of reasons, physician reimbursement has varied considerably based on geographic location. Some of the variance is legitimately based on differences in costs of living or provision of health care services. However, much of the variation is not fully understood or explained. In considering this issue, the Commission made the following recommendation:

> As an initial step to deal with geographic variation, the Commission recommends that Medicare pay an increment beyond approved charges for primary care services delivered in designated underserved areas. These additional increment payments would not affect coinsurance amounts and could be financed by a slight reduction in the MEI update factor.

In other words, the Commission recognized that reimbursement in certain geographic areas is low and in some instances barely covers the cost of providing services. By recommending that physicians practicing in these areas receive an incremental amount over and above the usual fee would make positive adjustments to their incomes. This, for the present, would make a somewhat favorable adjustment in the variance of reimbursement for services where payment is low versus those where it is high.

The variance has been estimated by multiple reports as being from 25% to 35%. Naturally, any fee-for-service schedule that might later be proposed and put into use by the Medicare program would take into account legitimate reasons for geographic variations, but it is hoped that it would eliminate factors that have no or little basis. This would be recognized primarily through a difference in the multipliers against the RVS, since it is assumed that the relative value for the services would be the same whether supplied in an urban or rural or underserved area.

The Consolidated Omnibus Budget Reconciliation Act (COBRA) of 1985 required the Secretary of the Department of Health and Human Services to promulgate regulations specifying criteria to determine inherent reasonableness regarding Medicare reimbursement. This legislation further requested that a process be established to identify services with allowed charges that are out of line with others. It would increase or decrease those allowed charges and place limits on services in which charges were decreased.

In the COBRA of 1986, Congress specified an approach to inherent reasonableness specified on actual charges when allowable charges are limited through inherent reasonableness. In particular, limits on actual charges for cataract surgery and associated anesthesia services were established. This issue led the Commission to make the following recommendation:

> The Commission endorses goals of inherent reasonableness to redress distortion in allowed charges that have arisen through the application of CPR reimbursement principles and to achieve short-term budget savings in ways that are more consistent with long-term policy directions than are across-the-board reductions in payments.
>
> However, for these goals to be reached, inherent reasonableness must be applied carefully through an open process that takes account of input from all interested parties.
>
> The Commission will test a consensus process as an alternative means of developing recommendations for changes in payments based on inherent reasonableness. If this process is successful, the results would provide the basis for recommendations to the Congress and to the Secretary of HHS on inherent reasonableness.

Without question, there are certain medical and surgical services for which charges are unreasonable. For this reason, excessive fees that fall into this category need to be addressed and reduced to some extent to bring the charges more in line with the costs of providing the services. This would make the charges more comparable with other services falling into similar categories.

It was this whole issue that led the Commission to make recommendations to Congress regarding certain services that appropriately should be considered as being unreasonable and that changes be made in their reimbursement for the 1988 federal and Medicare budgets. The services were identified by comparing several relative value scales that identified particular procedures as having unreasonable charges.

Among the operations are coronary artery bypass, total hip replacement, transurethral resection prostate, dilation and curettage, carpal tunnel release, and three ophthalmologic procedures. Subsequently, in the establishment of a fee schedule for physician reimbursement, it is presumed that all fees for services will be brought into line based on an acceptable relative value scale. Consequently, in the future there should be little or no reason to use the inherent reasonableness rule.

Since the inception of Medicare, HCFA has attempted several methods of encouraging physicians to participate in the Medicare program, to make expenditures more predictable, and to protect the costs to which the beneficiary might be exposed. Toward this end, the assignment and participating physician program has been developed:

> Since the inception of Medicare, physicians have been permitted to decide on a claim-by-claim basis whether to bill Medicare's carrier and accept the allowed charge as payment in full (the patient is to be billed only for the deductible and coinsurance), or to bill the patient for the full amount, with the patient also responsible for the difference between the billed charge and what Medicare allows. This difference is often referred to as a balance bill. Historically, physicians have accepted assignment for somewhat more than half

of all claims, though the percentage has increased sharply in recent years, to 68% in 1986.

This policy has left beneficiaries exposed to substantial financial risks. In 1985 Medicare-allowed charges were lower than billed charges on 85% of unassigned claims, with the difference for claims that were reduced averaging 26%. Unlike the deductible and coinsurance amounts, for which about two thirds of beneficiaries have purchased private supplemental insurance to limit risks associated with costly illness, balance-billed amounts are not covered by private insurance for most beneficiaries. According to the 1977 National Medical Care Expenditure Survey, only 41% of those covered by supplemental policies had any protection from the cost of additional charges for physicians' services delivered to inpatients, and 29% were protected for services performed outside of the hospital (Cafferata, 1984).

In 1987 approximately 30% of physicians participated in the program. However, on a voluntary basis about 70% of claims are assigned. Therefore physicians are voluntarily adjusting their billing practices to meet the needs of the patients. Even though this voluntary effort seems to be acceptable, there has been an ongoing effort on the parts of legislators in some states to make participation a requirement. The outstanding example of this is in Massachusetts, which now requires physicians to participate in the Medicare program as a contingency of licensure. A similar recommendation was placed to the vote of the citizens of the state of Washington and was soundly defeated. Other states are considering similar proposals. Undoubtedly, as more time elapses without a significant change in the administration of the Medicare program, other similar restrictions will be placed on physicians.

Among the recommendations of the Commission is the following:

> Continual attention needs to be given to ways to make it easier for participating physicians to have their Medicare claims processed and ways to increase beneficiaries' familiarity with the participating physician program.

Also, it is recommended that:

> HCFA and the Congress should undertake substantial efforts to monitor the impact of the recent policy changes affecting assignment and beneficiary liability for balance-billed amounts.

It is hoped that in the future, if a satisfactory fee-for-service schedule can be negotiated between the physician community and Medicare, the need for such arbitrary or compulsory programs will not be needed.

The rapid increase in Medicare payments to physicians during the latter part of the 1960s and the 1970s prompted a series of legislative actions to restrain these costs. One such action was the development of the Medicare economic index (MEI). It was anticipated that by the application of this index, physician fees would not advance more rapidly than inflation.

As stated in the Commission report, the MEI weighs physician's practice expenses and general earning levels relative to a base year. The weights are based primarily on a special HCFA survey of physician revenues and expenses and are periodically updated. The portion of the index related to practice expenses has a weight of approximately 40% spread among the following six components:

Salaries and wages of office employees	0.172
Office space	0.100
Drugs and supplies	0.040
Automobile expenses	0.028
Professional liability insurance	0.044
Other expenses	0.016

During the 10 years that the MEI has been applicable to physician reimbursement, the weights for the various factors have changed. For example, professional liability insurance has significantly increased and therefore represents a major factor in the cost of providing health care services on the part of the physician. In light of this and for other reasons, it is the Commission's position that the MEI should be rebased, and a more recent year should be used as the base year for computing adjusted prevailing charges.

When the Medicare program was enacted in 1965, the administration was placed in the hands of HCFA, which in turn has contracts with 35 different contractors, known as carriers, who are responsible for the administration of the program in 56 geographic sites. The carriers operate with relatively loose oversight by the Department of Health and Human Services. As a result, there is not entirely uniform performance among the carriers or the administration of the program in all geographic areas.

Recommendations of the Commission are that:

> Adequate funding for Medicare administration should be recognized as critical to protecting beneficiaries and containing benefit costs. Funding levels should reflect the complexity and scope of program requirements.

> HCFA should permit carriers greater flexibility in allocating administrative funds to the most productive uses.

> Strong standards for carrier claims processing—speed, accuracy, and service to beneficiaries and providers—should be a priority. Persistently poor performers should be eliminated from the program.

> HCFA should expand research to identify cost-effective utilization review and other techniques used by carriers, PROs, and private payers to manage benefit costs.

Certainly, to make administration of the Medicare program more efficient and effective would be of benefit to the overall program and may favorably affect the payout for health care services.

Future Concerns

In recent years the Current Procedural Terminology, fourth edition, commonly called CPT-4, is used by most physicians and carriers to identify services provided and charges made for those services. Originally, the CPT comprised 2000 separate codes, but over time, the number has increased to more than 7000. There are multiple modifiers that can be used, which increases the number of codes to more than 40,000. For medical record-keeping purposes, this coding system is excellent, because it does identify all of the medical services that are provided to the patient. From the medical standpoint, this is important information not only for the current care of the patient but for subsequent care that might be necessary.

Unfortunately, the coding system, when used for charge purposes, has led to certain abuses. One abuse is the unbundling of services, and a full charge applied to each part of a service (as described previously in this chapter).

Another abuse of the system is the upcoding of certain services. This is notably present in the coding of services where a higher code might be used for a service that in fact can be coded for a lesser amount. The magnitude of these abuses is not known, but they most likely add significantly to the overall cost of physician reimbursement in the Medicare program.

The 1986 COBRA directed the Secretary of HHS to study the potential for reducing the number of codes used by carriers for payment purposes, including merging of similar codes into a single category with one code. This could minimize inappropriate increases in the intensity or volume of services billed by reducing code distinctions that do not reflect substantial differences in services rendered. The law indicated that new groups of aggregated codes are to be instituted for payment purposes no later than July 1, 1990. The Commission concurred that the definition of codes for medical and surgical services including standardization of services governed by a global fee for surgery should be refined and standardized.

The issue of assistance at surgery is one that requires review, since in some instances payment for assistance at surgery is not justified.

This is often because assistance is not physically needed, or the level of assistance is not appropriate. The recommendation of the Commission regarding this is:

> Medicare limitations on part B payment for assistance at surgery should be supplemented by additional definitions and guidelines.
>
> Assistant at surgery should be defined as an individual who has the necessary qualifications to participate in the particular type of operation and who actively assists the surgeon in performing the surgical procedure. other situations should be evaluated on a case-by-case basis.
>
> Practical claims review guidelines should be specified so that carriers can assess the need for an assistant based on the complexity of the procedure, the possibility of patient complications, and the expected contribution of the assistant to the outcome.

Several issues require further indepth study by the Commission. Other governmental agencies and additional private groups within the medical community are considering many of these. Of high priority is the evaluation of quality of care for all Medicare beneficiaries and access to that care.

An additional issue is the study of variations of physician reimbursement among several specialties qualified to provide the same service but for which reimbursement varies. Likewise, there is the question of reimbursement between specialists and generalists providing similar services. The status of surgical second opinion programs requires further evaluation to determine whether such mandatory consultations have favorable or unfavorable effects on physician reimbursement.

The per-case or admission payment of radiologists, anesthesiologists, and pathologists (RAP) has been considered by the Commission and undoubtedly further discussions will take place. However, in the analyses to date, the Commission did not take a position in the RAP's proposal.

Finally, as mentioned earlier, the Commission favors more than one mechanism for physician reimbursement, even though it has recommended that a fee-for-service method be utilized primarily. It does not eliminate the fact that there should be multiple methods for reimbursement, and this implies consideration also of capitation. The discussion of capitation also involves investigation of a voucher approach to reimbursement.

Short-Term Recommendations

Although the Commission's responsibility is to make recommendations for long-term changes in physician reimbursement, it was asked to make short-term recommendations that might have an effect on current federal budgets, primarily that for reducing physician reimbursement costs. Previously mentioned has been the identification of nine surgical procedures that were considered outliers and for which it is recommended that a 10% reduction in those fees occur under the inherent reasonableness rule. Second, it recommends reducing the annual update of the prevailing charges by the MEI. This, in turn, would keep all fees at a lower level than if the full MEI was applied. Third, it recommends setting lower customary charge limits for new physicians. This would prevent physicians who are entering practice from establishing a higher profile than is currently permitted. Fourth, it recommends reducing prevailing charges for services in geographic areas where charges exceed the national or state averages by substantial margins.

Suggested Readings

American Association of Retired Persons: Medicare beneficiary liability for physician services: fact sheet, Washington, DC, 1987, Public Policy Institute Issue Brief, AARP.

American Medical Association: Equitable physician reimbursement under Medicare, Chicago, 1985, Internal memorandum, AMA.

American Medical Association: Socioeconomic characteristics of medical practice, Gonzalez ML and Emmons DW, editors, Chicago, 1986, American Medical Association.

Berenson R: Group decision-making methods. In J Hadley et al, Alternative methods of developing a Relative Value Scale of physicians' services: Year 1 report, Washington, DC, Feb 1983, The Urban Institute Press.

Blue Cross and Blue Shield Association: Medicare contractor budget for fiscal year 1984, Statement submitted to the Senate Committee on Appropriations, Subcommittee on Labor, Health and Human Services and Education, May 10, 1983.

Blumberg, MS: Provider price charges for improved health care use. In Chacko GK, editor: Health Handbook, North Holland, Amsterdam, 1979.

Bovbjerg RR: Medical malpractice on trial: quality of care is the important standard, Law and Contemporary Problems 49:321, 1986.

Burney I and Schieber G: Medicare physicians' services: the composition of spending and assignment rates, Health Care Finan Rev 7:81, 1985.

Burney I et al: Geographic variation in physicians' fees, JAMA 240:1368, 1978.

Burney, I et al: Medicare physician payment, participation, and reform, Health Aff 3:5, 1984.

Cafferata GL: Data preview 18: private health insurance coverage of the Medicare population, National Medical Care Expenditure Study, DHHS Pub No (PHS)84-3362, 1984 US Department of Health and Human Services, NCHSR.

Carter LE: Statement of the Medicare Administration Committee of the Health Insurance Association of America. Presented before the Subcommittee on Health of the Committee on Ways and Means, Washington, DC, April 22, 1986 US House of Representatives.

Congressional Budget Office, US Congress: Physician reimbursement under Medicare: options for change, Washington, DC, April 1986. Government Printing Office.

Davis K: Medicaid: Medigap for the poor elderly. Testimony before the Subcommittee on Health and the Environment, Washington, DC, March 26, 1986, US House of Representatives.

Dutton, BL and McMenamin P: The Medicare economic index: its background and beginnings, Health Care Finan Rev 3:137, 1981.

Dyckman ZY: Study of physicians' fees. Staff report prepared by the Council of Wage and Price Stability, Executive Office of the President, Washington, DC, 1978, US Government Printing Office.

Egdahl, RH and Manuel B: A consensus process to determine the relative complexity-severity of frequently performed surgical services, Surg Gynecol Obstet 160:403, 1985.

Etheredge, LM: The volume of Medicare physician services. In Holahan JF and Etheredge LM, editors: Medicare physician payment reform: issue and options, Washington, DC, 1986, The Urban Institute Press.

Federal Register 51:28710, August 11, 1986.

Federal Register 51:29321, August 15, 1986.

Federal Register 51:35693, October 7, 1986.

Fink A et al: Consensus methods: characteristics and guidelines for use, Am J Public Health 74:979, 1984.

Gordon NM: Congressional Budget Office. Statement before the Subcommittee on Health and the Environment Committee on Energy and Commerce, March 26, 1986. US House of Representatives.

Gornick M et al: Twenty years of Medicare and Medicaid: covered populations, use of benefits, and program expenditures, Health Care Finan Rev, annual supplement, 13, 1985.

Graduate Medical Education National Advisory Committee: Summary report of the GMENAC to the Secretary, Department of Health and Human Services, Vol 1, DHHS Pub No (HRA)81-651, Washington, DC, September 30, 1980. US Government Printing Office.

Hadley J and Berenson R: From a Relative Value Scale to a fee schedule. In Holahan JF and Etheredge LM editors: Medicare physician payment reform: issues and options, Washington, DC, 1986, Urban Institute Press.

Hadley J and Berenson RA: Seeking the "just" price: constructing Relative Value Scales and fee schedules, Ann Intern Med. (In press.)

Hadley J et al: Alternative approaches to constructing a Relative Value Scale. In Holahan JF and Etheredge LM, editors: Medicare physician payment reform: issues and options, Washington, DC, 1986, Urban Institute Press.

Harris JE: How many doctors are enough? Health Aff 5:73, 1986.

Health Care Financing Administration: Medicare directory of prevailing charges 1984, HCFA-10016, US Department of Health and Human Services, Washington, DC, 1984, US Government Printing Office.

Health Care Financing Administration: Report on Medicare participating physician/supplier claims workloads: July-September 1986, Baltimore, 1986, US Department of Health and Human Services.

Hsiao W: A national study of resource-based Relative Value Scales for physician services, Final proposal submitted to the Health Care Financing Administration, January 1986.

Hsiao W and Stason W: Toward developing a Relative Value Scale for medical and surgical services, Health Care Finan Rev Fall:23, 1979.

Jencks SF and Dobson A: Strategies for reforming Medicare's physician payments: physician diagnosis-related groups and other approaches, N Engl J Med 312:1492, 1985.

Juba D and Hadley J: Relative Value Scales for physicians' services, Health Care Finan Rev 6:93, 1985.

Juba D and Sulvetta M: Trends in Medicare payment for physician services. In Halahan, JF and Etheredge, LM editors: Medicare physician payment reform: issues and options, Washington, DC, 1986, The Urban Institute Press.

Keller, WE, Pennsylvania Blue Shield: A carrier's perspective on Medicare: administration, testimony before the Physician Payment Review Commission, Washington, DC, December, 1986.

Lubitz J and Pine P: Health care use by Medicare's disabled enrollees, Health Care Finan Rev 7:19, 1986.

Luft HS, and Arno P: Impact of increasing physician supply, Health Aff 5:31, 1986.

McMillan A, Lubitz J, and Newton M: Trends in physician assignment rates for Medicare services, 1968-85, Health Care Finan Rev 7:59, 1985.

Mitchell JB et al: Creating DRG-based physician reimbursement schemes: a conceptual and empirical analysis—Year 1 report, Chestnut Hill, MA, 1984, Center for Health Economics Research.

National Center for Health Statistics, US Department of Health and Human Service: Health United States, 1985, DHHS Pub No (PHS)86-1232, Hyattsville, MD, 1985.

National Center for Health Statistics, US Department of Health and Human Services: Unpublished data from 1985 Annual National Health Interview Survey, Hyattsville, MD.

Newhouse JP et al: Where have all the doctors gone? JAMA 247:2392, 1982.

Office of Technology Assessment, US Congress: Nurse practitioners, physician assistants, and certified nurse-midwives: a policy analysis (health technology case study 37), OTA-HCS-37, Washington, DC, December 1986, US Government Printing Office.

Office of Technology Assessment, US Congress: Payment for physician services: strategies for Medicare, OTA-H-294, Washington, DC, Feb 1986, US Government Printing Office.

O'Sullivan J: Medicare: FY88 budget, Issue Brief No. 1B87038, Washington, DC, Jan 1987, Congressional Research Service, US Congress.

Owens A: how much of your money comes from third parties, Med Econ 60:254, 1983.

Paringer L: Medicare assignment rates of physicians: their responses to changes in reimbursement policy, Health Care Financ Rev 1:75, 1980.

Pauly MV and Langwell KM: physician payment reform: who shall be paid? Med Care Rev 43:101, 1986.

Public Health Service, Health Resources and Services Administration, Bureau of health Professions, US Department of Health and Human Services: Fifth report to the President and Congress on the status of health personnel in the United States, DHHS Pub No (HRS)P-OD-86-1 or (HRP)09-06-767, March 1986.

Reinhardt UE: A framework for deliberations on the compensation of physicians, Statement before the United States Senate Special Committee on Aging, Washington, DC, March 16, 1984, Hearing on physician reimbursement.

Reinhardt UE: The compensation of physicians: approaches used in foreign countries, Quality Review Bulletin/Journal of Quality Assurance 11:366, 1985.

Reuter J, Stewart A, and Kline J: Medicare Part B: the Supplementary Medical insurance program, Report No 86-153 EPW, Washington, DC, Sept 1986, Congressional Research Service, US Congress.

Showstack JA et al: Fee for service payment: analysis of current methods and their development, Inquiry 16:230, 1979.

Sloan FA and Schwartz WB: More doctors: what will they cost, JAMA 299:766, 1983.

Sloan FA and Hay JW: Medicare pricing mechanisms for physician services: an overview of alternative approaches Med Care Rev 43:59, 1986.

Steinwald B and Sloan FA Determinants of physicians' fees, Business 47:493, 1974.

US Congress, Conference report to accompany HR 5300 of the 99th Congress: Providing for reconciliation pursuant to section 2 of the concurrent resolution on the budget for fiscal year 1987 (Report 99-1012), p. 158, 332.

US House of Representatives, Committee on Ways and Means: Physician reimbursement under Medicare: current policy, trends, and issues, WMCP 96-77, Washington, DC, Dec 23, 1980, US Government Printing Office.

US Senate, Special Committee on Aging, American Association of Retired Persons, Federal Council on the Aging, and the Administration on Aging: Aging America: trends and projections, Washington, DC, 1985-86. US Department of Health and Human Services.

US Department of Labor, Pension and Welfare Benefits Administration, Office of Policy and Research: Employer sponsored retiree health insurance, Washington, DC, May 1986, Unpublished paper.

US General Accounting Office: Medicare Contracting, (HRD)8648, Washington, DC, 1986.

Wagner J: The micro-costing approach. In Hadley J et al: Alternative methods of developing a Relative Value Scale of physicians' services: Year 1 Report, Washington, DC, Feb 1983, The Urban Institute Press.

Waldo DR and Lazenby HC: Demographic characteristics and health care use and expenditures by the aged in the United States: 1977-1984, Health Care Finan Rev 6:1-29, 1984.

Waldo DR, Levit KR, and Lazenby H: National health expenditures, 1985, Health Care Finan Rev 8:1, 1986.

West H, McMenamin P and Marcus GL: Development of MD-DRG algorithms, phase I final report, prepared for HCFA/ORD, Springfield, VA, August 15, 1986, Mandex, Inc.

Wilensky GR and Rossiter LF: Alternative units of payment for physician services: an overview of the issues, Med Care Rev 43:133, 1986.

RALPH W. SCHAFFARZICK

Ralph W. Schaffarzick received his AB degree from Stanford University in 1943 and his MD degree from the same institution in 1946. While engaged in the private practice of internal medicine in San Francisco from 1950 to 1977, he also held various clinical posts at Stanford University School of Medicine and is currently Clinical Professor of Medicine and Health Services Research. Since 1969 he has been Senior Vice-President and Medical Director, Blue Shield of California.

JOHN P. BUNKER

John P. Bunker is Professor of Health Research and Policy and of Anesthesia at Stanford University. He received his undergraduate degree (1942) and medical degree (1945) at Harvard University and his training in anesthesia at George Washington University and Massachusetts General Hospitals.

9

Regionalized Surgical Health Care

RALPH W. SCHAFFARZICK
JOHN P. BUNKER

During the past decade the health care system of the United States has been subjected to marked turbulence. The cost of health care has continued to escalate at a rate consistently greater than that of general inflation. In 1986, $458 billion was spent for health care: 10.9% of the Gross National Product (GNP) and $1620 per person.[17] The *Health Care Financing Review* has predicted that national health expenditures will reach $1.5 trillion by the year 2000: 15% of the GNP and $5500 per capita. Such costs have stimulated increasing concern among the purchasers of health care, both private and government. To date, all strategies to contain costs have been ineffective.

As more and more measures to reduce costs have been implemented, with consequent impediment to accessibility of services, the purchasers and public policy analysts have expressed worry that the quality of health care has suffered. Consequently, purchasers are now demanding objective data that can be used to document quality assessment and assurance.

A significant contributor to the cost and quality of health care, of course, is medical technology. The increasing costs and complexity of technologic advances in diagnosis and treatment have been accompanied by other important issues. They are often moral or ethical; they include the public's desire and determination to have access to these "high-tech" advances; and the quality and equity with which those advances are apportioned and applied must be addressed.[16]

In the Shattuck Lecture of 1978, Alain Enthoven, acknowledging the failure of purely regulatory attempts to contain the cost of health care, proposed a strategy to encourage competition—the Consumer-Choice Health Plan.[6] His goal was to stimulate the provision of cost-effective care by creating a vehicle in which groups of physicians and other providers would have incentives to compete with each other. Before this concept, the usual marketplace forces of supply and demand had not applied to the health care system.

In 1982 the California Legislature enacted AB-3480. This statute, in effect, made it possible for insurance companies and others to negotiate contracts with physicians and hospitals for the provision of health care services. At the same time, as a companion to AB-3480, the Legislature enacted a statute that cleared the way for the California Department of Health Services to negotiate contracts with hospitals for serving Medi-Cal (Medicaid) beneficiaries. The obvious purpose of this legislation was to reduce the strain of the Medi-Cal program on the state budget. Since then there has been an explosion of such contracting among all sorts of groups, individuals, and institutions, not only in California but also nationwide. The historical roles of physicians, hospitals, health care service plans, insurance companies, employers, and patients have been dislocated and scrambled. Physician-organized foundations for medical care have become for-profit companies and "gone public" on the stock exchange. Investor-owned hospital chains have entered the business of health insurance. Venture capital providers have solicited participation of doctors in nursing home chains, urgent-care centers ("Docs in the box"), third-party review organizations, and administrators. Insurance companies have flirted with the actual provision of health care delivery rather than confining their function to the financing of services. Major self-insured employers increasingly have negotiated directly with doctors and hospitals to attend the needs of their employees. Custodians of labor trust funds have done the same.

Alternative delivery systems (ADS) include health maintenance organizations, preferred provider organizations and exclusive provider organizations, in addition to the traditional fee-for-service health care service plans and indemnity insurance with managed care. Physicians and hospitals may have contracts with several different ADS entities. Almost all of these competitive groups include agreements for price discounts and varying degrees of restriction of access.

Another important element in the current environment, of course, is the surplus of physicians, particularly in the surgical specialties, and of hospital beds. In this era of competition, such surfeit of providers enhances the competitive atmosphere. As the number of potential patients per doctor and/or hospital diminishes, the providers are stimulated either to perform more services per patient or to demonstrate the excellence and economy of their services. (In 1987 there has been a surge in outpatient utilization, which has produced a serious drain on both Medicare part B and private health care financing. Although not yet completely analyzed, this surge in utilization is probably, in large measure, the result of physician surplus.) Marketing and advertising strategies are a way of life. Madison Avenue has a whole new field to exploit.

Thus we have a turbulent health care system, characterized by unrelenting escalation of cost, possible erosion of quality of care, proliferation of technology, intensifying competition with a profusion of contracting for professional and hospital services, and a surplus of hospital beds and medical specialists, particularly in metropolitan areas. In this milieu there are compelling reasons to examine the case for selective contracting or regionalization of certain surgical and other health care services.

TECHNOLOGY ASSESSMENT

Inextricably bonded to the development of a strategy for regionalization or selective coverage is the process of technology assessment (TA). This process is important in the determination of what is truly valuable in health care, and TA itself is emerging as a mature rigorous discipline.

As medical technology has proliferated almost exponentially in recent years, it has become imperative to be able to evaluate precisely and objectively both new and old procedures, devices, techniques, and other methods of diagnosis and treatment. Do they make significant contributions to the improvement in clinical outcomes? How can they be infused into health care in an orderly and cost-effective fashion? Are they truly a good investment for society? Who is qualified to use them and who is qualified to receive them?

Currently about 45 entities in the United States perform TA.[9] Within the government there is the Congressional Office of Technology

Assessment (OTA), and under the Public Health Service (PHS), the Office of Health Technology Assessment (OHTA) of the National Center for Health Services Research and Health Care Technology (NCHSRHCT), which draws on the findings of other federal resources such as the Food and Drug Administration (FDA), the National Institutes of Health (NIH), and the Center for Diseases Control (CDC).

In the private sector, TA is performed by entities such as the Clinical Efficacy Assessment Program (CEAP) of the American College of Physicians (ACP), the Diagnostic and Therapeutic Technology Assessment (DATTA) of the American Medical Association (AMA), the Technology Evaluation and Coverage (TEC) Department of the Blue Cross and Blue Shield Association (BCBSA), and several Blue Cross and Blue Shield plans.

In 1982 Bunker et al. reported their evaluation of medical technology strategies.[2] They found a lack of consistent and explicit policy regarding payment for new technologies; an absence of a single, organized, adequately funded program or agency responsible for generating data with which to evaluate technologies; a difficulty in establishing priorities for study; and a number of conflicts among the goals of insurers, practitioners, developers, evaluators, and government. To deal with this situation, they proposed the creation of a private nonprofit institute for health care evaluation that would be composed of representatives from both the private sector and the public sector. In 1983 the Institute of Medicine (IOM), for essentially the same reasons, recommended the establishment of a consortium that would assess medical technology.

Subsequently such an institute was created as the Institute of Medicine's Council on Health Care Technology. The Council was authorized by Congress in 1984 and established within the IOM in early 1986.[4] Its membership is distinguished, and there is good reason to be optimistic about its success.

The Process of TA

When a new technology is identified or when an established one is thought to have become obsolete, the first step is to perform a thorough literature search. All relevant reports published in peer-reviewed journals are collected. Preferable are reports of randomized clinical trials, double blind studies, and other controlled trials. Also included are review articles and reports of consensus development panels that have been conducted by authoritative bodies such as the NIH, and TAs performed by other respected entities such as the OTA, OHTA, or CEAP. Other evidence is solicited from relevant specialty societies and expert opinions from acknowledged experts.

When the evidence has been assembled, it is subjected to analysis, and preliminary conclusions are formulated. When the evidence is fragmentary or inconclusive (which frequently is the case), the technique of decision analysis or meta-analysis can be employed.[5,15]

Recently the BCBSA TEC Management Division, with the assistance of David Eddy, Director of the Center for Health Policy Research and Education, Duke University, and the Medical Advisory Panel (MAP), completed formulation of a set of TA criteria[1]:

1. The technology must have final approval from the appropriate government regulatory bodies.
   - A device, drug or biological product must have Food and Drug Administration approval to market for those specific indications and methods of use that Blue Cross and Blue Shield Association is assessing.
   - Approval to market refers to permission for commercial distribution. Any other approval that is granted as an interim step in the FDA regulatory process, e.g., an Investigational Device Exemption, is not sufficient.
2. The scientific evidence must permit conclusions concerning the effect of the technology on health outcomes.

- The evidence should consist of well designed and well conducted investigations published in peer-reviewed journals. The quality of the body of studies and the consistency of the results are considered in evaluating the evidence.
- The evidence should demonstrate that the technology can measure or alter the physiological changes related to a disease, injury, illness or condition. In addition there should be evidence or a convincing argument based on established medical facts that such measurement or alteration affects the health outcomes.
- Opinions and assessments by national medical associations, consensus panels or other technology assessment bodies are evaluated according to the scientific quality of the supporting evidence and rationale.
3. The technology must improve the net health outcome.
    - The technology's beneficial effects on health outcomes should outweigh any harmful effects on health outcomes.
4. The technology must be as beneficial as any established alternatives.
    - The technology should improve the net health outcome as much as or more than established alternatives.
5. The improvement must be attainable outside the investigational settings.
    - When used under the usual conditions of medical practice, the technology should be reasonably expected to satisfy criteria 3 and 4.

After the evidence is assembled and analyzed, and a preliminary conclusion is formulated, a recommendation is presented to the decision-making body such as the MAP of the BSBSA or the Medical Policy Committee (MPC) of Blue Shield of California (BSC).

MPC, a major committee of the Board of Directors, is composed of physicians and public members of the Board, augmented by health care economists, health policy analysts, and others. Expert oral testimony is presented to augment the written evidence. When, for example, the MPC was considering human heart transplantation (HT), Norman Shumway of Stanford, the leading pioneer, and other cardiac surgical authorities participated in the discussion. When liver transplantation (LT) was considered, Rudi Schmid, chairman of the NIH Consensus Panel, gave testimony. The meetings are conducted in open forum, and attendance is usually between 75 and 100 interested parties including the media. Debate is usually interesting, informative, occasionally impassioned, and rarely even enlivened by acrimony. The emphasis, however, is on the critical mass of objective evidence arrayed against the TA criteria (supra).

When the topic has been thoroughly discussed, the Committee decides whether the subject technology should be classified as "experimental," "investigational," or "accepted standard practice." The experimental classification indicates that the technology has been tested primarily in the laboratory, usually on animals. The investigational classification means that the technology is still in the process of clinical trials to determine efficacy and safety. In order for a technology to be "promoted" to accepted standard practice, it must satisfy the criteria set forth by the BCBSA.

Although the majority of technologies evaluated are new and emerging, a systematic review of older established procedures began in 1976. This review became formalized by the MAP of BCBSA as the initial "Medical Necessity Program," conducted in concert with the American College of Physicians, the American College of Surgeons, and other specialty colleges. In due process, numerous procedures have been declared to be obsolete, redundant, or of unproven value. Although some of these seem obvious, for example, BMR or icterus index tests, some have precipitated lively debate. In 1987, for example, the MPC found that chemonucleolysis for treatment of herniated nucleus pulposus had become obsolete. In this case the health care plan's claims experience provided useful evidence.

During the most recent 6 months, whereas 1289 claims for lumbar laminectomy had been submitted, there were only 13 chemonucleolysis. (Availability of data from claims is often useful as an adjunct to published reports of clinical trials.)

COVERAGE DETERMINATION

Only when a technology has achieved the status of accepted practice does it become eligible for coverage determination, that is, payable. In this process, factors other than purely scientific merit are considered. These include cost, cost effectiveness, allocation of resources, ethical and moral principles, legal implications, and contractual issues.

If, for example, the artificial heart should reach the status of accepted practice, the prohibitive cost might be greater than the purchasers of health care services would wish to pay. Other "staples" in the health care market basket might suffer in the process of reallocation of resources. Distributive justice would be difficult to attain. Some religious denominations might be offended by the replacement of a human heart with a mechanical pump. Some trial lawyers could find opportunities to press litigation for malpractice and bad faith. Special language would be required in contracts with health insurers.

Selective Coverage

Although covered procedures have historically been limited to those classified as acceptable standard practice, a new dimension has been introduced over the past three years—the device of selective coverage. Conscious of the need to promote the quality even more than the cost effectiveness of medical technology, the MPC has developed criteria for patient selection and requirements for provider qualification. These allow an emerging technology that is generally considered investigational to be covered when provided by certain innovators with documented and credible experience. Essentially, in the hands of such leaders a procedure may be deemed acceptable rather than investigational. In 1984, for example, the MPC determined that HT would be covered when performed at Stanford University or at any other institution that could document skill, resources commitment, and favorable clinical outcomes comparable with those at Stanford. Similarly, patient selection for HT must be consonant with the principles used by the patient selection committee at Stanford. The same selective coverage concept, based on the report of the NIH Consensus Development Panel,[12] was applied to LT.

This selective coverage approach promotes the improvement of clinical outcomes and the desirable goal of regionalization. If an institution and its physicians wish to be reimbursed for providing such complex services, they must be prepared to make a sustained commitment of time, skilled personnel, space, and money. Such an investment will presumably discourage undue proliferation of facilities and enhance the numbers of patients being treated in established institutions. This in turn can promote quality. Luft et al.[11] have reported the empirical relationship between surgical volume and mortality; for complex major surgery in particular, they found an inverse relationship between volume and mortality.

Another important advantage of selective coverage is less obvious. At a time when public and private sources of funding for research are less available, some of the cost of clinical inquiry can be defrayed by selective coverage. If a third-party payer is convinced that a new technology is potentially beneficial but not yet ready to be promoted beyond the investigational phase, it may decide to pay for the procedure when performed by specified investigators.

During 1987, for example, the MPC concluded that when performed at the University of California at San Francisco (UCSF) and at Los Angeles (UCLA), balloon embolization of intracranial aneurysms and fistulae are not investigational and, therefore, are eligible for payment. Also, when performed at UCLA and University of California at Irvine (UCI), selective posterior root ablation for spasticity of cerebral palsy is not investigational. By linking payment to TA and selective coverage, regionalization of services is evolving in response to the marketplace.

Modified Selective Coverage

Not infrequently, BSC receives claims or petitions for coverage of procedures and/or devices that are still in the investigational stage but that have the potential for effecting improved clinical outcomes at lower risk and lower cost. The scientific rationale may be valid, and preliminary clinical trials may be very encouraging. On the other hand, when a device is involved, it may not yet have FDA approval to market, and reports of sufficient clinical trials may not have been published in peer-reviewed journals. As a result, the technology must be classified as investigational and, therefore, not routinely covered.

Nevertheless, reimbursement for such procedures may occasionally be justified. A specific example of such an emerging technology is the ablation of abnormal conduction foci in the interior of the heart by means of electroshock delivered to the lesion through a heart catheter. The standard established treatment for such lesions is open heart surgery with surgical destruction of the offending tissue. If the treatment can be accomplished through a cardiac catheter, obviously the patient is not subjected to the risks, trauma, prolonged hospitalization, and cost of open heart surgery. In several centers clinical trials of the catheter technique are in progress, and the results so far are encouraging but not yet sufficient to assess fully the risks and benefits of this alternative approach. Another problem is that, while the catheter has FDA approval for the purpose of electrophysiologic mapping (study) (EPS), it has not been approved for the ablation procedure. Put another way, the catheter has been approved for purposes of locating the trouble but not for correcting the trouble. As a consequence, BSC can pay for the EPS, for open heart surgery to destroy the lesion(s) identified by EPS, and/or implantation of an automatic cardioverter/defibrillator but not for the catheter ablation.

Because the catheter ablation technique is still being perfected, even though in many cases it is successful, it does not always work, and the patient then must undergo open heart surgery. Thus while catheter ablation may sometimes replace the more formidable and expensive surgery, in other cases it may prove to be an additional source of risk and cost.

In order to promote the perfection of medical technology that has demonstrated genuine potential for producing clinical benefit, reduced risk, and lower cost but has not yet emerged fully from the investigational category, the concept of a modified form of selective coverage was considered by the MPC. (Probably the true nidation of the concept is found in the Code of Hammurabi.*)

When approached by an investigator of a procedure in this category, BSC might respond by suggesting an agreement to cover the professional and institutional costs of the procedure on eligible BSC subscribers when the clinical outcome is successful. If, on the other hand, the outcome is not successful, the investigator and hospital would absorb the cost and charge neither BSC nor the subscriber for any of the services related to the procedure.

In the case of the cardiac catheter ablation, for example, if the technique accomplished the purpose of correcting the cardiac arrhythmia, BSC would pay. If, however, the heart lesion failed to respond, and open heart surgery were required, the doctor(s) and hospital would charge no one for the attempted catheter ablation.

---

*"If a surgeon has operated with the bronze lancet on a patrician for a serious injury, and has caused his death, or has removed a cataract for a patrician, with the bronze lancet, and has made him lose his eye, his hands shall be cut off." Code of Hammurabi, 1950-1900 BC.[10]

QUALITY ASSESSMENT: VOLUME-OUTCOME

In 1978 Bunker et al., considering "Surgical Innovation and Its Evolution,"[3] suggested that early clinical trials should be concentrated in a relatively few institutions. This would result in improvement in treatment from greater experience and more reliable statistical information than can be achieved in larger series.

In 1979 Luft et al. asked "Should Operations be Regionalized?"[11] They examined mortality for 12 surgical procedures of varying complexity in 1498 hospitals to see whether there was a relation between a hospital's surgical volume and its surgical mortality. They found that the mortality after open heart surgery, vascular surgery, transurethral resection of the prostate, and coronary artery bypass graft (CABG) was markedly lower in hospitals with large numbers of operations. Hospitals in which 200 or more of these operations were performed annually had death rates, adjusted for case mix, that were 25% to 41% lower than those of hospitals with lower volumes. For other procedures, for example, total hip replacement, the mortality curve flattened at lower volumes. They were not able to resolve the question of whether the volume-outcome relationship represented the effect of experience ("practice makes perfect") or whether it is the result of attraction of more patients to centers having better than average results.

In 1987 Showstack et al., confirming the association of volume with outcome for coronary artery bypass graft, concluded that:

> Empirical evidence suggests that mortality rates for coronary artery bypass graft (CABG) surgery are lower in hospitals that perform a higher volume of the procedure. In recent years, the criteria for CABG surgery have been expanded to include patients with a wide variety of co-morbidities. To address the question of whether the volume-outcome relationship continues to exist for this new group of patients, discharge abstracts for 18,986 CABG operations at 77 hospitals in California in 1983 were analyzed using multiple-regression techniques. Higher-volume hospitals had lower in-hospital mortality (adjusted for case mix); this effect was greatest in patients who might be characterized as having "non-scheduled" CABG surgery. Higher-volume hospitals also had shorter average postoperative lengths of stay and fewer patients with extremely long stays. The results of this study suggest that the greatest improvement in average outcomes for CABG surgery would result from the closure of low-volume surgery units.*

Based on this study performed by BSC and the Institute for Health Policy Studies, UCSF, the Office of Inspector General (OIG), Department of Health and Human Services, conducted an inspection to ascertain the national significance of the findings for the Medicare program and future beneficiaries subjected to CABG. Gottlober, Purvis, and colleagues published the findings of this inspection in August 1987.[8] They had conducted extensive interviews with 44 cardiovascular surgeons and cardiologists, surveyed 38 Medicare carriers, and reviewed hospital and payment records for more than 200 Medicare beneficiaries.

The major OIG findings were:

> Hospitals and surgical teams that perform more than 200 CABG surgeries per year have better outcomes in terms of mortality rates, lengths of stay and charges. Contracting with selected high volume surgeons and facilities would assure that Medicare beneficiaries receive the highest quality of care in the most efficient and economical settings.
>
> Some of the most prominent cardiac surgeons and medical centers are offering package prices for CABG surgery. If the Health Care Financing Administration (HCFA) negotiated similar rates for Medicare, more than $192 million could be saved each year in hospital and medical insurance reimbursement. Many health maintenance organizations and other payers have taken ad-

---
*Showstack JA et al, JAMA 257:785, 1987. Copyright 1987, American Medical Association.

vantage of these offers or have negotiated package prices on their own initiative.

There is considerable controversy surrounding the medical necessity of coronary bypass surgery for certain patients.

Medicare reasonable charge allowances for the primary surgeon are often inconsistent and inequitable. The allowances do not consider the economies of the marketplace. Furthermore, if the reasonable charge allowance for the primary surgeon's fee were limited to the amount paid for three grafts, at least $5 million would be saved each year. If separate payments for assistant surgeons and anesthesiologists were eliminated, $69 million could be saved annually.

The implementation of the HCFA Common Procedure Coding System (HCPCS), which added three codes for CABG surgery, has increased Medicare outlays for CABG surgery.

Carrier utilization controls and payment guidelines for services associated with CABG surgery are inconsistent. This costs Medicare at least $4 million annually. Some carriers have implemented utilization screens to limit the costs associated with CABG surgery and prevent fragmentation of the global fee.

As evidence of provider willingness to participate in the contracting process, the OIG report cited the initiative of the Texas Heart Institute (THI). From 1980 to 1985, this prestigious center had experienced a reduction in the annual number of cardiac surgeries from about 3500 to 2500. In a proposal to HCFA, the THI offered a package price of $13,800 for CABG for Medicare and non-Medicare patients. The package price included hospitalization, professional fees, and all customary laboratory tests. At the time of the offer from the THI, the national Medicare mean allowance for the same set of services was $24,588.

In the fall of 1987 Freeland et al. examined some of the prospects, problems, and unanswered questions concerning selective contracting for hospital care based on volume, quality, and price.[7] They issued the caveat that although selective contracting has the potential to reduce duplication of services, to reduce cost, and to lower mortality and morbidity for some patient groups, care must be taken to preserve continuity in care and reasonable access to care. Their analysis of outcome data on 37 metropolitan hospitals performing CABG led to the conclusion that outcome data based on statistical norms should be viewed as no more than a first step in evaluating quality and price performance.

SUMMARY AND CONCLUSIONS

Efforts to regionalize medical care in the past have been unsuccessful. Recent evidence, demonstrating that for complex procedures, high volumes are associated with better results, together with the incentives for cost-effective care of the new competitive environment, has given new life to the movement to regionalize. Selective coverage, implemented privately, by state governments, and now by the federal government, for heart transplants is rapidly moving tertiary care surgery towards de facto regionalization, as hospitals not favored with contracts are forced to eliminate selected services or possibly to close entirely.

Regionalization via selective coverage can be expected to occur incrementally, with specific procedures being examined and accepted for selective coverage based on frequency of performance, complexity, and cost. Cardiac surgery (CABG in particular) has received the greatest attention and is currently being groomed for early implementation of selective coverage. Institutions with lower mortality, fewer complications, and lower costs and charges will be those that succeed in winning contracts, with a gradual weeding out of those cardiac programs with poorer results and higher costs. Not only hospitals but cardiac surgeons with poorer results will be squeezed out.

A major concern has been that regionalization will limit access to care, particularly in rural areas. This has been examined in detail by Robinson et al.[14] These authors have surveyed the geographic distribution, surgical volume, and mortality after CABG for all hospitals in the United States. More than 80% of hospitals carrying out fewer than 200 such procedures a year were in geographic areas with at least one and usually many more hospitals equipped for open heart surgery within 15 miles. Closure of such hospitals will not, therefore, limit access for patients served by the majority of those hospitals.

Access to cardiac surgical services for the population, largely rural, served by those hospitals performing fewer than 200 bypass operations a year need not be jeopardized, for selective coverage will, in most cases, not attempt to limit such services. Selective coverage is designed expressly to eliminate duplicative and less cost-effective services. No purpose would be served by attempting to limit coverage for patients served by isolated rural hospitals.

The closing of surgical and other facilities not selected for coverage will inevitably put some surgeons and cardiologists out of work. It can be assumed that these will be physicians who have experienced poorer results. Some such physicians may, of course, be well qualified. These will, in most cases, be physicians practicing in urban areas overcrowded with specialists, and some, perhaps many, of these physicians will choose to relocate in rural areas or in the urban ghetto, helping, as a result, to improve overall access rather than the reverse, as feared.

Regionalization of organ transplantation is already a fact.[13] CABG, as we have discussed, is next in line. Other prime candidates for selective coverage and regionalization are total hip and other joint replacement, oncology, neurosurgery, neonatal intensive care, and rehabilitation services. It can be assumed that regionalization that develops for selected procedures such as these, based on the quality as well as on the cost of services, will advance the public health.

References

1. Blue Cross and Blue Shield Association: Letter of transmittal, Dec 1986.
2. Bunker JP, Fowles J, and Schaffarzick RW: Evaluation of medical-technology strategies, N Engl J Med 306:620, 687, 1982.
3. Bunker JP, Hinkley D, and McDermott WV: Surgical innovation and its evaluation, Science 200:937, 1978.
4. CHCTA, Newsletter of the Council on Health Care Technology/Institute of Medicine/National Academy of Sciences 1, 1986.
5. Eddy D: Personal communications, 1976 to present.
6. Enthoven AC: Consumer-choice health plan, N Engl J Med 298:650, 709, 1978.
7. Freeland MS, Hunt SS, and Luft HS: Selective contracting for hospital care based on volume, quality, and price: prospects, problems, and unanswered questions. Health Polit Policy Law, 12:409, 1987.
8. Gottlober P et al: Coronary artery bypass graft (CABG) surgery: assuring quality while controlling Medicare costs, Office of Inspector General, Department of Health & Human Services, Aug 1987.
9. Jannssen TJ and Norris CK: Technology assessment and coverage decisionmaking in the Department of Health and Human Services. Final report submitted to office of the Assistant Secretary for Planning and Evaluation, US DHHS, Aug 1984, Macro Systems.
10. Knoles GH and Snyder RK: Readings in Western Civilization, Philadelphia, 1951, JB Lippincott Co.
11. Luft HS, Bunker JP, and Enthoven A: Should operations be regionalized? N Engl J Med 301, 1364, 1979; see also Bunker JP, Luft HS, and Enthoven A: Should surgery be regionalized? Surg Clin North Am 62:657, 1982.
12. National Institutes of Health: Consensus Development Conference on Liver Transplantation, January 23, 1983.
13. Renlund DG et al: Medicare-designated centers for cardiac transplantation, N Engl J Med 316:873, 1987.
14. Robinson JC, Garnick DW, and McPhee SJ: Market and regulatory influences on the availability of coronary angioplasty and bypass surgery in US hospitals, N Engl J Med 317:85, 1987.
15. Sacks HS et al: Meta-analyses of randomized controlled trials, N Engl J Med 316:450, 1987.
16. Schaffarzick RW: Health care technology and quality of care, American College of Utilization Review Physicians 2:84, 1987.
17. The Medical-Economic Digest, Charlottesville, Virginia, Oct 15, 1987, Kelly Communications.

LYNN R. GRUBER

Lynn R. Gruber is the Vice President of the Center for Managed Care Research at InterStudy. Ms. Gruber received her degree in law from Hamline University School of Law (1978) in St. Paul, Minn.

SUSAN HARTWELL

Susan Hartwell is a senior research associate at InterStudy and project director of their study on rural health care. She received her MS degree from Cornell University (1983) with a concentration in human service studies.

CYNTHIA L. POLICH

Cynthia L. Polich is the president of InterStudy and director of their Center for Aging and Long-Term Care. She received her MA degree in 1978 from the Humphrey Institute of Public Affairs, University of Minnesota, with a concentration in gerontology.

10

The Impact of Managed Health Care Systems on Surgeons

LYNN R. GRUBER
SUSAN HARTWELL
CYNTHIA L. POLICH

THE RISE OF HMOs AND MANAGED HEALTH CARE

President Nixon declared a crisis in medicine in the early 1970s when health care costs soared to new, unfamiliar, and unwelcomed heights.[15] Since then, proponents of organizational change in health care in the United States have been busy stimulating market forces to improve the system by challenging the traditional financial incentives embodied in the fee-for-service reimbursement methodology and by investigating the way in which health care services were being delivered—largely inside hospitals. Ironically, George Bernard Shaw, the British playwright, was berating the logic of fee-for-service payment to physicians in 1911 in "Preface on Doctors" from *Doctors' Dilemma*:[13]

> It is not the fault of our doctors that the medical service of the community, as at present provided for, is a murderous absurdity. That any sane nation, having observed that you could provide for the supply of bread by giving bakers a pecuniary interest in baking for you, should go on to give a surgeon a pecuniary interest in cutting off your leg, is enough to make one despair of political humanity. But this is precisely what we have done. And the more appalling the mutilation, the more the mutilator is paid. Scandalized voices murmur that . . . operations are necessary. They may be. It may also be necessary to hang a man or pull down a house. But we take good care not to make the hangman and the housebreaker the judges of that. If we did, no man's neck would be safe and no man's house stable.

The time was ripe for change. Paul Ellwood, a physician from Excelsior, Minn., firmly believed that a new prepaid delivery vehicle was needed to spark competition in health care on the basis of cost effectiveness and quality. He won the ear of Nixon's health care administrators and convinced them to support health maintenance organizations (HMOs) as a means to provide comprehensive health services for a fixed prepaid amount through a single entity arranging and coordinating all services. The HMO industry took off in 1974 and is still growing in 1988 with total enrollment of nearly 31 million.[6]

Significant differences exist between traditional insurance and HMOs (the most well-known managed care product). Traditional indemnity insurance companies establish premiums by experience rating various groups of insureds.

165

The insured is offered a policy that generally contains benefit limitations, such as no preventive services and a fixed number of home health visits, but the chief feature is patient freedom of choice regarding selection of physicians and hospitals. Additionally, most traditional indemnity policies require the insured to pay initial deductibles and copayments for services less than $1000, and the insured is fully responsible for the cost of pharmaceuticals. Generally the insured must fill out a claim form in order for the provider to receive payment. Physicians are paid under the "usual and customary" fee-for-service method.

HMOs offer comprehensive health care, including preventive services, that is, routine eye examinations, history and physical examinations unrelated to symptoms, immunizations, and family planning services, drugs for a minimal copayment ($2.50 to $5), no claims filing paperwork, and more uniform premiums established through the community rating process, not by group experience rating.

The HMO organizes the delivery of services through special contracts with physicians, hospitals, home health agencies, and other vendors of allied services, HMO enrollees are required to select providers with whom the HMO has contracted; therefore selection is limited.

Physicians who sign HMO provider contracts and formally become part of the HMO's organized delivery system are legally bound to follow administrative policies established by the HMO management office. Such policies relate to compensation, utilization control mechanisms, use of contract institutions and vendors, and reporting requirements.

Competition in the marketplace has produced other forms of alternative delivery systems besides HMOs. The most common one is the preferred provider organization (also known as preferred provider arrangements). A PPO has been described by the National Health Lawyers Association as "a health care financing and delivery program which provides financial incentives to consumers to utilize a select panel of preferred providers."[7] Physicians are usually paid by negotiated discounted fee-for-service. PPOs emphasize their provider networks and tend not to have the organized systems of care featured in HMOs.

In our estimation, managed care plans are those entities offering comprehensive healthcare benefits for a prepaid fee delivered through organized systems of administration (provider contracting, provider payment, utilization control techniques and analysis and management report generation) and coordinated systems of care (management of patient's total needs—primary care, specialty home healthcare) to achieve cost-effective, quality health care.

For the purposes of this chapter, the focus will be on HMOs as the most sophisticated managed care plan options. HMOs pioneered the application of utilization control protocols and the development of systems for the financing and delivery of care. In addition, nearly 30 million persons are enrolled in HMOs throughout the United States.

THE GROWTH OF MANAGED CARE

A managed care plan should have the following features to be considered an HMO:
- Offers prepaid, comprehensive health coverage for both hospital and physician services
- Requires members to use participating providers
- Enrolls members for specific time periods

Although the structural and organizational features of various HMOs differ significantly, they are generally categorized according to four model type definitions. These are operationally defined as follows:

Staff: An HMO that delivers health services through a physician group that is controlled by the HMO unit. Historically, the providers are salaried staff members of the HMO who treat only HMO patients.

Group: An HMO that predominately contracts with one independent group practice to provide health services. The group is usually compensated on a capitation basis for its HMO enrollees. Participating physicians frequently provide services to non-HMO members on a fee-for-service basis.

Network: An HMO that contracts with two or more independent group practices, possibly including a staff group, to provide health services. While a network may contain a few solo practices, it is predominately organized around group practices.

IPA: An HMO that contracts directly with physicians in independent practices; and/or contracts with one or more associations of physicians in independent practice; and/or contracts with one or more multispecialty group practices (but the plan is predominately organized around solo/single specialty practices).

The major growth of HMOs began in the mid-1970s with the support and funding of the federal government. Because HMOs generally require several years from inception to implementation, it is not surprising that the rapid proliferation of the mid-1980s lagged a number of years behind the enabling legislation (Table 10-1). The steady growth in the number of HMOs began accelerating in 1984. Between June 1984 and June 1985 the number of plans increased by 28.4% and in the next year, a record-breaking 51.4% increase was realized. Since mid-1986 HMO start-ups have slackened considerably, as noted by the modest 11.3% growth between 1986 and 1987. Growth in enrollment accelerated in 1985 and 1986, and by mid-1987 more than 28.5 million people belonged to HMOs.

Several observations are noteworthy in regard to HMO model types (Table 10-2). It appears there is a clear trend toward IPAs. In June 1987, for example, nearly two thirds of all HMOs were IPAs versus only 35% of the total as recently as 1983. Notably, some of the oldest HMOs are group or staff models; until recent years these have accounted for a sizable proportion of HMO enrollment.

IPAs have become increasingly popular among both providers and consumers for a variety of reasons. To providers, IPAs are perceived as offering more freedom in the practice of medicine than group or staff plans. Consumers often prefer the opportunity to choose from a broad panel of physicians, possibly including the physician(s) they visited even before joining the HMO. This preference toward IPAs is clearly evidenced by HMO enrollment figures. In 1983 IPAs ac-

Table 10-1. HMO growth, 1980-1987

	Number of HMOs		HMO Enrollment	
	Number of HMOs	% Growth from previous year	HMO enrollment	% Growth from previous year
June 1980	236	—	9,099,858	—
June 1981	243	3.0	10,266,172	12.8
June 1982	265	9.1	10,826,729	5.5
June 1983	280	5.7	12,490,780	15.3
June 1984	305	9.3	15,140,756	21.2
June 1985	393	28.4	18,893,607	24.8
June 1986	595	51.4	23,663,626	25.2
June 1987	662	11.3	28,587,119	20.8

Table 10-2. Growth in number of HMOs by model type, 1980-1987

	Staff		Group		Network		IPA	
	Number of HMOs	Percent of total	Number of HMOs	Percent of total	Number of HMOs	Percent of total	Number of HMOs	Percent of total
June 1980	63	26.7%	76	32.2%	*	—	97	41.1%
June 1981	44	18.1	88	36.2	21	8.6	90	37.0
June 1982	57	21.5	80	30.2	31	11.7	97	36.6
June 1983	59	21.1	86	30.7	36	12.9	99	35.4
June 1984	53	17.3	70	22.9	57	18.6	126	41.2
June 1985	55	14.0	71	18.1	86	21.9	181	46.0
June 1986	71	11.9	86	14.5	93	15.6	345	58.0
June 1987	64	9.7	74	11.2	107	16.2	417	63.0

*The Office of Health Maintenance Organizations (OHMO) collected the 1980 model type data. OHMO did not break out network plans from the group category.

counted for only 15% of all HMO enrollment, but by 1987 this proportion had increased to nearly 40% (Table 10-3).

Since 1985 InterStudy has collected data on the number of for-profit versus nonprofit HMOs. Between 1985 and 1987 there was a significant increase in the proportion of plans that are for-profit: from 36% to 66%. It should be noted in interpreting this statistic that many nonprofit HMOs are operated by for-profit management companies, because some state regulations prohibit HMOs from being for-profit entities. Thus the 66% for-profit figure for 1987 may not even reflect the full involvement of for-profit firms in the ownership and/or operation of HMOs. Nevertheless, the for-profit plans represent more than half of all HMO enrollment.

The substantial growth of HMOs in the 1980s has resulted in the distribution of HMOs to all regions of the nation. When HMOs first began, they were primarily a West Coast phenomenon, with some slight presence in parts of the Midwest. By June 1987 HMOs were operational in all states but Alaska and Mississippi. The following 10 states had 20 or more HMOs in 1987: California, Colorado, Florida, Illinois, Michigan, New York, Ohio, Pennsylvania, Texas, and Wisconsin. These states also accounted for 63% of total HMO enrollment. For several of these states, the strong HMO penetration can be quite readily explained. California, for example, has been the home of the Kaiser Foundation Health Plan since the mid-1940s. Kaiser has thus experienced nearly 4 decades of growth, compared with less than 10 years' growth for most other plans. Florida consistently has had substantial HMO penetration, in part because of the enrollment of many senior citizens in HMOs with Medicare contracts. One reason Wisconsin and Illinois both have large HMO enrollments is because of strong participation in the state HMO Medicaid programs.

In contrast to these states, a number of others have experienced relatively little HMO growth. Providers in the southern states have historically demonstrated the most resistance to HMOs as they have sought to preserve their traditional way of practicing medicine. In other states, such as Vermont and South Dakota, there has been an insufficient population base and a relative dearth of the midsized and large employers needed to support an HMO. With the exception of their involvement in the senior market, HMOs gain most of their enrollees through contracts with employers. In the absence of enough potential customers, relatively few HMOs have passed the

Table 10-3. Growth in HMO enrollment by model type, 1980-1987

	Staff		Group		Network		IPA	
	HMO enrollment	Percent of total	HMO enrollment	Percent of total	HMO enrollment	Percent of total	HMO enrollment	Percent of total
June 1980	1,673,401	18.4	5,732,255	63.0	*	—	1,694,202	18.6
June 1981	1,137,332	11.1	6,702,370	65.3	844,795	8.2	1,581,675	15.4
June 1982	1,618,231	14.9	5,969,625	55.1	1,772,831	16.4	1,470,542	13.6
June 1983	2,145,072	17.2	6,286,369	50.3	2,170,579	17.4	1,888,760	15.1
June 1984	2,066,742	13.6	6,597,783	43.6	3,531,298	23.3	2,944,933	19.5
June 1985	3,211,913	17.0	4,345,530	23.0	3,589,785	19.0	7,746,379	41.0
June 1986	3,135,830	13.3	7,118,377	30.1	4,955,262	20.9	8,454,157	35.7
June 1987	3,079,308	10.8	7,285,902	25.5	6,895,375	24.1	11,326,534	39.6

*The Office of Health Maintenance Organizations (OHMO) collected the 1980 model type data. OHMO did not break out network plans from the group category.

feasibility stage in some of the less populous states.

In the early days of HMOs most plans were freestanding entities not affiliated with any other HMOs or organizations. The impetus for founding HMOs usually came from providers, consumers, and/or employers in local communities. In the last several years there has been a great upsurge in start-ups and buyouts by national HMO firms. For this chapter we will define a national HMO firm as a company that owns and/or manages HMOs in two or more states (Table 10-4).

The first major surge of national firm activity, reaching its peak in 1985, consisted mostly of new plan start-ups by national HMO management firms. Having achieved some success in local communities, various regional and national firms duplicated their efforts in a number of target markets around the nation. These start-ups met with mixed results. While some of the new plans prospered, others found it difficult to remain operational long enough to break even.

More recently, much of the national firm activity has centered around mergers, acquisitions, and joint ventures. These have included some major shake-ups in the industry and have resulted in the emergence of several major national players. Maxicare Health Plans, Inc. became the second largest national HMO firm when it acquired the HMO holdings of HealthAmerica Corporation and HealthCare USA in 1986. In August 1987 Maxicare was operating 37 HMOs in 25 states. United Healthcare Corporation grew to be the fifth largest firm in terms of membership when Peak Health Care, Inc. and Share Development Corporation became divisions of the firm—boosting enrollment beyond 900,000 through 28 HMOs. A new company, Equicor, was formed in 1986 when Equitable Life Assurance Society of the United States merged its group life and health lines and combined with the HMO base of Hospital Corporation of America. Equicor now operates 21 HMOs in 13 states. Not surprisingly, many of these national firms are diversifying into the full spectrum of managed care so that they can maximize their market penetration. It seems likely that national firms will remain as a major presence in the marketplace.

UTILIZATION MANAGEMENT

One of the distinguishing characteristics of a managed care health plan is its use of utilization review techniques to control health care costs. Presumably the object of this aspect of managed

Table 10-4. HMO affiliation with national firms, 1980-1987

	1980	1981	1982	1983	1985	1986	1987
Number of national firms	7	8	10	14	24	42	41
Number of HMOs in national firms*	26	36	60	81	156	310	320
Number of enrollees in national firms† (in millions)	4.6	5.1	5.9	7.1	11.1	15.6	18.0

*Figures for 1980, 1981, and 1985 are from June; 1982 and 1983 figures are from March; 1986 figure is from December.
†Figures for 1980, 1981, and 1985 are from June; figures for 1982 and 1983 are from December 1981 and 1982, respectively. National firm data are not available for 1984.

care is to prevent unnecessary care and to see that the needed services are rendered in the most cost-effective settings.

Common utilization review techniques are: preadmission screening of potential elective hospitalizations, concurrent review of admissions by nurse reviewers, estimation of length of stay for admissions, designation of certain procedures that are to be performed in an outpatient setting, discharge planning that is coordinated by health plan utilization review personnel, and second opinion programs for surgical procedures.

Other utilization control/cost control techniques utilized by HMOs and other managed care health programs include: mandatory drug formularies, primary care physician gatekeepers, and select case management of potential high-cost cases. Drug formularies are lists of drugs that have been determined to be less expensive than comparable brand-name pharmaceuticals. Primary care physician gatekeeping is a method of motivating the primary care physician to coordinate all the patient's health care needs, especially specialty care services, to ensure that only medically necessary services are provided. Typically, an enrollee of a gatekeeper-managed health plan is required to select one medical office out of the plan's finite list of offices from which he/she must receive his/her care. The enrollee assumes the financial risk of receiving health services from other providers for whom a referral authorization has not been preapproved by the primary care physician gatekeeper.

Case management of potential high-cost cases goes a step beyond primary physician gatekeeping and introduces additional personnel, that is, registered nurses, social workers, rehabilitation experts, who monitor the case day by day and coordinate the care plan with the physicians involved.

Health maintenance organizations are not the only managed care plans that make use of the array of utilization review techniques. Third-party administrative firms sometimes use a telephone utilization review process to ask the admitting physician whether a new admission meets the insurance companies' admission criteria. In other instances, a non-HMO managed care plan may utilize retrospective review of claims looking for lengths of stay out of the norm and patterns of care that raise the issue of inappropriateness. Preferred provider organizations have adopted some of the common utilization review techniques as well. For-profit review organizations have emerged to serve self-insured companies and independent third-party payer organizations.

Whether the institution of utilization review

techniques has a deleterious impact on patients needs thorough research. Siu et al.[14] conducted a randomized trial of hospital utilization for discretionary and nondiscretionary medical and surgical conditions for 122 traditional fee-for-service insurance plan patients and 122 HMO patients (from Group Health Cooperative of Puget Sound). The study covered a 5-year span—1976 to 1981. Researchers were seeking "to determine whether the HMO accomplished savings in hospital use by avoiding discretionary admissions alone or by avoiding nondiscretionary ones as well." The researchers concluded:

> The rate of discretionary surgery was lower in the HMO, while the rate of nondiscretionary surgery was equivalent in the two systems. For medical admissions, rates of discretionary and nondiscretionary admissions were lower in the HMO. There were no observable adverse effects on health from the lower rates of nondiscretionary hospitalization either because the net effect on health was small or because the HMO substituted appropriate ambulatory services. We conclude that HMO reductions in hospitalization rates do not occur "across the board", discretionary surgery is selectively avoided.

On this last point, the researchers explained that when "surgery was inappropriate or potentially avoidable, surgery was less likely to occur at the HMO."

Caution is advised against making the assumption that this research is generalizable to other managed care plans, and one must ponder whether the application of more recently validated admission appropriateness criteria would produce different results than the Siu study. In any event, more research is certainly needed for cases undergoing utilization review in the late 1980s.

Some health care experts believe that our swiftly changing health care delivery scene calls for "a second generation review system"[17] to link with management information systems, claims processing, and provider reports. Coupling this sentiment with the amazing growth of HMOs and other managed care plans, it is quite apparent that the practice of medicine will undergo even greater intrusions by buyers aimed at achieving their cost-containment goals.

As more chipping away at the mountain of medical sovereignty[15] takes place, is the territory of one medical specialist more encroached upon than another's by utilization review? Certainly, in the gatekeeper model, managed care plans' primary care physicians (family practitioners, internists, obstetricians, and pediatricians) are on the front line with respect to obtaining preadmission certification for elective surgeries, compliance with health plan mandated drug formularies, screening referrals to specialists and maintaining close communication with the specialists to whom they refer cases, and cooperating with health plan utilization review coordinators in the discharge planning task.

Considering a generally accepted fact that primary care physicians actually see a greater volume of HMO and managed care plan patients than surgical specialists, one can conclude that primary care physicians must deal with the array of utilization control protocols more frequently than surgical specialists.[10]

This is not to say that surgeons can distance themselves from utilization processes altogether. If the surgeon is the admitting physician, he/she will be communicating with the health plans's utilization review personnel regarding the reasons the admission is necessary. Once preadmission certification has been approved, the surgeon and/or primary care physician on the case will be questioned about the length of stay if the patient is not discharged according to the estimated length of stay guidelines adopted by the patient's health plan. If the surgeon is operating within the confines of a gatekeeper health plan, he/she may be asked to communicate during the course of the case with the patient's primary care physician, particularly about discharge plans. If the surgeon prescribed drugs, and the health plan utilizes a drug formulary list, he/she will be expected to select formulary drugs unless there is a specific medical reason that necessitates a "dispense as written" order.

Two utilization controls that affect surgeons in particular are second opinion surgery programs and ambulatory surgery procedure lists. Despite a lack of proven efficacy for second opinion programs, major employers (and soon the federal government through PROs) tenaciously promote the programs, as evidenced by the more than 25 million persons currently mandated to comply with the perceived cost saving process.[2] Typically, the programs require patients who have been told they need surgery by one surgeon to obtain the opinion of a second surgeon before the managed care health plan will approve surgery. Most second opinion programs do not allow the second surgeon consulted to perform the surgery in an effort to ensure an unbiased opinion. A minority of companies, however, do allow the physician rendering the second opinion to perform the operation if the patient desires that surgeon, to allow patients full choice of provider.

On the one hand, surgeons who consult for second opinion programs have a new source of income; on the other, there is more intrusion into their once singularly closed profession.

In the late 1970s rapidly escalating health care costs set the stage for bold moves by third-party payers, such as Blue Cross/Blue Shield plans, to contain costs through policies prohibiting payment for duplicative diagnostic tests and the development of ambulatory procedure lists. Formerly performed only in the inpatient hospital setting, procedures on these lists were to be performed in an ambulatory setting to reduce costs. Physician advisory committees and local specialty societies were consulted in the formation of the lists. Shortly thereafter, familiar procedures like tonsillectomies and D&Cs were removed to outpatient surgical suites. The adjustment factor was greater for the patients than it was for the surgeons involved. But surgeons and their auxiliary staff had new responsibilities determining which patients could safely withstand the outpatient procedures and preparing those who can for the home recovery. Ambulatory procedure lists have undergone many revisions through the 1980s and are firmly entrenched as a staple of managed care plans.

The solid acceptance of ambulatory surgery has given rise in the 1980s to construction of freestanding "surgi-centers" by hospitals and groups of entrepreneurial physicians not only as a means to produce less costly services but also as a convenience measure in response to market demand.

With the marked shift to render services in the ambulatory setting, managed care plans must create processes to ensure that the procedures scheduled are truly necessary, will be performed by efficient qualified providers, and can be accomplished at a less costly rate than if done in a hospital. A concomitant quality concern raised by the increase in ambulatory procedures is sufficiency of patient instructions about recovery and care at home after the procedure. Here the attending physicians and allied health care staff should agree, in advance, about the content of the instructions and which member of the staff explains them to the patient.

Utilization management began during the cost-containment crisis of the late 1970s and has expanded and been embraced in the present decade by large health care organizations that have as their aim the mastery of managed health care. Physicians, once loath to accept interference with their established hospital practice patterns and professional judgment, by now seem to accept, if not somewhat reluctantly, utilization control protocols and utilization review personnel as integral parts of medical practice in the new age of managed health care.

COMPENSATION UNDER MANAGED HEALTH CARE PLANS

Discussion of compensation for physicians and surgeons who participate in HMOs and other managed health care plans begins with an understanding of the various models of health plans fitting into the managed care genre. With regard to HMOs, model types include: staff, group practice, network, and the individual practice association (IPA). Preferred provider organizations and preferred provider arrangements evolved after the early growth of the HMO industry in the mid-1980s and are generally considered the other major players in the managed care industry.

There are three basic methods of physician payment in the four HMO model types described above: fee-for-service, capitation, and salary. Under a fee-for-service payment methodology, the managed care plan will either purchase or develop its own fee schedule, based on historical charges. The plan will typically select a percentile, such as 80th percentile, from the range of fees, procedure by procedure, and reimburse physicians that amount.

As a cost-containment incentive, HMOs using this payment method often hold back a certain percentage of the tabulated reimbursement and place the amounts into escrow funds. At year end, physicians' utilization performances are compared with the HMO's preestablished utilization goals, that is, days of hospitalization per 1000 enrollees and hospital admissions per 1000 enrollees. The amount of payment withheld, or escrowed, as a portion thereof, will be paid to the physicians depending upon their individual performance or the performance of the group they are in, such as all family practice physicians in the plan.

The rudiments of capitation are (1) determination of a fixed monthly amount to be paid to the physician group for various categories of enrollees (non-Medicare adult, pediatrics, and Medicare) to cover their total health needs as specified in the HMO's benefit package (ambulatory care—provided by primary care physicians and specialists, hospital care, and home health care); and (2) risk sharing levels between the contracted provider groups and the health plan. For instance, some HMOs have multiple provider contracts with varying levels of risk for the physician groups to assume. Often, contracting groups of large size (in terms of members of physicians in the group, number of enrollees signed up with their office, and percentage of revenue received in a particular HMO) will negotiate substantial levels of risk, that is, 100% for physician group, 0% for the HMO, based on the group's ability to absorb negative risk. If an HMO is recruiting a small primary care office network, it may offer a shared risk arrangement, such as, physician group responsible for 50% of positive and negative risk—HMO same level of risk in the first 24 months of the contract to ensure that the physician group is financially and philosophically capable of dealing with the uncertainties of case mix and resultant utilization rates.

Capitation is the most complicated of the three payment methodologies from the standpoint of data collection, claims payment–pool allocation, and contracting. A criticism of capitation is that it holds the greatest temptation for underserving enrollees.

Staff model HMOs employ the salary method of physician reimbursement. Quite often a base salary is offered with bonus potential based on the financial state of the HMO at the end of the year. Some HMOs also tie bonuses to physician performance based on HMO-established criteria.

PPOs make greatest use of the fee-for-service approach. Three strains of fee-for-service reimbursement have been identified:[7]

1. Straight discounting from established fee schedules: physician fee schedules are established by the PPO or purchaser with physicians paid typically the lower of their charge or the established fee schedule.

2. Usual, customary and reasonable fees based on preestablished conversion factors: a number of conversion factors are utilized in attempting to standardize fees paid to specialists for similar services. A comprehensive study of current physician fee schedules is typically a condition precedent to effective utilization of this reimbursement methodology.

3. Usual and customary fees with holdback arrangements provide utilization management incentives: targets are set up for utilization of services, which serve as the basis for disposition of amounts withheld from physician fees. If utilization targets are achieved by physicians, a return of the withhold or a portion thereof is affected. Failure to reach utilization targets will result in retention of all or a portion of the withheld amounts.

FINANCIAL INCENTIVES

Traditional undiscounted fee-for-service produces incentives two ways. A positive incentive is created for the fee recipient to supply more services than are possibly needed. Except for a physician's ethical[12] or individual commitment to be conservative when taking inventory of the patient's needs, fee-for-service also represents a disincentive to be prudent in the production and ordering of services.

A variety of financial incentive arrangements exist in HMOs and other managed care plans. Commonly, these are bonus, fee withhold, bonus and withhold, full risk, no risk, and shared risk.[3] The principle behind managed care plan incentives is that they stimulate physicians to be cost conscious. The realization of plan-established utilization goals will result in greater compensation for the physician.

In addition to financial incentives is the more intangible incentive of exemplary performance in the eyes of the physician's peers through production of quality health care. As the surplus of physicians continues to be felt in the United States, and competitive market forces accelerate, the incentive to achieve "preferred" status in the eyes of consumers, purchasers, and recruiters of physicians may be the greatest prize of multiple incentives.

Currently, the emphasis of the public at-large and physician opponents of prepaid health care seems to be a concern that compensation incentives produce a singular serious conflict of interest for physicians—which interest shall they serve, their own or their patient's? Arnold S. Relman, MD, editor of *The New England Journal of Medicine,* presents the position that physicians must not abandon the traditional physician/patient relationship and the corollary principle that the patient's interest takes precedence over all other considerations. Dr. Relman writes:

> The essential features of that special relation are, first of all, that except in emergencies, a physician is free to choose whom he will serve. But once he accepts responsibility to serve a patient, the physician is obligated to act as the trustee for the patient's interest, and whenever possible, with the patient's informed consent. In serving as the patient's trustee, the physician is expected to apply generally accepted professional standards of care, always for the patient's benefit. The patient's interest takes precedence over all other considerations—certainly over any financial or other personal interests of the physician.

In an exhaustive study of 302 HMOs regarding financial incentives for physicians, Alan L. Hillman, MD, writes:[5]

> The question is where to draw the line. At what point does a financial incentive create a conflict of interest, in which physicians' behavior may be motivated substantially by pecuniary self-interest rather than by the patient's best interest? At one end of the spectrum are incentives that reward or penalize an individual physician substantially for the parsimony of his or her approach to individual patients. At the other end are programs that tie moderate incentives to the experience of groups of physicians with pools of patients. Whereas incentives that encourage the use of resources have always existed in traditional fee-for-service practice, cost has not been a concern in the past, and our society has valued an approach to health care that relies on the heavy use of resources. Potential conflicts of interest have been less of a concern under this arrangement, as long as practitioners have acted on behalf of the patient. In contrast, incentives that favor the conservation of resources ignite much opposition and concern about their potential effect on the quality of patient care. As HMOs continue to grow and as more physicians continue to

sign contracts with them, these concerns will intensify.

Financial incentives may take the form of penalties, rewards, or both. Physicians may be at risk of losing a percentage of their payment that is withheld in the case of deficits, or they may be rewarded with bonuses in the case of surpluses. In addition, capitation payments—with physicians guaranteeing a comprehensive range of defined services for a fixed price—have inherent risks. But is there a conflict of interest?

Dr. Hillman ends his written description of the research by stating:

> In conclusion, HMOs use a wide variety of contractual obligations to encourage cost-conscious behavior by primary care physicians. HMOs that use certain strong financial incentives, especially in combination, should be examined to determine whether physicians affiliated with those HMOs are able to act in the best interests of the patient. Certainly, physicians' natural inclination is to act on behalf of the patient, and they react to other stimuli than the purely economic. Nonetheless, we must structure financial incentives carefully so as to avoid encouraging physicians to conserve health care resources excessively, thus creating a conflict of interest.

LEVEL OF COMPENSATION

To thoroughly assess the impact of managed health plans on physician income levels, one must consider: the specialty of the physician, the physician's office overhead, and percent of business (or percent of patient load) that can be attributed to each managed care plan in which the physician participates and the types of managed care plans to which the physician belongs.

As a general rule, independent surgical specialty groups are not paid by the capitation method (except in some multispecialty groups) but are most often paid via discounted fee-for-service or salary, if they are part of a staff model plan.

Goodman and Swartwout published a report in 1984 on the effects of financial arrangement and organizational setting on the socioeconomic aspects of four health care delivery systems that they described as: solo fee-for-service, group fee-for-service, independent practice association, and prepaid group practices.[4] A portion of their findings reveal:

> On average, patient care physicians earned $80,800 after expenses in 1979. Physicians in group FFS arrangements had the highest average net incomes (29% higher than physicians in PGP, who had the lowest net incomes). Professional expenses were highest in group FFS practices and lowest in PGPs; physicians in PGPs had approximately one-half the expenses of group FFS physicians. The significant differences in professional expenses provide an interesting "organizational effect" between individual physician practices and group arrangements. On the one hand, physicians in solo practice arrangements, regardless of payment system, are responsible for their own professional expenses. On the other hand, physicians in group arrangements are less likely to monitor their own expenses, because expenses are, in general, proportionally allocated among all members or partners in the group.

> These data indicate that income maximization is clearly not a goal of physicians in PGPs; physicians in this delivery system tend to emphasize the nonpecuniary aspects of medical practice. Two alternative explanations are equally plausible. First, physicians in PGPs are significantly younger than physicians in other arrangements and may not have established a financially viable medical practice. Second, the lack of practice opportunities in alternative delivery systems, coupled with competitive pressures from an increasing supply of physicians in certain locations, may compel physicians to join closed panel groups with a guaranteed, although significantly lower, professional remuneration for services.

The authors conclude:

> We have examined the socioeconomic aspects of four health care delivery systems. Differentials between solo FFS, group FFS, PGP, and IPA practitioners were almost all statistically significant

with respect to individual physician characteristics, personal practice preferences, medical practice economics, health system organization, and area market characteristics. On the one hand, physicians in solo FFS practice were more likely than physicians in other practice arrangements to be older, to be non-board-certified, to be graduates of a foreign medical school, to prefer autonomy over earnings or practice location, to have more patient visits, longer hours, and shorter waits for an appointment, to provide more services to patients without health insurance coverage, and to locate in more rural areas. On the other hand, PGP practitioners could be characterized as being younger, preferring a specific practice location and a predictable schedule to high earnings, having lower incomes and expenses coupled with fewer patient visits, shorter work weeks, and substantially longer patient waiting times, and locating in high medical resource areas, SMSAs, and communities with a relatively affluent patient population.

Given the limitation of our data, we were able to determine several organizational and payment effects between systems. However, a consistent differential between health care systems regarding organizational setting or financial arrangement did not emerge.

The authors call for more research, particularly because of the fast-changing competitive environment, which in 1984 prompted the emergence of for-profit health care organizations and the growth of IPAs and preferred provider organizations.

A national survey of physicians indicates that in 1985 office-based physicians with HMO affiliations grossed a median of $202,330, which was 11% more than the $182,260 median for all the physicians surveyed.[10] But the "income superiority" was restricted to those practices that had fewer than 40% HMO patients. Physicians whose practices had 60% to 100% HMO patients had a median gross income 40% below the median of all physicians surveyed. Family physicians and pediatricians received the biggest proportions of gross income from HMOs at 13%. Plastic surgeons were at the low end of the scale with a median of only 5% of gross income derived from HMOs.

Looking at size of practice, the median for physicians in large groups (50 or more physicians) was 23% of gross income from HMOs. This compares with 9% for two-doctor practices. Single-specialty groups grossed 9%, while multi-specialty groups achieved 15% of gross income from HMOs.

Since 1985 enrollment in HMOs nationwide has grown from 21 million people to almost 29 million as of September 30, 1987.[6] Growth in other managed care products, such as PPOs and "open-ended" HMOs, has grown as well. The impact of this growth on physician income levels is hard to project without having access to research precisely on point.

Nevertheless, a national survey on physician earnings reveals a significant increase in 1986 income for 13 specialties.[11] Surveyed physicians' median individual profits from practice for 1986 rose 10% ($10,270) to $112,790. It was indicated that this amount represents "the biggest annual dollar gain ever registered and the biggest percentage increase since 1979 when median practice net leaped 12.8%." With the inflation rate slowing from 13.3% to 1.1% in that 7-year period, the authors posit an increase in physician purchasing power. They quickly point out, however, that these positive events are tempered by an increase in professional expenses—up to 10.6% in 1986. Median patient visits per week dropped to 102 from 103 in 1985, according to survey data, and the authors conclude that "doctors owe their latest income gains mainly to higher charges." They cite the 1986 Consumer Price Index to support this, noting that charges for physician services rose 7.8% overall for 1986, when the index for all services increased by only 4.4%.

A more recent national survey reviewing 1987 physician fees revealed "hefty fee hikes" in primary care and "examples of notable restraint in the surgical specialties." Reasons cited for the fee increases in primary care specialties included a movement toward more appropriate charges for services that had been undervalued and the appearance in the office of patients with more complex maladies who previously would have been cared for in the hospital. Survey analysts speculate that fee restraint on the part of surgical specialists may be a result of competitiveness for referrals and a conscious effort to be price sensitive.[8]

PHYSICIAN SATISFACTION

The Henry J. Kaiser Family Foundation sponsored a survey on the attitudes of physicians, employers, and the public towards health maintenance organizations (HMOs) in 1980. A second survey was conducted in 1984, and the results were published in 1986.[16]

With the growth and penetration of HMOs in the marketplace, the authors of the survey noted a change in attitude of physicians from hostility in 1980 to a much more positive overall attitude in 1984:

> In the past, many doctors and leaders of organized medicine were extremely hostile to prepaid practice. Now the nation's physicians are becoming increasingly positive about HMOs. By 1984, 50% of the country's physicians said they were at least somewhat favorable to HMOs. IN 1981, only 36% had been favorable. Many of the country's physicians still have deep reservations about HMOs, but the trend is clear. Physicians are becoming steadily more positive about prepaid plans.

The survey also revealed that HMO subscribers were generally well pleased with the medical care they received. Ninety percent of HMO members surveyed were satisfied with the quality of their doctors, and 76% were satisfied with the quality of hospital care. Level of satisfaction among HMO members slightly exceeded that of patients who received care on a fee-for-service basis.

In 1988 growth in HMOs continues to march on. Enrollment is expected to exceed 30 million persons, compared with 17 million in 1984. As prepaid health care becomes a bigger part of a physician's practice, it is difficult to predict what direction physician attitudes will take. We know that physicians who participate in managed care plans have had a variety of significant changes thrust upon them and that these changes have prevailed outside the reach of physician control and anti-HMO rhetoric. Areas of change include: payment methodology, that is, capitation, discounted fee-for-service, plus withholds, a shift away from extended hospital stays toward ambulatory services, growth of for-profit health care corporations managing HMOs, an emphasis on cost containment, and delayed competition on the basis of quality.

In certain parts of the nation, particularly where HMO markets are mature, some physician groups have expressed noisy dissatisfaction with the corporatization of medicine. In Minneapolis two major fights have erupted. A dissident group of physicians who contracted with Physicians Health Plan (PHP) objected in 1986 to PHP management officials' decision to limit enrollees' choice of hospital by stratifying PHP premiums according to amount of choice desired. The dissident group had a long history of objections to management activity and eventually effected an out-of-court settlement. Election of a new board of directors resulted, with a member of the dissident physician group taking over as chairman of the board—the struggle for more physician control apparently having been achieved.

Park Nicollet Medical Center, a 275-physician multispecialty group and chief supplier of MedCenters Health Plan, recently sued MedCenters over allegedly insufficient fees. The matter proceeded to binding arbitration where the decision of the arbitration panel (in support of the physicians) has been challenged by the State Commissioner of Health as too dangerous to the survival of the health plan.

The New England Journal of Medicine featured

an article titled "The Physician Rebellion" in its February 5, 1987 issue.[9] The Minneapolis situation was noted as well as similar developments in other metropolitan areas where HMO enrollment is significant, namely: Los Angeles, Honolulu, West Palm Beach, Florida, and San Antonio.

The authors muse:

> Although much of this conflict centers on HMOs, the issue is not that simple. In many ways the conflict would be much easier to resolve if it concerned only HMOs. Rather, it is a multifaceted issue involving the degree of an individual clinician's control over patient care versus control by some organizational entity, local versus national and physician versus nonphysician ownership and management of those organizations, the degree to which the organization uses professional measures rather than bureaucratic manipulation (or bureaucratic stalling) to influence physicians' practice styles, and the distribution of income to clinicians rather than to administration and overhead...
>
> Regardless of physicians' motives, the conflict generated by these changes is by and large predictable and indeed useful. The practice of medicine is shifting to large-scale organizations. Those organizations are functioning in a highly constrained economic environment and thus are controlling resource use at every level, including day-to-day clinical decisions. Good or bad, this shift parallels the changes that have taken place in virtually every other profession and reflects the realities of the current stage of the life cycle of the field of medicine. As in other fields, this massive change is accompanied by a great deal of uncertainty, and some entrepreneurs are taking advantage of this uncertainty to amass considerable wealth. Also as in other fields, the professionals most affected often try to ignore or block the change rather than take a leadership role, and thus they unwittingly enhance the opportunities for outside entrepreneurs with short-term profit motives.

The authors endorse multispecialty group practices as the medium physicians should consider to gain optimum satisfaction in the existing competitive corporate environment for the following reasons:

> In the long run, physicians must either gain control over premium dollars and take responsibility for the health plans or work for those who do control the plans. Moreover, assuming responsibility for a health plan means assuming financial, organizational, and clinical responsibility for the health of a population.

Finally, physician satisfaction, or lack thereof, might be gauged by current interest in doctors "unions".[1] Since 1980 membership has jumped from 14,000 to 43,000 in the largest physician union in the country—Union of American Physicians and Dentists (UAPD). Physicians Who Care, founded in 1985 in San Antonio, has attempted to expand nationally and the head count is 2000. Independent Doctors of America, with 1000 members, was established in 1986 by a general surgeon from Whittier, Calif., Dr. Frank Rogers.

The thrust of these loosely named "unions" is to more forcefully represent physician interests than organized medical societies can in the present environment of outsider control. The common goal of these organizations is to ensure the survival of private practice. Sanford A. Marcus, the general surgeon who founded UAPD, is not optimistic. He believes fee-for-service will disappear, and major unemployment of physicians will develop. Leaders of the other two "unions" disagree. They believe the public needs to be educated about fee-for-service and the existence of health insurance that offers them free choice of physicians and hospitals. But significant support by the majority of physicians does not exist for doctor "unions." Dr. Marcus himself has admitted that doctors must pick a side in today's "increasingly polarized health care environment":

Either you'll sell out to management and become part of the mechanism that oppresses and exploits your colleagues, or you'll stand together with other worker doctors.... Physicians cling to this entrepreneurial, go-it-alone thing out of pure nostalgia and vanity.[1]

CONCLUSION

This chapter has attempted to summarize the changes managed care has imposed upon physicians in the United States and on surgeons in particular. It is evident that the future holds even more significant changes for surgeons than the present impact of managed care. For surgeons, changes will be forthcoming in these areas: compensation (HCFA is considering implementation of the relative value scale developed by Harvard economist William Hsiao to eliminate the inequity in payment rates for surgical and diagnostic procedures. Medicare payment for many surgical fees will be reduced if Hsiao's plan is adopted); the cognitive/procedural debate will boil over; efficacy of surgical procedures will be closely scrutinized in the attempt to measure quality; quality of surgeon's performance—moving beyond technical competence and including rapport with patients—will emerge; and an examination of the holistic approach to health care will receive greater airing as consumers become more savvy about their bodies and the influence of nonphysical factors on their health.

The successful and content surgeons will be those who understand the necessity of change, who are open to new approaches, and who seek to be involved in the process.

References

1. Bumle D: Where doctor unions are finding new life, Med Econ, Dec 21:63, 1987.
2. Crane M: Second opinions: where are the savings? Med Econ, Feb 2:174, 1987.
3. Gold M: Physician incentive arrangements in prepaid managed care plans (briefing materials presented at Jan 1988 Legislative Conference of Group Health Assoc. of America, Washington, D.C.)
4. Goodman LJ and Swartwout JE: Comparative aspects of medical practice: organizational setting and financial arrangements in four delivery systems, Med Care 22:255, 1984.
5. Hillman AL: Financial incentives for physicians in HMOs: is there a conflict of interest? N Eng J Med 317:1743, 1987.
6. InterStudy: The InterStudy Edge, Excelsior, MN Winter 1987.
7. Johnson JM, editor: Introduction to alternative delivery mechanisms: HMOs, PPOs and CMPs, Washington, DC, 1986, National Health Lawyers Association.
8. Kircher M: Are doctors pushing fees to a breaking point? Med Econ, Oct 5:81, 1987.
9. Kralewski J et al: The physician rebellion, N Eng J Med 316:339, 1987.
10. Owens A: What's prepaid care worth to doctors? Med Econ 64:202, 1987.
11. Owens A: Doctors' earnings on the rise again, Med Econ Sept 7:212, 1987.
12. Relman AS: The future of medical practice, Health Aff Summer: 5, 1983.
13. Shaw G: Doctors dilemma, Harmondsworth Middlesex, England, Penguin Books, Ltd.
14. Siu AL et al: Use of the hospital in a randomized trial of prepaid care, JAMA 259:1343, 1988.
15. Starr P: The social transformation of American medicine, New York, 1982, Basic Books, Inc.
16. Taylor H and Kagay M: The HMO report card, Health Aff Spring:81, 1986.
17. Trauner J: The next generation of utilization review, Business and Health, Feb 1987.

Suggested Readings

Barr JK: Physicians' view of patients in a prepaid group practice: reasons for visits to HMOs, J Health Soc Behav 24:244, 1983.
Barr JK and Steinburg MK: Professional participation in organizational decison making, J Community Health 8:160, 1983.
Barr JK and Steinburg MK: A physician role typology: colleague and client dependence in an HMO, Soc Sci Med 20:253, 1985.
Barr JK and Steinburg MK: Organization structure and professional norms in an alternative health care setting: physicians in health maintenance organizations. In Isershein AW, editor: Challenge and innovation in US health care, Boulder, CO, 1981, Westview Press, Inc.
Berenson RA: Capitation and conflict of interest, Health Aff Spring: 141, 1986.
Boggs HG: Health maintenance organizations: improvement in the regulatory environment, Health Care Manage Rev Spring: 45, 1986.
Daniels N: Why saying no to patients in the United States is so hard, N Engl J Med 314:1380, 1986.

Data Watch: Medicare risk contracting: promise and problems, Health Aff Spring: 183, 1986.

Demkovich L: Are HMOs what the doctor ordered? Modern Maturity Dec: 120, 1984.

Eisenberg JM: The state of research about physicians' practice patterns, Med Care 23:461, 1985.

Ellwood P: Forecast for change: health care organizations and the new medical leadership, J Med Assoc Ga 73:299, 1984.

Fielding SL: Organizational impact on medicine: The HMO concept, Soc Sci Med 18:615, 1984.

Fincham JE and Wertheimer AI: Predictors of patient satisfaction in a health maintenance organization, J Health Care Marketing 6:5, 1986.

Fink R: What does it mean to be an HMO physician? Paper presented to Medical Directors Conference, Group Health Association of America, Washington, DC, Jan 6, 1984.

Freeborn DK: Physician satisfaction in a prepaid group practice HMO, GHAA Journal 6:3, 1985.

Freeborn DK et al: Determinants of medical care utilization: physician's use of laboratory services, Am J Public Health 62:846, 1972.

Freeborn DK, Johnson RE, and Mullooly JF: Length of service, leadership, and outpatient resource use among HMO physicians, GHAA Journal 8:63, 1987.

Ginsburg PG and Hackbarth GM: Alternative delivery systems and Medicare, Health Aff Spring: 6, 1986.

Greenlick MR: The impact of prepaid group practice on American medical care: a critical evaluation, Ann Am Acad Polit Soc Sci 339:100, 1972.

Greifinger TB and Bluestone MS: Building physician alliances for cost containment, Health Care Manage Rev 11:63, 1986.

HMO chains grow faster than independent plans, Hospitals, April 5, 1986.

HMO, PPO growth booms, Am Med News, January 3, 1986.

Hornbrook M and Berki S: Practice mode and payment method: effects on use, cost, quality and access, Med Care 23:507, 1985.

Iglehart JK: Health policy report: Medicare turns to HMOs, N Eng J Med Jan: 132, 1985.

Johnson D: Doctors dilemma: unionizing, New York Times, July 13, 1987.

Johnson RE, Freeborn DK, and Mullooly JP: Physicians' use of laboratory, radiology and drugs in a prepaid group practice HMO, Health Serv Res, 20:525, 1985.

Kahn L: A physician's view of managed care, Health Aff, Fall: 90, 1987.

Kirchner M: Can IPAs save small practices? Medical Econ, July 22, 1985.

Kohrman CH: Medical practice where HMOs dominate: the perspective of physicians in Minneapolis-St. Paul, J Med Prac Manage, 2:81, 1986.

Kosterlitz J: The government health experts, Wall Street pinning their hopes on HMOs, National Journal, November 23, 1985.

Levinson DF: Toward full disclosure of referral restrictions and financial incentives by prepaid health plans, N Eng J Med 317:1729, 1987.

Lichtenstein R: Measuring the job satisfaction of physicians in organized settings, Med Care 22:56, 1984.

Luft H: Assessing the evidence on HMO performance, Milbank Mem Fund Quart 58:501, 1980.

Luft H: Health maintenance organizations: dimensions of performance, New York, 1981, John Wiley and Sons, Inc.

Marcus AC and Stone JP: Mode of payment and identification with a regular doctor: a prospective look at reported use of services, Med Care 22:647, 1984.

McElrath D: Perspective and participation of physicians in prepaid group practice, Am Soc Rev 26:596, 1961.

Mechanic D: The organization of medical practice and practice orientations among physicians in prepaid and non-prepaid primary care settings, Med Care 8:189, 1975.

Mott PD: Hospital utilization by health maintenance organizations: separating apples from oranges, Med Care 24:398, 1986.

Pasternak DP, Tuttle WC, and Smith HL: Physician satisfaction in group practice: a comparison of primary care physicians with specialists, GHAA Journal 7:50, 1986.

Peck P: HMOs: physicians' experience explored, Physicians Management 27:97, 1987.

Peterson ML: Physicians' forecasts of medical practice: why is the glass half empty? Ann Intern Med 97:778, 1982.

Phillips RR and Dorsey JL: A look inside: some aspects of structure and function in forty prepaid group practice HMOs, GHAA Journal 1:16, 1980.

PPOs luring enrollees from HMOs, Modern Healthcare, June 6, 1986.

Proter LW et al: Organizational commitment, job satisfaction, and turnover among psychiatric technicians, J App Psychol 19:475, 1974.

Pinealut R: The effect of prepaid group practice on physicians utilization behavior, Med Care 14:121, 1976.

Reagan MD: Physicians as gatekeepers: a complex challenge, N Eng J Med 317:1731, 1987.

Reece RL: The corporate transformation of medicine in Minnesota: the accelerating industrialization of health care in the Twin Cities, First in a series, Minn Med 66:667, 1983.

Reece RL: The corporate transformation of medicine in Minnesota: the struggle by independent physicians for a place in the Twin Cities, Sixth in a series, Minn Med 67:473, 1984.

Renaissance of the HMO, Boston Consulting Group: Health Care Industry Strategy Series, January 1986.

A report card on HMOs 1980-84, Henry J. Kaiser Foundation, 525 Middlefield Road, Suite 200, Menlo Park, CA 94025.

Savitz S and Roberts P: Some notes on the development of an IPA model HMO, J Ambulatory Care Manage, 9:33, 1986.

Schroeder JL, Clarke JT, and Webster JR: Prepaid entitlements: a new challenge for physician-patient relationships, JAMA 254:3080, 1985.

Smith HL: Quality of working life in a health maintenance organization, J Ambulatory Care Manage 3:37, 1980.

Stein J: How HMOs adapt: a prospective from the inside, Business and Health, Oct 1986.

Tarlov AR: HMO enrollment growth and physicians: the third component, Health Aff Spring: 23, 1986.

Wolinsky FD and Corry BA: Organizational structure and medical practice in health maintenance organizations. In Goldbarb E, editor, Profile of medical practice, Chicago, 1981, AMA, 1982.

Wolinsky FD and Marder WD: Spending time with patients: the impact of organizational structure on medical practice, Med Care 20:1052, 1982.

Wolinsky FD and Marder WD: Waiting to see the doctor: the impact of organizational structure on medical practice, Med Care 21:531, 1983.

MARK SCHLESINGER

Mark Schlesinger received his MS (1981) and PhD (1984) in economics from the University of Wisconsin. At Harvard University, Dr. Schlesinger is currently lecturer in Public Policy at the John F. Kennedy School of Government. He is also the assistant director of The Center for Health and Human Resources Policy.

BRIGID GOODY

Brigid Goody received an MBA from Boston College and an MPH from Boston University. She is currently a doctoral student in the Department of Health Policy and Management at Harvard University's School of Public Health.

11

For-profit Health Care and the Practice of Surgery

MARK SCHLESINGER
BRIGID GOODY

The past 15 years have seen a dramatic growth in the number of investor-owned health care facilities. Few ongoing changes in medicine in the United States have caused as much controversy. Profit making in health care evokes reactions that are both ideological and emotional. For many observers, the distinction between for-profit and nonprofit enterprise goes beyond the legal requirement that individuals who control a nonprofit enterprise cannot share in its financial surpluses. For them, the distinction is viewed as one between private markets and public service, between commercial transactions and "care-giving" relationships.

These broad assessments rest on more specific, though often unstated, predictions about how proprietary ownership affects the behavior of health care providers. The rapidly growing academic literature studying for-profit health care is filled with seemingly contradictory links between ownership form and socially valued outcomes, such as access to services for the poor or adequate quality of care. Some studies suggest that investor-owned facilities are more efficient and as socially responsible as their private nonprofit counterparts. Others with equally sound methodology conclude that health care in for-profit institutions is more expensive and of lower quality. Additional research finds that ownership is essentially irrelevant to the delivery of health care services.

This chapter is intended to clarify the relationships between ownership form and organizational performance as well as to assess their consequences for surgical practices. It identifies a set of mediating factors that shape these relationships and suggests how changes in these mediating factors over time have altered the ways in which institutional ownership affects clinical decision making.

A HISTORY OF THE NONPROFIT AND FOR-PROFIT FORMS OF MEDICINE IN THE UNITED STATES

The relative importance of nonprofit and for-profit medical facilities in the United States has fluctuated considerably over time. Services that are now dominated by nonprofit institutions, such as acute care hospitals, were at one time predominantly investor-owned. Services that now have a substantial proprietary sector, including health maintenance organizations and renal dialysis facilities, were only 15 years ago almost exclusively delivered by nonprofit and public agencies.

These historical fluctuations in market share

have been accompanied by corresponding changes in the role and nature of nonprofit and for-profit health care providers. Three distinct periods emerge from this history.

1900-1950: The Institutionalization of Health Care and the Dominance of Nonprofit Organizations

Throughout most of the nineteenth century, medical care was largely a "cottage industry." Hospitals were principally facilities for treating the sick poor; those with higher incomes were treated at home by physicians. Hospitals and physicians coexisted, the former supported by religious organizations and government subsidies and the latter by fees from patients.[47,68,70] Because of their religious affiliations, most of the hospitals established during this period were nonprofit.

Toward the end of the nineteenth century, the practice of medicine became more complex. Medical education became increasingly specialized, and hospitals evolved into a primary setting for treatment of the very ill. In this evolution, for-profit and nonprofit hospitals retained many of the distinctions that had previously existed between doctors and hospitals. For-profit facilities were generally operated by a single doctor or a small group of physicians and catered to richer patients.[68] The nonprofit hospitals, typically larger, continued to rely heavily on philanthropic support.

As the country grew to the West during the late nineteenth century, there was a rapid proliferation of proprietary hospitals and medical schools. This occurred in large part because nonprofit facilities were scarce in these high-growth regions. State and local governments had withdrawn their subsidies that had been previously available to nonprofit facilities, slowing the expansion of these institutions.[70] By 1900 the growth of proprietary institutions had significantly changed the ownership of medicine in the United States: half of the medical and dental schools as well as 60% of the hospitals were operating under proprietary auspices.

The subsequent 50 years brought increased formalization, standardization, and institutionalization to medicine in this country. The increased complexity raised the cost of both medical training and treatment, creating a greater need for subsidization from private philanthropy.[68] This favored the growth of nonprofit institutions, which could tap religious affiliations,[72] offer deductions from income taxes in return for donations, and which were largely exempt from growing government regulation.[44] By the mid-1920s, there were virtually no proprietary medical schools, only a handful of for-profit dental schools were still in operation, and the proportion of investor-owned hospitals had declined to just more than a third of all facilities.[5,20,72] The remaining for-profit institutions were almost exclusively in fast growing areas, where demand increased faster than philanthropic voluntarism could supply new capital.[69]

This trend was reinforced in the short run by the introduction of health insurance during the 1930s. Faced by proposals for national health insurance and by financially stressed hospitals, the American Medical Association abandoned its earlier opposition to hospital insurance. With the cooperation of the American Hospital Association and enabling legislation passed by state governments, Blue Cross and later Blue Shield were established as nonprofit insurance plans, offering hospital and medical insurance, respectively.

The growth of Blue Cross and Blue Shield initially enhanced the dominant position of nonprofit organizations in health care. By the early 1940s, these nonprofit plans controlled more than three fourths of the health insurance market. Blue Cross negotiated reimbursement rates that were lower for proprietary hospitals than for their nonprofit counterparts.* This exacerbated

---

*This practice has persisted to the present. A recent study using 1979 data found that proprietary hospitals paid discounts to Blue Cross that were 1% to 6% larger than those paid by comparable nonprofit hospitals.[64]

the decline of investor-owned facilities, which by 1946 represented less than 10% of all hospitals.* Nevertheless, the growth of insurance under the auspices of Blue Cross and Blue Shield was to sow the seeds of the eventual rebirth of proprietary health care institutions.

1950-1975: Public Subsidies and the Reemergence of Proprietary Health Care

After World War II, federal policymakers became increasingly concerned with encouraging access to medical care. To this end, legislation was passed subsidizing the delivery of health services to particular groups of patients and parts of the country. Many funding programs made funds available either exclusively or preferentially to nonprofit or public agencies.

However, because nonprofit agencies were relatively slow to expand their capacity, their market share increased only marginally as a result of these preferential subsidies.[36,72] Federal subsidies actually produced a much larger expansion of health care facilities operated by state and local governments. In doing so, these federal policies indirectly altered, and to some extent undermined, the traditional role of private nonprofit health care. The growth of public health care facilities shifted much of the responsibility for caring for the poor to these institutions and away from their private nonprofit counterparts.[25] This shift, coupled with the availabilty of public funds for capital projects, reduced the apparent need for donative financing, one of the chief justifications for nonprofit status.[13]

In the 1960s and continuing through the mid-1970s, governmental subsidies shifted from the "supply side" to the "demand side," from vendor payments to health insurance. The passage of Medicare and Medicaid in 1965 and further amendments to the Social Security Act in 1972 and 1974 reflected this trend and had a significant impact on the mix of ownership in medicine in the United States. By increasing demand far more rapidly than nonprofit organizations could respond, these public programs created a new niche for proprietary facilities. The initial passage of Medicare and Medicaid boosted the market share of investor-owned hospitals and nursing homes. Subsequent expansion of Medicare benefits in 1972 and 1981 encouraged the growth of for-profit renal dialysis centers and home health agencies, respectively. Increases in the market share of investor-owned psychiatric facilities occurred as a result of expanded public contracting with private agencies as well as the spread of state-mandated coverage of mental illness under private insurance.*

Stimulating the growth of proprietary institutions, however, was not the only important legacy of the Medicare/Medicaid legislation for the relative roles of nonprofit and for-profit providers of medical care. This legislation shaped in several ways the health care system and popular attitudes toward medicine in this country. These indirectly but profoundly affected views toward different forms of ownership.

First, by adopting a cost-based system for reimbursing hospital treatment and a generous depreciation allowance for capital purchases, Medicare reinforced existing incentives favoring increased health care spending. The inflation rate for medical services grew dramatically after Medicare's enactment,[38] and national health care expenditures as a percentage of the gross national product virtually doubled between 1960 and 1980.[23] By the late 1970s the magnitude of these costs had become a pressing concern for both private and public purchasers of health insurance. High costs were perceived to result, at least in part, from providers' predisposition toward unnecessarily elaborate and expensive treatments. This disillusionment with

---

*Recent studies have found that investor-owned hospitals to this day are less common in states "in which Blue Cross penetration was high or its discount deep."[49]

*Although short-term growth of proprietary providers occurred for all these services, for some, such as hospitalization, the growth of for-profit facilities has been far more pronounced over the longer term.[66]

professional norms sharpened the debate about the appropriate role for nonprofit organizations in health care,[13] with some observers believing that investor ownership would beneficially reduce physician control over delivery of services.*

Second, the passage of Medicare and Medicaid led to a panoply of regulation. These were at best only partially successful at accomplishing their objectives and appeared least successful at controlling health care costs.[9,12,67] The perceived failure of these regulatory initiatives encouraged policy makers to seek other mechanisms, particularly market-based competition, for achieving socially valued goals. Because proprietary organizations were perceived to be more sensitive to market forces, this shift in policymakers' perspectives encouraged greater acceptance of investor-owned medical facilities.

1975-1985: The Era of Cost Containment and Competition.

Growing concerns about costs have encouraged a number of changes in the health care system including the growth of prospective payment and pre-paid health plans. More important as an influence on the roles of nonprofit and for-profit health care providers has been the increased price competition among suppliers of medical services.

This competition has taken a number of forms. A variety of negotiated arrangements including "preferred provider" and "exclusive provider" agreements have been established to channel patients to particular providers in return for price discounts.[24] Price-cutting pressures on all providers have eroded their ability to cross-subsidize particular services or patients.[27,58]

Price-based competition has significant implications for the role of private nonprofit providers. On one hand, diminished cross-subsidization of patients and services has reduced the ability of nonprofit institutions to offer unprofitable services.* On the other hand, the loss of cross-subsidization and increased dumping of the sickest patients from private facilities has threatened the financial stability of many public institutions.[19] Between 1977 and 1985, 235 short-term hospitals operated by state and local governments were closed, a decline of 13%. Ironically, the need for a charitable role for private health institutions seems to be growing at exactly the time when nonprofit organizations are least able to meet that need.

At the same time there has been a subtle shift in popular expectations about the roles and responsibilities of health care providers in the local community. In the past, patients placed considerable trust in providers' competence and willingness to act in their behalf. This trust has seemingly eroded as a more commercially oriented ethic has developed among providers. These changes have been accompanied by a loss of professional authority and autonomy. A portion of the power previously held by physicians has been shifted to those who previously had acted in supporting roles—the financial and operating officers of hospitals, administrators of group practices, and public and private insurers.

Increased competition and lessened professional autonomy have reduced or eliminated some of the goals and practices that once distinguished nonprofit and for-profit providers of health care. Administrators of nonprofit facilities are advised that, for the good of their institutions and the general public, they must increasingly

---

*For example, a recent survey revealed that 60% of corporate executives and benefits managers favored for-profit over nonprofit prepaid health plans, anticipating that the former would have lower health care costs.[40]

*Recent research has found that when nonprofit hospitals face competition from for-profit hospitals, they discourage admissions by uninsured patients. This competitive effect was as large as the measured difference between nonprofit and for-profit hospitals in their willingness to treat uninsured patients.[51,58]

emulate their proprietary counterparts.* Consequently, nonprofit institutions often mirror the institutional structure of their investor-owned competitors, establishing holding companies, for-profit subsidiaries, multifacility chains, and more overtly hierarchical organizations that create a stronger role and added discretion for nonphysician managers.[17]

Summary: Historical Perspectives on the Role of Nonprofit and For-profit Health Care Providers

This historical review suggests that there is a "life cycle" in the role of nonprofit providers. As new services develop through technologic or social innovation, the initial pioneers are almost exclusively private nonprofit agencies. This occurs in part because new services are typically expensive and require subsidization from donations or other sources. In addition, innovators in health care have traditionally been motivated in large part by nonpecuniary goals, and these may be more compatible with the goals of nonprofit as compared with for-profit agencies.[75]

As a health service gains broader acceptance, it enters a second developmental stage represented by two major changes. First, the demand for services by private purchasers increases.† If this increase is sufficiently rapid, it will outstrip the capacity of existing nonprofit providers, forcing those who seek services to turn to alternative sources. Because proprietary organizations can rapidly acquire capital from investors, many of the new entrants are organized under for-profit auspices.

The second change involves a shift in public policy. As private demand expands, access to the service is increasingly viewed as a "right", and policymakers become concerned with ensuring adequate access for those unable to pay for care. This concerns leads them to subsidize public agencies to provide services to the poor and uninsured, reducing the apparent need for philanthropically oriented medical providers.

The growth of demand and changing perceptions of appropriate access create pressures that, in the third stage of a service's life cycle, encourage a convergence in behavior between nonprofit and for-profit providers. The resulting entry of proprietary institutions during the second stage eliminates excess demand and forces providers to compete for patients. Increased competition, by reducing institutional surpluses and leading purchasers to be more sensitive to price, lessens the potential for discretionary spending by providers and forces all facilities, whatever their ownership, to be more responsive to the dictates of the market. The growth of the public sector during the second stage reduces the importance of charity care by nonprofit agencies and changes the popular views about the appropriate role of these organizations in the local community. These shifting attitudes reinforce the convergence in performance created by competition.

To understand the complex interaction of nonprofit and for-profit health care providers, it is thus important to understand where a particular service lies in this developmental cycle. For the health care sector as a whole, there will be some services at early stages, some at intermediate, and some at later stages. HMOs, for example, are just moving from the first to the second stage; hospitals are entering the third stage. There may

---

*A recent article addressed to hospital administrators, for example, contained the following advice: "We are all familiar with the stories of hospitals on their last legs that were turned around in short periods of time after being sold to investor-owned corporations. . . . The new leaders didn't see the hospital as a community trust. The change of ownership transformed an otherwise stagnant institution from a care-providing into a consumer satisfying organization. . . . A similar shift in focus for a voluntary hospital that chooses to retain its existing form of ownership will be more difficult. Recent experience suggests that it can take from two to five years. But the necessary changes in focus can be made."[50]

†Most health insurance plans, for instance, do not cover the costs of "experimental" procedures. It is only when such care is provided on a sufficiently widespread basis that it is covered and thus affordable to most individuals.

also be interactions among services. A large proprietary share for one service can speed the evolutionary process for other services as proprietary corporations diversify out of their original markets into new types of care.

COMPARATIVE STUDIES OF NONPROFIT AND FOR-PROFIT HEALTH CARE
Ownership and Health Care Costs

There have been two substantial sets of empirical studies of the relationship between ownership and economic performance: the first focusing on short-stay general hospitals, the second on nursing homes. Investigations of the hospital industry have found only small and inconsistent differences in reported costs of proprietary and nonprofit facilities. Cost per day is generally higher in for-profit hospitals. Because of shorter length of stay, however, cost per admission in investor-owned institutions is estimated to be lower by some studies, higher by others, and about equal in the rest.* Recent studies of the HMO industry indicate there is no evidence that proprietary ownership is associated with the more efficient delivery of services. In particular, HMOs owned by commercial insurance companies, which are almost all proprietary, have higher costs per enrollee. Other system-affiliated plans, however, have significantly lower total costs. This supports the theory that organizational factors other than profit status are important determinants of costs in these organizations.[53,56]

In contrast, studies comparing the average cost of care in nonprofit and for-profit nursing homes have found that for-profit homes have average costs 5% to 15% lower than their nonprofit counterparts.† This research suggests ownership-related differences in costs in facilities where physicians' roles are relatively attenuated, as in nursing homes,[51,72] but not where there is a stronger professional presence. Research on facilities delivering other types of services confirms this pattern. For-profit agencies have lower costs in the provision of laboratory services and health insurance but equal or higher costs for renal dialysis services. Physicians play an important role in the latter service, but not in the former.[21,29,53]

This pattern suggests that professional norms in some way mitigate some of the incentives for cost reduction that might otherwise be found in for-profit settings. Exactly how this occurs is unclear. Professionals may simply be difficult to manage, as a result of their training, their disposition, or the nature of their tasks. Alternatively, professional training may imbue providers with values that limit the extent to which they are willing to reduce costs of care in ways that may lower quality.*

Ownership and Access to Health Care

Health care providers can avoid unprofitable patients in four ways. First, facilities can simply be located away from low-income areas. Second, they can choose not to provide services used disproportionately by the uninsured or underinsured. Third, they can choose not to participate in public programs that provide services to high-risk populations. Fourth, they can actively screen for and discourage admission to those unable to pay for care. Evidence from studies suggests that for-profit providers are more likely to use these methods and that this occurs both in facilities in which physicians play an important role and in those in which they do not.

Screening and the location of the facility. To the extent that facilities avoid patients with limited ability to pay, one would expect them to locate in affluent areas. If for-profit providers are more sensitive to these incentives, they

---

*References 6, 14, 18, 37, 45, 49.
†About half of these are reviewed and summarized in Bishop.[7] Since that review was published, additional research has been completed by a number of investigators.[11,22,28,34,52,71]

*Analysis of cost savings found in proprietary nursing homes show that about three quarters of the savings resulted from cuts in spending on patient (nursing) care.[28]

would provide a higher proportion of services in these areas than in less profitable localities.

Most studies of the relationship between ownership and choice of location examine the location patterns of short-stay general hospitals. These studies have found that the share of services provided under proprietary auspices is highest in states with high per capita income,[35] with rapidly increasing levels of income,[69] and with extensive insurance coverage.[4] These patterns persist whether one focuses on all for-profit hospitals or just those associated with multifacility chains.[42] Similar patterns exist within states where investor-owned facilities locate disproportionately in counties that have relatively few Medicaid patients.[31]

The determinants of location for other types of health care facilities have been less carefully studied, but here too, for-profit providers appear more sensitive to regional differences in ability to pay for care. The proportion of care provided by proprietary psychiatric hospitals is more than 3 times as high in those states with mandated inpatient psychiatric benefits than in those states without such mandated benefits. Proprietary home health agencies are almost 3 times as prevalent in states with "generous" Medicaid programs as in states with lower Medicaid payments.[39]

Screening and selection of services. To screen out patients with limited ability to pay, a facility can be expected to avoid offering two types of services: services that are not reimbursed or underreimbursed by insurance plans and services that are used disproportionately by patients who are uninsured or covered by Medicaid.[64]

Psychiatric hospitals provide several good examples of the first type of service. Emergency telephone and suicide prevention services are generally unreimbursed, since the client is often unidentified and therefore cannot be billed. Home care and day care programs tend, for historical reasons, to be underreimbursed by insurers.[55] Facilities screening on ability to pay would tend to avoid such services, and indeed, surveys of psychiatric hospitals show that for-profit institutions are 4 to 5 times less likely to offer such services than are either their private nonprofit or public counterparts.[55]

Investor-owned hospitals are also less likely to offer services that are used disproportionately by indigent patients, even if those services offer widespread benefits to the local community.[15,32,59,62] The difference between for-profit and nonprofit facilities, however, is less pronounced when each is affiliated with a multihospital corporation.[59,61]

Screening and participation in public programs. Health care providers may avoid high-risk populations by choosing not to participate in public programs that provide services to these populations. Hospitals have never considered nonparticipation in the Medicare program an option, since the program is the source of approximately 30% of their revenue and, until recently, reimbursed them on the basis of costs incurred providing services to beneficiaries.

Health maintenance organizations are, however, faced with a decision of whether to participate in the Medicare Program. If a decision is made to participate, the organization accepts the entire risk associated with the large variability inherent in the health care expenditures of individual elderly enrollees. Two recent studies have examined the hypothesis that for-profit HMOs would be less likely to accept this risk than their non-profit counterparts. In both studies, profit status was not a significant factor in the decision to participate in the program.[1,46]

Screening and admissions policies. Admissions policies can influence the average ability to pay in a facility in two ways. First, exclusionary policies can be used to screen out particular classes of payers, such as the uninsured or those covered by Medicaid. Second, by providing services at a reduced charge, facilities can encourage the patronage of lower-income patients. Facilities that seek more profitable patients can be expected to adopt the former policies but avoid the latter.

For-profit institutions appear significantly more likely to fit this pattern. A 1984 survey of physicians found that investor-owned hospitals are 2 to 3 times more likely than comparable nonprofit hospitals to adopt policies to "discourage admissions" of uninsured or Medicaid patients.[58] A survey of long-term care facilities, including nursing homes, psychiatric hospitals, and institutions for the mentally handicapped, found that proprietary facilities were one half to one quarter as likely to offer sevices at reduced charge as were their nonprofit counterparts.[39]

Net effects of ownership on access to care. Although studies indicate that the greater sensitivity of for-profit organizations to financial considerations reduces access to care for low-income patients, there may sometimes be countervailing effects. Studies have shown that for-profit facilities are quickest to move into rapidly growing regions.[36,42,69] This would promote access in otherwise underserved areas.

It is difficult to assess the net impact of these various aspects of access. The additional uncompensated care provided by private nonprofit hospitals equals about 1% to 2% of their total revenues nationwide, though it is as much as 3% to 4% in some parts of the country.[32,65] Comparable statistics are not available for other types of health care facilities. It is striking, however, that for the various measures of access to care reported here, ownership-related differences appear whether or not health care professionals have strong influence in the facility.

There are several possible explanations for this contrast between studies of access and those of cost reported earlier. To some extent, access to care may be managed without directly interfering with the prerogatives of private practitioners. As stated, though, there is evidence that administrators of for-profit facilities explicitly try to alter the admitting practices of some physicians. Perhaps admission decisions are simply less governed by professional norms and thus more susceptible to influence through administrative controls or financial incentives.

CLINICAL DECISION MAKING IN THE FOR-PROFIT HEALTH CARE SECTOR

The growth of proprietary facilities has raised serious questions about the consequences for treatment decisions made by physicians. These concerns take two forms. First, it has been suggested that physicians who share in ownership of a medical facility will make clinical decisions based, in part, on the financial health of the facility, as opposed to the well-being of their patients.[48] Certainly this potential exists. However, physicians have always been guided to some extent by a concern for the facilities in which they practice—they have too much invested in their affiliation to do otherwise. Whether nonprofit or for-profit, a hospital filled with empty beds will evoke some response from its medical staff—most likely an effort to find more patients. Profit-sharing may lead to less appropriate responses, but this remains largely a matter of conjecture.

The debate over the appropriateness of profit-making in health care strikes closest to home for physicians when it focuses on a second concern—the potential for institutions to influence clinical decision making. Many observers believe that for-profit institutions are more oriented toward the "bottom line" and thus more willing to intrude on physicians' decisions in the interest of the institution's financial condition.

> The truth is that when a for-profit public corporation takes over the ownership of a hospital, a subtle yet profound change takes place in the entire system of health care dispensation . . . the reasons have something to do with the entire network of decision making—decision making on the highest level and therefore affecting the very nature of medicine in the land—being shifted from within the professional domain itself to the backrooms, usually the accounting rooms, of corporate command.[74]

The prospect of institutional constraints on physician behavior has become salient as the market for institutional services has become more competitive and the nature of proprietary ownership of facilities has changed over the past decade. In this environment the only major opportunity for creating or maintaining an institutional surplus lies in reducing costs, which, in many cases, involves altering the extent or ways in which medical care is provided. With motive comes opportunity. The past several years have witnessed the development of sophisticated systems to monitor physician practices and provide feedback on performance to individual practitioners.

Two trends in the nature of proprietary ownership also may explain the growing concern of physicians about potential interference with their practices. First, for-profit facilities are no longer owned solely by the physicians who practice in them. During the past decade the proportion of investor-owned community hospitals that are operated by large corporations grew from 32.7% to 66.9%;[42] corporate ownership of for-profit psychiatric hospitals reached 85% in 1982.[55] Corporate ownership can shift authority from the medical staff or individual physician to the central office, often far removed from their practice. Second, proprietary ownership has expanded from laboratories or drug companies to organizations such as health maintenance organizations and kidney dialysis centers, which have for-profit market shares of 62%[33] and 40%[53] respectively. This extends profit-making incentives and corporate control more directly into the mainstream of medicine in the United States. It creates at least the potential for greater influence over direct patient care.

Organizations may pursue various strategies to realign physician practices with organizational objectives. These strategies include financial incentives, administrative contraints, and shifts in the availability of supportive services. If these strategies are successful in altering physician practices, differences in treatment decisions should be observed between those institutions choosing to implement these strategies and those that do not. There is little empirical evidence of a direct link between ownership and treatment decisions, but this reflects more a paucity of studies than it does negative findings from research.

Physicians' Influence on Health Care Organizations

The relative authority of physicians in health care institutions depends, in part, on their ability to collectively influence a facility's governance. This could take several forms, including membership on the board of trustees, input into budgetary decisions, or participation in management. There has been relatively little research on the links between ownership and physician influence: that which exists is limited almost exclusively to short-stay general hospitals. Nonetheless, several interesting findings emerge from these studies.

Authority is clearly more concentrated in for-profit than in nonprofit organizations. Surveys conducted by the American Hospital Association in the mid-1970s revealed that boards of directors were considerably smaller in for-profit hospitals and were composed almost exclusively of either local businessmen or physicians.[63] Average board size of proprietary facilities ranged from 5.7 to 8.9 members, depending upon the facility's bed size. In comparison, the average board size of voluntary hospitals ranged from 10.2 to 30.4 members. Boards of nonprofit hospitals included representatives of a broader spectrum of the local community, with a commensurately smaller role for medical providers. The average percentage of physician board members in proprietary facilities ranged from 51.7 in incorporated facilities to 63.4 in unincorporated facilities. For non-profit facilities, averages ranged from 4.2% for government nonteaching facilities to 23.7% for religious nonteaching facilities. Sloan concluded from this data that boards of proprietary hospital were probably more efficient decision-making groups.[63] All else equal, this should lead them to intervene to a greater extent in the management of the facility.

Whether this fosters or inhibits physician authority is uncertain. If more aggressive boards reflect the values of their physician members, this could lead to greater authority for the medical staff. If, on the other hand, they are dominated by their representatives in the business community, physician authority would decline. The only published study comparing the relative authority of the medical staff in nonprofit and for-profit hospitals found no significant differences related to ownership, suggesting that either representations on boards had little relationship to true influence over the organization or that increased influence of medical and business interests on proprietary boards effectively offset one another.[10]

Because the expansion of proprietary ownership has been, to a large extent, tied to the growth of multifacility corporations, it is important to consider how system affiliation interacts with ownership in shaping physician influence over health care facilities. Studies of system-affiliated hospitals have concluded that hospitals of the same ownership status are more similar along several dimensions of hospital performance and managerial strategy than hospitals of the same system-affiliation status.[49] For-profit system-affiliated hospitals seem to follow a pattern similar to that of independent investor-owned facilities. They generally have greater physician representation on boards of directors than do their nonprofit counterparts. Physicians on for-profit boards are also more likely to have voting privileges and participate on the board's executive committee.[2,63]

On the other hand, physicians in system-owned proprietary hospitals participate less in managerial activities than do physicians in other hospitals. A recent study examined physician participation in hospital management along several dimensions. Results indicate that physicians in investor-owned system hospitals are less likely than physicians in other types of system hospitals to hold salaried positions as part of the hospital's administrative team. The medical staff in a proprietary hospital is only half as likely to be involved in committees concerned with long-range planning for the facility.[2] The consequences of these differences for the relative authority of physicians have not been carefully studied and remain a topic of considerable debate.[18]

Health Care Organizations' Influence on Physician Practices

A second aspect of the link between ownership and clinical practice involves physician autonomy. As noted previously, organizations may seek to influence physician decision making and circumscribe clinical discretion in two ways: by providing financial incentives and by establishing administrative constraints or rationing of medical resources. In either area, ownership may affect either facilities' willingess or ability to influence physicians' practices.

Financial incentives. By giving physicians an economic stake in an institution, organizations can use financial incentives to realign physicians' practices to match institutional goals. If, for example, the institutional focus is on reducing expenses, incentives might take the form of sharing in cost savings. If the institutional focus is on increasing volume, incentives might be based on a share of the facility's gross revenues. Incentives may also be indirect, created by giving physicians an equity interest, that is, share of ownership, in the organization.

Both hospitals and health maintenance organizations frequently compensate physicians based on the organization's economic performance. For hospitals, these payments are often based on net or gross departmental billings. A recent study showed that physicians associated with for-profit chain hospitals are most likely to receive payments as a percentage of net or gross departmental billings.[43] Little is known about the consequences of these payment policies for clinical decision making, though research has found that physicians paid by a hospital on the basis of gross or net departmental revenues have a significantly smaller proportion of uninsured patients in their office-based practice.[8] Performance-based compensation arrangements thus appear to affect physicians' patient selection criteria. Whether they also affect treatment decisions is unknown.

Health maintenance organizations use a variety of performance-based compensation, ranging from salary with performance bonuses, to fee-for-service, or capitation with a "holdback." Under holdback arrangements, a portion of primary care physician payments is withheld and put into a risk pool. The amount of money redistributed to physicians depends on the cost of the treatment for the plan's patients. The amount of risk transferred to the physician depends on the details of the reimbursement system. Individual physicians can be held accountable for the costs of their own panel of patients or an entire medical group can be held accountable for the collective experience of its patients. Performance can be measured in terms of utilization of primary care services only or all medical care paid by the plan. The most risk is transferred to an individual physician when he is held financially accountable for all aspects of the care of his patients.

Although there do not appear to be ownership-related differences in methods of reimbursing physicians (salary, fee-for-service, or capitation), a higher percentage of for-profit plans (70%) use a withholding account than do their nonprofit counterparts (59%). For-profit plans withhold a larger percentage of payment than nonprofits: 59% of for-profit plans withheld more than 10% of the payment compared with 46% of the nonprofit plans.[30] For-profit plans (23%) are also more likely than non-profit plans (9%) to base the distribution of the risk pool on the experience of individual physicians.[30] Thus, when physicians practice in for-profit plans, they are more likely to face strong financial incentives to restrict the use of medical services by their patients.

The potential effect of these arrangements can be inferred from a recent study by Welch. Modern individual practice associations (IPAs) that put individual physicians or small medical groups at risk had substantially lower hospitalization rates (363 days per 1000 enrollees) than did foundation plans that do not put individual physicians at risk (483 days per 1000 enrollees).[73] These results suggest that financial incentives do affect primary care physician decisions to hospitalize their patients. Whether these reductions in treatment led to inadequate care or simply eliminated unnecessary institutionalization has not been determined.

Physicians' decision making may also be shaped by their ownership of medical facilities. There are many types of physician ownership. The physician may be the sole investor, may be part of a joint venture with the hospital, or may operate franchise operations that are built by investor-owned organizations that take local physicians as minority partners. These may even occur under the auspices of a nonprofit firm that has established proprietary subsidies.

A study of hospital ownership by Musacchio et al. indicates that only 10% of physicians with their primary privileges at for-profit hospitals hold ownership in that facility. The study did, however, find that physician ownership was more prevalent among physicians affiliated with independent for-profit hospitals (22%) than those affiliated with chain hospitals (6%).[43] This suggests that as the proportion of proprietary facilities that are chain affiliated increases fewer physicians will have an ownership interest in their hospital. Physician ownership is, however, more common in other areas of the delivery system. For example, more than three quarters of all free-standing kidney dialysis centers are investor-owned, many of which are owned wholly or partly by physicians.[54]

To the extent that a portion of a physician's income is derived from his investment in a health care facility, there is a potential for conflict between the role of the physician as investor and his role as caregiver. The nature of this conflict will depend upon the proportion of a physician's income that is derived from this investment and his relationship to the facility as either a practicing or referring physician.

Research suggests that physicians' decisions are shaped in part by the financial consequences of ownership. For example, physicians who own laboratory or diagnostic testing facilities order between 30% and 50% more tests than do their colleagues who are not owners.[32] A recent study of kidney dialysis centers offers some indirect evidence on the effects ownership incentives have on clinical decision making. At the time the data were collected for this study in 1983, it was generally more profitable to treat a patient with renal failure in the facility than to provide the patient with either home dialysis, peritoneal dialysis, or a kidney transplant. Controlling for characteristics of patients and the dialysis facility, investor-owned centers were shown to have lower rates of both homes and peritoneal dialysis than were non-profit centers.[54] This suggests that physician ownership did in fact affect treatment decisions, though, again, there is no conclusive evidence that the medical care received in for-profit centers is less appropriate than that received at other facilities.[54]

Administrative controls and resource availability. In addition to providing financial inducements, organizations frequently implement administrative controls over physicians practices. These controls include the granting and revoking of privileges, monitoring of physician practice patterns, and allocating support services. Complex modern administrative systems, which include utilization review and preadmission screening, enable organizations to monitor physician decisions to admit and discharge patients and to order particular services. In the hospital setting the information gathered can be used to restrict or revoke admitting privileges. Likewise, in a health maintenance organization, this information can be used as the basis of salary reviews or contract renewals. Such sanctions are, however, fairly extreme: merely monitoring serves as a reminder that the appropriateness of practice patterns are being judged, in part, by whether they have an adverse effect on the institution's financial performance.

Although empirical evidence concerning the relative prevalence of administrative controls in the proprietary and nonprofit sectors is sparse, there is some sketchy information on hospitals' behavior. Investor-owned system hospitals appear to apply similar criteria for granting privileges as do other hospitals. The same proportion of investor-owned system hospitals require board certification as a requirement of medical staff membership.[41,63] Investor-owned hospitals also appear to take the same time to review physician performance before awarding privileges.[41] There are some sketchy and somewhat contradictory descriptive data collected by the AMA concerning the monitoring of physician practice patterns in proprietary and non-profit hospitals. A slightly higher percentage of proprietary hospitals (83%) formally review clinical decisions than do nonproprietary hospitals (79.8%), whereas a slightly lower percentage of proprietary hospitals set guidelines to reduce length of stay (65.9% versus 71.8%) and review length of stay after discharge (84.9% versus 90.1%).[3] None of these results suggest that proprietary hospitals use administrative controls much more extensively than do nonprofit hospitals.

Proprietary facilities may, however, use controls more aggressively or effectively. Physicians were asked as part of a 1984 AMA survey whether "physicians have greater, less, or the same amount of clinical discretion at a for-profit hospital as they do at a not-for-profit hospital." Nine percent reported that there was greater discretion in for-profit settings, but 28% indicated that discretion was less. Interestingly, by a 3 to 1 margin, physicians affiliated with for-profit facilities also felt that for-profit ownership was associated with reduced clinical discretion.[43]

Physician discretion is also affected by the quality and availability of nursing staff and the operating room schedule.[60] In fact, these types of support services may be more affected by ownership-related considerations. Although decisions about which services to offer are generally made by local boards of trustees with physician input, decisions concerning the nursing staff and operating room schedules are generally made by lower-level administrators. Musacchio et al. asked physicians to compare their primary hospital with other hospitals with which they are familiar along three dimensions: nursing support, responsiveness of hospital administration, and technical resources. Significant differences related to hospital ownership emerged in only one dimension—responsiveness of hospital administration. Physicians at proprietary facilities more frequently reported that administrators were responsive to their needs than did their colleagues at nonprofit facilities.[43]

As the health care system becomes more competitive, however, more ownership-related differences may emerge. A recent study of services provided by nonprofit and for-profit hospitals found that nonprofit and for-profit hospitals in uncompetitive regions were equally likely to offer unprofitable service (as measured by services for which uncompensated care is provided). However, in more competitive areas the proportion of proprietary hospitals offering unprofitable services fell markedly, though services in nonprofit hospitals remained essentially unchanged.[62] This suggests that unprofitable support services in proprietary facilities may become more limited as competition increases. But this will probably occur selectively, since under prospective payment arrangements such as DRGs, different hospitals will judge different types of services to be unprofitable.

Although there appear to be few differences in the administrative constraints on treating patients within nonprofit and for-profit facilities, getting the patients admitted is another matter. As noted earlier, investor-owned facilities are significantly more likely to restrict admissions of unprofitable patients. Surveys conducted by the AMA in 1984 found that 43% of the physicians in independent for-profit hospitals "discouraged admissions" of uninsured patients. This compared with 20% in independent nonprofit hospitals and 14% in independent public hospitals. Physicians (52%) who practiced at system-affiliated proprietary hospitals were significantly more likely to report restricted admissions than were those in independent for-profit facilities.[58]

DISCUSSION AND CONCLUSION

To what extent will the expanding number of investor-owned healthcare facilities affect surgeons' practices? To date, no studies have focused specifically on this question, but the results of more general research provide a basis for speculation. This research suggests three ways in which changing ownership might affect surgeons: the settings in which surgery is performed, the financial incentives offered to surgeons, and the volume of referrals from other physicians.

The potential for profits has already transformed the settings in which surgeons practice. In recent years the number of surgical procedures performed in freestanding ambulatory centers has grown dramatically to an estimated 900,000 procedures in 1986.[17] The opportunity for a high return on investment has clearly encouraged this growth. Most of these facilities are operated on a proprietary basis, more than half by individual or small groups of physicians and about a quarter by larger corporations.[17] In terms of the "product life cycle" described earlier, ambulatory surgical centers appear to be moving from the first to the second developmental stage as ambulatory surgery practices become more standardized and more widely reimbursed by insurance. Precedent suggests that this transformation will be accompanied by a continued rapid expansion of these centers, an even greater influx of investor capital, and a further consolidation of the industry under the auspices of large corporate chains (similar to dialysis centers in the late 1970s). A much greater number of surgeons will find themselves operating in for-profit, freestanding facilities. This will raise new questions for the profession about how to maintain standards of care and physician discretion in these newly developed medical "franchises."

As more surgery is performed in proprietary facilities, both hospital-based and freestanding, surgeons are likely to be increasingly exposed to compensation arrangements that incorporate financial incentives based on the facilities profitability. At present, surgeons are relatively unexposed to incentive-based compensation arrangements: as of 1984 only 11% of all surgeons were compensated by such arrangements, making them among those specialities least commonly paid in this manner (less, surprisingly, than were primary care physicians). As a result, surgeons have had less experience dealing with these incentive arrangements. Both individually and collectively, surgeons will need to develop standards defining the conditions under which incentive payments are appropriate and when they might be viewed as unsuitably affecting clinical decisions.

Finally, surgeons depend to great extent on other physicians to provide patients to them through referrals. Increasingly, these other providers will be practicing in facilities that may provide them with economic incentives that discourage referrals. Studies of the treatment of end-stage renal disease, for example, have found that patients treated at for-profit kidney dialysis centers are less often referred for kidney transplantation. These reductions were not extremely large, about 5% to 10%, but could nonetheless significantly reduce the need for transplant surgeons. As the number of proprietary facilities in health care increases, similar issues will undoubtedly arise in the context of different types of procedures. This is particularly likely as proprietary systems integrate vertically along a continuum of care, channelling patients only to those providers affiliated with the system.

Most important, surgeons' interactions with patients and other providers result in their being affected by the norms and organizational arrangements of the entire heath care system. This makes the answers to broad-based questions relevant to the practices of individual surgeons. Is proprietary ownership transforming surgery in the United States? Does it represent a threat to clinical autonomy? Will it undermine good quality health care? These are all important questions and, at this point, none can be answered conclusively. On the basis of available evidence, we can, however, make some preliminary assessments: the last of these questions seems the least likely to be true, the second somewhat more likely, and the first virtually inevitable.

In facilities where surgeons practice, there is no evidence that ownership has any significant effects on health outcomes,[26] at least as we can crudely measure them at this point.* Physicians' professional norms appear to provide an appropriate safeguard against many of the more egregious forms of profiteering in health care.

But these norms provide neither comprehensive nor uncompromised protection. Surgeons who practice in proprietary settings do operate with more nonclinical influences and intrusions on their decision making. They face significantly greater financial inducements to offer more of some services and less of others. They may have somewhat less discretion, particularly involving patient admissions. When the facility is part of a larger proprietary corporation, physicians are less likely to participate in the day-to-day administration of the facility.

Combined, these factors will almost assuredly reduce clinical autonomy for surgeons affiliated with for-profit facilities. This will not affect all surgeons, nor will it alter the surgical care for the majority of patients. It will, however, produce changes in overall medical care. These will be greatest for services for which professional norms are weakest, for example, laboratory tests or chronic illness; for those aspects of care least

---

*This is, however, not true of all health care facilities. Investor-owned nursing homes, for example, are disproportionately among the lowest quality facilities and, in some cases, unacceptably bad.[57]

related to professional criteria, such as decisions about whether to admit unprofitable patients to the hospital; and for those surgeons whose incomes are most closely linked to the financial performance of the institutions where they practice.

Even if these changes directly affect only a relatively small proportion of the total surgical care provided in the United States, their consequences will be felt more widely. By increasing the relative importance of financial incentives and reducing the influence of the community in the governance of health care facilities, proprietary ownership raises questions about whether the services provided to individual patients are in the best interests of that patient and about whether facilities are being operated in the best interests of the community in which they are located. These doubts can drive a wedge between surgeon and patient, one that is likely to be felt throughout the medical profession. In this sense, for-profit ownership will transform surgery in the United States by altering patients' perceptions and reducing their level of trust. These are not changes that can be readily addressed by remedial public policies. But they are ones that will require some response by surgeons, both in their individual practices and their professional associations.

References

1. Adamache K and Rossiter L: The entry of HMOs into the Medicare market: implications for TEFRA's mandate, Inquiry 23:349, 1986.
2. Alexander J, Morrisey M, and Shortell S: Physician participation in the administration and governance of system and freestanding hospitals: a comparison of ownership types. In Gray B, editor: For-profit enterprise in health care, Washington, DC, 1986, National Academy Press.
3. American Medical Association: SMS Report 3, 1984.
4. Bays C: Patterns of hospital growth: the case of profit hospitals, Med Care 21:850, 1983.
5. Bays C: Why most private hospitals are nonprofit, J Policy Analysis Manage 2:366, 1983.
6. Bays C: Cost comparisons of forprofit and nonprofit hospitals, Soc Sci Med 13:219, 1979.
7. Bishop C: Nursing home cost studies and reimbursement issues, Health Care Financing Rev 2:47, 1980.
8. Blumenthal D: Physician services for the uninsured: who cares, how much and why? Cambridge, Mass, 1987, Working Paper, Center for Health Policy and Management, John F. Kennedy School of Government, Harvard University.
9. Blumstein J: The role of PSROs in hospital cost containment. In McKinlay J, editor: Economics and health care, Cambridge, Mass, 1981, The MIT Press.
10. Carper W and Litschert R: Strategic power relationships in contemporary profit and nonprofit hospitals, Academy Manage J 26:311, 1983.
11. Caswell R and Cleverly W: Cost analysis of the Ohio nursing home industry, Health Serv Res 18:359, 1983.
12. Christianson J: Long-term care standards: enforcement and compliance. Journal Health Polit Policy Law 4:414, 1978.
13. Clark R: Does the nonprofit form fit the hospital industry? Harvard Law Review 93:1416, 1980.
14. Coelen C: 1986. Hospital ownership and comparative hospital costs. In Gray B, editor: For-profit enterprise in health care, Washington, DC, 1986, National Academy Press.
15. Cromwell J and Kanak J: The effects of prospective reimbursement on hospital adoption and service sharing, Health Care Finan Rev 4:89, 1983.
16. Danzon P: Hospital 'profits': the effects of reimbursement policies, J Health Econ 1:29, 1982.
17. Ermann D and Gabel J: The changing face of American health care: multihospital systems, emergency centers and surgery centers, Med Care 23:410, 1985.
18. Ermann D and Gagel J: Multihospital systems: issues and empirical findings, Health Aff 3:50, 1984.
19. Feder J, Hadley J, and Mullner R: Falling through the cracks: poverty, insurance coverage, and hospital care for the poor, 1980 and 1982, Milbank Mem Fund Quart 62:544, 1984.
20. Fraundorf K: Organized dentistry and the pursuit of entry control, J Health Polit Policy Law 8:759, 1984.
21. Frech H: Health insurance: private, mutual or government. In Clarkson K and Martin D, editors: The economics of nonproprietary organizations, Greenwich, Conn 1980, JAI Press, Inc.
22. Frech H and Ginsburg P: The cost of nursing home care in the United States: government financing, ownership and efficiency. In Van Der Gaag J and Perlman M, editors: Health, economics and health economics, New York, 1981, North Holland.
23. Freeland M and Schendler C: Health spending in the 1980s: integration of clinical practice patterns with management, Health Care Finan Rev 5:1, 1984.

24. Gabel J and Ermann D: Preferred provider organizations: performance, problems and promise, Health Aff 4:24, 1985.
25. Gage L Impact on the public hospital, Bull Acad Med 61:75, 1985.
26. Gaumer G: Medicare patient outcomes and hospital organizational mission. In Gray B, editor: For-profit enterprise in health care, Washington, DC, 1986, National Academy Press.
27. Hadley J and Feder J: Hospital cost shifting and care for the uninsured, Health Aff 4:67, 1985.
28. Hawes C and Phillips C: The changing structure of the nursing home industry and the impact of ownership on quality, cost and access. In Gray B, editor: For-profit enterprise in health care, Washington, DC, 1986, National Academy Press.
29. Held P and Pauly M: An economic analysis of the production and cost of renal dialysis treatments. Working paper No 3064-03, Washington, DC, 1982, The Urban Institute Press.
30. Hillman A: Financial incentives for physicians in HMOs, N Engl J Med 317:1743, 1987.
31. Homer C, Bradham D, and Rushefsky M: Investor-owned and not-for-profit hospitals: beyond the cost and revenue debate, Health Aff 3:133, 1984.
32. Institute of Medicine: For-profit enterprise in health care, Washington, DC, 1986, National Academy Press.
33. Interstudy Edge, Excelsior, MN, 1987, Interstudy.
34. Koetting M: Nursing-home organization and efficiency, Lexington, Mass, 1980, Lexington Books.
35. Kushman J and Nuckton C: Further evidence on the relative performance of proprietary and nonprofit hospitals, Med Care 15:189, 1977.
36. Lave J and Lave L: The hospital construction act, Washington, DC, 1974, American Enterprise Institute for Public Policy Research.
37. Lewin L, Derzon R, and Marguiles R: Investor-owneds and nonprofits differ in economic performance, Hospitals 56:52, 1981.
38. Marmor T: Political analysis and American medical care, New York, 1983, Cambridge University Press.
39. Marmor T, Schlesinger M, and Smithey R: Nonprofit organizations and health care. In Powell W, editor: The nonprofit sector: a research handbook, New Haven, Conn, 1987, Yale University Press.
40. Montgomery E. and Paranjpe A: A report card on health maintenance organizations: 1980-1984, New York, 1985, Louis Harris and Associates.
41. Morrisey M, Alexander J, and Shortell S: Medical staff size, hospital privileges and compensation arrangements: a comparison of system hospitals. In Gray B, editor: For-profit enterprise in health care, Washington, DC, 1986, National Academy Press.
42. Mullner R and Hadley J: Interstate variation in the growth of chain-owned proprietary hospitals, 1973-1982, Inquiry 21:144, 1984.
43. Musacchio R et al: Hospital ownership and the practice of medicine: evidence from the physician's perspective. In Gray B, editor: For-profit enterprise in health care, Washington, DC, 1986, National Academy Press.
44. Nielsen W: The endangered sector, New York, 1979, Columbia University Press.
45. Pattison R and Katz H: Investor-owned and not-for-profit hospitals: a comparison based on California data, N Engl J Med 309:347, 1983.
46. Porell F and Wallach S: HMO responses to TEFRA regulations, Working paper, Health Policy Center, Waltham, Mass, 1986, Heller Graduate School at Brandeis.
47. Raffel M: The U.S. health system: origins and functions, New York, 1980, John Wiley and Sons, Inc.
48. Relman A: The new medical-industrial complex, N Engl J Med 303:963, 1980.
49. Renn S et al: The effects of ownership and system affiliation on the economic performance of hospitals, Inquiry 22:219, 1985.
50. Robinette T: Adapting to the age of competition: a paradigm shift for voluntary hospitals, Hosp Health Serv Admin 7:8, 1985.
51. Ruchlin H: An analysis of regulatory issues and options in long-term care. In La Porte V and Rubin J, editors: Reform and regulation in long-term care, New York, 1979, Praeger Publishers.
52. Schlenker R and Shaughnessy P: Case mix, quality, and cost relationships in Colorado nursing homes, Health Care Finan Review 6:61, 1984.
53. Schlesinger M, Blumenthal D, and Schlesinger E: Profits under pressure, Med Care 24:615, 1986.
54. Schlesinger M, Cleary P, and Blumenthal D: The ownership of health care facilities and clinical decision-making: the case of the ESRD industry, Med Care, 1988 (forthcoming).
55. Schlesinger M and Dorwart R: 1984. Ownership and mental-health services: a reappraisal of the shift toward privately owned facilities. N Engl J Med 311:959, 1984.
56. Schlesinger et al: Economic performance of HMOs: the role of ownership and other organizational factors. Paper presented at the annual meeting of the American Public Health Association, New Orleans, LA, 1987.
57. Schlesinger M, Marmor T, and Smithey R: Nonprofit and for-profit medical care: shifting roles and implications for health policy, J Health Polit Policy Law 12:427, 1987.
58. Schlesinger M: The privatization of health care and physicians' perceptions of access to hospital services, Milbank Mem Fund Quart 65:25, 1987.

59. Schlesinger M et al: Multihospital systems and access to health care. In Rossiter L et al., editors: Advances in health economics and health services research, Greenwich, Conn, 1987, JAI Press, Inc.
60. Shortell S: Physician involvement in hospital decision making. In Gray B, editor: The new health care for profit, Washington, DC, 1983, National Academy Press.
61. Shortell S et al: The impact of multi-institutional systems on service provision. In Rossiter L et al., editors: Advances in health economics and health services research, Greenwich, Conn, 1987, JAI Press, Inc.
62. Shortell S et al: The effects of hospital ownership on nontraditional services, Health Aff 5:97, 1986.
63. Sloan F: The internal organizations of hospitals: a descriptive study, Health Serv Res 15:294, 1980.
64. Sloan F and Beckner E: Cross-subsidies and payment for hospital care, J Health Polit Policy Law 8:660, 1984.
65. Sloan F, Valvona J, and Mullner R: Identifying the issues: a statistical profile. In Sloan F, Blumstein J, and Perrin J, editors: Uncompensated hospital care: rights and responsibilities, Baltimore, 1986, Johns Hopkins University Press.
66. Sloan F and Vraciu R: Investor-owned and not-for-profit hospitals: addressing some issues, Health Aff 2:25, 1983.
67. Smith D: Long-term care in transition: the regulation of nursing homes, Washington, DC, 1981, AUPHA Press.
68. Starr P: Social transformation of American medicine, New York, 1982, Basic Books, Inc, Publishers.
69. Steinwald B and Neuhauser D: The role of the proprietary hospital, J Law Contemp Prob 35:817, 1970.
70. Stevens R: 'A poor sort of memory': voluntary hospitals and government before the depression. Milbank Mem Fund Quart 60:551, 1982.
71. Ullman S: The impact of quality on cost in the provision of long-term care, Inquiry 22:293, 1985.
72. Vladeck B: Unloving care: the nursing home tragedy, New York, 1980, Columbia University Press.
73. Welch W: The new structure of individual practice associations, J Health Polit Policy Law 12:723, 1987.
74. Wohl S: The medical industrial complex, New York, 1985, Harmony Books.
75. Young D: If not for profit, for what? Lexington, Mass, 1983, Lexington Books.

STEVEN SIEVERTS

Steven Sieverts has been Vice President, Health Care Finance, of Blue Cross and Blue Shield of the National Capital Area since 1985. Before that, he held a similar position for 10 years with Empire Blue Cross and Blue Shield in downstate New York. He previously served as the general director of the Northern Division of the Albert Einstein Medical Center in Philadelphia in the early 1970s after 8 years as head of the Hospital Planning Association in Pittsburgh. Born in Germany, he was raised in Wisconsin and is a graduate of Haverford College (1956). Mr. Sieverts has an MS in hospital administration from Columbia University (1961).

12

Surgical Second Opinion Programs

IRA M. RUTKOW
STEVEN SIEVERTS

It is rare that the appearance of a single article in a medical journal stimulates fundamental changes in the health care delivery system. This chapter begins with one such paper and goes on to discuss the effects of surgical second opinion programs in the United States.

HISTORY OF SECOND OPINION PROGRAMS

In 1974 McCarthy and Widmer presented the results of an investigation concerning the effects of screening by consultants on recommended elective surgical procedures.[46] They assessed the need for elective operations previously recommended to a group of 1356 union members by reexamining them with board-certified surgical specialists. They found that approximately 24% of all procedures previously recommended were not confirmed by the specialists. Another 2% were confirmed but did not require hospitalization. McCarthy and Widmer reported operating costs that were about one eighth of the estimated savings from hospitalizations not required. Because of the purported cost savings and the demonstrated high percentage of operations not approved, they advocated the implementation of presurgical screening programs. So was born the concept of surgical second opinion programs, which appeared of substantial benefit to any medically insured population.

In the mid-1970s there was growing concern about a rapid rise in rates of elective surgical operations. Some papers stated that the increase from 1971 to 1978 approached 25%.[41] Other research was contradictory, but nonetheless, there was a sense that measures needed to be taken to control rates of surgical procedures and health care expenditures.[53,54,57,60] Because the high cost of hospitalization and surgery is borne in part by employee health plans, the application of an innovative management technique, that is, surgical second opinion programs, to decrease surgical rates and expenses by reducing unneeded procedures seemed logical.

It was not without some precedent that such work was initiated. Historically, the first attempt at a surgical second opinion program occurred in the mid-1950s by the United Mine Workers Union. However, because of organized medicine's vociferous and vehement opposition in eastern Kentucky, western Pennsylvania, and West Virginia, the program was never implemented. Little more was heard about second opinion programs until the early 1970s when the Storeworkers Health and Welfare Fund in New York began seeking ways to reduce "unnecessary" surgery among its members. This interest was passed along to Cornell University Medical College and its Department of Public Health. With labor management welfare funds supplying monetary backing and McCarthy and his associates at Cornell providing program consultation and evaluation, a bold experiment began.

It was this investigation and its eventual presentation in the *New England Journal of Medicine* that provided the impetus for the proliferation of other second opinion programs throughout the United States. At present, it would be the exception to find a consumer who has not heard of the concept of formalized surgical second opinions.

The rationale behind the early programs was not only financial considerations but also enhancement of the quality of care. It was hypothesized that a board-certified second opinion consultant could act effectively to contain costs by screening out potentially inappropriate surgery. In addition, properly educated consultants could presumably shift many surgical operations from an inpatient basis to a less costly outpatient basis merely on the strength of their recommendation.

Although the concept of referrals to specialists was obviously not new, what was radically different was the manner in which these new consultations were being structured. They were stimulated and often arranged by those involved in payment for medical services, such as, corporations, government, insurance companies, unions, and labor management funds, as opposed to those receiving or providing the services. The consumer and his payer assumed a more active role than ever in the physician/patient relationship. On a practical level, the consumers became better educated and informed about their conditions as well as about the implications of alternative treatments.

Initial Response by Surgeons

As could be expected, the reaction of the medical community to such programs was far from enthusiastic.[14] Surgeons, whose training is extensive, were reluctant to have their clinical decision making challenged. Many considered the programs to be an invasion of the surgeon/patient relationship. Others felt that the programs did little more than quantify perfectly acceptable clinical disagreements between physicians in a way that promoted antagonism toward the surgeon.

It was the latter concern that became a major stumbling block in attempts to mollify physicians to accept second opinion programs. How and why a surgeon arrives at a specific therapeutic decision are complex questions. It is known that even highly skilled and experienced surgeons examining the same patient will often disagree regarding the findings. Such disagreements, which may do little more than reflect the imperfect reliability of clinical methods and data, are the foundation of surgical second opinion programs. What remains unknown is how this disagreement affects the care eventually rendered to the patient.

Although surgical second opinion programs were not designed to quantify differences of clinical opinion, in effect this is what they accomplished. A major concern arose when some made these rates of disagreements the equivalent of amounts of "unnecessary surgery." After all, how reliable and reproducible is the surgical decision making process?

RELIABILITY AND REPRODUCIBILITY OF SURGICAL DECISIONS

In order to more completely comprehend the controversies that surround surgical second opinion programs, it is important that studies on the reliability and reproducibility of the surgical decision-making process be understood.[56] The reliability of observations or judgments is defined as "do surgeons agree with one another about a similar patient or clinical situation."

Intraobserver Agreement

The reliability of clinical decision making, however, differs from its accuracy. The findings of two surgeons may agree, that is, be reliable, and yet be incorrect when compared with an independent standard of accuracy. For example, two surgeons may agree that a patient is in need of an exploratory laparotomy for presumed appendicitis. Yet they may be proved wrong when the appendix is exposed and found to be pathologically normal. Such agreements, regardless of being correct or incorrect, are termed interobserver agreement. The term intraobserver agreement denotes a physician's consistency with himself or herself about a patient or clinical situation over the course of time.

Koran, in a review of studies on the reliability of clinical methods, data, and judgments, stated[29]:

> The unreliability of clinical methods and data and the physician's judgments regarding indicated treatments must be acknowledged in any fair review process. Moreover, the limited dependability of physician's evaluations of quality of care suggests that the reliability and accuracy of the reviewing process should itself be repeatedly assayed.

The concept of error or variation on the part of the observer is not new. In 1646 Sir Thomas Browne in his book *Pseudodoxia Epidemica* described several sources of human error that are still present today. These included false deductions, credulity, adherence to tradition and authority, and misapprehension. In the early 1930s the variability of surgical judgment was studied when a random sample of 1000 school children from New York City were chosen to undergo examination for tonsil disease.[8] Of the 1000 students, 611 had had previous tonsillectomies. Of the remaining 389, 174 were told they needed to have their tonsils removed at once. The 215 with so-called healthy tonsils were examined by a second group of school physicians who felt that 99 of them were in need of tonsillectomies. Still another group of doctors examined the remaining 116 children, of whom an additional 51 were recommended for removal of their tonsils. By the end of four examinations by different physicians, only 65 of the original 1000 children had tonsils that were not removed or recommended for removal. Variation in the surgical decision-making process with regard to the choice of a treatment plan was clearly established.

A study from 1964 showed that the preoperative diagnosis of the presence or absence of cervical metastases by palpation of the neck was accurate for only 72% of the palpable nodes and for only 72% of the nonpalpable nodes.[61] In other words, experienced head and neck surgeons were wrong in 28% of the patients when they stated, on the basis of cervical palpation, that no metastatic nodes were present. In addition, they were also incorrect in 28% of the patients when they stated that metastatic disease was present on the basis of cervical palpation. Similarly, a report from Great Britain documented a 45% variation among surgeons in recording the presence or absence of axillary nodes in women who had breast lesions and a 55% discrepancy in sizing the primary lesion.[65]

Articles by Graham et al. and Geffen et al. demonstrated a significant amount of interobserver variation in the interpretation of physical signs and overall treatment plans in patients with ulcerative colitis.[22,26] Two surgeons examining the same patients for inguinal hernia, correctly identified the indirect type only 77% of the time and the direct form only 59% of the time.[51] More important, there was only 50% agreement between the two surgeons with regard to each other's findings.

An additional method to investigate surgical decision making is through the use of fictional patient vignettes. Such studies by Lazaro et al. have demonstrated the extent of interobserver surgical disagreement with regard to the management of carcinoma of the colon and rectum, arterial insufficiency of the lower extremities, abdominal sepsis, and breast carcinoma.[31-35] Vayda et al. showed considerable divergence of opinion regarding need for surgery in Canadian patients.[67,68] Clarke, in a rather sophisticated approach to clinical surgical reliability, demonstrated marked inconsistency in the manner in which surgeons arrive at therapeutic decisions.[11,12]

Rutkow reported several randomized and controlled surveys of surgical specialists that defined patterns of agreement/disagreement (interobserver) in surgical decision making for various elective surgical procedures.[56,58,59] He asked board-certified general surgeons and surgical specialists from Maryland and the District of Columbia to evaluate case vignettes as if they were second opinion consultants and to indicate whether they would or would not perform the procedures under question. Of 19 surgical vignettes, only one showed more than 90% agreement among the respondents. Seven demonstrated from 80% to 89% agreement, three from 70% to 79%, four from 60% to 69%, and four from 50% to 59%.[59]

Two years later in an attempt to define patterns of intraobserver agreement/disagreement, Rutkow followed the first study by sending to the same surgeons another study of exactly the same patient vignettes on which they had previously commented. Analysis of the individual surgeons' responses revealed a substantial number of changed clinical judgments. Of the 19 cases, only 2 demonstrated less than 10% reversal. Five showed from 10% to 19% change, 8 from 20% to 29%, 3 from 30% to 39%, and 1 more than 40%. As in the first study, there remained a considerable divergence of opinion regarding the necessity for surgery, indicating substantial continued interobserver disagreement.[55,56]

In a third investigation Rutkow measured surgical decision making on an international basis. A total of 4687 surgeons from Canada, England, and the United States were asked to assess the need for surgical intervention in fictional patient vignettes. Significant differences were noted in the way surgeons from one country answered the vignettes when contrasted with surgeons in another country. As expected, there was much disagreement within countries.[58]

All of these studies demonstrate that for some common elective surgical situations, opinions differ to a major degree from one surgeon to the next, and for the individual practitioner, change with time. The impact of second opinions on the doctor and patient surgical decision-making process is crucial to understanding both the theoretical basis of second opinion programs and their real end results.

TYPES OF PROGRAMS
Voluntary Plans

Although surgical second opinion programs have assumed numerous hybrid forms, there are two basic types: voluntary and mandatory. The former relies on the individual's initiative to seek the second opinion consultation. Typically, less than 5% of a population pool will take advantage of this benefit, and usually it is those individuals who are faced with major medical problems or those who already have misgivings about their particular procedure or about surgery in general. Some of these patients may be motivated by irrational fears of surgery that are unrelated to whether the specific surgical proposal is medically advisable.

It stands to reason, however, that the small proportion of patients who seek a surgical second opinion do so mostly because of reasonable doubts or well-founded questions. This may reflect ambiguity in the patient's understanding of the surgeon's actual proposal or an actual ambiguity in that proposal. The patient may also have valid knowledge about debates among physicians concerning surgical criteria for this procedure or for a wide range of surgical operations. Significantly, it may reflect intelligent doubts about whether this surgery is right for this patient. In any case, it seems inevitable that patients, whether well-informed or not, who voluntarily choose a second opinion are more likely to display clinical findings about which surgical consultants disagree than are a randomized cross-section of elective surgical patients who get second opinions in order to conform to a mandatory program's dictates. Moreover, the fact that this patient has come to this consultant with questions about what another doctor proposes seems likely subtly to stimulate a second opinion that differs from the initial proposal, at least in some respects. Indeed, one wonders whether that patient raised the same questions with the original surgeon and, if he or she had done so, how that doctor might have altered the surgical proposal. It stands to reason, at any rate, that the actual second opinion in a voluntary program will differ from the second opinion in a mandatory program.

If the patients' insurance benefits are not affected by obtaining a surgical second opinion before an elective operation, much less by what the consultant recommended, relatively few individuals will seek second opinions. Those who do will be more likely to receive nonconfirming opinions than those under mandatory programs.

It is thus not surprising that the rates of nonconfirming second opinions are much higher in voluntary programs than in mandatory ones. A 1985 report on surgical second opinion programs issued by the federal government's Health Care Financing Administration (HCFA) summarized findings from 11 mandatory and 10 voluntary programs.[50] The nonconfirmation rates among the mandatory programs ranged from 7.5% in a Wisconsin Medicaid project to 18.7% in one of McCarthy's programs. Nonconfirmation rates among the voluntary programs went from 16% in Prudential Insurance Company of America's experience to more than 34% in two experimental programs involving Pennsylvania Blue Shield and Michigan Blue Cross and Blue Shield, respectively, the latter being restricted to Medicare beneficiaries.

Mandatory Plans

Mandatory plans require that each member of the group obtain a second opinion in order to assure basic hospitalization and physician financial coverage for the procedure. Therefore, a more representative cross section of the insured population can be screened. In addition to the more complete representation of eligible cases, mandatory plans offer a distinct secondary effect: some patients fear that they will insult or upset their surgeons if second opinions are sought voluntarily. However, in a mandatory program the patient can explain to the physician that the payer's organization is mandating a second opinion to be scheduled, thereby placing the blame on the administrative party.

In 1987, of 78 Blue Cross/Blue Shield plans nationwide, 60 offered mandatory surgical second opinion programs.[15] More than 25 million people in the United States are now bound by such programs. That number is certain to increase if HCFA proceeds with plans to implement second opinion programs for Medicare patients. At least 17 states have second opinion programs for Medicaid recipients, and it can be assumed that those states that do not require them will be the next target.

Recently The Wyatt Company issued the seventh of its biannual reports on the benefits plans of business firms in the United States, based on surveying a sample of 1418 small, medium, and large companies.[69] A factor in this analysis was that 85% of employers in 1986 included in their health benefits plans a provision encouraging employees and covered family members to obtain second surgical opinions: this was an increase from 61% in 1984.

Almost one half of the second opinion programs were mandatory. That is, these programs impose penalties involving reductions in benefits if a covered individual undergoes a nonemergency surgical procedure without having an acceptable second opinion before the operation. Indeed, some go beyond the simple requirement that a second opinion be obtained by decreasing benefits for the procedure if the second opinion consultant had recommended against the procedure, unless a third opinion favored the operation.

Regardless, because only a very small percentage of elective surgical patients take advantage of a voluntary second opinion program, even a remarkably high rate of nonconfirming consultations with significant behavior-changing impacts cannot appreciably affect the overall health care cost experience of the enrolled population. For instance, HCFA's report discussed the relatively successful Medicare surgical second opinion demonstration project conducted by Blue Cross and Blue Shield of Greater New York. After estimating that only 2% of Medicare elective surgery patients in downstate New York utilized this voluntary program despite vigorous publicity efforts, it was calculated that the program's entire effect on the rate of surgical operations among those few who did obtain second opinions was a 3% net deduction. For the entire body of Medicare elective surgery patients including those who didn't use the program, however, that amounts to a net reduction of less than one fifth of 1%. It is not inconceivable that a few days of inclement weather could have had an equal or greater effect in lowering the number of elective surgeries that year.

Findings of this kind have led third-party payers and the purchasers of health insurance to concentrate on the mandatory approach. Voluntary programs are a nice complement to any benefits package, but their effects are extremely limited other than to help a few people make better-informed decisions about their own care.

At present at least one state's department of health (Maryland) now mandates hospitals to assure that their patients obtain second opinions before any of the following operations: anorectal surgery, appendectomy, arthroplasty with total joint replacement, cataract extraction, cholecystectomy, coronary artery bypass, diagnostic arthroscopy, diskectomy, hernia repair for children younger than 2 years, hysterectomy, intestinal bypass or gastric stapling for obesity, laminectomy, radical or modified radical mastectomy, revascularization of lower extremity, spinal fusion, tonsillectomy, and transurethral resection of the prostate.[3] Not surprisingly, major third-party payers in Maryland have incorporated that list into their mandatory second opinion programs.

Typical Mandatory Plan

The following is a brief overview of how a typical mandatory second opinion program works. The third-party payer incorporates new provisions into an existing plan to reduce benefits by a fixed percentage (ranging from 20% to 50%) if the insured patient fails to get a second opinion in the prescribed manner. The covered charges subject to the penalty invariably include the surgeon's fee, anesthetic fee, and assistant surgeon's fee. Occasionally the facility's charges are likewise subject to a benefit reduction, either in toto or only with respect to ancillary services related to the operative procedure. This means that in some mandatory programs the penalties for neglecting to conform may be rather severe.

A list of specified procedures is usually issued that tells the beneficiaries when they should obtain a second opinion to avoid the risk of incurring prescribed insurance penalties. The lists vary in length and content among programs. This list can also be of use to the surgeon, who has both an economic interest and, often, a sense of responsibility for the patient's welfare in making certain that the mandatory program's rules are followed. In some preferred provider plans and health maintenance organizations it is the surgeon's responsibility rather than the patient's to assure completion of a second opinion. This shifts the potential payment reduction to the surgeon, who then has no further recourse in charging the patient the amount of the penalty.

A cadre of general surgeons and surgical specialists is recruited to provide the second opinions. This is known as the surgical panel and involves a special enrollment of geographically distributed physicians in all surgical specialties. These surgeons meet specific criteria, such as board certification or board eligibility, and are prepared to execute agreements controlling the insurance plan's payments, waiving their rights to accept the second opinion patient as their own patient and agreeing not to provide surgical second opinions to the patients of doctors with whom they are closely affiliated. Some second opinion programs do function without specifically enrolled panels of consultants, relying instead either on a list of doctors who are regular participants in the insurance plan or even on local physician directories. Both the Blue Cross and Blue Shield Association and the Health Insurance Association of America have developed nationwide panels of second opinion consultants.

The insurance plan sets up a telephone center. This is either a direct operation of the plan or is established through a contract with an external firm. Typically staffed by nurses, these centers receive the patients' calls asking for the second opinion consultation. After ascertaining the nature of the proposed surgery, the center's staff commonly recommends three surgical consultants at locations convenient for the caller. The consultants are almost invariably in the same surgical specialty as the surgeon who proposed the operation. It is usually then incumbent on the patient to arrange for an examination with one of the three consultants. In a few programs the center assists in arranging an appointment with the second opinion consultant whom the patient independently selects.

The insurance plan builds steps into its administrative processing system that can identify both claims for surgical procedures on the second opinion list and claims for the surgical second opinions. The plan can then clear for regular payment the surgical and related claims if it is shown that the required consultation was obtained. If no second opinion claim has been received, investigation becomes necessary. Was there in fact a surgical second opinion, but the claim has not yet been transmitted, or was the case nonelective, which would lead to nullification of the penalty? Did the second opinion telephone center waive the requirement for the second opinion, perhaps because the patient had already obtained one or more independent surgical consultations, because the surgery was not elective or simply because the operation was to be performed on an outpatient basis? More important, did the patient neglect to call for and then obtain the second opinion? Only in the latter circumstance would the penalty be imposed. It should be noted that a few insurance plans impose the penalty automatically if they have no record of the second opinion, and investigate and readjudicate only those claims that generate an appeal from the insured person whose benefits were reduced.

Unfortunately, in many instances if the patient is unaware of the need for a second opinion or is negligent about following the rules, it then becomes the problem of the surgeon. This is because the patient receives a decreased insurance benefit, and the surgeon in turn must bill the patient to compensate for the unexpected decrease. This may place the surgeon in an uncomfortable role between the patient and his or her insurance company. In the final analysis, the patient has undergone a surgical operation, the insurance company pays a lesser amount than it normally would, and the party who must solve the problem is the physician.

Finally, there is a subset of mandatory surgical second opinion programs in which benefits will be reduced or denied if the second opinion consultant did not confirm the need for the surgery, unless a third opinion overrules the second opinion. McCarthy et al. have dubbed such programs as "double C."[45] In "double C" programs, consultation and confirmation are both required as distinct from "single C" programs, in which just obtaining the confirmation suffices.

PREVALENCE OF PROGRAMS

Clearly, second opinion programs are being taken seriously by most of those in the private sector who pay the bills for health care insurance. Second surgical opinion benefits are almost as common in employee health benefit plans as are provisions to pay for diagnostic tests in advance of elective hospital admissions and to pay for surgery performed in ambulatory care facilities. They have become more widespread than benefits for home health care, hospice care, and annual routine physical examinations.

At present it would seem that insurance companies, to remain competitive, are almost obligated to offer second opinion programs as part of any benefits package. In this country the public increasingly expects to receive second opinions, and payers are under pressures to provide such programs. It is of some interest that few if any insurance companies have come forth in recent years to expound the virtues of second opinion programs or to provide financial information on their effectiveness in cost containment.

The commitment to second opinion programs is not limited to the private sector. Seventeen states have put mandatory second opinion provisions into their Medicaid programs, and there have been experimental programs involving Medicare recipients. Unfortunately, in the context of Medicaid "savings" a major way in which this is achieved is seemingly by delaying surgery until the person is no longer Medicaid-eligible.

It is commonly accepted that poor people often carry a burden of ignorance and ill health that is greater than that of those living in better circumstances. The rules of a second opinion program may be difficult for many low-income persons to grasp and follow. If an educated relatively affluent individual has difficulty understanding how a second opinion program works and when it is to be utilized, how is an indigent person, perhaps of limited literacy or with limited English language comprehension, going to use a Medicaid mandatory surgical second opinion program? It is no wonder that such programs show savings of health care dollars by decreasing numbers of surgical operations. In truth, they may have done so more by erecting barriers that the beneficiaries have trouble overcoming than by screening out questionable cases, and more by delaying surgery until the person is no longer covered by Medicaid than by actually reducing the amount of surgery.

IMPACT ON PATIENT CARE

With the proliferation of surgical second opinion programs there has been a growing body of periodical literature that has assessed the impact of such programs. The majority of the initial research was conducted by McCarthy's group with little other published confirmation, and almost all of the more recent papers originate from that source.

Publication of McCarthy's first paper was followed by a considerable amount of public confusion.[1,4,16,30] In early 1976 a Congressional subcommittee report on unnecessary surgery stated there were more than 2 million such operations performed yearly.[13] This figure was determined by extrapolating the 17.6% nonconfirmation rate in McCarthy's study to the entire surgical experience of the United States. McCarthy is the first to admit that the results from second opinion studies cannot be used to justify such an estimate of unnecessary surgery in this country. Even if the cases in a second opinion program were a perfect cross section of all surgery, it would be foolish to equate surgical procedures that are not confirmed by second opinions with surgical procedures that are definitely unjustified or unwarranted.

Follow-up data by McCarthy and his staff have been considerable and include in-depth evaluations of their second opinion programs for general surgery, orthopedic surgery, pediatric surgery, and urology.* The group has actually published two books on managing such programs.[38,43] From 1972 through 1980, their mandatory programs had an 18.7% nonconfirmation rate. This ranged from a low of 11.1% for general surgery to 19.9% for ophthalmology, and as much as 32.9% for orthopedic surgery. Of the

---

*References: 19, 20, 37, 39, 40, 42, 44, 45, 52.

aggregate of 18.7% who were not confirmed by the second opinion consultant, follow-up data showed that 48.6% of this group did not have the surgery within 24 months of their initial consultations. Therefore the 18.7% who were not confirmed were reduced to 9.1% who did not have surgery. Of those patients who were not confirmed and who did not have surgery, approximately one fourth remained under medical supervision for the condition involved. Consequently, the overall figure representing those patients who were not confirmed for surgery and who no longer required medical attention was slightly less than 7% after 2 years.

Perhaps the most startling of McCarthy's data was that approximately 5% of the individuals who were confirmed for operation by both the first and second opinion consultants elected not to undergo the procedure. The reasons given by the individuals for not having the surgery performed included: judged surgery to be postponable, thought surgery too risky, felt condition was tolerable, condition improved, feared surgery, or followed the advice of a third consultant. In effect, this finding suggests that there is a population of "walking wounded." What effect this has on persons needing surgical care but avoiding it despite medical advice remains uncertain.

Grafe and McSherry assessed their participation as general surgical consultants in McCarthy's program and showed 15% of the cases they reviewed were not confirmed for surgery.[25] Their reasons for not endorsing the proposed surgery were in five main categories: no pathology demonstrated, medical treatment was preferable, surgery should be deferred pending results of medical treatment, surgery approved on an ambulatory basis only, and surgery was contraindicated.

In gynecology McCarthy et al. reported almost half of the procedures not recommended for surgery were hysterectomies.[40] The reasons for nonconfirmation include: symptoms not severe enough to warrant surgery, further evaluation needed, no pathology evident, medical treatment preferable, alternate procedure recommended, and surgery deferred pending medical tests.

A review of elective orthopedic surgery showed that 75% of nonrecommended surgery was for either foot surgery, knee surgery, or bunionectomy.[42] Among the major reasons for nonconfirmation were cast, brace, or footwear preferable; symptoms not severe enough to warrant surgery; physical therapy preferable; further evaluation needed; and medical treatment preferable. Investigation into a second opinion podiatry program revealed an 18% nonconfirmation rate.[19] However, the confirmation rate among those seeing a podiatrist serving as consultant was 94%, whereas the confirmation rate of those seeing an orthopedist serving as consultant was 50%.

Regarding urologic surgery, a recent report revealed a 26% nonconfirmation rate.[63] Among those urologic operations with the higher nonconfirmation rates are transurethral resection of the prostate, cystourethropexy, pyelolithotomy/ureterolithotomy, and internal spermatic vein ligation. Urologic consultants' reasons for nonconfirmation included surgery deferred pending results of medical tests, medication preferable to surgery, symptoms not severe enough to warrant surgery, regular examinations preferable to surgery, and different diagnosis made.

In McCarthy's "double C" program a total of 30 of 142 patients with nonconfirming second opinions sought third opinions.[45] Of the 30 third opinions, 87% disagreed with the second opinion, recommending instead that the original surgeon's proposal for surgery had been appropriate. Quite clearly, this result was indicative of the problem with inter-observer reliability in the surgical decision-making process. The result suggests that in a situation in which the patient was distressed by the second opinion that did not confirm the need for surgery, the third opinion consultant may tend to agree with the alternative preferred by the patient.

Perhaps the most significant finding from second opinion studies was enumerated by McCarthy and Finkel in their evaluation of such programs over time.[37] They enunciated the concept of the sentinel effect. When the existence of a second surgical opinion program becomes known to both the consumer and the physician, the rate of total surgical claims (even those procedures outside the program) seems to diminish. Regardless of whether physicians and patients are directly affected by the second opinion program, there appears to be a secondary effect on all individuals that decreases rates of surgical operations. This presumably comes about because the program creates a perception of stronger surveillance and peer review that leads to more cautious approaches to surgery.

Studies other than from McCarthy's group have sometimes not been as sanguine about second opinions. Although there was immediate political and public acceptance of the concept, several reports gave mixed reviews. Paris et al. showed that voluntary use of a second opinion program was extremely low (2%) and that a detailed analysis of the consultants' narrative suggestions for patient care firmly rejected surgical intervention in only 8% of the cases.[49] Nonconfirmation rates were found to be unsatisfactory measures of program success in preventing potentially unnecessary surgery. The key benefit of such programs may be to facilitate and to encourage communication between patients and physicians.

Gertman et al. studied the mandatory Medicaid second opinion program of Massachusetts.[23] They noted that a negative second opinion was reversed by a third consultant in 70% of the cases. Overall, surgery was rejected by the second and third opinion consultants for only 7.7% of the participating patients. They concluded that the substantial savings in medical expenditures anticipated by proponents of second opinion programs were unlikely to be realized. However, their data did indicate that the programs influence the patients who actually have surgery and might influence patterns of health care.

To demonstrate the confusion surrounding the evaluation of second opinion programs, Martin et al. studied the same Medicaid program as Gertman.[36] On the contrary, they found that the mandatory program saved Medicaid $3 to $4 for every dollar spent. The decline in surgery rates was attributed both to a direct effect on patients referred to the program and to a sentinel effect whereby fewer operations were proposed. What the effect was of persons losing Medicaid eligibility during the extended second opinion process was not addressed.

Beginning in 1976 Blue Cross and Blue Shield of Greater New York conducted a massive voluntary second opinion program.[64] There were few questions as to why the program was begun. Sieverts and other executives of the insurance company were clearly impressed by McCarthy's findings and sought his counsel at the outset. However, it was the plan's findings that proved unexpected. The group discovered that after nearly 5 years of large-scale experience, the ways in which people respond to surgical second opinions were far more complex than was initially perceived. The original simple formulation was not wrong—that some persons who have been inappropriately recommended for operation will be dissuaded from getting that inappropriate operation by nonconfirming second opinion. It was correct but only for a small percentage of individuals who receive surgical second opinions. For the remainder of those who used the programs, the results were more complicated. Only about 2% of their subscribers having elective operations used the program. However, interestingly, this was in the face of an enormous advertising campaign and a good deal of media attention.

The administrators of the program came to the unexpected conclusion that rather than reducing surgical utilization, the second opinions may actually have increased the number of patients who follow their surgeons' recommendation for operation. Sieverts speculated[64]:

Logic suggests that if nonconfirming second opinions deter some patients from elective surgery that they would otherwise have undergone, then confirming second opinions must persuade some patients to go through with procedures that they would otherwise have rejected. This plainly results in something of an increase in elective surgical procedures. Is the increase great enough to equal or surpass the decrease that results from nonconfirming second opinions? No sure answer exists to that question, but because confirming opinions outnumber nonconfirming ones, it seems sensible to wonder whether the overall impact of the second opinion program could actually be to increase the volume of elective surgery.

It was further hypothesized that even though the program may not actually save money, there may be some savings if early surgical intervention prevents some complications or avoids costly interim care before a probable later operation. Sieverts also suggested that the program had positive effects by strengthening peer review and by helping patients make better-informed decisions about their medical care.

The Blue Cross and Blue Shield of Greater New York report aroused considerable controversy. That same month *The New York Times* ran an editorial on second opinion programs that questioned the supposed monetary savings from such programs but supported the indirect benefits[6]:

> Even if it turns out that second opinions don't save much, allowing or requiring them may still be wise on medical grounds. They almost certainly discourage some frivolous surgery; and they probably encourage some hesitant patients to undergo operations they badly need. And that kind of operation will probably also save money in the long run. Patients who postpone needed surgery now almost always face complications and higher costs later.

Numerous others studies have been published, all of which tend to confirm the previously noted mixed findings.* A review of this collected experience narrows the subject to several basic issues: overall usage rates, nonconfirmation rates, patient compliance, effects on surgical rates and patient outcomes, program costs and benefits, and relative merits of voluntary versus mandatory programs.[9]

There is a dearth of studies, however, of the dynamics of how patients respond, in general, to proposals for elective surgery. How many, for example, simply do not comply? This may be like patients who do not get prescriptions filled or patients who do not return for scheduled follow-up visits. Clearly, second opinions have effects, but in the absence of knowledge of how patients respond without getting second opinions, how does one assess the differences generated by the second and third opinions?

Participation in voluntary programs has been consistently low, usually around 1% to 3% of eligible beneficiaries. The problem of low utilization has most often been analyzed in relationship to promotional efforts, since lack of knowledge about programs is the most often cited reason for low usage rates. However, even when advertising and direct mail have been significant, usage remains low. The attitude of patients toward their physicians may largely account for the low utilization rates. Patients often seem unwilling to question their physicians or feel no need to ask.

The highest nonconfirmation rates have been found for elective orthopedic, gynecologic, podiatric, and ophthalmic operations. Frequently the nonconfirming opinion, however, does not unequivocally reject an operation but proposes a more cautious wait and see approach. What is certain is that nonconfirmation rates emphasize inter-observer disagreement in the surgical decision-making process. In and of themselves, however, the rates do not measure to any degree the amount of unnecessary surgery.

---

*References: 2, 5, 7, 9, 10, 14, 15, 17, 18, 21, 24, 27, 28, 47, 48, 62, 66.

In general, the opinion of the consulting physician appears to influence the patients' decisions.[15] Most patients in a nonconfirmed group not having operations state it is because the consultants had recommended against surgery, although this may be partly a rationalization for those who were already ambivalent. The influence of the consulting surgeons' opinions on the patients' decisions whether to have operations has obvious implications for any cost/benefit analysis of surgical second opinion programs. Most analyses implicitly assume that patients who undergo surgery would make the same surgical decisions whether or not they participated in second opinion programs. This assumption ignores the reinforcing effect of the second physicians' opinions. Because there are many more confirming second opinions than nonconfirming ones, it is possible that second opinion programs promote surgical treatment rather than reduce it, by encouraging patients who are fearful or sensibly reluctant to go ahead with what had been proposed and confirmed.

Whether second opinion programs truly decrease rates of surgical operations is uncertain. Similarly, it remains unknown whether they change the quality of care and ultimate morbidity/mortality for a given disease process. Without a doubt, they have identified a proportion of patients who need surgery but refuse, no matter how many doctors try to persuade them. This group is worthy of further study.

Because of these many unknown factors, any cost/benefit analysis of second opinion programs is statistically troublesome and presents dilemmas to accountants. It is only McCarthy's group that has claimed consistent cost reductions, perhaps because their persistence in advocating and administering these programs is unparalleled.

CONCLUSIONS

It is difficult to reach definitive conclusions regarding surgical second opinion programs. In many aspects they have been helpful to the surgeon. They have made patients more cognizant of the surgical credentialing process including board certification. At the same time they have been instrumental in reinforcing the many positive aspects of patient autonomy that have affected medicine in the United States. Whether they have, as originally designed, increased the overall quality of surgery is unresolved. It is also uncertain if surgeons have suffered financially from their presence.

Second opinion programs were also intended to curb health care costs. There is no solid evidence this has occurred. For many elective operations, it is clearly redundant to require second opinion. Consultations for obvious inguinal hernias, stones in the gallbladder, or cancer of the uterus, for example, represent duplication of individual effort and dollars expended to obtain needless and often pointless second opinions.

Unfortunately, there is little published research that attempts to investigate the current impact of matured second opinion programs. One wonders why the major insurance companies and the federal and state government have not published any recent reports on the favorable aspects of surgical second opinion programs.

Because of interobserver variation in the surgical decision-making process, it would seem that second opinion programs, while they do give patients more information, do not necessarily represent a process to give them reliably better information and advice than they received from the surgeon who originally proposed surgery. This in and of itself is hardly an argument against such programs, because the "incorrectness" of original surgical recommendations is presumably about the same as the "incorrectness" of the second and third opinions. It is not unreasonable to propose that the value of second opinions is significant, precisely because competent and conscientious surgical specialists do come up with different answers to the same question. Therefore they give the wise individual a broader information base on which to make a decision that may have utmost importance in his or her health, comfort, and quality of life.

Surgical second opinion programs have been shown to have both positive and negative benefits from various viewpoints. Which ones outweigh the others is uncertain. It is doubtful, at this point, whether they have truly achieved their intended dual goals of containing health care costs and raising quality of surgical care. They have clearly been successful in focusing public awareness on how to choose a surgeon and enhancing consumerism in health care in this country. Their ultimate survival will probably be determined by their impact on health status.[10] Rigorous evaluations of the effects of second opinion programs on long-term surgical morbidity and mortality need to be conducted as does research on surgical decision making by patients. In the short term, decreasing health care expenditures may have appeared most important. However, in the long run, improving the quality of surgical care, protecting the overall health status of individuals recommended for surgery, and ensuring social equity to the United States' health care delivery system remain most significant.

References

1. Second opinion program reduces surgical procedures, produces no net savings, Employee Benefit Plan Rev 32:53, 1977.
2. Second surgical opinion programs: status report, Conn Med 47:363, 1983.
3. Section 10.07.01 of Title 10, Department of Health and Mental Hygiene of the State of Maryland, 1985 (under Health - General Article S19-319(d)(3) of the Annotated Code of Maryland).
4. Status report on second surgical opinions, Conn Med 43:307, 1979.
5. Status report on second surgical opinion programs, Conn Med 49:537, 1985.
6. Third thoughts on second opinions (editorial), The New York Times, January 29, 1981.
7. Alsup PA: Medicaid's second surgical opinion program, J Tenn Med Assoc 77:537, 1984.
8. American Child Health Association: School health influence on tonsillectomy, In: Physical defects-the pathway to correction, New York, 1934, American Child Health Association.
9. American College of Surgeons: Second surgical opinion programs: a review and progress report. Chicago, March 1982.
10. Brook RH and Lohr KN: Second-opinion programs: beyond cost-benefit analyses, Med Care 20:1, 1982.
11. Clarke JR: Surgical judgment using decision sciences, New York, 1984, Praeger Publishers.
12. Clarke JR: A comparison of decision analysis and second opinions for surgical decisions, Arch Surg 120:844, 1985.
13. Cost and quality of health care: unnecessary surgery. Report by the Subcommittee on Oversight and Investigations of the Committee on Interstate and Foreign Commerce, Washington, DC, 1976.
14. Crane M: Second opinions: the cost-saving program that isn't, Med Econ, July 1982.
15. Crane M: Second opinions: aren't they saving money yet? Med Econ, June 1987.
16. Culliton BJ and Waterfall WK: Second opinion on surgery, Br Med J 1:1267, 1979.
17. Cuniff CL: The Blue Shield of New Jersey second surgical opinion program, J Med Soc NJ 80:821, 1983.
18. Dunham MH and Hunt VB: Second surgical opinion programs: evaluation deficiencies, Wis Med J 83:23, 1984.
19. Finkel ML, McCarthy EG, and Miller D: Podiatric surgery: the need for a second opinion, Med Care 20:862, 1982.
20. Finkel ML, McCarthy EG, and Ruchlin HS: The current status of surgical second opinion programs, Surg Clin North Am 62:707, 1982.
21. Friedlob AS: Medicare second surgical opinion programs: the effect of waiving cost-sharing, Health Care Finan Rev 4:99, 1982.
22. Geffen N et al: Signs of ulcerative colitis: assessment of their reliability by means of observer variation studies, Gut 109:19, 1973.
23. Gertman PM et al: Second opinions for elective surgery: the mandatory Medicaid program in Massachusetts, N Engl J Med 302:1169, 1980.
24. Graboys TB et al: Results of a second-opinion program for coronary artery bypass graft surgery, JAMA 258:1611, 1987.
25. Grafe WR et al: The elective surgery second surgical opinion program, Ann Surg 188:323, 1978.
26. Graham NG, DeDombal ET, and Goligher JC: Reliability of physical signs in patients with severe attacks of ulcerative colitis, Br Med J 1:746, 1971.
27. Joffe J: Evaluating a voluntary second surgical opinion program, Eval Health Prof 3:421, 1980.
28. Kirchner M: How much will second opinions cut patient loads? Med Econ April 1980.
29. Koran LM: The reliability of clinical methods, data and judgments, N Engl J Med 293:642, 1975.

30. Lance R and Haug JN: An update on second surgical opinion programs, Bull Am Coll Surg 63:26, 1978.
31. Lazaro FJ and Rush BF: Controversies in the management of carcinoma of the colon and rectum, J Med Soc NJ 72:93, 1975.
32. Lazaro FJ and Rush BF: Controversies in the management of aterial insufficiency of the lower extremities, J Med Soc NJ 73:45, 1976.
33. Lazaro FJ, Rush BF: Controversies in the management of abdominal sepsis, J Med Soc NJ 74:234, 1977.
34. Lazaro FJ and Rush BF: Controversies in the management of cancer of the breast, J Med Soc NJ 74:943, 1977.
35. Lazaro FJ and Rush BF: Changing attitudes in the management of cancer of the breast, Surgery 84:441, 1978.
36. Martin SG et al: Impact of a mandatory second-opinion program on Medicaid surgery rates, Med Care 20:21, 1982.
37. McCarthy EG and Finkel ML: Second opinion elective surgery programs: outcome status over time, Med Care 16:984, 1978.
38. McCarthy EG and Finkel ML: Fundamentals of second opinion programs for elective surgery, Brookfield, 1979, International Foundation of Employee Benefit Plans.
39. McCarthy EG and Finkel ML: Second opinion elective surgery program: a concept whose time has come, Employ Benefits J 4:34, 1979.
40. McCarthy EG and Finkel ML: Second consultant opinion for elective gynecologic surgery, Obstet Gynecol 56:403, 1980.
41. McCarthy EG and Finkel ML: Surgical utilization in the USA, Med Care 18:883, 1980.
42. McCarthy EG and Finkel ML: Second consultant opinion for elective orthopedic surgery, Am J Public Health 71:1233, 1981.
43. McCarthy EG, Finkel ML, and Ruchlin HS: Second opinion elective surgery, Boston, 1981, Auburn House Publishing Co.
44. McCarthy EG, Finkel ML, and Ruchlin HS: Second opinions on elective surgery, Lancet 1:1352, 1981.
45. McCarthy EG, Tucker J, and Astor L: The use and value of third surgical opinions, Health Cost Manage 4:12, 1987.
46. McCarthy EG and Widmer GW: Effects of screening by consultants on recommended elective surgical procedures, N Engl J Med 291:1331, 1974.
47. McIntosh HD: Second opinions for aortocoronary bypass grafting are beneficial, JAMA 258:1645, 1987.
48. Moore FD: What to do when physicians disagree: a second look at second opinion, Arch Surg 113:1397, 1978.
49. Paris M, Salsberg E, and Berenson L: An analysis of nonconfirmation rates; experiences of a surgical second opinion program, JAMA 242:2424, 1979.
50. Poggio EC: Second surgical opinion programs: an analysis of public policy options, Washington, DC, 1985, Department of Health and Human services, Health Care Financing Administrations, Office of Research and Demonstrations.
51. Ralphs DN, Brian AJ, and Grundy DJ: How accurately can direct and indirect inguinal hernias be distinguished? Br Med J 280:1039, 1980.
52. Ruchlin HS, Finkel ML, and McCarthy EG: The efficacy of second opinion consultation programs: a cost-benefit perspective, Med Care 20:3, 1982.
53. Rutkow IM: Delivery of surgical health care in the United States, Arch Surg 116:963, 1981.
54. Rutkow IM: Rates of surgery in the United States: the decade of the 1970s, Surg Clin North Am 62:559, 1982.
55. Rutkow IM: Surgical decision making: the reproducibility of clinical judgement, Arch Surg 117:337, 1982.
56. Rutkow IM: The reliability and reproducibility of the surgical decision-making process, Surg Clin North Am 62:721, 1982.
57. Rutkow IM: Surgical operations in the United States, 1979 to 1984, Surgery 101:192, 1987.
58. Rutkow IM and Starfield BH: Surgical decision making and operative rates, Arch Surg 119:899, 1984.
59. Rutkow IM, Zuidema GD, and Gittelsohn AM: Surgical decision making: the reliability of clinical judgment, Ann Surg 190:409, 1979.
60. Rutkow IM and Zuidema GD: Surgical rates in the United States: 1966 to 1978, Surgery 89:151, 1981.
61. Sako K et al: Fallibility of palpation in the diagnosis of metastases to cervical nodes, Surg Gynecol Obstet 118:989, 1964.
62. Schachter M et al: Evaluation of a surgical second opinion program, Quart Rev Bull 9:11, 1983.
63. Schlossberg SM et al: Second opinion for urologic surgery, J Urol 131:209, 1984.
64. Sieverts S: The effects of surgical second opinions, Bull Am Coll Surg 66:6, 1981.
65. Smiddy FG: Observer variation in recording clinical data from women presenting with breast lesions, Br Med J 2:1196, 1977.
66. Tyson TJ: The evaluation and monitoring of a Medicaid second surgical opinion program, Eval Program Plan 8:207, 1985.
67. Vayda E, Mindell WR, and Mueller CB: Use of hypothetical cases to investigate indications for surgery, Can J Surg 24:19, 1981.
68. Vayda E, Mindell WR, and Mueller CB: Measuring surgical decision making with hypothetical cases, Can Med Assoc 127:287, 1982.
69. Wyatt Company's Research and Information Center: The 1986 group benefits survey, Washington, 1987.

PART THREE

Quality of Surgical Care

13. QUALITY ASSURANCE AND UTILIZATION REVIEW
    Charles K. McSherry
14. EVALUATION OF SURGICAL THERAPIES
    Darryl T. Gray
    Peg Hewitt
    Thomas C. Chalmers
15. LARGE DATABASES AND RESEARCH ON SURGERY
    Leslie L. Roos
    Noralou P. Roos
16. THE HIGH-COST SURGICAL PATIENT
    William R. Drucker
    J. William Gavett
17. COMMERCIAL CONSTRAINTS ON SURGICAL QUALITY
    Francis D. Moore
18. IMPLICATIONS OF FEDERAL LEGISLATION FOR SURGICAL PRACTICE
    Paul A. Ebert

CHARLES K. McSHERRY

Charles K. McSherry is a professor in the Department of Surgery, Mount Sinai School of Medicine, and Director of Surgery, Beth Israel Medical Center, New York. He received his doctorate from Cornell University Medical College in 1957. After internship and residency at The New York Hospital, Cornell Medical Center, he completed a fellowship in surgical research. He currently serves as Chairman of the Governors Committee on Socioeconomic Issues, American College of Surgeons Board of Governors.

13

Quality Assurance and Utilization Review

CHARLES K. McSHERRY

HISTORICAL PERSPECTIVE

It is almost axiomatic that no one has difficulty recognizing or appreciating "quality." However, there is little consensus when one attempts to define it in precise terms. To the trained observer, good medical care, like great works of art, is easy to recognize but hard to characterize. There does not yet exist a measure of quality that can be applied to medical care that both enjoys a scientific basis and is widely accepted. Perhaps, for purposes of the present discussion, quality is best expressed as "degree of excellence."

Our inability to define precisely what is quality of surgical care does not mean that surgeons have failed to assess the results of their efforts. References to quality of care date back to the Edwin Smith papyrus[5] (circa 2000 BC) and the code of Hammurabi[7] (circa 1700 BC). The physicians of ancient Greece relied on the honor and dignity of the individual practitioner and not legal sanctions to guarantee quality of care. In what may have been the first attempt at delineation of privileges, practitioners of the Hippocratic school (400 BC) tried to influence the quality of surgical care by restricting the performance of certain procedures to those practitioners trained in the technique, for example, lithotomists.

In this century, Groves[20] in England in 1908 and Codman[10] of Boston in 1914 suggested that the way to measure quality is to look at what happens to the patient after treatment. Although simple in form, this technique is still the cornerstone of our efforts to evaluate quality.

In 1912 a committee of the American College of Surgeons reported the need for standardization of hospitals and in response to this need established a committee to accredit, survey, and inspect hospitals. In 1951 the need for more broad-based support and representation became obvious, and the Joint Commission on Accreditation of Hospitals (JCAH) was founded. The American College of Surgeons was joined by the American Medical Association, the American College of Physicians, and the American Hospital Association in this effort to establish standards of hospital care. In 1987 the role of the JCAH was expanded to include other health care facilities, such as ambulatory surgery centers and nursing homes. In keeping with this expanded role, the name of the organization has been changed recently to the Joint Commission on Accreditation of Health Care Organizations.

With the advent of federal legislation that established the Medicare and Medicaid programs in the mid-1960s, the role of the JCAH expanded in both scope and importance. With federal money came federal regulation, initially in the form of utilization review and then medical audit. Collectively, these programs constituted the basis of the hospitals quality assurance programs.

More recently the quality of care has been considered in relation to cost. With the increasing costs of medical care in the face of declining national resources, there is greater need to justify the expenditures for all facets of health care delivery. Indeed the Secretary of Health and Human Services, Otis R. Bowen,[4] stated in the 1987 Shattuck Lecture, "The supreme challenge today is to contain costs without lowering the quality of care." Some would argue that these goals are mutually exclusive. Others point to the tremendous discrepancies that exist on a regional and national basis with respect to such parameters of health care delivery as average lengths of stay, costs per admission, and professional fees as evidence that there is a great deal that can be accomplished to improve quality and cost containment.

Within the framework of quality and cost are fundamental questions related to societal needs and expectations that remain unchallenged. The cost and perhaps quality of medical care could be improved if legislators and health care administrators would address such controversial issues as the provision of expensive high-technology care to patients who have obvious terminal illnesses and brief life expectancy. One must ask why the government and private insurance carriers continue to pay for outmoded, unproven, or otherwise questionable therapeutic endeavors. How many millions of dollars have been misspent and continue to be spent for the use of some chemotherapeutic agents of little or no value in the treatment of patients who have metastatic cancer? Medical care could be vastly improved if reimbursement was limited in cancer patients to those individuals enrolled in approved protocols or those being treated with drugs that offer significant and proven enhancement of the quality of life or prolonged survival. In patients with AIDS, one wonders what benefits are to be achieved by the aggressive treatment of pneumocystitis pneumonia or Kaposi's sarcoma. It is perhaps unrealistic to believe that these types of issues will ever be addressed by a society that is so responsive to pressures exerted by special interest groups.

At the beginning of the 1980s the federal government appeared to be entering into an era of deregulation. In many industries there has been significant movement in that direction with improved efficiency and economy. Unfortunately, medicine has not only failed to participate in that effort but has been subjected to increased regulation. Utilization review and medical audit continue to be the cornerstones of quality assurance. Tissue review, a time-honored but marginally effective activity, has been expanded to include those operations in which no tissue is removed. The activities related to the credentialing process have vastly expanded in an effort to document that the individual physician or surgeon possesses the skills to perform those activities and procedures that he or she proposes to accomplish. Continuing medical education activities now constitute an increasingly important part of the hospital appointment process. Risk management experience must now also be factored into the decision regarding privileges. Finally, there has been increasing demand that hospital trustees participate in a more meaningful and active way in the quality assurance programs.

VALUE OF UTILIZATION REVIEW

Utilization review, initiated in 1966, was the first major technique introduced to formalize the quality assurance programs as they now exist. Its stated purpose was to measure the efficiency of use of hospital facilities and services. Its goals included assurance to patients that they received no more or less care than they needed and assurance to purchasers of that care (government and other third-party payers) that it was both medically necessary and delivered in the most economical manner. In the first 10 years of this program, Gertman[17] reported that more than 1 million hours of physician time had been spent each year on hospital utilization activities. There is every reason to believe that this effort probably increased in the second decade of the program.

Data to support the continued effort in surgical utilization review are at best anecdotal and for the most part nonexistent. To the best of my knowledge and after a recent computer library search, there are no reports in peer/reviewed surgical journals that demonstrate these programs to be cost effective on a local or national basis. In 1976, Gertmand and Egdahl[17] reported on 22,000 admission and extended stay reviews in 44 Massachusetts hospitals during a 2-week period. The continued stay in the hospital of 2120 patients was questioned, and the utilization review committee formally terminated continued health insurance benefits in 84 cases (0.4%). The median age of these patients exceeded 80 years, and their medical problems were for the most part chronic illnesses. Their continued stay in acute care facilities reflected the relative unavailability of chronic care beds. The introduction of the concept of "alternate level of care" in the acute care facilities for patients waiting for post discharge placement has been a positive step in decreasing the costs of medical care. However, one may ask with justification if the money spent to identify these patients might not have been better utilized to provide for post discharge care in the form of, for example, homemakers or nursing home beds, and thus reduce the need for in-hospital care.

In 1976, I reported on my experience as chairman of the Utilization Review Committee at a major urban university hospital.[24] Approximately 9500 charts were reviewed annually to identify an average of six patients per year who required the intervention of the utilization review committee because of unnecessarily prolonged length of stay. The cost of identifying each patient was $34,212—clearly not cost effective.

Although these studies are now more than 10 years old and perhaps relatively outdated, they were, until recently, the only ones reported. In May 1988 Feldstein and associates reported the effects of utilization review programs on cost containment in 222 groups of employees insured by a private insurance carrier. Compulsory utilization review procedures reduced admissions by 12.3%, inpatient days by 8%, hospital expenditures by 11.9%, and total medical expenditures by 8.3%. The savings to cost ratio was highly favorable, approximately 8 to 1.[15] Undoubtedly, the cost effectiveness of utilization review needs to be studied on a regional and national basis by an agency of the federal government, such as the General Accounting Office, to establish the continued need for this activity.

There is no doubt that the average length of hospital stay for virtually every disease category has decreased during the past 20 years, and this decrease has been beneficial. The extent to which utilization review has contributed to this decrease is unknown. Many factors and new programs have contributed to it. Ambulatory and same-day surgery as well as preadmission testing are but a few examples of the more efficient use of hospital services. Whether these programs would have been implemented in the absence of utilization review committees is unknown.

Recent efforts by the federal government to reinforce utilization review programs have included PSRO (professional services review organizations) and more recently PRO (professional review organization) activities. These agencies are committed by virtue of their own survival to further reduce both the number and lengths of hospital stays. To achieve this, reimbursement to hospitals is denied for time or services deemed to be inappropriate (carve-out days). In order to minimize the financial loss of these carve outs, hospitals have responded by increasing their utilization review staff to insure the quality of the medical record. The 962-bed hospital that I am now associated with has 27 FTEs (full-time equivalents) devoted to quality assurance. In the final analysis it is the documentation in the medical record that is the basis for financial sanctions and, in return, the hospital's appeal process. The end result in perhaps a simplistic view is that the government is funding two cadres of people—one whose energy is devoted to the denial of payment for medical care and the other to ensure, in so far as possible, the payment for medical care. Utilization review, now 21 years old, has reached maturity and seems destined to live to a ripe old age. It has become an entity unto itself, and its survival without proof of cost benefit is a tribute to the durability of bureaucracy.

Since their inception 3 years ago, PROs have become increasingly active with respect to both cost containment and quality of care. Using generic quality screens, approximately 19,000 physicians nationwide have had inquiries from Medicare PROs during the past 18 months regarding the quality of care they had provided. The overwhelming majority of these concerns were resolved by further documentation or explanation.

PROs recommended sanctions against 133 physicians as of the end of 1987 because of quality concerns. The Department of Health and Human Resources suspended the participation of 58 physicians in the Medicare program for periods as long as 10 years, levied fines on 24 doctors, and rejected 52 recommendations for sanction. Other cases are still waiting disposition.

PRO activities are scheduled to expand in 1988 to include reviews of outpatient surgery and nursing home and home health care, and due process rights have been protected for the sanctioned physicians by organized medicine.

Peer review activity was inhibited in 1987 by the $2.1 million award to a physician after his successful suit against 11 fellow peer review physicians. The physician alleged bad faith and an anticompetitive intent (Patrick versus Burget). This decision was reversed by the U.S. Court of Appeals but has been sustained by the U.S. Supreme Court.

MEDICAL AUDIT

Medical audit is a program designed to measure the care received by patients as judged by professional standards. The program compares some aspects of the actual medical care received by groups of patients with standards judged to be commensurate with high quality care for each group. The program evolved during several years of trial and error and was firmly entrenched by 1973. During the past 2 to 3 years the rigid format of these studies was relaxed to permit more local input into both the subjects audited and the format of the audit.

Medical audit was conceived in response to the perception that there were serious and widespread deficiencies in the delivery of health care. Regulatory agencies and third-party payers insisted that their payment for medical services entitled them, indeed obligated them, to assure their clients that the medical care purchased was of the highest possible caliber. The perceived deficiencies about surgery are related to two concerns: namely, the indications and therefore the necessity for surgery and the caliber of the services performed. The latter relates to operative mortality and morbidity and to a lesser extent, long-term survival.

The Charge of "Unnecessary Surgery"

The issue of "unnecessary surgery" has been the focal point of public debate during the 1970s and 1980s. This debate was preceded by a number of publications that first appeared in the scientific literature and then, often distorted and sensationalized, in the lay press that suggested that certain operations were being performed without proper indications. In 1970 Bunker[8] reported the much higher utilization of surgical services in the United States compared with that in England and Wales. Reports by Doyle[13,14] in 1952 and 1953 declared 47% of oophorectomies and 39% of hysterectomies to be unnecessary. Trussell[29] in 1962 studied the medical care received by a sample of families of members of a teamsters union in the New York City area. Approximately 30% of the hysterectomies performed in this cohort were judged retrospectively to be unnecessary.

Concern over the issue of unnecessary surgery led McCarthy[23] and his associates in 1974 to reexamine the issue of second opinions as part of the presurgical screening process. These programs relied on a board-certified surgeon's evaluation of the necessity for elective surgery after the patient had been advised to undergo an operation. Since their inception, they have become widely accepted in the insurance industry and are especially popular with union health plans. These programs are questionably cost effective.[27] Unfortunately, McCarthy's data on the incidence of nonconfirmed indications for surgery were grossly distorted by both *The New York Times* and the Moss subcommittee of the House of Representatives. The data were unjustifiably extrapolated to declare that there were 12,000 needless deaths in the United States in 1974 because of unnecessary surgery. This conclusion could not be supported by any of the published data on second opinion programs.

Concern over the indications for surgery also were a result of the reports of the variations in the rates of surgery in different localities and the variations between fee-for-service and prepaid health care delivery systems. Variations of as much as 1000% in the patterns of use of nine common surgical procedures in Vermont and Maine were reported by Wennberg and Gittelsohn.[30] Similar discrepancies in Wisconsin have been noted by Detmer and Tyson.[11]

There is convincing evidence that the method of physician payment influences surgical rates. Most studies suggest that enrollees in prepaid insurance plans undergo less surgery than do patients in a fee-for-service system. For example, Gaus et al.[16] reported a surgical admission rate of 24 per 1000 population in a prepaid group and 82 per 1000 in a fee-for-service group. LoGerfo et al.,[22] in a similar study, found that the frequency of appendectomy, tonsillectomy, cholecystectomy, and hysterectomy was higher in a prepaid independent practice setting in which surgeons were reimbursed on a fee-for-service basis compared with a large prepaid group practice with salaried physicians.

The above data have contributed to the increasing popularity of HMOs. The federal government now mandates that certain segments of the population be given a choice between fee-for-service and prepaid health plans. The latter of course lend themselves to capitation agreements and thus relieve the government of much of its direct involvement in health care delivery. Under the capitation agreement the provider is given a fixed sum of money to pay for the health care needs of each subscriber. The success or failure of the provider organization thus depends on its ability to deliver such care in an efficient and economical manner. This system has attracted a whole new group of entrepreneurs to the health care industry. These individuals are best epitomized by the recent graduates of the nation's leading business schools, for example, the Harvard MBAs. By putting together large prepaid groups such as HMOs, PPOs, and IPAs (independent practice organizations), some have become instant millionaires. Their success can be attributed to the oversupply of physician manpower and the competitive greed of a substantial segment of the medical profession. As experience increases, the deficiencies of many of these alternate health care delivery plans is becoming evident. More and more patients are beginning to question the validity of a health care system that rewards those who fail to provide care as opposed to those who deliver it. Although alternate health care delivery systems are associated with lower surgical rates, one must ask if the denial of surgical care is always in the best interest of the patient. How has the reduced frequency of surgery affected the patient's life-style and long-term survival? In spite of large federal subsidies, some HMOs have clearly failed to provide for the health care needs of their subscribers and have declared bankruptcy. This is particularly evident in Florida. By promoting capitation the federal government has destroyed one of the most effective means of assuring the quality of care, namely, the patient's ability to choose his own physician.

Preferred providers. Frustrated by their inability to seriously affect physician behavior and to achieve cost-control targets, the federal government has taken a "meat ax" approach to the issue by publishing raw data on hospital mortalities. This was first done in 1986 and proved to be both a disservice to the public and an unfair attack on those hospitals whose statistics were displayed without the opportunity for effective public explanation. A similar public release occurred in late 1987 but only after the hospitals were permitted to study and prepare critiques of their statistics. It is hoped that this will permit these institutions to factor in the important severity-of-illness issue that is essential to a meaningful interpretation of this data. On an individual basis the government is planning to publish its own "preferred provider" list of physicians. Presumably, Medicare beneficiaries would be advised to select these "providers" because of their track record on low fees and hospital services utilization. This approach might well prove to be an embarrassment for both the government as well as the "preferred providers" because exclusion from the list might imply that physicians not included on the list are more interested in the welfare of their patients than the economic goals and targets of the funding agencies.

Process Audits

Traditionally, medical audit has been concerned with structure, process, and outcome in relation to the delivery of health care. Structure concerns the physical plant of the health care facility. Process deals with the issues of record keeping, the administration of medication, the provision of nursing care, and the written protocols for all major facets of inpatient care. Outcome concerns mortality and morbidity.

Until recently the principal focus of medical audit was process. Process audits analyzed the methodology involved in the delivery of care and the end results—the final outcome of such care. The latter assumed greater importance as studies demonstrated that the standards for good process of care were not verified by proof of better outcome for patients. The essential feature of medical audit evolved into the degree of compliance with preestablished criteria of elements of care that could be documented in the medical records of individual patients. The quality of the medical record assumed great importance for the success of these audits, since events or data not recorded were presumed to be absent or deficient.

Numerous reports attest to the willingness and cooperation of physicians to comply with the need for process audits. Goldstone and Way[18] at the University of California, San Francisco, conducted audits in the form of conferences attended by surgical residents, faculty members, and students. Strauch[28] approached medical audit in two community hospitals of Stamford, Connecticut, by establishing a single audit committee to review the medical records of all patients with problems in the fields of general, thoracic, vascular, pediatric, and plastic surgery. In the United Kingdom other techniques have been employed. Blanchard and Downs[3] employed weekly on-the-ward capture of complications and deaths with immediate feedback to the involved surgeons. Retrospective peer review of surgical deaths judged the process of patient care in terms of treatment, investigation, and documentation.

Impact on Patient Care

Irrespective of the method employed, the results of medical audit studies have had little impact on patient care. On the positive side, Ashbaugh and Lung[1] reported favorably on the effect of studies evaluating medical care in their community hospitals in Boise, Idaho. They cited educational benefits, compliance with JCAH requirements, increased percentage of surgery performed by qualified surgeons, and the establishment of an effective mortality and morbidity conference as some of the advantages that have resulted from their audits. Gruer et al.[19] in Scotland reported significant decreases in the number of reoperations for intraabdominal complications, retained gallstones, arterial grafts, and amputations during a 5-year period attributed, at least in part, to audits.

Most reports, however, of the results of medical audit have been unfavorable and unenthusiastic about its accomplishments. In 1974 Cayten et al.[9] reported the results of six audits and observed that in both process and outcome, relatively little change occurred as a result of these studies. In 1976 McSherry[24] reported on the results of 15 audits and noted the failure of these studies to alter physician practices and behavior. Additional evidence that medical audits do not improve the performance of physicians has been presented by Devitt and Ironside.[12] In a 1975 study of patients undergoing cholecystectomy, these authors commented on the multitude of factors that can affect the data used to measure physician performance. Using the criteria of complication rate and mean length of postoperative stay, it was not possible to distinguish end results among a group of surgeons. More recently Berry[2] reported an analysis of the problems encountered in the performance of an audit of patients operated on for resection of colon disease. The criteria developed for this audit revealed unclear objectives, controversial clinical material, problems in terminology, ineffective audit technique, and unnecessary work for the audit committee members. After 20 years of enforced process audits, a recent Rand Corporation study by Brook and Lohr[6] concluded, "There are, at best, only a handful of clinically validated criteria or standards, either in the process or the outcome domain, that can simply be taken off a shelf and applied. Indeed, the bookcase in which to place the shelf has yet to be built."

Although unstated, one can assume that the failure of medical audits to affect the quality of patient care has prompted the Joint Commission's "Agenda for Change." The goal of this project is to develop an outcome-oriented monitoring and evaluation process. Instead of simply measuring an organization's "capacity" to provide high quality care, it will permit the organizations to actually evaluate their performance. At present this new approach is being tested in 17 hospitals nationwide and, if successful, will be expanded to 100 hospitals in 1989.

During the past few years computer-based data systems have been developed in an effort to classify patients according to the severity of their illnesses. The data entered relies on findings from the physical examination, laboratory findings, radiologic examination, and pathologic findings obtained during the first 48 hours of hospitalization. This leads to a severity score that is independent of the diagnosis and that can be reevaluated as treatment progresses. An expected clinical outcome can then be ascertained and compared with the actual outcome to evaluate the effectiveness of therapy. The most widely used of these computer-based systems is the Medical Illness Severity Grouping System (MedisGroups) developed by Charles M. Jacobs, an attorney with a long-standing interest in the quality of health care. There is considerable interest in these computer-based systems, and they are in use in hundreds of hospitals throughout the country.

If these systems can indeed control for the severity of illness, it should be possible to generate provider practice profiles and identify who has the best results at the lowest cost. Such information may be used by third-party payers to reward "quality" institutions and providers at the expense of less productive facilities. Severity adjusted data may also be used as a partial guide to cost-reimbursement plans.

Until such time as there exists a meaningful and effective audit system, the careful, complete, and fair-minded peer review of all deaths and complications occurring in the surgical setting will continue to be the basis for effective quality assurance.

The measurement of quality in surgical practice is difficult, time-consuming, and enveloped in an enormous bureaucracy. However, the goal is a worthy one that deserves our support and cooperation. Surgeons should support new approaches to ensure quality of care, but they should also be permitted to discard those techniques that have proven ineffective. Systems of audit imposed by legislative or administrative fiat that fail to exert a meaningful improvement in the quality of surgical care will continue to be frustrated by physicians' lack of interest and passive resistance.

CREDENTIALS AND DELINEATION OF PRIVILEGES

A recent survey by Jenson and Larson[21] of 500 physicians indicated that the quality of care at hospitals was primarily determined by the quality of the physicians serving on its staff. This observation has important implications for hospital governing bodies and credentials committees who are charged with the responsibility for staff membership and delineation of privileges. All new applicants to the medical and dental staff of the hospital must be subject to an extensive background check to verify their training and experience. In addition, and perhaps more important, their moral and ethical standards must be scrutinized. In this age of substance abuse and chemical dependency, physicians are not immune to these problems and deserve the same scrutiny as any other hospital worker.

With respect to delineation of privileges, board certification has been considered the benchmark of preparedness for specific inpatient activities. In some areas, experience and specialized training must be used to judge qualifications. An example of the latter is endoscopy, in which a variety of interests converge and agreed on standards of training are lacking. Each institution must decide its own criteria for granting privileges to perform new techniques.

The scope of a physician's privileges should be reviewed at reasonable intervals to ensure their continued appropriateness. The institutional experience with procedures should be monitored, and the experience of the individual physician should be compared with that of his or her peers. The involvement of trustees at this level of governance is appropriate and helpful. By enforcing the bylaws of the institution, they can protect both the public and the individual physician by ensuring due process.

In 1976 Mitchell[25] described an approach to the problem of how to deal with alleged incompetence or malfeasance on the part of an individual practitioner. With minor modifications this is the approach employed by many hospitals. In the face of allegations that a staff member is rendering poor care, the hospital governing body must decide on the merits of the events precipitating the situation. The individuals who are the source of the charges of the alleged deficiency on the part of the practitioner should have personal knowledge of the facts and the expertise to raise questions of professional performance. The allegations should be investigated carefully and documented by appropriate superiors (department chief) or peers as the situation merits. In some instances it may be advisable to secure an independent review of the problem by an outside consultant. This removes the issue of personal animosity or competitive jealousy from the allegations. There must be ample opportunity for a fair hearing, and the physician should be given a written statement that specifies the charges against him or her. Here again the trustees must be involved and must be the final arbiters of the in-house review process.

Individuals judged to be guilty of gross incompetence or malfeasance should be dismissed from the hospital staff and also be reported to the appropriate state regulatory agency. The latter is empowered to revoke the practitioner's license to practice, if that is necessary to protect the public. Where criminal activities are suspect, for example, the illicit prescription and distribution of drugs, the appropriate law-enforcement agency should also be notified. One of the major criticisms of organized medicine is that it fails to identify and "weed out" the incompetent and unethical physicians. This criticism is partly justified, but the climate has changed dramatically in the past decade, and the number of physician licenses revoked has increased significantly.

Corrective action short of dismissal may be considered in three categories of increasing severity, namely, education/feedback, surveillance, and restriction of privileges. Education/feedback must be directed to the needs of the individual physician and his or her deficiency if it is to be successful. Less-focused efforts directed at continuing medical education programs for the entire staff are usually ineffective. Examples of such recommendations include goal-oriented and specific continuing medical education courses, special tutoring, selected readings, or a "voluntary" request for consultation in certain clinical situations. Monitoring should accompany the education to assure that the necessary improvements have been achieved.

Surveillance measures may include mandatory consultation with designated peers before the performance of certain procedures or a requirement for a co-surgeon, approved by the governing body, for any major surgery by the physician.

Restriction of privileges may include discontinuing the physician's privileges for a certain procedure shown to have been performed without the requisite skill. Suspension of all operative procedures would be appropriate in circumstances where the surgeon's motivation and ethical standards have violated hospital and community norms.

DEPARTMENTAL LEADERSHIP

Perhaps the most important but ill-defined factor in quality assurance and the delivery of surgical care is the quality of leadership of the departments. The activities of the staff, and particularly the residents, usually reflect the interests, goals, and ethical standards of the chairman. It is the latter's interest and dedication to high quality professionalism that sets the tone for the other members of the staff. Unfortunately, because this is difficult to quantify, it is never factored into the review process by the regulatory agencies.

Ravitch[26] in 1981 outlined the measures he employed at the Montefiore Hospital in Pittsburgh to assure quality of care. Weekly review of all deaths and complications, discussion of cases selected at random from the operative schedule, rounds with medical students and house staff, informal review and inspection of operative procedures in progress, and informal discussions with the pathologist-in-chief when necessary were among the measures he routinely used to ensure the safety and well-being of the patients admitted to his department. This list with minor modifications and local variations embodies much of the constellation of factors and attributes that constitute a "good" department of surgery.

Clearly, the governing body of each hospital has the obligation to seek out and appoint to positions of leadership only those individuals capable of setting high standards of patient care. Continued appointment as chairman should be contingent upon successful outside peer review at intervals of approximately every 5 years. Although this is not mandated by any regulatory agency, it should be implemented on a voluntary basis to ensure high-quality leadership and patient care.

References

1. Ashbaugh DG and Lung JA: Benefits of an intensive community surgical audit program, Arch Surg 112:389, 1977.
2. Berry RE: Unfulfilled objectives: critique of criteria from an actual audit of colon resection, QRB 5:6, 1979.
3. Blanchard RJW and Downs AR: Clinical audit of surgery in a large teaching hospital, Can J Surg 23:278, 1980.
4. Bowen OR: Shattuck Lecture—what is quality care? N Engl J Med 316:1578, 1987.
5. Breasted JH: Edwin Smith Papyrus, 2 vols, Chicago, 1930, University Press.

6. Brook RH and Lohr KN: Monitoring quality of care in the medicare program, JAMA 258:3138, 1987.
7. Buckingham WB and Tabatabai C: Assuring the quality of surgical outcomes in the ancient world, QRB 4:9, 1978.
8. Bunker JP: Surgical manpower: a comparison of operation and surgeons in the United States and England and Wales, N Engl J Med 282:185, 1970.
9. Cayten CG et al: Surgical audit using predetermined weighted criteria, Conn Med 38:117, 1974.
10. Codman EA: The product of a hospital, Surg Gynecol Obstet: 18:491, 1914.
11. Detmer DE and Tyson TJ: Regional differences in surgical care based upon uniform physician and hospital discharge abstract data, Ann Surg 187:166, 1978.
12. Devitt JE and Ironside MR: Difficulties in applying patient care audit to surgeons, Bull Am Coll Surg 60:18, 1975.
13. Doyle JC: Unnecessary ovariectomies, JAMA 148:1105, 1952.
14. Doyle JC: Unnecessary hysterectomies, JAMA, 151:360, 1953.
15. Feldstein PJ et al: Private cost containment: the effects of utilization review programs on health care use and expenditures, N Engl J Med 318:1310, 1988.
16. Gaus CR, Cooper BS, and Hirschman C: Contrasts in HMO and fee-for-services performance, Soc Secur Bull 39:3, 1975.
17. Gertman PM and Egdahl RE: The dynamics of utilization review: a case study of 44 Massachusetts hospitals, Ann Surg 188:544, 1978.
18. Goldstone J and Way LW: The use of medical audits in surgical education, Surgery 84:25, 1978.
19. Gruer R et al: Audit of surgical audit, Lancet 1:23, 1986.
20. Hey Groves EW: Surgical statistics: a plea for a uniform registration of operation results, Br Med J 2:1008, 1908.
21. Jensen J and Larson S: Physicians say quality of care at hospitals depends on the quality of doctors—survey, Modern Healthcare, p 64, May 22, 1987.
22. LoGerfo, JP et al: Rates of surgical care in prepaid group practices and the independent setting: what are the reasons for the differences? Med Care 17:1, 1979.
23. McCarthy EG and Widner G: Effects of screening by consultants on recommended elective surgical procedures, N Engl J Med 291: 1331, 1974.
24. McSherry CK: Quality assurance: the cost of utilization review and the educational value of medical audit in a university hospital, Surgery 80:122, 1976.
25. Mitchell WE Jr: How to deal with poor medical care, JAMA 236:2875, 1976.
26. Ravitch MM: Bureaucracy is bureaucracy, is bureaucracy, Surg Rounds 4:13, 1981.
27. Ruchlin HS, Finkel ML and McCArthy EG: The efficacy of second-opinion consultation programs: a cost-benefit perspective, Med Care 20:3, 1982.
28. Strauch GO: Problem-oriented surgical audit in the community hospital, Am J Surg 129:401, 1975.
29. Trussell, RE, Morehead MA, and Ehrlich J: The quantity, quality and costs of medical and hospital care secured by a sample of teamster families in the New York area, New York, 1962, Columbia University School of Public Health and Administrative Medicine.
30. Wennberg J and Gittelsohn AM: Small area variations in health care delivery, Science 182:1102, 1973.

DARRYL T. GRAY

Darryl T. Gray is currently a Teaching Fellow and doctoral candidate in epidemiology at the Harvard School of Public Health. A native of the New York City area, Dr. Gray received his AB magna cum laude from Harvard College in 1974. After working in health planning and in the design of clinical algorithms, he received his MPH from the University of Washington (Seattle) in 1981. Dr. Gray received his MD from Case Western Reserve University in 1984 and completed a transitional internship at St Luke's Hospital (Cleveland) in 1985.

PEG HEWITT

Peg Hewitt is Research Librarian with the Technology Assessment Group, Department of Health Policy and Management, at the Harvard School of Public Health in Boston, Massachusetts. She received her MS in Library and Information Science from Drexel University in Philadelphia and has held positions in Harvard libraries and in her own information brokerage.

THOMAS C. CHALMERS

Thomas C. Chalmers is Distinguished Physician, Boston Veterans Administration Medical Center, and Lecturer in Health Policy and Management at the Harvard School of Public Health working with the Technology Assessment Group. His clinical training in internal medicine, gastroenterology, and clinical research was with the Harvard Medical Services at Boston City Hospital. Dr. Chalmers was Chief of Medical Services at Lemuel Shattuck Hospital, Boston, for 13 years while serving as a Lecturer at Harvard Medical School and Professor of Medicine at Tufts. He later was Chief of Research and Education for the Veterans Administration Central Office and then Associate Director for Clinical Care and Director of the Clinical Center, National Institutes of Health. He previously served for 10 years as President and Dean at Mt. Sinai Medical Center, New York.

14

The Evaluation of Surgical Therapies

DARRYL T. GRAY
PEG HEWITT
THOMAS C. CHALMERS

Among investigators conducting clinical therapeutic research, there is general agreement that randomly assigning patients to experimental or control therapy is the best way to obtain valid and/or reproducible results. Articles advocating the use of randomized control trials include A. Bradford Hill's classic 1953 paper[64,65] and need not be referenced here. Published objections and suggestions of alternative evaluation strategies are few* and focus mostly on treatment for cancer or cardiovascular disease or on surgery as a whole. This review of the evaluation of surgical therapies will focus on randomized control trials (RCTs) and on non-randomized comparisons (NRCs) of surgical treatments. Although not explicitly concerned with the socioeconomic theme of this book, the proper evaluation of therapy has broad socioeconomic as well as ethical and clinical implications.

DEFINITIONS

For the purposes of this chapter, the term "trial" refers to a study of the effects of one or more clinical interventions in which patient selection criteria, measures of outcome, and any associated hypotheses to be tested were determined before patients were actually treated.[47] Trials of single procedures used in consecutive or selected series of patients with no controls are outside the scope of this discussion. Prospectively designed trials evaluating the relative merits of two or more treatments generally use some random method to assign therapy, and these studies are termed RCTs.

The general term comparison encompasses RCTs but also includes other study designs in which the investigator has equal control (or lack of it) over treatment assignment in all patients or has equal access to data on patients already treated with the modalities of interest. Investigators would have less information on controls obtained from the literature or from disease registries than they would on patients or patient records they had actually seen. Therefore we did not include studies comparing outcomes in individual patients with those from such "external" controls.[1] Theoretically, a prospectively planned comparative trial could involve nonrandom allocation, but such studies are rarely conducted. The more frequently encountered NRCs involve reviews of results of patients previously treated

---
*References 9, 10, 51, 53, 96, 118, 120.

with the therapies of interest. Patients may have received the different treatments at different institutions and/or in different time periods. In situations in which both treatments were potentially available at the same time and place, allocation presumably was made on the basis of convenience or clinical judgment. Although all types of NRCs are prone to bias, comparisons of treatments allocated on clinical grounds are especially prone to "confounding by indication"[57,83] a situation in which selection effects cannot be completely separated from therapeutic effects.

BACKGROUND

The majority of research on cancer therapies is conducted by the various cooperative groups whose definitive studies are almost exclusively RCTs. Although one group maintains that there are advantages to using historical controls, those investigators also employ randomization.[50,51] For comparing treatment outcomes in cardiovascular disease, some suggest that careful analysis of information contained in clinical databases may reduce the need for prospective clinical trials.[96] This point, however, is disputed by Byar.[14,56] Clinical databases are useful only to the extent that the information contained allows for adequate adjustment for the biases and confounders invariably in operation when the data were collected. Finally, some surgeons have claimed that surgery presents a special problem with regard to randomization and that the evaluation of surgical operations should not be done via the RCT mechanism.[9,10,118]

Using the RCT as a "gold standard," several studies have provided direct evidence of bias in the selection of patients receiving experimental

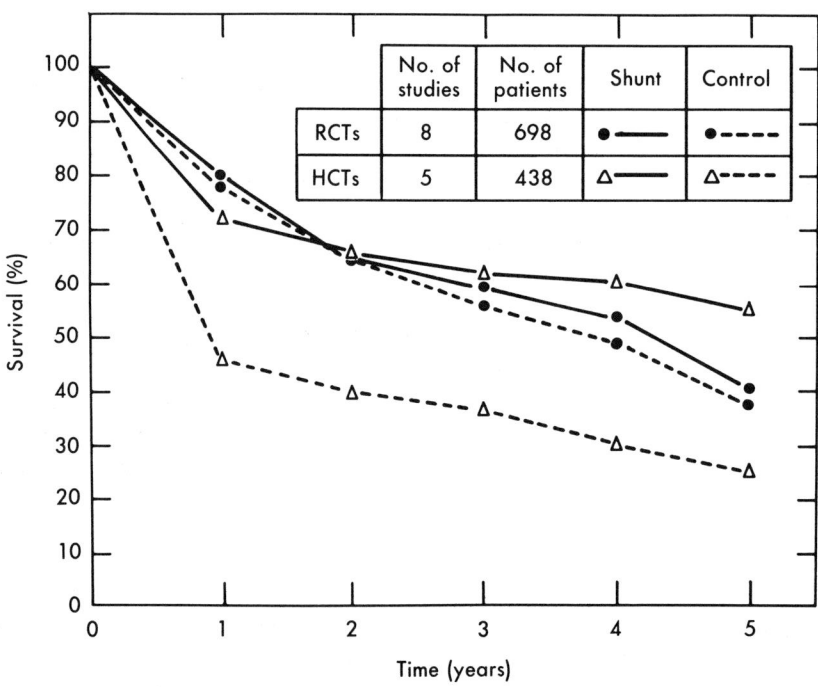

Figure 14-1. Survival of treated and control groups in clinical trials of shunt surgery for cirrhosis and esophageal varices. (From Sacks H et al: Am J Med 72:233, 1982.)

and control therapies in NRCs.* Two meta-analyses,[25,103] a new term for research that combines data from different studies,[102] have compared RCTs with historically controlled comparisons (HCCs) of surgery and medical therapy. In the case of portacaval shunt surgery, survival of the patients assigned to surgery and medical treatment in the RCTs and to surgery in the HCCs was the same, but the medically treated controls in the HCCs had considerably higher mortality (Figure 14-1). In the case of one RCT and one HCC of coronary artery surgery, the two surgical groups and the randomly assigned medical group had similar outcomes, but the historical controls assigned to medical therapy had significantly worse outcomes (Figure 14-2). Historical controls are not usually treated with a research purpose in mind and do not usually go through the selection process of signing informed consent documents.

Evidence of misleading information coming from the use of nonrandomized controls has been reiterated in a classic book on surgery and its evaluation.[2,12a,52] However, the message is clearly not accepted by all because NRCs continue to be published. Discussion of the objections to randomization in surgery is warranted.

---

*References 23, 36, 82, 84, 103, 104.

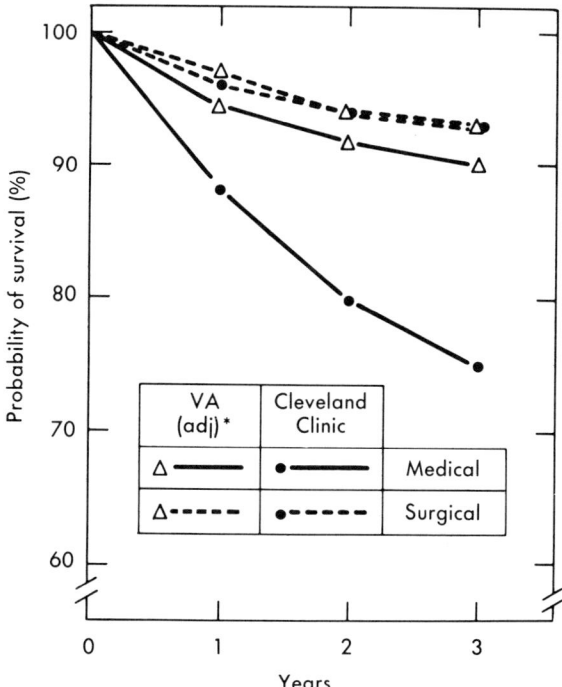

*Adjusted for relative frequency of one-, two-, and three-vessel diseases.

Figure 14-2. Three-year survival curves of surgical (*broken lines*) and medical (*solid lines*) treatment of coronary artery disease. From the Veterans Administration Cooperative Trial (*triangles*) and the Cleveland Clinic experience. Curves redrawn to adjust for different frequences of one-, two-, and three-vessel disease. (From Chalmers TC: Clin Res 26:230, 1978.)

CONTROVERSIES CONCERNING RCTS IN SURGICAL EVALUATION

Bonchek has previously written about the role of the randomized control trial in the evaluation of new operations.[10] He reviewed the quality requirements of a good trial and agreed that randomization was eminently applicable to the comparison of one operation with another. However, he detailed several reasons why RCTs could not be employed to compare new operations with nonoperative therapy. These and other issues of contention are considered in the following section.

Biased Selection of Patients for Randomization

Bonchek correctly points out that, in the case of operations variably accepted as effective, there is often haphazard and possibly biased selection of patients who will be assigned at random to surgical or medical therapy. Once the operation has been described in detail, some patients may be withheld from randomization by referring physicians or by surgeons who do not believe in it. Conversely, others will be withheld from randomization and will be treated with surgery by those who believe strongly that the procedure should be carried out in their particular patients.

This problem has hampered the proper conduct of adequate comparisons of surgery and nonoperative therapy since the first trials of prophylactic portacaval shunt therapy.[29,49] These early RCTs of surgical versus nonoperative treatment provided two valuable lessons. First, the patients randomized were clearly shown to have survival rates different from those patients who refused permission for study (Figure 14-3) or those who were considered for the study but not included because they were felt to be poor operative risks. The patients randomized were different from the population as a whole because

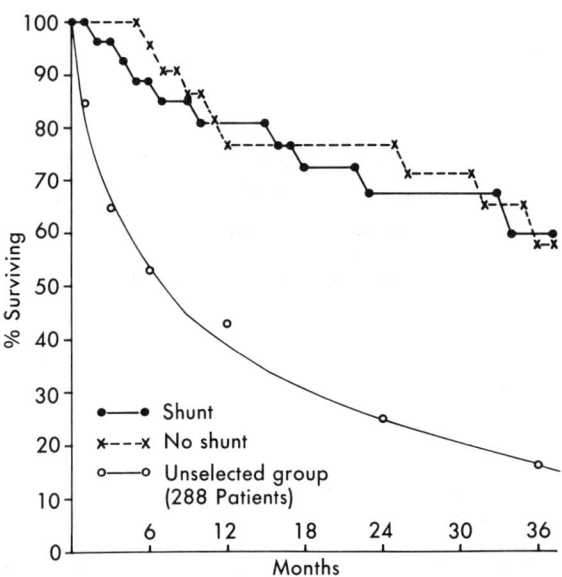

Figure 14-3. Survival from onset of varices of patients randomized to portacaval shunt or medical therapy compared with a group of patients considered and not selected for randomization. (Reprinted, by permission of *The New England Journal of Medicine*, 270:496, 1964.)

investigators believed that even if the operation proved to be effective, the sickest patients would not be operated on as a matter of policy in most circumstances and, therefore, should not be included in the study. Some patients refused to give consent for the study, and these may also have been more severely ill. It is difficult to standardize the subtle influences involved in ethical issues such as the obtaining of informed consent.

Second, the social class of randomized subjects may have differed from that of patients more often seen in private practice. The Boston Inter-Hospital Liver Group, which conducted two of the trials of portacaval shunt surgery, consisted of physicians and surgeons from eight teaching hospitals in the Boston area. The group collaborated in preparing the protocol and presumably continued to participate in the study by seeking patients to be randomized. In the study of prophylactic shunts[49] and a subsequent evaluation of therapeutic shunts,[95] almost all of the trial patients came from public hospitals in which patients found to have varices did not have private physicians. In the other teaching hospitals in which most of the patients had private physicians, few were included in the trial. Consequently, 100% of the patients in the study were alcoholics with cirrhosis, and no information was obtained on the management of varices in nonalcoholic patients. To date, no one has done a trial in nonalcoholics, and the physicians caring for such patients must still make management decisions without adequate data. One could ask whether it is ethical to continue to experiment on such patients in an uncontrolled manner[19,20,22,112] when information could have been obtained so long ago by the proper conduct of a controlled trial. Unencumbered by the referral patterns, which, according to Bonchek,[10] so strongly influence the decisions of surgeons, evaluation of care for alcoholic patients was readily performed. Because survival was unchanged by operation, the patients randomly assigned to nonoperative therapy were the lucky ones.

"Crossovers": Patients Reassigned to Different Treatment Groups After Randomizing

"Crossovers" are a major problem plaguing some medical and surgical trials. They can be diminished by carefully obtaining adequate informed consent before randomization and by randomizing just before surgery so that the uncertainty of the investigator or the natural qualms of the patient or changes in the patient's clinical status will not lead to a change of mind after a commitment to surgery has been made.

In patients who drop out before surgery or who later have surgery after having been assigned to medical therapy, Bonchek rightfully argues for analyzing patients in the group to which they were originally assigned.[10] However, he erroneously states that the Veterans Administration cooperative trial comparing coronary artery bypass grafting (CABG) with medical therapy[86] only counted crossover patients in the group in which they finally were treated. In fact, the VA study analyzed its data in all possible ways. "Intention to treat," that is, analyzing patients according to the group to which they were originally randomized, was the primary scheme. In separate secondary analyses, outcomes in crossover patients were (1) counted only until they crossed over, (2) excluded from the analyses entirely, or (3) counted in the group to which they crossed over. The last is the least desirable method of analysis when it stands alone, but when there are large numbers of crossovers, it should also be performed to determine their effect on the results. In the VA study the method of handling the dropouts did not affect the conclusion that surgery had no appreciable impact on survival. As the patients have been followed for the past 10 years or longer, a clinically and statistically significant benefit from surgery has appeared and then disappeared.[40] If analysis both by intention to treat and by the treatment actually received produces no difference in the conclusions, a study is more credible. If there is a difference, the study needs to be carefully examined and possibly expanded or repeated.[6]

The "Learning Curve" Problem

One of Bonchek's objections to RCTs of surgical versus medical therapy deserves careful consideration from an ethical standpoint. The following quote is pertinent and follows a logic that has been espoused by many others: "In contrast, new operations are introduced tentatively with uncertain indications and high risk."[10]

Clearly, new operations should be performed as well as possible whether they are compared with randomly assigned nonsurgical therapy or not. However, there should be no double standard regarding the ethical conduct of research.[19,21,112] An RCT cannot be started until a protocol describing in detail exactly what will be said to the patients volunteering to be randomized has been approved by an institutional review board. Patients should be told that one or the other treatment is experimental, that they have every right not to volunteer, and that they instead may decide specifically which therapy they would prefer. Is similarly detailed, informed consent ever obtained in the uncontrolled development of new surgical techniques? Does the informed consent form in uncontrolled series state specifically that randomization is being postponed because a higher death rate or complication rate is expected in the early use of the new operation? Bonchek and others argue that it would be unfair to the study if patients were randomly assigned to a new operation at a point in its development when patients are likely to do badly or not survive. How many patients would volunteer for uncontrolled pilot trials if they were adequately informed that this was the reason for not randomizing? When a new operation is first attempted, it is entirely possible that things will go well and that the operation will prove to be better than medical therapy or than the standard operation. In that case, the patients randomized to the experimental treatment will have received the better treatment. On the other hand, if there is a "learning curve," and the early patients have less favorable outcomes, the patients randomized to the standard therapy will have been more fortunate. It seems logical that if such a situation were explained adequately, most patients would opt for early randomization. It is ethically untenable to decide that early patients should be "sacrificed" while the operation is perfected so that it can be more successfully compared with standard therapy later on. The natural inclination of the surgeon to try the new operation in everyone who seems suitable is understandable but should be rejected in favor of testing the procedure in a proper trial from the beginning. Uncontrolled pilot studies are unethical in that they deprive patients of the 50/50 chance of getting what could be the better therapy, and they deprive future patients of the opportunity to be better treated because the new therapy was properly evaluated from the beginning. Allowances for technical modifications resulting from accumulated experience can still be incorporated into the protocol for a surgical RCT. Prior planning can allow separate analyses of modifications, and these changes can be better evaluated if they occur as part of a controlled trial.

Proficiency of Surgeons

Another argument against RCTs is that surgeons participating in them may not be as well trained in the specific operation at issue as are the originators of the operation. Some evidence of the effect of experience is presented in a meta-analysis of papers on proximal vagotomy[8] in which it was shown that the recurrence rate was proportional to the number of authors of the reporting paper. This study implies that, when several surgeons perform a procedure and author the paper, individuals may have fewer opportunities to perfect their surgical techniques. Conversely, lower recurrence rates in series compiled by fewer investigator clinicians may reflect the favorable impact of individuals each having more cumulative experience. This paper is not an argument against RCTs but rather an argument encouraging adequate training of practitioners, whether they are treating patients surgically or medically and whether those patients are part of a trial or not.

One of the major objections to the VA coronary artery surgery study was that the published surgical operative mortality was higher than that obtained in private hospitals.[111] However, a survey of nonpublished operative mortality data from New York state revealed that the average mortality in unpublished trials performed at the time of the VA study was identical to that of the VA study[25] (Figure 14-4). This is one example of "publication bias,"[35,109] which results in the publication of good operative mortality statistics more often than bad ones. Interpretation of the results of trials should be performed in light of the average local mortality rather than the idealized statistics that may appear in the literature.

"Negative" RCTs

When to decide that a new therapy is not a useful advance has always been a difficult problem. Proving a negative, that is, establishing with statistical validity that a treatment does not work, is much more difficult than proving a positive, that is, that it probably does work. In the negative situation the decision depends on the magnitude of the smallest effect that the investigator wishes not to miss. The closer to zero the size of the difference, the closer to infinity the number of

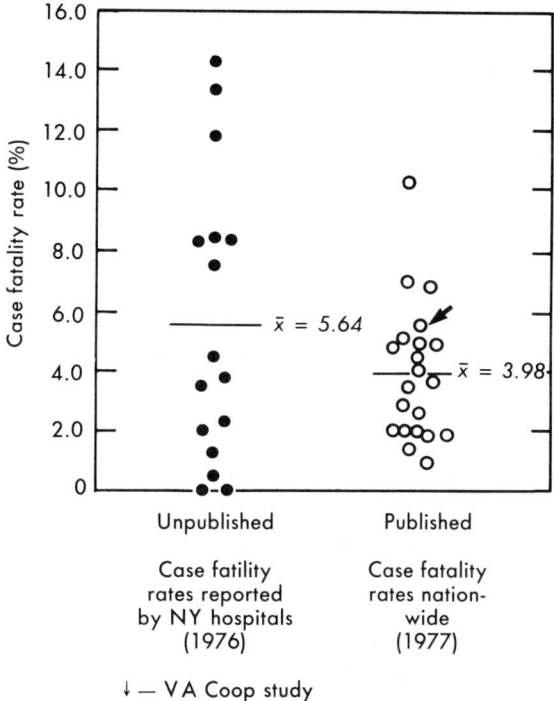

Figure 14-4. Operative fatality rates for coronary artery bypass graft surgery as reported in the literature and as unpublished during the same period. (From Chalmers TC: Clin Res 26:230, 1978.)

patients required to avoid a beta or type II error. This situation was discussed in a survey of 71 trials in which the authors concluded that the test therapy did not work but had samples too small to establish that clinically important differences in treatment effect were still feasible.[48]

Recent Controversies

Trials concluding that a popular therapy does not work usually generate a storm of protest from those who like the treatment. In a classic example that demonstrates that this is not just a surgical problem, the University Group Diabetes Program concluded that oral hypoglycemic agents shorten rather than prolong life in patients with adult-onset diabetes.[117] In response, a large body of diabetologists and pharmaceutical firms stimulated a reaction[44,108] to which there was adequate response[30] but that delayed for 15 years the inclusion by the FDA of a warning label on such agents. In that case the freedom to use a convenient drug rather than an established operation was at issue.

When the Veterans Administration cooperating surgeons and cardiologists reported that there was no apparent prolongation of life 5 years after coronary artery bypass surgery,[86] there was an almost equal response.[111] In that case the initial impression was reversed for a while. Two other studies have confirmed that in some classes of patients with severe coronary artery disease, lives are prolonged and anginal symptoms relieved by surgery.[16,17,31,71] However, there is still a group of patients with one vessel disease, some of whom are asymptomatic, whose lives may be shortened by surgery.[16,40]

The latest example of a flood of protests raised when popular therapy was shown to be ineffective was the EC/IC study,[42] comparing extracranial-intracranial arterial bypass with medical therapy. This also represents a recent example of the effect of not randomizing patients who should be included in an RCT. According to the protocol followed predominantly by Canadian neurologists, neurosurgeons, and vascular surgeons, surgery was found to be no more effective than medication. Because of its large sample size, this trial had a small type II error term, indicating sufficient statistical power to detect a clinically interesting difference if it truly existed. As RCTs go, the study was an excellent one. When analyzed by a scoring system devised by one of the authors of this chapter,[26] the study was found to have a quality score of .93, the highest figure among the 265 RCTs analyzed by this method thus far.[93] Admittedly, the original version of the paper submitted to the *New England Journal of Medicine* was reviewed by one of the originators of the scoring system, and some of the reporting deficiencies were corrected before final publication. Nonetheless, it was hard to find fault with the study as it was designed and executed. An accompanying editorial recognized that the study's design, execution, and analysis made incontrovertible its conclusion that the operation should be abandoned.[91]

The whole subject was reopened with a bang 1½ years later. This was after the publication of a survey of neurosurgeons who had participated in the study,[114] an investigation by a committee of the Association of Neurological Surgeons,[53] and an editorial in the *New England Journal of Medicine*,[94] as well as a detailed response by the original investigators to the criticisms that had been made.[3] This flurry of papers then resulted in another series of letters in the *New England Journal of Medicine*[39] and an editorial published in *The British Medical Journal* by a surgeon.[38] A synopsis highlighting the clinical trials aspect of the controversy can be found in a discussion of generalizability of clinical trials.[60] In general, the conclusions of these communications have followed subspecialty lines, with surgeons protesting the study's conclusions most strongly and nonsurgeons defending them. The problem was similar to that described earlier for the study performed by the Boston Inter-Hospital Liver Group: too many patients had apparently been withheld from randomization and were either operated on or not, depending on the choices of the attending physicians. Although the exact number is debated, numerous patients were operated on during the course of the EC/IC study by neurosurgeons who were ostensibly participating in the study but who did not report the nonstudy operations as had been required by the protocol.

Controversy persists as to what the study would have concluded had the neurosurgeons participating in the study not "shot themselves in the foot" and instead had included even most of the eligible patients. One editorial has suggested that the excluded patients should be followed post hoc to determine their outcome, but this information could be as biased as that of any study with historical or concurrent nonrandomized controls.* Three courses of action seem possible. First, the neurosurgeons who mistrust the study could operate, but in view of the quality of the study and its negative conclusions, to do so would raise ethical and medicolegal problems. Second, those who believe the study could withhold surgery from all future patients but might do so with a gnawing feeling of uncertainty because of the large number of patients who were not randomized. Finally, a logical next step is for those who do not believe the study to organize another one and to start randomizing, immediately, patients such as those whom they think would have demonstrated the superiority of surgery had they been included in the original study.

In contrast, a few RCTs have followed eligible patients who declined randomization and were therefore treated according to patient or physician preference. In the Coronary Artery Surgery Study (CASS),[18] 780 patients with angina pectoris or prior myocardial infarction were randomized to medical therapy or coronary artery bypass grafting (CABG) after a diagnostic cardiac catheterization. An additional 1315 clinically eligible patients treated at the same 11 participating institutions were not randomized after catheterization. Instead, they and/or their physicians elected individually to use medical or surgical therapies. Of these 1315 patients, 43% underwent surgery within 90 days of catheterization, whereas 57% were managed medically for at least 90 days after catheterization.

The eligible (but not randomized) patients treated medically had less extensive coronary disease than did the RCT patients randomized to medical therapy. The surgically treated nonrandomized patients had more extensive coronary disease than did the patients randomized to surgery. Thus among the nonrandomized patients, those undergoing surgery had more extensive disease than those managed medically, whereas the patients randomized to surgery were presumably similar to their medical counterparts. By the fifth year of follow-up, 22% of the eligible but *not* randomized medical patients had "crossed over" to surgery, whereas 24% of the patients originally randomized to medicine had received bypass surgery. Aggregate 5-year survival was 92% for both eligible and randomized medically managed groups, and prognostically stratified subgroups also had similar outcomes. Five-year survival for randomized surgical patients was 95% compared with 94% for their nonrandomized counterparts. Thus although the nonrandomized medical and surgical patients differed prognostically from the randomized patients, 5-year survival figures indicate similar outcomes for all groups.

More important, this is one of the few trials that included careful follow-up of eligible but nonrandomized patients.[18] Thus the investigators could address directly the issues of comparability of randomized and nonrandomized patients as well as the degree to which the RCT results could be generalized to the average patient fitting the clinical criteria for inclusion in the trial. Findings of similar mortality experience

---

*References 23,82,84,103,104.

in the randomized and nonrandomized cohorts strengthened conclusions about the generalizability of the results, but different outcome rates would also have been informative. The published study did not discuss whether observed differences in quality of life among the patients randomized to surgery versus medicine[17] were also observed in those not randomized, presumably because of lack of data for the nonrandomized patients. The parallel follow-up performed in this study sets an example to be emulated wherever possible in all randomized trials. It is an expensive process but is much less costly than continuing to treat patients without valuable information that might help determine optimal management. Such follow-up of nonrandomized patients offers considerable information about the generalizability of RCT results but contributes no information about the relative effectiveness of the procedures under consideration.

Carotid endarterectomy is an operation soon to stimulate arguments similar to those involving EC/IC. Introduced 30 years ago, this procedure was evaluated in only two randomized trials, which were reported as "negative" but had too small sample size.[45,107] Ironically, more than 100,000 of the procedures are performed each year in the United States.[121] A recent report by the Rand Corporation indicated that only 23% of the patients operated on would have been considered appropriate when reviewed by a panel of experts.[80] In 32% of the 107 cases examined, the experts could not agree. It is hoped that the RCT of carotid endarterectomy now in progress should answer some questions about the procedure's usefulness. Had such trials been performed 30 years ago, there might be no need for them now. However, they were not, and while awaiting the RCT results, we must try to determine optimal patient care by convening a group of experts from various fields to review specific cases.[11,27] This is an interesting approach but not one on which much money should be spent. Inconclusive results are quite likely compared with what could be learned by early and properly conducted randomized control trials.

CROSS-SECTIONAL SURVEY OF CURRENT CLINICAL TRIALS IN SURGERY
Survey Goals and Exclusion Criteria

To determine the proportion of surgical treatment comparisons currently using a randomized approach, a cross-sectional survey was made of the English language literature published between January 1985 and September 1987. The goal was to identify comparisons of outcomes for two or more treatment approaches in which at least *one* arm included surgery (here defined as a diagnostic or therapeutic intervention involving a skin incision). There were no specific prior hypotheses, although it was felt that the majority of comparisons would probably be nonrandomized. Excluded papers included review articles, letters and discussions, studies not directly comparing outcomes from different therapeutic regimens, comparisons of outcomes of the same procedure used in different clinical settings, comparisons not involving at least one surgical modality, animal studies, and papers not published in English. Excluded comparisons also included preliminary findings for which subsequently published results were also available, comparisons restricted to minor procedures (such as the choice of central versus peripheral vascular access lines), those involving direct comparisons of medication (for example, intraoperative antibiotics) or nutritional (for example, hyperalimentation) regimens administered in a surgical context, and comparisons of materials or devices in which the choice would not significantly alter the intraoperative procedure. For example, comparisons of different types of prosthetic heart valves or cemented versus noncemented hip prostheses were excluded. However, comparisons of the use of synthetic vascular prostheses versus saphenous vein grafts for arterial bypasses were included, because the process of "harvesting" saphenous veins alters significantly the way in which the surgical procedure was performed. Comparisons in which the only procedure was the ophthalmologic or gynecologic use of lasers were excluded, as were all obstetrical procedures, including procedures performed to restore or eliminate female fertility.

Search Strategies

To identify randomized trials in MEDLINE, (Computerized Version of *Index Medicus*), the following search strategy was used: explode SURGERY, OPERATIVE (includes approximately 225 surgical procedure terms) and (explode RESEARCH DESIGN [includes DOUBLE-BLIND METHOD; RANDOM ALLOCATION or CLINICAL TRIALS or [the root text word] random: [with any ending, from the title or abstract] or COMPARATIVE STUDY).*

This strategy generated 492 citations, of which 360 were rejected. Title or abstract description of a study as "randomized" was accepted although such descriptions are not always accurate. Ten of the 492 citations were described in the abstract as nonrandomized comparisons and were, therefore, included among the NRCs rather than the RCTs. Among studies rejected from the surgical RCT group, 65% compared drug regimens with one another. However, many studies could be rejected for multiple reasons, and no specific classifying hierarchy was used.

For nonrandomized comparison studies, the explode SURGERY, OPERATIVE and COMPARATIVE STUDY terms, with the addition of explode LONGITUDINAL STUDIES (includes FOLLOW-UP STUDIES, PROSPECTIVE STUDIES, RETROSPECTIVE STUDIES) were used to search the literature. Some 958 citations were obtained, and 832 were rejected. Two RCTs identified in the NRC search of 958 postings were included in the RCT group. The majority (60%) of studies rejected as inappropriate NRCs had no internal comparison group; most were case series describing results from a single treatment approach with vague, if any, reference to results in an implied control group. Several papers not addressing a treatment choice, for example, studies comparing results of older versus younger patients, were also excluded. Again, no attempt was made to categorize formally the excluded studies.

These search strategies were deliberately "permissive," thereby increasing the number of citations subsequently rejected in order to avoid missing citations that should be included. For both randomized and nonrandomized comparisons, the title, key words, and abstract (if originally provided) were used to include or exclude studies when possible; only in cases of uncertainty were the actual articles obtained. In only two cases did studies have to be excluded because sufficient information—a detailed abstract or the actual article—could not be obtained.

Results

Table 14-1 describes the 270 included studies, which were first grouped by surgical specialty. Surgical procedures involving the vertebral column were listed separately, because they are often performed by both neurosurgeons and orthopedists. The specialty areas are ranked in decreasing order of proportion of all comparisons that are RCTs. Within each specialty the studies were then classified by type of comparison, that is, procedure-procedure, procedure-medication, procedure-radiation, presence or absence of prophylactic procedure, or exploratory surgical versus imaging procedure performed for diagnostic purposes. No studies actually compared surgery alone with radiation therapy alone; in this category some single modality was used in all patients, and an adjuvant modality was classified as either surgical or radiotherapeutic in nature.

---

*The strategy is given as one logical formula, although *and* and *or* statements are not permitted in the same search statement in the MEDLARS system (Medical Literature Analysis and Retrieval System).

Table 14-1. Survey of randomized trials and nonrandomized comparisons published between 1985 and 1987

Surgical Field	Types of Interventions Compared	RCTs	NRCs	Total	%RCT
Cardiovascular	Procedure versus procedure*	6	4	10	60.0
	Procedure versus medication	12	0	12	100.0
	TOTAL	18	4	22	81.8
Breast	Procedure versus procedure	7	4	11	63.6
	Procedure versus radiation	4	0	4	100.0
	TOTAL	11	4	15	73.3
General (GI)	Procedure versus procedure	31	8	39	79.5
	Procedure versus medication†	11	8	19	57.9
	Prophylactic procedure versus no prophylactic procedure	1	0	1	100.0
	Exploratory procedure versus diagnostic imaging	0	6	6	0.0
	TOTAL	43	22	65	66.2
Urology‡	Procedure versus procedure	18	12	30	60.0
	Procedure versus medication	2	5	7	28.6
	Procedure versus radiation	2	0	2	100.0
	Prophylactic procedure versus no prophylactic procedure	2	0	2	100.0
	TOTAL	24	17	41	58.5
Ophthalmology	Procedure versus procedure	5	4	9	55.4
Other GYN	Procedure versus procedure	5	9	14	35.7
	Procedure versus medication	4	0	4	100.0
	Procedure versus radiation	2	1	3	66.7
	TOTAL	11	10	21	52.4
Neurosurgical§	Procedure versus procedure	1	3	4	25.0
	Procedure versus medication	2	1	3	66.7
	TOTAL	3	4	7	42.3
Head and neck‖	Procedure versus procedure	5	15	20	25.0
	Procedure versus medication	1	1	2	50.0
	TOTAL	6	16	22	27.3
Other thoracic	Procedure versus procedure	0	3	3	0.0
	Procedure versus medication	2	0	2	100.0
	Procedure versus radiation	0	1	1	0.0
	Exploratory procedure versus diagnostic imaging	0	2	2	0.0
	TOTAL	2	6	8	25.0

Continued.

Table 14-1.—cont'd Survey of randomized trials and nonrandomized comparisons published between 1985 and 1987

Surgical Field	Types of Interventions Compared	Number of Studies Performed			
		RCTs	NRCs	Total	%RCT
Miscellaneous	Procedure versus procedure	1	2	3	66.7
	Procedure versus medication	0	1	1	0.0
	TOTAL	1	3	4	25.0
Orthopedics	Closed versus open procedure	5	7	12	41.7
	(Other) procedure versus procedure	5	17	22	29.4
	Procedure versus medication	0	10	10	0.0
	TOTAL	10	34	44	22.7
Vertebral column	Procedure versus procedure	0	8	8	0.0
	Procedure versus medication	0	4	4	0.0
	TOTAL	0	12	12	0.0
GRAND TOTALS	Prophylactic procedure versus no prophylactic procedure	3	0	3	100.0
	Procedure versus radiation	8	2	10	80.0
	Procedure versus medication	34	30	64	53.1
	Procedure versus procedure	89	96	185	48.1
	Exploratory procedure versus diagnostic imaging	0	8	8	0.0
	TOTAL	134	136	270	49.6

*Includes procedures on thoracic vessels.
†Includes sclerotherapy for esophageal varices.
‡Includes male and female renal or adrenal surgery but excludes GYN procedures.
§Includes cerebrovascular procedures but excludes vertebral column surgery.
‖Includes ear, nose, and throat procedures.

Similarly, a prophylactic surgical procedure was either performed or omitted in the context of an already planned intervention, for example, performing or not performing a prophylactic appendectomy during a therapeutic cholecystectomy.

The results of Table 14-1 indicate that approximately 50% of surgical comparisons are RCTs and that there may be significant variation among specialties in the proportion of studies using this design. The relative overall frequency of studies performed within different specialties reflects a multitude of factors, including disease prevalence, numbers of actively publishing investigators, availability of journals accepting such publications, and current areas of clinical controversy. The high proportion of RCTs among cardiovascular surgery evaluations includes those addressing controversies surrounding the use of bypass grafting when compared with medication or angioplasty for treating arterial occlusive disease. The frequency with which RCTs appear in evaluation of gastrointestinal

(GI), genitourinary (GU), breast, and other gynecologic (GYN) surgery reflects the common use of this study design in evaluations of all oncology regimens. It is unclear why RCTs are much less commonly used to evaluate vertebral column surgery and other orthopedic procedures.

The breakdown by type of comparison is also informative, although the numbers of studies in some categories are small. Two thirds (185/270) of the studies compared one procedure with another. It is encouraging to note that, of these, almost half (48%) were RCTs. This figure compares favorably with estimates based on casual review of the earlier literature. Despite Boncheck's[9,10] claim that the RCT is not appropriate for comparing surgical with medical therapy, 34 of 60 such comparisons published in the 33 months of observation were randomized. Cardiovascular surgery (12 RCTs, O NRCs) and gastrointestinal surgery (11 RCTs, 8 NRCs) accounted for the bulk of the RCTs; these areas appear to have made increasing use of randomized designs in recent years.

That all three studies of "prophylactic" procedures were RCTs probably reflects that adding such a procedure to an already planned operation is generally not a major therapeutic decision. Thus patients and physicians are less likely to object to randomization in this situation. Although performing an adjuvant surgical procedure versus a radiotherapeutic procedure has more serious implications, six of eight studies comparing these options were RCTs. This is not surprising because such a choice generally occurs in oncology, a field in which RCTs are frequently performed. It is difficult to interpret the fact that of the eight identified comparisons of the use of exploratory surgery (including peritoneal lavage) versus imaging procedures for diagnosis, none were randomized.

Discussion

Any conclusions to be taken from Table 14-1 must be drawn cautiously. Within any specialty the specific clinical questions addressed by RCTs may differ from those examined in NRCs, making it difficult to interpret the proportion of studies using randomized designs. Furthermore, it is unclear to what degree this survey adequately represents the range of surgical evaluation research. For RCTs, there is some evidence that "publication bias" preferentially results in submission and publication of studies favoring new treatments relative to studies indicating no difference in treatment effect or the superiority of conventional therapy.[4,5,35,109] This phenomenon may be even more pronounced for retrospective nonrandomized comparisons in which the smaller effort required to perform the studies may make investigators feel less compelled to publish what they consider to be "uninteresting" results.[4] There may also have been residual misclassification concerning actual use of randomized designs. This could only have been detected (if then) by obtaining all 270 articles.

Furthermore, much of the surgical evaluation literature still consists of the results of a single mode of treatment described without an internal comparison group.[1] Such studies were not included in this survey. One study sampling the 1976 contents of the *Journal of the American Medical Association,* the *Lancet,* and the *New England Journal of Medicine* found that 5% of the articles were RCTs, 6% were NRCs (apparently excluding papers with literature or registry controls) and 10% were uncontrolled case series of greater than 10 patients.[47] Although this survey contains estimates from 10 years ago and includes no surgical journals, it is reasonable to expect that case series still comprise a significant proportion of the surgical evaluation literature.

One study[34] indicates that computerized searching of the MEDLINE database may identify fewer than half of the published clinical trials on a given topic. However, for this general survey of surgical trials, more exhaustive searching (involving, for example, perusal of reference citations and *Current Contents*) would have been impractical. Furthermore, a cross-sectional survey of MEDLINE may be more representative than a review of the contents of selected medical and surgical journals that may preferentially publish certain types of articles. The survey was concerned primarily with the relative frequencies of RCTs and NRCs within surgical specialty areas. There is no particular reason to suspect that bias in MEDLINE retrieval would distort the relative frequencies obtained.

DETAILED COMPARISONS
Subject Choice

From among the several surgical management questions that had each been addressed by both RCTs and NRCs in the 1985 to 1987 published literature, three were chosen for more extensive review. These were: orchiectomy versus hormonal therapy in prostatic cancer, early surgical excision with immediate autografting versus spontaneous separation with late grafting in deep burns, and various combinations of tonsillectomy, adenoidectomy, and antibiotics for recurrent ear, nose, and throat infections. They were chosen because of the number of RCTs and NRCs available, the distribution of surgical specialties and ages represented, and our experience with the subject matter. We had no recollection of the concordance of conclusions of the RCTs versus NRCs so this could not influence our choices of topics. Gastric "freezing" for duodenal ulcer was added as an example of a manipulative therapy that had been originally popularized by uncontrolled trials but was later abandoned after definitive RCTs that failed to demonstrate an effect.

Result Classification

For these four topics Tables 14-2 to 14-9 summarize the RCTs and NRCs that considered clinical (as opposed to just laboratory) outcome. The authors' conclusions were summarized on a five-point scale. For each outcome considered, the study was considered to have favored one treatment or another if it demonstrated a treatment effect that was both statistically significant and, apparently to the author, clinically important. The study was considered to have indicated a trend favoring one treatment over the other if it demonstrated a clinically important difference that was not statistically significant. We considered the results of the comparison to be equivocal if the study demonstrated no difference of interest to the authors. Trends and statistically significant differences in favor of the control complete the five-point scale. It should be recognized that most of the authors' conclusions about treatment differences (or their absence) are based on inadequate numbers of patients; our superficial reviews were performed merely to illustrate the apparent findings of RCTs and NRCs in selected areas. They did not utilize the "blinded" study critiques and careful interpretation and weighted averaging of results that characterize our formal meta-analysis procedure[102] and should not be considered a valid substitute for such an analysis.

Specific Comparisons

Orchiectomy versus hormonal therapy. The comparison between orchiectomy and hormonal therapy for advanced prostate carcinoma is unusual in that the largest study addressing the question is a randomized trial. The Veterans Administration Cooperative Urological Study Group trial, which enrolled patients until 1968, (Table 14-2) demonstrated equivalent overall mortality for patients treated with all combinations of orchiectomy, estrogen, and placebo. Because of persistent hormonal secretion, orchiectomy, a procedure with some risk in older patients and some possible psychologic side effects, did not decrease death from cancer progression as well as did estrogen therapy. However, medical treatment increased the risk of death from cardiovascular disease such that overall mortality for the two approaches in most randomized and nonrandomized studies have been equal. More recent studies comparing orchiectomy with hormonal therapy have not demonstrated improved outcomes using analogs of luteinizing hormone releasing hormone (LHRH) or

Table 14-2. Orchiectomy versus hormonal therapy for prostatic carcinoma: randomized control trials

Authors (Year)	Number of Patients Orch	Hormonal	Inclusion Criteria	Authors' Conclusions
Jordan et al.[67] (1977)	469	475 Estrogen	Advanced (stage III or stage IV) prostatic carcinoma*	Equivocal for overall mortality, clinical progression
Tolis et al.[116] (1984)	29 randomized to ORCH or LHRH analog		"Advanced" prostate carcinoma	Equivocal for clinical progression at 2 years
DeSy et al.[33] (1986)	13	37 LHRH analog	"Histologically proven carcinoma for which orchiectomy would be conventional treatment"	Equivocal for clinical progression, mortality, testosterone level
Haapiainen et al.[58] (1986)	131	146 Estrogen	Histologically or cytologically proven prostate cancer (various stages)	Equivocal for overall mortality; Favored orchiectomy for cardiovascular events; Favored hormones for cancer progression, cancer mortality at 2 years
Henricksson & Edhag[61] (1986)	50	50 Estrogen	Newly diagnosed prostate cancer "judged appropriate for orchiectomy"; no history of prior cardiovascular events	Favored orchiectomy for cardiovascular events
Parmar et al.[88] (1987)	49	55 LHRH analog	Untreated, histologically proven metastatic cancer; expected survival >3 mos	Equivocal for biochemical and clinical outcomes, mortality, side effects at 2 years

*This large cooperative trial also included patients with local disease not requiring orchiectomy, as well as patients with advanced disease randomized to a combination of orchiectomy and estrogen therapy.

other compounds in place of estrogens (Tables 14-2 and 14-3); studies directly comparing different hormonal therapies are beyond the scope of this analysis.

If the early RCT had conclusively favored one treatment or the other, the current controversy would not exist, and there might be no comparisons still performed. Given the high prevalence of prostatic cancer and the absence of widely accepted treatment, there is strong justification for performing another cooperative RCT comparing various combinations of orchiectomy, LHRH analogs, and (possibly) estrogen therapy. The apparent similarities in clinical outcome make attainment of adequate sample size, either through initial collaboration or through meta-analysis of results of small trials, especially important.

There were two instances in which RCTs appear to have been later distorted by the addition to both arms of patients whose treatment had been determined by some nonrandom mechanism. Even though minimally increasing sample size, this procedure weakens a study's conclusions by including patients whose treatment might have been chosen for clinically important reasons. Although one study did analyze results with and without the additional patients (finding no significant change), the practice of combining randomized and nonrandomized patients in the same study should be discouraged. Also, of six studies reported as having been randomized, one allocated patients using a poorly described combination of birth dates and staging, and another demonstrated such unequal numbers (13 patients receiving orchiectomy versus 37 patients receiving the investigational LHRH analog) that strict adherence to randomization is doubtful (Table 14-2). Two studies published in less well-known journals could not be included because no information beyond the titles and indexing terms could be obtained.

Tonsillectomy versus nonsurgical treatment. Tonsillectomy and adenoidectomy are excellent examples of the dearth of good studies in the surgical literature (Tables 14-4 and 14-5). Both operations were undoubtedly overused in the past, and there have been sharp decreases in their recent performance.[85,122] In the past 20 years there have been at least 10 RCTs and 7 NRCs of tonsillectomy and/or adenoidectomy. These trials were confined to the era of MEDLINE and modern antibiotics. However, two large RCTs carried out in the early 1960s are included because they seem to be the only RCTs to have been performed with sufficient numbers.

Table 14-3. Orchiectomy versus hormonal therapy for prostatic carcinoma: nonrandomized comparisons

Authors (Year)	Number of Patients		Inclusion Criteria	Authors' Conclusions
	Orch	Hormonal		
Koutsilieris[69] (1986)	17	42 Buselerin	Advanced disease (stage D_2)	Equivocal for relapse, side effects, overall mortality at 3 years; Equivocal for hormone levels at 8 weeks
Labrie[70] (1986)	13 also received Flutamine	118 LHRH analog	Untreated advanced disease (stage D_2)	Unclear for comparative effectiveness

Both indicate a clinically significant reduction in illness from the combined operation in enough patients to make the mean differences statistically significant. Differences in the number of days lost from school are less impressive, and, surprisingly, the treatment groups do not count the days lost because of the operation. Because there are more than 100,000 people annually who have tonsillectomies and adenoidectomies in the United States,[66] there continues to be a need for a properly conducted study that is large enough to sort out the potential benefits for subgroups of patients.

Some trials compared T&A with nonsurgical

Table 14-4. Tonsillectomy and/or adenoidectomy: randomized control trials

Authors (Year)	Treatment and Number of Patients		Inclusion Criteria	Authors' Conclusions
Rynnel-Dagöö[101] (1978)	A* No operation	37 39	Frequent URI and otitis media	"Still an open question"
Roydhouse[98] (1980)	A No operation	49 50	Otitis media with effusion in children	No benefit from A
Fiellau-Nikolajsen[46] (1986)	A No operation	21 21	Chronic otitis media	No difference in middle ear status
Black[7] (1986)	A No operation	50 50	"Glue ear" in children	"Similar responses to treatment"
Maw[75] (1986)	A T&A No operation	47 47 56	Chronic otitis media	A helped hearing, but T added nothing
Bulman[12] (1984)	A Grommet insertion and paracentesis	46+ 46+	Glue ear, bilateral deafness in children	Hearing improved significantly at 3 & 6 months, and not at 1 year
Paradise[87] (1984)	T±A No operation	43 48	Recurrent sore throats without airway obstruction	Significant reduction in throat infection at 1, 2, but not 3 years
Stafford[113] (1986)	T Antibiotics	20 20	Adults with recurrent sore throat	"Adequate medical treatment equally good in majority of patients"
Mawson[76] (1967)	T&A Nonoperative treatment	202 202	Children with chronic tonsillitis excluding very severe and mild	"Noticeable reduction in frequency of attacks"
McKee[78] (1963)	T&A Nonoperative treatment	231 182	Same as Mawson	Children under 5 years most helped

*T = tonsillectomy; A = adenoidectomy.

treatment; others were three-way trials designed to compare each operation independently with the other as well as with nonoperative treatment. The proper way to have conducted these studies would have been by a 2x2 factorial design.[15,24] This is a very useful experimental design in which two treatments can be compared with each other and simultaneously, each with a no-treatment group. It can be performed with half the number of patients necessary for two separate treatment/no-treatment studies if there is no suggestion of an interaction between the two treatments. An interaction exists when one treatment works better or worse when given with the other than when given alone. If there is a suggested or real interaction, the number of patients required may be twice as large as in an individual treatment design. However, there is no other way to prove the existence of an interaction than by the 2x2 design, and an interaction may be of critical clinical importance. That is most certainly the case with tonsillectomy and adenoidectomy.

Early surgical excision versus conservative debridement for deep burns. Surgical excision of nonviable tissue with immediate autografting early in the postburn period is an aggressive approach to care of deep burns. It may be compared with the more conservative procedure of late debridement and grafting areas that

Table 14-5. Tonsillectomy and/or adenoidectomy; nonrandomized comparisons

Authors (Year)	Treatment and Number of Patients		Inclusion Criteria	Authors' Conclusions
Hibbert[63] (1978)	T* alone T&A	32 32	"Children with usual symptoms"	"Adenoidal" symptoms equally reduced
Marshak[74] (1980)	A* Tympanostomy	29 29	Children with chronic mucoid middle ear effusion	Tympanostomy better with respect to return of hearing
Potsic[92] (1986)	T&A Age-matched normal controls	100 50	Children with partial airway obstruction	"Far-ranging benefit"
Widemar[123] (1985)	A + Paracentesis Paracentesis alone	24 35	Chronic secretory otitis media in children	Equivocal
Fairbanks[43] (1984)	T and/or A Nonoperative treatment	101 ?	Snoring children and adults	"Amenable to surgical therapy"
McCurdy[77] (1977)	Early T Interval T	28 34	Peritonsillar abscess in adults	Duration of illness less with early
Roydhouse[97] (1970)	T&A "Waiting List" Normal controls	251 175 173	Children with recurrent respiratory infections	Favored T&A in reduction of URI
Paradise[87] (1984)	T ± A No surgery	52 44	Patients whose parents chose treatment instead of randomization	Throat infection significantly reduced at 1, 2, and 3 years

*T = tonsillectomy; A = adenoidectomy.

have remained necrotic. The increased operative risks associated with early excision may be justified by the reduced likelihood of infections and other complications, more rapid wound closure, and shorter length of stay. Early excision is one of the few advances in trauma surgery to have been evaluated in both RCTs and NRCs (Tables 14-6 and 14-7). Most studies of both types agree that early excision confers some benefit in most circumstances although the NRCs favor it more strongly. Unfortunately, most of the NRCs and RCTs suffered from serious methodologic and statistical weaknesses that would tend to favor early excision. In the NRCs, decisions concerning whether to excise early seem to have been influenced by severity of burn and other factors affecting burn prognosis. Therefore, comparisons of outcome were susceptible to considerable "confounding by indication" that severely hampered attempts to identify the influence of treatment on outcome. Historically, controlled NRCs could have been biased by secular changes in various other aspects of burn management.

Proper randomization would presumably have eliminated this potential bias in the RCTs, but many of these studies appeared to have had

Table 14-6. Early excision versus conservative debridement of deep thermal burns; randomized control trials

Authors (Year)	Number of Patients Excision	Number of Patients Debridement	Inclusion criteria	Authors' Conclusions
Salisbury et al.[105] (1976)	7	8	Patients with noncharred hands with digital burns	Trend favored excision for digital salvage, function
Salisbury and Wright[106] (1983)	8	12	Patients with third-degree or deep second-degree hand burns	Equivocal for function at 12 mo
Engrav et al.[41] (1983)	22	25	Patients with burns of <20% TBSA* of indeterminate depth (second- versus third-degree)	Favored excision for LOS†; equivocal for late function, cosmetics
Sørensen et al.[110] (1984)	73	76	Patients >6 years old, <24 hours postburn, no isolated face or hand burns	Favored excision for infection; trend favored excision for LOS; equivocal for mortality
Kalaja[68] (1984)	52	50	Patients from Sørensen (1984) who survived 3 years	Equivocal for function, cosmetics
Thompson et al.[115] (1987)	25	25	Patients with ≥30% TBSA, admitted <5 days postburn, no multisystem injury	Uninterpretable‡ for mortality >50% TBSA; equivalent for mortality, LOS in other groups

*Percent of total body surface area receiving second- or third-degree burn.
†Length of hospital stay.
‡Result favored excision but was confounded by age distribution.

flawed or, at best, inadequately described randomization. Also, most of the RCTs and NRCs had small sample sizes, inadequate assessment of the distribution of prognostic factors, variable and poorly described follow-up, and other problems. Patients and their treating physicians obviously could not be blinded to the surgical regimen used, and such knowledge should not have influenced assessment of outcomes such as mortality. However, subsequent functional, cosmetic, or even clinical outcomes could have been assessed by observers unfamiliar with each patient's treatment. Without such blinding, it is possible that knowledge of the treatment received influenced assessment of these subjective outcomes in all studies. Analysis of results was also often quite limited, with minimal consideration of the possible effects of potential biases and small sample sizes. In one of our experiences, coinvestigators' perceptions of journal space constraints and of the audience's orientation have limited discussions of important methodologic and statistical issues. Deficiencies of design and analysis in the burn studies raise serious questions about the usefulness of conclusions to be drawn form improperly performed RCTs relative to those of NRCs. However, studies of both designs demonstrated a need for significant improvement.

Gastric freezing. Gastric freezing for relief of intractable duodenal ulcer is one of a small number of new procedures that was abandoned with relatively little fanfare after double-blind clinical trials conformed suspicions that the ini-

Table 14-7. Early excision versus conservative debridement of deep thermal burns; nonrandomized comparisons

Authors (Year)	Number of Patients Excision	Number of Patients Debridement	Inclusion Criteria	Authors' Conclusions
Burke et al.[13] (1976)	76	76	Patients with hand burns	Favored excision for function, cosmetics, reconstruction
Gray et al.[55] (1982)	23	24	Patients with burns of 20%-40% TBSA*, no major comorbidity time	Favored excision for infection, graft take, LOS†; equivocal for mortality, other complications, operative adjusted costs
Goodwin et al.[54] (1983)	67	31	Patients with hand burns	Equivocal for mortality, function in deep burns; trend favored debridement for function in shallow burns
Pietsch et al.[90] (1985)	20	33	Children with burns >25% TBSA, no major comorbidity	Favored excision for complications, LOS; trend favored excision for mortality
Herndon et al.[62] (1986)	32	32	Children with burns >45% TBSA	Favored fascial excision for LOS, number of operations; equivocal for mortality, blood loss, operative time
Mahler et al.[73] (1987)	253 hands	154 hands	Patients with deep hand burns	Favored excision for infection, healing time, scarring

*Percent of total body surface area receiving second- or third-degree burn.
†Length of hospital stay.

Table 14-8. Gastric freezing versus sham cooling for duodenal ulcer: randomized control trials

Authors (Year)	Number of Patients "Freeze"	"Sham"	Inclusion Criteria	Authors' Conclusions
Perry et al.[89] (1964)	20 (50 min at inflow temp of −20° to −17°C)	20 (50 min at inflow temp of +5°C)	Male VA patients with "clear-cut" evidence of recurrent ulcer	Trend favored sham for complications, gastroscopic changes, ulcer recurrence at 6 months
Wangensteen et al.[119] (1965)	30 (6 min at inflow temp of −20° to −17°C)	30 (6 min at inflow temp of −5°C)	Patients with x-ray-proven ulcer refractory to medication; no other GI disease or changes; surgical risk factors	Favored freezing for symptom relief at 1 to 6 months; trend favored sham for gastroscopic
Harrell et al.[59] (1967)	28 (50 min at inflow temp of −20° to −15°C)	24 (50 min at inflow temp of −20% to −15°C, but no liquid in stomach)	Patients with x-ray-proven chronic nonobstructive duodenal ulcer with peptic ulcer pain not relieved by standard therapy	Trend slightly favored Freezing for symptom relief at 18 months; Equivocal for later surgery
Zikria et al.[124] (1967)	8 (6 min at inflow temp of −20° to −17°C)	8 (6 min at inflow temp of +5° to +10°C)	Patients 20-60 years old with ≥ normal secretion, x-ray evidence and symptoms of ulcer refractory to treatment; no GI bleed, pyloric destruction, or gastric stasis	Equivocal for pain at 1 week and 18 to 24 months; Unclear for need for surgery by 18 to 24 months
Ruffin et al.[100] (1969)	82 (5 min at outflow temp of −10°C)	78 (5 min with proximal coolant but with gastric balloon temp of +37°C)	Patients ≥ 18 years old, recurrent symptoms, and x-ray evidence or secretory pattern consistent with ulcer	Trend slightly favored freezing for symptom relief at up to 24 months; equivocal for GI complications, GI sequelae

tial enthusiasm about the procedure might have been unwarranted (Tables 14-8 and 14-9). The procedure appeared to be based on sound physiologic principles: cooling of the stomach in animals reduces both the quantity and digestive activity of gastric secretions and should, therefore, slow the progressive ulcer disease. The gastric freezing procedure required patients to swallow a balloon that was then cooled to -20°C to -15°C using a circulating solution. This seemed like an attractive alternative to chronic often unsuccessful use of symptom-directed medication or surgery, which entailed some risk without guarantee of success.

Encouraging preliminary results published by several investigators including the respected surgeon who had developed the procedure stimulated widespread popularity of this approach among physicians and patients.[81] Gastric freezing machines became standard hospital equipment, and although this approach had not been advocated as an office procedure, it was also being done in such settings. In a panel discussion at the 1963 American Gastroenterological Association meeting, it was estimated that approximately 300 machines had been used to perform about 4000 such procedures.[99]

Doubts about the efficacy of gastric freezing and concerns about possible associated cardiac and GI complications were expressed at the same meeting. This prompted the conduct of one NRC and 5 RCTs of clinical outcomes, all of which employed control groups receiving "sham freezing." Use of a sham control group to estimate a possible placebo effect of gastric "freezing" was a relatively benign procedure and provoked less controversy than had use of sham surgery in the 1958 and 1959 RCTs of internal mammary artery ligation for angina pectoris.[28,37]

One nonrandomized study of 188 outpatients compared clinical results of gastric freezing with and without medical therapy with those of a sham procedure (see Table 14-8 and 14-9). This trial did not specify patient treatment allocation criteria, but like the RCTs, indicated no difference in gastric secretion or clinical outcome for as long as one year later among the five treated subgroups. Of the five RCTs (see Table 14-8), only one indicated some relative benefit among patients who received "freezing." The others, which included a five-center collaboration enrolling 160 patients, generally indicated equivalent long-term clinical results for the two treatments. For most studies the variable initial differences in treatment effect disappeared over time, and there was no correlation between gastric secretion and clinical outcomes. Consequently the "freezing" procedure was abandoned without much protest.

CONCLUSIONS
Study Results

Although randomization is generally accepted as the preferable scheme for comparing competing treatment modalities, its adoption in surgical

Table 14-9. Gastric freezing versus sham cooling for duodenal ulcer: nonrandomized comparison

Authors (Year)	Number of Patients		Inclusion Criteria	Authors' Conclusions
	"Freeze"	"Sham"		
Lubos et al.[72] (1966)	171 (1 hr at inflow temp of −20° to −17°C)	17 (1 hr at inflow temp of +10° to +15°C)	Outpatients with x-ray and clinical evidence of active ulcer disease	Equivocal for clinical response at 12 months

evaluation has been slow in coming. Justifications presented by Bonchek and others do not appear valid, and failure to randomize has prolonged clinical controversies that should have been settled earlier. Our study demonstrated that randomization was employed in almost half of the comparative studies involving one or more surgical modalities. However, there is considerable variation among surgical specialties and among the different types of comparisons.

In-depth review of the RCTs and NRCs used to settle specific clinical controversies indicated a surprising concordance of results. For comparisons of orchiectomy with hormonal therapy for prostatic cancer, the observed equivalence of mortality found in all study designs probably indicates that the occasional failure of surgical castration or LHRH analogs to halt disease progression is balanced by increased risk of cardiovascular events associated with estrogen use. There appear to be real benefits associated with the use of early excision for deep burns in some circumstances. However, both the RCTs and NRCs suffer from considerable methodologic weaknesses that seem to favor excision in most instances. Small sample sizes and limited analyses of results weaken many of these studies as was the case in other clinical questions we reviewed. The placebo effect of surgery and other therapeutic manipulations may be appreciable, and comparisons of procedures with medication should acknowledge this phenomenon. Although carefully performed, analyzed, and interpreted NRCs may be helpful, the advantages of well-conducted RCTs make this the preferable evaluation approach. There can be no substitute for minimizing the play of chance and biased treatment assignment in the conduct of comparative clinical trials.

Key Features of Good Trials

While stating a preference for randomized control trials, we wish to emphasize that they should be properly executed.[26] A good trial is minimally more expensive and time-consuming than a poorly conducted one. The many aspects of a good trial are reviewed elsewhere,[26,79] but six essentials can be reiterated here:

1. All patients who might be treated according to the study protocol should be included and a log kept of all patients considered for the study and not randomized. Parallel follow-up of patients who were eligible for randomization but were treated outside of trials is a commendable feature that should be performed whenever possible.
2. The randomization process should be blinded so that there is no hint of the next assignment when the next patient is chosen and informed consent sought.[23]
3. Interpretation of therapeutic outcome should be blinded when possible.
4. Withdrawals, dropouts, and crossovers should be handled so that they do not bias the results.[6] Follow-up should be pursued equally in all groups.
5. Participating physicians should be blinded as to developing trends in the data so that they do not become biased as the study progresses. Studies stopped because of premature "results" would be extremely difficult to repeat.
6. Published reports should consider the effects of any sample size requirements caused by the smallness of the clinical effect of interest or restrictions on the number of patients available.

Adhering to these and other principles will enable investigators to perform reproducible RCTs that should better approach the truth than any other method of clinical evaluation.

References

1. Bailar JC III et al: Studies without internal controls, N Engl J Med 311:156, 1984.
2. Barnes BA: Discarded operations: surgical innovation by trial and error. In Bunker JP, Barnes BA, and Mosteller F, editors: Costs, risks, and benefits of surgery, New York, 1977, Oxford University Press.
3. Barnett HJ et al: Are the results of the extracranial-intracranial bypasss trial generalizable? N Engl J Med 316:820, 1987.

4. Berlin JA, Begg CB, and Louis TA: Assessing the magnitude of publication bias in clinical trials. Controlled Clin Trials 301:180, 1987.
5. Berlin JA, Begg CB, and Louis TA: An assessment of publication bias using a sample of published clinical trials, J Am Stat Soc (in press).
6. Bhaskar R et al: Loss of patients in clinical trials that measure long-term survival following myocardial infarction, Controlled Clin Trials 7:134, 1986.
7. Black R: Tonsillectomy and adenoidectomy: a review. Aust Fam Physician 15:714, 1986.
8. Blum AL, Popein J, and Bauerfeind: Decisions in a case of recurrent duodenal ulcer. In Chalmers TC, editor: Data analysis for clinical medicine: the quantitative approach to patient care, Rome, 1988, International University Press.
9. Bonchek LI: Are randomized trials appropriate for evaluating new operations? N Engl J Med 301:44, 1980.
10. Bonchek LI: The role of the randomized clinical trial in the evaluation of new operations, Surg Clin North Am 1982 62:761, 1982.
11. Brook RH and Lohr KN: Monitoring quality of care in the Medicare program: two proposed systems, JAMA 258:3138, 1987.
12. Bulman CH, Brook SJ, and Berry MG: A prospective randomized trial of adenoidectomy vs grommet insertion in the treatment of glue ear, Clin Otolaryngol 9:67, 1984.
12a. Bunker JP, Barnes BA, and Mosteller F, editors: Costs, risks, and benefits of surgery, New York, 1977, Oxford University Press.
13. Burke JF et al: Primary surgical management of the deeply burned hand, J Trauma 16:593, 1976.
14. Byar DP: Why data bases should not replace randomized clinical trials, Biometrics 36:337, 1980.
15. Byar DP and Piantadosi S: Factorial designs for randomized clinical trials, Cancer Treat Rep 69:1055, 1985.
16. CASS principal investigators and their associates: coronary artery surgery study (CASS): a randomized trial of coronary artery bypass surgery: survival data, Circulation 68:939, 1983.
17. CASS principal investigators and their associates: Coronary artery surgery study (CASS): a randomized trial of coronary artery bypass surgery: quality of life in patients randomly assigned to treatment groups, Circulation 68:951, 1983.
18. CASS principal investigators and their associates: Coronary artery surgery study (CASS): a randomized trial of coronary artery bypass surgery: comparability of entry characteristics and survival in randomized patients and nonrandomized patients meeting randomization criteria, J Am Coll Cardiol 3:114, 1984.
19. Chalmers I: Minimizing harm and maximizing benefit during innovation in health care: controlled or uncontrolled experimentation? Birth 13:155, 1986.
20. Chalmers TC: Ethical aspects of clinical trials, Am J Ophthalmol 79:753, 1975.
21. Chalmers TC: Informed consent, clinical research and the practice of medicine, Trans Am Clin Climatol Assoc 94:204, 1982.
22. Chalmers TC: Randomized clinical trials in surgery. In Varco RL and Delaney JP, editors: Controversies in surgery, Philadelphia, 1976, WB Saunders Co.
23. Chalmers TC et al: Bias in treatment assignment in controlled clinical trials, N Engl J Med 309:1358, 1983.
24. Chalmers TC et al: Treatment of acute infectious hepatitis in the Armed Forces: advantages of ad lib bed rest and early reconditioning, JAMA 159:1431, 1959.
25. Chalmers TC et al: In defense of the VA randomized control trial of coronary artery surgery, Clin Res 26:230, 1978.
26. Chalmers TC et al: A method for assessing the quality of a randomized control trial, Controlled Clin Trials 2:31, 1981.
27. Chassin MR et al: Does inappropriate use explain geographic variations in the use of health care services? A study of three procedures, JAMA 258:2533, 1987.
28. Cobb LA et al: An evaluation of internal-mammary-artery ligation by a double-blind technic, N Engl J Med 260:1115, 1959.
29. Conn Ho and Lindenmuth WW: Prophylactic portacaval anastomosis in cirrhotic patients with esophageal varices: preliminary report of a controlled study, New Eng J Med 266:743, 1962.
30. Cornfield J: The University Group Diabetes Program: a further statistical analysis of the mortality findings, JAMA 231:583, 1975.
31. Coronary-artery bypass surgery in stable angina pectoris: survival at two years: European Coronary Surgery Study Group, Lancet 1:889, 1979.
32. Reference deleted in proofs.
33. De Sy WA et al: A comparative study of a long acting luteinizing hormone releasing hormone agonist (Decapeptyl) and orchiectomy in the treatment of advanced prostatic cancer: preliminary report, Acta Urol Belg 54:221, 1986.
34. Dickersin K et al: Perusing the literature: comparison of MEDLINE searching with a perinatal trials database, Controlled Clin Trials 6:306, 1985.
35. Dickersin K et al: Publication bias and randomized control trials, Controlled Clin Trials, 8:343, 1987.
36. Diehl LF and Perry DJ: A comparison of randomized concurrent control groups with matched historical control groups: are historical controls valid? J Clin Oncol 4:1114, 1986.

37. Dimond EG, Kittle CF, and Crockett JE: Evaluation of internal mammary artery ligation and sham procedure in angina pectoris, Circulation 18:712, 1958.
38. Dudley HA: Extracranial-intracranial bypass, one; clinical trials, nil, Br Med J 294:1501, 1987.
39. The EC-IC bypass study: letters to the editor, N Engl J Med 317:1030, 1987.
40. Eleven-year survival in the Veterans Administration randomized trial of coronary bypass surgery for stable angina: The Veterans Administration Coronary Artery Bypass Surgery Cooperative Study Group, N Engl J Med 311:1333, 1984.
41. Engrav LH et al: Early excision and grafting vs. inoperative treatment of burns of indeterminant depth: a randomized prospective study, J Trauma 23:1001, 1983.
42. Failure of extracranial-intracranial arterial bypass to reduce the risk of ischemic stroke: results of an international randomized trial, The EC/IC Bypass Study Group, N Engl J Med 313:1191, 1985.
43. Fairbanks DN: Snoring: surgical vs. nonsurgical management, Laryngoscope 94:1188, 1984.
44. Feinstein AR: Clinical biostatistics. VIII: an analytical appraisal of the University Group Diabetes Program (UGDP) study, Clin Pharmacol Ther 12(2 part I):167, 1971.
45. Fields WS et al: Joint study of extracranial vascular occlusion, part 5 (prognosis following surgical or non surgical treatment for transient cerebral ischaemic attacks and cervical carotid artery lesions), JAMA 211:1993, 1970.
46. Fiellau-Nikolajsen M: Audiological aspects on treatment of SOM: Indications and results, Scand Audiol Suppl 26:77, 1986.
47. Fletcher RH and Fletcher SW: Clinical research in general medical journals: a 30-year perspective, N Engl J Med 301:180, 1979.
48. Freiman JA et al: The importance of beta, the type II error and sample size in the design and interpretation of the randomized control trial: survey of 71 "negative" trials: N Engl J Med 299:690, 1978.
49. Garceau AJ et al: A controlled trial of prophylactic portacaval-shunt surgery: N Engl J Med 270:496, 1964.
50. Gehan EA: Design of controlled clinical trials: use of historical controls, Cancer Treat Rep 66:1089, 1982.
51. Gehan EA and Freireich EJ: Non-randomized controls in cancer clinical trials, N Engl J Med 290:198, 1974.
52. Gilbert JP, McPeek B, and Mosteller F: Progress in surgery and anesthesia: benefits and risks of innovative therapy. In Bunker JP, Barnes BA, and Mosteller, F, editors: Costs, risks, and benefits of surgery, New York, 1977, Oxford University.
53. Goldring S, Zervas N, and Langfitt T: The extracranial-intracranial bypass study: N Engl J Med 316:817, 1987.
54. Goodwin CW et al: Prospective study of wound excision of the hands, J Trauma 23:510, 1983.
55. Gray DT et al: Early surgical excision versus conventional therapy in patients with 20 to 40 percent burns: a comparative study, Am J Surg 144:76, 1982.
56. Green SB and Byar DP: Using observational data from registries to compare treatments: the fallacy of omnimetrics: Stat Med 3:361, 1984.
57. Greenland S and Neutra R: Control of confounding in the assessment of medical technology, Int J Epidemiol 9:361, 1980.
58. Haapiainen R, Rannikko S, and Alfthan O: Comparison of primary orchiectomy with oestrogen therapy in advanced prostatic cancer; A 2-year follow-up report of a national prospective prostatic cancer study, Br J Urol 58:528, 1986.
59. Harrell WR et al: Gastric hypothermia for duodenal ulcer: a long-term controlled study, JAMA 200:290, 1967.
60. Hawkins B: Perusing the literature: generalization of clinical trials, Controlled Clin Trials 8:255, 1987.
61. Henriksson P and Edhag O: Orchiectomy versus oestrogen for prostatic cancer: cardiovascular effects, Br Med J [Clin Res] 293:413, 1986.
62. Herndon DN and Parks DH: Comparison of serial debridement and autografting and early massive excision with cadaver skin overlay in the treatment of large burns in children, J Trauma 26:149, 1986.
63. Hibbert J and Stell P: Critical evaluation of adenoidectomy, Lancet 1:489, 1978.
64. Hill AB: Observation and experimentation, N Engl J Med 248:995, 1953.
65. Hill AB: Principles of medical statistics, ed 9, New York, 1971, Oxford University Press.
66. Hospital Discharge Data. Detailed diagnoses and procedures for patients discharges from short-stay hospitals. Vital and Health Statistics, Series 13(90). [DHHS Publication (PHS) p 7-1751]. Hyattsville, Md, 1987, US National Center for Health Statistics: 170.
67. Jordan WP Jr, Blackard CE, and Byar DP: Reconsideration of orchiectomy in the treatment of advanced prostatic carcinoma, South Med J 70:1411, 1977.
68. Kalaja E: Acute excision or exposure treatment? Secondary reconstructions and functional results, Scand J Plast Reconstr Surg 18:95, 1984.
69. Koutsilieris M et al: Objective response and disease outcome in 59 patients with stage D2 prostatic cancer treated with either Buserelin or orchiectomy: disease aggresivity and its association with response and outcome. Urology 27:221, 1986.

70. Labrie F et al: Advantages of the combination therapy in previously untreated and treated patients with advanced prostate cancer, J Steroid Biochem 25:877, 1986.
71. Long-term results of prospective randomized study of coronary artery bypass surgery in stable angina pectoris, European Coronary Surgery Study Group, Lancet 2:1173, 1982.
72. Lubos ME, Viril LC, and Klotz AP: A controlled study of outpatient gastric freezing, Am J Dig Dis 11:266, 1966.
73. Mahler D et al: Treatment of the burned hand: early surgical treatment (1975-85) vs. conservative treatment (1964-74): a comparative study. Burns Incl Therm Inj 13:45, 1987.
74. Marshak G and Neriah ZB: Adenoidectomy versus tympanostomy in chronic secretory otitis media, Ann Otol Rhinol Laryngol [Suppl] 89(3 Pt Suppl 68):316, 1980.
75. Maw AR and Herod F: Otoscopic, impedance, and audiometric findings in glue ear treated by adenoidectomy and tonsillectomy: a prospective randomized study, Lancet 1:1399, 1986.
76. Mawson SR, Adlington P, and Evans M: A Controlled study evaluation of adeno-tonsillectomy in children, J Laryngol Otol 81:777, 1967.
77. McCurdy JA Jr: Peritonsillar abscess: a comparison of treatment by immediate tonsillectomy and interval tonsillectomy, Arch Otolaryngol Head Neck Surg 103:414, 1977.
78. McKee WJE: A controlled study of the effects of tonsillectomy and adenoidectomy in children. Brit J Prev Soc Med 17:49, 1963.
79. Meinert CL: Clinical trials : design, conduct, and analysis, New York, 1986, Oxford University Press, Inc.
80. Merrick NJ et al: Use of carotid endarterectomy in five California Veterans Administration medical centers, JAMA 256:2532, 1986.
81. Miao LL: Gastric freezing: an example of the evaluation of medical therapy by randomized clinical trials. In Bunker JP, Barnes BA, Mosteller F, editors: Costs, risks, and benefits of surgery, New York, 1979, Oxford University Press.
82. Micciolo R, Valagussa P, and Marubini E: The use of historical controls in breast cancer: an assessment in three consecutive trials, Controlled Clin Trials 6:259, 1985.
83. Miettinen OS: The need for randomization in the study of intended effects, Stat Med 2:267, 1983.
84. Miller JN, Colditz GA, and Mosteller F: How study design affects outcomes in comparisons of surgical treatments (manuscript in preparation).
85. Mindell WR, Vayda E, and Cardillo B: Ten-year trends in Canada for selected operations, Can Med Assoc J 127:23, 1981.
86. Murphy ML et al: Treatment of chronic stable angina: a preliminary report of survival data of the randomized Veterans Administration cooperative study, N Engl J Med 297:621, 1977.
87. Paradise JL et al: Efficacy of tonsillectomy for recurrent throat infection in severely affected children: results of parallel randomized and nonrandomized clinical trials, N Engl J Med 310:674, 1984.
88. Parmar H et al: Orchiectomy versus long-acting D-Trp-6-LHRH in advanced prostatic cancer: Br J Urol 59:248, 1987.
89. Perry GT et al: Gastric freezing for duodenal ulcer, Gastroenterology 47:6, 1964.
90. Pietsch JB et al: Early excision of major burns in children: effect on morbidity and mortality, J Pediatr Surg 20:754, 1985.
91. Plum F: Extracranial-intracranial arterial bypass and cerebral vascular disease, N Engl J Med 313:1221, 1985.
92. Potsic WP et al: Relief of upper airway obstruction by adenotonsillectomy, Arch Otolaryngol Head Neck Surg 94:476, 1986.
93. Reitman D, Sacks, HS, and Chalmers TC: Technical quality assessment of randomized control trials (RCTs), Controlled Clin Trials 8:282, 1987.
94. Relman AS: The extracranial-intracranial arterial bypass study: what have we learned? [editorial], N Engl J Med 316:809, 1987.
95. Resnick RH et al: A controlled study of the therapeutic portacaval shunt, Gastroenterology 67:843, 1974.
96. Rosati RA et al: Problems and advantages of an observational database approach to evaluating the effect of therapy on outcome, Circulation 65(7 Pt 2):27, 1982.
97. Roydhouse N: A controlled study of adenotonsillectomy, Arch Otolaryngol Head Neck Surg 92:611, 1970.
98. Roydhouse N: Adenoidectomy for otitis media with mucoid effusion, Ann Otol Rhinol Laryngol [Suppl] 89(3 Pt 3 Suppl 68):312, 1980.
99. Ruffin JM: Gastric "freezing": the life and death of a myth, Hosp Pract 5:57, 1970.
100. Ruffin JM et al: A cooperative double-blind evaluation of gastric "freezing" in the treatment of duodenal ulcer, N Engl J Med 281:16, 1969.
101. Rynnel-Dagöö B, Ahlbom A, and Schiratzki H: Effects of adenoidectomy: a controlled two-year follow-up, Ann Otol Rhinol Laryngol 87(2 Pt 1):272, 1978.
102. Sacks et al: Meta-analyses of randomized control trials, N Engl J Med 316:450, 1987.

103. Sacks HS, Chalmers TC, and Smith H Jr: Randomized versus historical controls for clinical trials, Am J Med 72:233, 1982.
104. Sacks HS, Chalmers TC, and Smith H Jr: Sensitivity and specificity of clinical trials: randomized vs historical controls, Arch Intern Med 143:753, 1983.
105. Salisbury RE, Taylor JW, and Levine NS: Evaluation of digital escharotomy in burned hands, Plast Reconstr Surg 58:440, 1976.
106. Salisbury RE and Wright P: Evaluation of early excision of dorsal burns of the hand, Plast Reconstr Surg 69:670, 1982.
107. Shaw DA et al: Carotid endarterectomy in patients with transient cerebral ischaemia, J Neurol Sci 64:45, 1984.
108. Shor S: The University Group Diabetes Program: a statistician looks at the mortality results, JAMA 217:167, 1971.
109. Simes RJ: Publication bias: the case for an international registry of clinical trials, J Clin Oncol 4:1529, 1986.
110. Sørensen B et al: Acute excision or exposure treatment? Final results of a three-year randomized controlled trial, Scand J Plast Reconstr Surg 18:87, 1984.
111. Special correspondence: a debate on coronary bypass, N Engl J Med 297:1464, 1977.
112. Spodick DH: The surgical mystique and the double standard: controlled trials of medical and surgical therapy for cardiac disease: analysis, hypothesis, proposal, Am Heart J 85:579, 1973.
113. Stafford N et al: The treatment of recurrent tonsillitis in adults, J Laryngol Otol 100:175, 1986.
114. Sundt TM Jr: Was the international randomized trial of extracranial-intracranial arterial bypass representative of the population at risk? N Engl J Med 316:814, 1987.
115. Thompson P et al: Effect of early excision on patients with major thermal injury, J Trauma 27:205, 1987.
116. Tolis G et al: Advanced prostatic adenocarcinoma: biological aspects and effects of androgen deprivation achieved by castration or agonistic analogues of LHRH. Med Oncol Tumor Pharmacother 1:129, 1984.
117. The University Group Diabetes Program: A study of the effects of hypoglycemic agents on vascular complications in patients with adult-onset diabetes, Diabetes 19(Suppl. 2):747, 1970.
118. van der Linden W: Pitfalls in randomized surgical trials, Surgery 87:258, 1980.
119. Wangensteen SL et al: Gastric "freezing": a double blind study, Am J Dig Dis 10:420, 1965.
120. Weinstein MC: Allocation of subjects in medical experiments, N Engl J Med 291:1278, 1974.
121. Wennberg JE: Setting outcome-based standards for carotid endarterectomy, JAMA 256:2566, 1986.
122. Wennberg JE et al: Changes in tonsillectomy rates associated with feedback and review, Pediatrics 59:821, 1977.
123. Widemar L et al: The effect of adenoidectomy on secretory otitis media: a 2-year controlled prospective study, Clin Otolaryngol 10:345, 1985.
124. Zikria BA et al: Gastric "freezing"—a clinical double-blind study, Am J Gastroenterol 47:208, 1967.

LESLIE L. ROOS

Leslie L. Roos, born and raised in San Francisco, graduated from Stanford University in 1962. Dr. Roos received his doctoral degree in political science from Massachusetts Institute of Technology in 1967. Before coming to the University of Manitoba in 1973, he held faculty positions at Brandeis, Northwestern, and Indiana Universities. He has held a National Health Scientist Award from the Research Programs Directorate, Health and Welfare Canada since 1982. Dr. Roos is a member of the Department of Business Administration (Faculty of Management) and the Department of Community Health Sciences (Faculty of Medicine) at the University of Manitoba.

NORALOU P. ROOS

Noralou P. Roos, born in Chino, California, and raised in Riddle, Oregon, graduated from Stanford University in 1963. Dr. Roos received her doctoral degree in political science from Massachusetts Institute of Technology in 1968. Before coming to the University of Manitoba in 1973, she taught at MIT and at Northwestern University. She has held a National Health Scientist Award from the Research Programs Directorate, Health and Welfare Canada since 1975. Dr. Roos teaches in the Department of Community Health Sciences (Faculty of Medicine) and in the Department of Business Administration (Faculty of Management) at the University of Manitoba.

15

Large Databases and Research on Surgery

LESLIE L. ROOS
NORALOU P. ROOS

Health care databases of varying scope and quality exist in a number of different settings; they are held by research groups, hospitals, insurers, and governmental agencies. Of particular interest are the data currently generated by health insurance systems in North America, Europe, Australia, and New Zealand. Large numbers of patient discharge abstracts filed by hospitals are produced, and investigators are increasingly aware of the research potential of these systems. Thus the National Institute of Medicine (Committee for Evaluating Medical Technologies in Clinical Use, 1985) has recommended strengthening methods to evaluate medical practice by the use of existing databases. Feinleib[16] has stressed the number of investigations possible when rich high-quality databases are made more accessible. Researchers, administrators, and practitioners are increasingly facing an information-rich environment, if they only knew what to do with the data! This chapter addresses questions of (1) how administrative databases should be constructed to facilitate surgical research and (2) how existing data can best be analyzed.

THE IDEAL DATABASE

What would be the characteristics of an ideal database to research surgery? First, coverage of an entire population would permit looking at utilization epidemiologically, attributing use to individuals according to their place of residence, no matter where the services are provided. Populations could then be compared in terms of the amount used of any given resource. Such population-based data can be adjusted for age, sex, and other characteristics to facilitate comparisons.

In this ideal data set each person should be specified by a unique number or combination of identifiers. When individuals are so identified, usage can be cumulated for them wherever they receive care. This database should capture all contacts with the health care system for each individual (with the unique identifier available to facilitate tracing). Among contacts that might be recorded are all hospital care, both inpatient and outpatient, services in free-standing surgery centers, activities in physician offices, entry to a nursing or personal care home, health care received in the home setting, and prescription drug use. Thus an individual who has surgery in one setting and is readmitted to a second institution will have both contacts captured by the system.

Finally, tracking when each individual's coverage begins and ends and why is useful. Such a registry or enrollment file is necessary to answer the question: if an individual has no recorded contact with the health care system, was he resident within the jurisdiction and indeed had no contact? Alternatively, has he left or has he died?

Such a database would facilitate not only comparative studies of utilization in different medical market areas, but also longitudinal research on utilization by groups of individuals (defined in many different ways). This type of nonintrusive follow-up has a number of advantages over follow-up by more labor-intensive methods.[38] Such follow-up can greatly aid research directed toward understanding the outcomes of various surgical interventions. Longitudinal designs are also essential for tracing the history of certain medical conditions, both those that result in hospitalization and those that do not.

Administrative data are particularly well suited for studying major health outcomes: death, nursing home admission, and hospitalization. Other outcomes resulting in contacts with the health care system can be traced; in many cases the proportions of individuals enjoying "intervention-free survival"—survival without any contact with the health care system—can also be ascertained.

Because many databases are maintained and updated for administrative purposes, the researcher, after obtaining access, may be able to analyze the database for a relatively small marginal cost. Major costs would already have been underwritten by the agency that uses the data for management purposes, and a variety of analyses would be possible. The number of years (of treatments or other events) can be increased either by bringing in more recent years of data or by going back further in time. This facilitates the long-term follow-up of individuals and the studies of rare events; more mundanely, adding extra years leads to a larger number of cases, which will increase the statistical power of any analysis.

Database Limitations

Even such an "ideal" database may have problems. First, the quality of the information that has been recorded must be assessed. Several Canadian provinces have databases that have been used extensively for research purposes.[3,75] For example, in Manitoba both the surgical procedures performed in hospitals and discrete billable items (even if not major events, for example, Pap smears) appear to be reliably captured in the claims system.[43,46] The accuracy of diagnostic data depends on both the physicians and the clerks recording the diagnoses. United States' Medicare data appear to record procedures performed fairly accurately, particularly if the "order of procedure" is ignored. Medicare data quality may have improved since the introduction of the prospective payment system (PPS), but diagnostic information may not be as accurate as in the Manitoba files.[12,74] Medicare data also suffer from not including outpatient information in the hospital file.

Diagnoses on hospital records are likely to be more accurate than diagnoses on claims generated by physicians' visits. In Manitoba diagnoses are noted with reasonable accuracy and specificity in the hospital system, reflecting the professional training of medical records technicians. A comparison of diagnoses recorded on hospital records with those reported in the claims showed 95% correspondence in gallbladder disease, and 89% to 92% correspondence (representing identical diagnoses) in a study of acute myocardial infarction patients.[45,46] Manitoba currently records as many as 16 diagnoses on every hospitalized patient, using the internationally standardized ICD-9-CM system. Diagnoses from an ambulatory care system are useful but at a much more generalized level. One approach that has proved fruitful in Manitoba is to group diagnoses available from physician claims (for example, those reflecting contacts for gynecologic problems in a study of women undergoing hysterectomy and those reflecting gallbladder disease—

abdominal pain for a study of contacts before and after gallbladder surgery) rather than to attempt fine diagnostic distinctions.[49,51]

Another problem relates to the detail of the coding conventions used. The widely used ICD-9-CM coding system does not distinguish procedures performed on the left side of the body from those on the right side. This presents difficulties in assessing the results of orthopedic surgery; a second hip or knee replacement operation on someone who has already had one means either a reoperation on the same extremity or an operation on the other one.[52]

No matter how much is provided in any database, specific items desired for a given study may not be available. Additional information may or may not be contained in other sources that permit linkage to an existing database. In particular, administrative databases often do not include the performance of certain tests or x-ray examinations if they are not billable; the results of tests are frequently not included. Information on medical treatment, such as drugs used, is typically not available, which makes it difficult to compare medical and surgical alternatives in the treatment of many conditions.

Finally, the individual rather than the researcher initiates contact with the system generating the data. Thus a person who is ill but has no contact with the health care system does not produce a record that contains information on this particular episode of illness or chronic condition. The degree to which this affects health status measurement will vary both with certain system characteristics, such as the extent of insurance coverage, and with individual characteristics (care-seeking behavior). Given universal insurance, relatively few ill individuals do not have contact with the health care system.[30] In fact, during a 4-year period, 91% of Manitoba adults contact a physician at least once.

The uniform hospital discharge data set is likely to be available in many political jurisdictions. The following data seem commonly available on hospital claims collected in almost all Canadian provinces and in many US settings.

Such items include:
- Date of birth
- Sex
- Place of residence
- Identifying number (individual or family)

Other items for analysis include:
- Discharge diagnoses (several)
- Procedures performed in hospital (several)
- Hospital
- Date of admission
- Date of discharge
- Discharge code (for example, death, another hospital, and home)

Secondary items:
- Admitting physician identifying number
- Physician performing each procedure (identifying number)

As noted above, the following important information may or may not be available in a given data set:
- Coverage of an entire population
- Unique identifying number (or combination of identifiers)
- Enrollment or registry file specifying when coverage begins and ends

RESEARCH DESIGNS

Given variation both in the questions researchers wish to ask and in the characteristics of the data to be accessed, Table 15-1 highlights the information required for different types of studies of cost control, quality of care, and treatment outcomes. The designs form a continuum from relatively simple to relatively complex, according to the data requirements imposed by each design. In this table, level is identified on the basis of what can be done with the data. Thus the most comprehensive information (level 1 data) permits all the analyses possible using simpler level 2 and level 3 data, as well as supporting research that cannot be done using less complete data

Table 15-1. Data requirements and types of studies using hospital data

Level	Data Requirements	Types of Studies
Simple—level 3	Need hospital discharge abstracts	In-hospital mortality (volume-outcome comparisons, monitoring of individual hospitals); length of stay; small area analyses
Intermediate—level 2	Need hospital discharge abstracts and consistent individual identifiers	Timely longitudinal research: short-term readmissions; volume-outcome comparisons, monitoring of individual hospitals; quality assurance and cost control
Comprehensive—level 1	Need hospital discharge abstracts, consistent individual identifiers, and enrollment file	Highest quality longitudinal research: short-term and long-term outcome studies; identification of incident cases, volume-outcome comparisons, monitoring of individual hospitals; choice of treatment studies; small area analysis by person

sets. The simpler the data requirements are for a given design, the more the political units, such as states and provinces, will have collected information to permit this particular type of research.

Designs with Simple Data Requirements (Level 3 Data)

The data requirements for some designs are relatively simple. If both a consistent individual identifier and an enrollment file are lacking, three types of cross-sectional studies are common. Such studies build on the information in the hospital discharge abstracts without trying to trace individuals. The data sets involved in such studies tend to be large and generally permit comparisons across many hospitals. The hospital-focused studies of mortality and length of stay described below often are not population-based; thus controls for case mix are especially important.

Luft and his collaborators[26,27,60] have used data from hospitals subscribing to the Commission on Professional and Hospital Activities (CPHA) to demonstrate the importance of hospital volume as a variable affecting survival after complex surgical procedures. For many procedures, patients operated on at hospitals where a greater number of procedures are done, on average do better than those operated on at hospitals where fewer procedures are done. Although Sloan et al.[61] present 1972 to 1981 data from 521 CPHA hospitals to argue that an adequate statistical basis for setting minimum volume standards does not exist, the bulk of evidence supports the volume-outcome relationship.[28] These cross-sectional analyses are limited to such outcomes as "mortality within the hospital stay in which surgery took place." Although better data will permit more long-term outcome studies, ongoing research suggests that, for many common surgical procedures, studies concentrating on in-hospital mortality capture enough of the deaths that occur within 3 months of surgery to permit useful research.

Another type of study uses information on the

Table 15-2. Admission rates, length of stay, and total days per capita for coronary artery bypass graft surgery for residents of Manitoba's seven regions (1979-1984)

Region	Direct-adjusted Admission Rate per 10,000 Adults	Mean Length of Stay	Total Days per 10,000 Adults
Central	2.93	22.32	65.42
Eastern	3.73	21.47	80.22
Interlake	4.06	18.80	76.36
Northern	5.15	20.67	106.38
Parkland	3.28	19.47	63.83
Western	2.40	20.47	49.05
Winnipeg	5.04	20.64	104.01

hospital discharge abstract to classify patients into diagnosis related groups (DRGs). Patients in a given group are assumed to have similar processes of hospital care and services provided.[17] Hospitals can be compared DRG by DRG to determine which hospitals' patients have longer lengths of stays; an overall case mix adjusted length of stay index can be computed for each hospital. Legislation in the United States that mandates the use of DRGs as part of the Medicare prospective payment system has made such studies important for ongoing monitoring of hospital utilization. Length of stay is being used heavily by hospital managers "as a surrogate measure for cost."[63] The application of DRGs has generated considerable controversy; a number of efforts to improve on this method of controlling for case mix are underway.[10,20,64]

Small area analyses also have relatively simple data requirements, but they do require a population base. Hospital market areas are defined to include "any geographic subunit in which more of the people living there use that particular hospital than any other one (a 'plurality rule')."[6] Such a population base provides a denominator (counting all individuals living in an area) and permits age and sex adjustment of the utilization experience of the population, thus removing one of the most important patient-related contributions to variation in utilization rates.[54] All health care utilization by persons in the area is counted, regardless of where it takes place.

Combining length of stay and small area analyses can highlight the most effective way to control utilization. Treatments are likely to differ in terms of whether the DRG approach, which emphasizes length of stay, or the small area approach, which focuses on admission per capita, is most suitable for understanding the overall variation in total days spent in hospital.[72] Analyses from Manitoba dramatically illustrate this difference. Coronary artery bypass graft surgery is centralized in Manitoba with all procedures done in two Winnipeg teaching hospitals. The physicians in western Manitoba refer relatively few patients to Winnipeg for coronary angiography and subsequent bypass surgery. Table 15-2 shows how variation in the bypass procedures per capita are more important than differences in lengths of stays for bypass patients in understanding regional differences in overall utilization. The right-hand column presents total days/utilization per 10,000 adults for the seven planning regions of Manitoba. This column is the product of the direct adjusted rate per 10,000 adults and the mean length of stay per admission for bypass surgery.

From a policy perspective, both strategies—reducing admissions and shortening length of stay—can be effective in cost control. Both have played a role in the recent slowing of increase in American hospital costs.[57] Such analyses are particularly important because admission rates for most medical and surgical hospitalizations vary among hospital market areas. Major differences are found even between Boston and New Haven, sites of major teaching centers linked to Harvard and Yale, respectively.[71] Because large differences in illness rates cannot adequately explain the differences in hospitalization rates seen in small area studies,[54,70] this variation is increasingly the focus of attention.[72] Feedback has sometimes been successful in reducing rates that are very high.[73] These rate data are also essential for payment systems based on capitation, which are being vigorously promoted by the United States' Medicare program.[22]

Designs with Intermediate Data Requirements (Level 2 Data)

Intermediate designs are suitable when consistent individual identifiers are included in the data set, but enrollment files are not readily available. Hospital claims can be sorted by date and identifying number to generate hospitalization histories for each individual. Without an enrollment file, the time when coverage began and ended for an individual cannot be incorporated into the analysis. A focus on short-term outcomes—both morbidity and mortality—is therefore appropriate with these designs. Such short-term outcomes might include readmission for particular complications, readmission after time periods of interest (48 hours, 7 days, 6 weeks from original discharge), or mortality (when present on a subsequent hospital abstract). In many cases, if the time interval is fairly short (to a year or so after surgery), loss to follow-up (because of migration or in the United States because of change of insurer) can be ignored without significantly biasing the results. In the United States this appears to be true for Medicare recipients but not for Medicaid recipients.[24,70] Designs that do not depend on an enrollment file allow for outcome research more efficiently and quickly than those that involve linking utilization and enrollment files. This may be important in providing rapid feedback for audit committees overseeing quality of care.

A computer algorithm using a combination of "time after surgery" and "diagnosis at time of readmission" for classifying hospital readmissions as postsurgical complications would be useful for monitoring. Recent work with hysterectomy, cholecystectomy, and prostatectomy has shown the feasibility of developing computer algorithms for such classification; results produced using these algorithms closely corresponded with those from physician panels.[47] Such studies of short-term outcomes may involve printing out cases for more detailed investigation; a listing that identifies individuals who were readmitted to hospital because of certain diagnoses or during a particular period after surgery can significantly reduce the amount of paper that quality assurance committees must confront. Thus the computer can act as a first screen; hospital records can then be pulled for further investigation.

Population-based (as compared with hospital-based) data help improve these intermediate designs. If individuals have an identifying number assigned by a single hospital, only readmissions to this hospital will be captured. If, however, unique identifying information is assigned by a larger geographically based insurance plan, such as some Canadian provincial plans and United States' Medicare, data for a given patient can be aggregated across all providers reimbursed by the plan. This is especially important for capturing readmissions of rural patients who have had surgery in an urban hospital; many of their readmissions will be in small hospitals in their home areas. For example, 45% of Manitoba rural patients readmitted for complications after cholecystectomy entered hospitals other than ones in which they had surgery.[47] Thus when system-wide data are not available, record reviews will systematically underestimate postsurgical complication rates.

Designs with Comprehensive Data Requirements (Level 1 Data)

If both consistent individual identifiers and an enrollment file are present, loss to follow-up can be estimated. Longitudinal studies that meet various criteria desirable for high-quality cause-effect research can be conducted.[21] The ability to develop person-based longitudinal histories permits identifying the number of new (first-time) occurrences in a population. This identification of incident cases is important in generating a relatively homogeneous group for study; a second operation or recurrence of a condition can be distinguished from new events. Outcome studies can be markedly improved by such information: because a second bypass operation may well be riskier than the first such operation, analyzing the two separately is helpful. In similar fashion, valve replacement surgery after a bypass operation can be distinguished from valve surgery with no patient history of major operations.

In a system with national health insurance, short-term studies incorporating an enrollment file will be only slightly more accurate than those without such a file.[41] When coverage is not universal (at least within a given age group, that is, the elderly), checks against an enrollment file will be necessary.[24] Migration in and out of a given insurance plan may be large enough to substantially affect results.

Such long-term outcomes as reoperations, nursing home entry, and mortality are particularly suitable for study using comprehensive databases. As noted previously,[56] information from an insurance system that provides complete coverage for a population regardless of where they are treated may uncover problems that are undetected in research based on data from a single hospital. As time passes, patients become increasingly likely to have received care in more than one hospital; single hospital data sets drift into increasing rates of error.

Research on both efficacy and effectiveness is greatly facilitated by system-wide data. Studies of efficacy, of results in the so-called "best" situation (generally a teaching hospital), have usually been reported in studies of technology assessment.[5] However, research on the efficacy of many procedures is lacking.[34] The relative paucity of solid outcome studies seems to support physician uncertainty as to choice of treatment, which may underlie much of the data on small area variation.[68] Moreover, community hospital practices and medical care outcomes may differ from those publicized by researchers at academic centers. Effectiveness studies, studies that present outcome results from representative samples of all hospitals and all physicians, have seldom been done.

Recent studies of prostatectomy can serve as a model for longitudinal studies of a common surgical procedure.[53,74] Data from Maine and Manitoba were combined to follow men for as long as 8 years who had prostatectomies. Combining data from these two jurisdictions helped generate a larger number of cases. This in itself can be important because some outcomes, particularly postoperative mortality, are relatively infrequent, and the numbers of providers are relatively small. Both morbidity (as judged, for example, by revisions or by readmissions because of complications) and postoperative mortality were measured. Overall, adverse outcomes (both deaths and nonfatal complications) were more frequent than had been noted in the literature. The database facilitated the capture of admissions to hospitals other than where surgery was done; this and the longer period of follow-up no doubt contributed to the higher rates of adverse outcomes found in this study compared with other studies (most of which were based in teaching hospitals). The wide range of outcomes among different hospitals reinforced the need for such studies of effectiveness. The adjusted odds ratios for mortality within 3 months of surgery ranged from 0.48 to 4.79 among individual hospitals. In one hospital the mortality was one half as high as in the baseline hospital; in another institution the rate was almost 5 times as great. One particular subgroup, men in nursing homes, was found to have especially high mortality.

Cohort data can sometimes be used to compare the outcomes of two types of surgery or of medical versus surgical treatment. The prostatectomy research discussed above found statistically significant differences between the outcomes of open and transurethral procedures.[40] These differences are being investigated more fully. In another example, administrative data proved especially useful in accumulating a sufficient number of cases of infective endocarditis for analysis. Alternative treatments for this condition, which requires hospitalization on diagnosis, have been analyzed using a cohort design.[1]

Other comparisons of treatment options have dealt with more common conditions. Manitoba cohort studies of tonsillectomy focused on patient variables, such as age, sex, and the number of preoperative episodes of respiratory illness in the treated and untreated groups. Because operated and unoperated siblings could be compared using the database, family variables were also considered.[37,39] Sensitivity testing estimated the accuracy of the analysis of tonsillectomy outcomes. Postoperative outcomes of a subset of Manitoba patients—those matching the Pittsburgh randomized trial of tonsillectomy criteria of a preoperative history of seven episodes in the year before surgery—could be compared with outcomes of patients enrolled in the Pittsburgh trial. With patients equated for preoperative history, the Manitoba results (from the cohort comparisons) were quite similar to those from the Pittsburgh randomized trial. Manitoba and Pittsburgh patients showed similar magnitudes of improvement after tonsil surgery; the surgical patients experienced between one and one and a half fewer episodes of respiratory illness than did the nonsurgical groups.

SUBSTANTIVE ISSUES

A number of issues are relevant across data sets and research designs. First, in addition to focusing on the patient, administrative databases can be fruitfully used to examine various aspects of physician behavior. This is important, since physicians are responsible for decisions that govern how as much as 90% of each health care dollar is spent.[14] Although some research can be carried out using cross-sectional data, most work on physician behavior will depend on comprehensive level 1 data. Doctors enter and leave geographic areas and insurance plans; data on physician enrollment are a necessity for many studies.

Existing databases should have an increasing impact on the burgeoning field of clinical decision analysis.[35] Abrams et al.[1] note that "decision analysis has helped to clarify the structure of some management controversies, balancing the risks and benefits of different strategies in a quantitative fashion." Decision analytic techniques estimating the probabilities associated with alternative treatment choices call out for better information on outcomes. Such data are sketchy for many treatments, even those that have been in general use for a number of years. Combining decision-analysis with claims databases seems "useful as an alternative or precursor to randomized trials," especially when the difficulties of performing such trials are great.[1] Longitudinal data—level 1 or possibly level 2 data—are required for such studies.

Relatively complete data sets are invaluable in estimating the limitations of less complete data bases. Analyses of comprehensive level 1 data can provide a practical "gold standard" with which other data can be compared. This permits estimating the practicality of a particular study in a jurisdiction with less comprehensive data. Eventually, feeding back results to those responsible may lead to changes in data collection. Both the section on case mix and the subsequent one comparing hospital-based and population-based approaches use the more complete data sets to highlight problems with the less complete.

Physician Behavior

Small area and hospital analyses imply a concern about physician practice patterns.[13] If physician identifiers (admitting physician, physician performing surgery) are available, physicians can be studied with the same techniques used for analyzing hospitals. Both volume-outcome relationships and the monitoring of individual physicians are legitimate areas of research and policy interest using administrative data bases.[48,64a]

Physician referral behavior also deserves more study. In several Canadian provinces and several of this country's states, more complicated cases are routinely referred from rural areas and small towns to urban tertiary centers distant from the patient's home.[25] As discussed earlier, some differences in surgical rates across areas are shown to be caused by differences in the rate of referral to tertiary centers.[55] Such findings supported the hypothesis that having a small number of centrally located physicians perform a particular procedure may contribute to the maintenance of regional variation; Manitoba data indicate that differences in referral behavior may continue over long periods. Because of the previously cited findings "of an inverse relation between the number of patients treated with specific diagnoses or procedures in a hospital and subsequent adverse outcomes,"[29] policies directed toward centralization must deal with the possibility of adversely affecting equity of access.

A surgeon's hospitalization practice style is a third research topic facilitated by existing databases. Because "only a small proportion of hospitalizations fit a model based on medical need,"[67] researchers typically assume that significant differences in physician practice patterns are the primary reason for small area variations in both surgical and nonsurgical hospitalization usage rates.[18] Although these assumptions about physician practice style and patient need have seldom been tested directly, they have important implications for health planners. If need can be met with more cost-effective medicine, health care spending can be restricted without rationing.[67]

The comprehensive Manitoba data have facilitated developing an index of physician hospitalization style based on:
1. Identifying physicians' primary patients
2. Calculating the expected rate of hospitalization for these primary patients over a 2-year period, controlling for differences in health status
3. Comparing each physician's expected rate of hospitalizing his patients with the observed (actual) hospitalization patterns of his primary patients[55]

This index is being used to assess the influence of physician style on the utilization of hospitals, to test the stability of practice style over a long-term period, and to look at the reasons for and outcomes of hospitalization for patients of "hospitalization-prone" and "nonhospitalization-prone" physicians. Both overall hospitalizations and surgical hospitalizations can be studied using this methodology.

Clinical Decision Analysis

The field of clinical decision analysis can benefit greatly from the information in existing databases. For example, a clinical decision analysis of treatment alternatives for infective endocarditis has provided insights into how to use retrospective chart reviews from a single hospital in tandem with large claims database.[1] Probabilities derived from the two data sources were remarkably similar, given the relatively low numbers for both the single hospital (16 cases) and provincial hospital claims data (127 cases). The use of the Manitoba database, aggregating cases over a 5-year period—(1979 to 1984), made feasible the analysis of survival and the comparisons of alternative treatments.

Researchers in clinical decision analysis have developed sophisticated methods of sensitivity testing. Given that the individuals in different "arms" of a cohort study (that is, those having a particular operation at different hospitals, those receiving different treatments) are not randomly assigned, such sensitivity testing is very useful in establishing a particular difference in outcomes in the face of possible measurement error.

Clinical decision analysis also needs to incorporate the previously discussed research showing major differences among providers in case mix adjusted outcomes after surgery. The probabilities for different outcomes clearly vary among hospitals and surgeons; data on such variation are now available for about six surgical procedures.[28] Decision analyses might present "high-quality treatment" and "low-quality treatment" decision trees. Although such results might be controversial, they may accurately reflect the real world.

Case Mix Adjustment

Controlling for possible differences in patient characteristics is critical for comparing treatments and providers. Deciding what types of data are necessary for adequate controls to study length of stay, death, disability, and rehospitalization is not simple. As Jencks and Dobson[23] pointed out, "severity adjustments that predict outcome are not identical to those that predict cost." Research on this topic is timely because decisions about expenditures for additional data collection are being made. Thus Pennsylvania Health Care Cost Containment Council has recently required extra data (collected by Medis-Groups) to be added to the hospital discharge abstract to facilitate more detailed risk adjustment for quality assessment.[23] The necessity of such expensive prospective data for case mix adjustment needs to be established.

If cross-sectional data can provide enough information for case mix controls, large-scale studies of in-hospital mortality after surgery will be relatively easy to conduct. Researchers have to establish empirically the extent to which information from claims at each level is sufficient for case mix controls:

Level 3   Cross-sectional
Level 2   Intermediate (longitudinal without an enrollment file)
Level 1   Comprehensive (longitudinal with an enrollment file)

Different outcomes may well require different types of controls.

As noted, considerable effort has been—and is being—exerted to try to cost-effectively improve measurement of case mix using cross-sectional data. Age, sex, and comorbidity data from the surgical hospitalization have been used to control for interhospital differences in Luft's and his collaborators' research.[27,60] Using information on the claim for each hospital stay, DRGs often control for age, sex, and (sometimes) comorbidity. Jencks and Dobson[22] believe "no available measure of severity of illness" would markedly improve the accuracy of Medicare payments "if used to supplement or replace the system of diagnosis related groups."

When consistent individual identifiers are present, additional covariates can be obtained from data available from the period preceding the index hospitalization, that is, the hospitalization of surgery. A methodology for conducting outcomes research using covariates from prior claims is being developed.[40,74] Such covariates are not subject to the potential biases of covariates derived from cross-sectional data. For example, in a cross-sectional study the diagnosis of "myocardial infarction" may represent a preexisting condition or an event that occurred after surgery but during the surgical hospitalization.[4]

The availability of an enrollment file helps ensure that individuals whose coverage began just before surgery will not be confused with those having more complete histories. Such a file is desirable; its necessity depends on the population being studied. For Medicaid recipients in two states, only between 54% (Georgia) and 63% (Michigan) were enrolled for a full 6 months before and after hospital admission for one of eight selected surgical procedures.[24] When a system of universal health insurance is in place, the results of considerable sensitivity testing show that an enrollment file is not essential when the presurgical period is short (up to 2 years) and migration is comparatively low.[45] Thus longitudinal analyses of follow-up using Medicare data suggest case mix adjustment without checking an enrollment file is unlikely to present major problems.

The appropriate strategy for developing measures of case mix adjustment needs attention. Because of the relatively few adverse outcomes, large data sets are highly desirable for case mix adjustment. Some strategies, such as the "condition/treatment" model proposed by Wennberg,[69] depend on using a number of dichotomous independent variables, for example, presence or absence of prior cancer, as separate predictors; however, for most surgical and medical treatments comparatively few cases of specific conditions, such as presence of cancer, are available. Without a very large number of cases, combining some of the independent variables into an index of comorbidity or illness severity may be essential for case mix adjustment.

Mosteller et al.[31] note that the "potential gain from measurement offers one reason for developing scales of measurement." Indices and scales offer the promise of both increased reliability and use of a metric rather than a dichotomy; consequently, the required sample size can be smaller. Charlson et al.[7] have developed and validated a method of classifying comorbidity to estimate risk of death. Because the Charlson Index was constructed from hospital medical records, it should also be possible to use either cross-sectional claims data or claims recorded during the presurgical period to generate the index. For several common surgical procedures, hospital claims alone provide almost as good case mix adjustment as does linking information from hospital claims with that taken from physician visits or from more costly survey information.[30,56] Ongoing work suggests that using both the claims recorded before the surgical hospitalization and those generated by this hospitalization provides the best case mix adjustment.

In the previously cited prostatectomy research, case mix was measured using all available hospital claims—both those in the 6 months before surgery and those for the individual at the time of surgery.[74] Relevant items from the 6 months before prostatectomy included: hospitalized with cancer (except prostate), hospitalized with cardiovascular diagnoses, and resident of a nursing home. Associated diagnoses at the time of surgery included: cancer of prostate (not previously diagnosed), cancer (except prostatic), cardiovascular diseases, and other associated diagnoses (more than one diagnosis given). In addition to comparing hospitals, this study has also compared open versus transurethral prostatectomy with regard to postoperative mortality. Because transurethral procedures are generally thought appropriate for patients too ill to undergo open procedures, developing adequate covariates to adjust across the two groups was clearly key.

To address this problem, claims data were combined with data collected prospectively from one Manitoba hospital.[8,9] In this hospital every surgical patient was interviewed by a nurse who collected information about preoperative drug use (the number of drugs used as well as the specific drugs, for example, digitalis) and the number of preoperative conditions that affected the patient, such as obesity or respiratory problems. In addition, the anesthesiologists rated each patient using the American Society of Anesthesiologists' Physical Status Classification (ASAPS).[33] This 5-point scale runs from 1, healthy normal patients, to 5, those not expected to survive surgery.

Two logistic regression models were developed for predicting the occurrence of death in the period after surgery. One model included variables derived from administrative data alone; the second model added prospectively collected data, such as ASAPS, to the variables available from administrative data. Two of the variables collected prospectively (ASAPS and being on digitalis) entered the equation with significant coefficients, replacing four of the six variables derived from claims data. The model that included prospective data had only slightly better predictive power; both models fit the data reasonably well. Moreover, the coefficient indicating the association of type of surgery with postoperative mortality was identical in the two models, suggesting that administrative data provided useful controls for case severity.[50] These analyses are being conducted across a number of surgical procedures. If the prostatectomy findings are generalizable, they will provide strong evidence that claims data can do almost as well in providing measures of comorbidity as can measures based on expensive primary data collection.

When are administrative data "good enough" for distinguishing the better of two treatments, for testing hypotheses about the relationship between surgical volume and treatment outcomes, and for identifying hospitals with particularly poor (or especially good) outcomes? In studying the link between volume and outcomes, one needs only to show that the average case mix in high-volume hospitals is no different than that in their low-volume counterparts. Statistical adjustments are much more likely to be necessary when comparing treatment alternatives and monitoring individual hospitals. Both because the true differences in case mix are not known and because there is a limit to how much case mix can be adjusted with present knowledge, the results of any technique must be compared with a standard of what can be done given the best available techniques.

As seen, improving on what can be done using administrative data is often difficult. Given the costs of gathering data on risk factors prospectively, extensive data collection seems hard to justify by the available evidence. Prospective data collection for a small number of hospitals may be helpful in gathering risk factor data plus information on postoperative condition or on possible causal factors associated with particular outcomes.

Hospital-Based versus Population-Based Data

Analyses of outcomes of care are facilitated by population-based data on all deaths and all readmissions, not just events occurring in the hospital of surgery. On the other hand, data from the hospital of surgery may be more widely available and easier to analyze, facilitating more timely feedback and monitoring of quality of care. Analyses that are hospital-centered (either because the investigators are based at a single hospital or because the individuals being studied are identified by a number specific to one hospital) may miss important events in following the patient population.

Such work is particularly timely because of the concern that Medicare's prospective payment system might encourage such short stays that quality of care would be adversely affected. If this were so, readmissions and mortality that might be avoidable could be missed or assigned to the wrong hospital by a monitoring system. Comprehensive data facilitate improvement of outcome analyses. Cross-sectional hospital-based analyses that do not depend on individual identifiers or enrollment files can be compared with longitudinal population-based analyses capturing all readmissions and all deaths within a specified period. Thus the more comprehensive data (typically available from fewer jurisdictions) can indicate for which procedures and for which types of patients in-hospital mortality is an adequate measure of mortality in the period after surgery and for which it is not. Preliminary analyses suggest that for certain procedures (coronary artery bypass graft surgery, valve replacement surgery) deaths during the surgical hospital stay represent a high proportion of deaths in the 3 months after surgery. For other procedures and conditions (prostatectomy, hip fracture), this is not the case.

PRACTICAL CONSIDERATIONS

Two practical issues confronting researchers wishing to use administrative data are (1) how can I get better (more comprehensive, more detailed) data and (2) what kind of software can help efficiently analyze these data? This section discusses the application of record linkage techniques to produce better data and the characteristics of software to work with existing databases.

Record Linkage

Record linkage has often been used in research on occupational health[62] to add mortality information to data on workers' exposure to possible health hazards. Other linkages with mortality data have involved disease cohorts, lifestyle/risk factors, clinical trials, and general population cohorts. When enough identifying variables are available, record linkage permits generating level 1 data for studies of survival. However, record linkage can also be used more generally to merge administrative data with other studies.[66] The statistical techniques on which record linkage rests have been treated extensively elsewhere. This discussion notes how record linkage as a way of thinking may suggest opportunities otherwise overlooked. Given a unique identifier (or a set of other identifiers), bringing in additional research (based on, for example, surveys or hospital record reviews) to augment the information on each individual is often possible. For example, the Manitoba Longitudinal Study on Aging has retrospectively linked survey information and claims to provide a fuller picture of the relationship between self-reported health status and utilization.[56] Cancer registry data and vital statistics records have also been combined with Manitoba Health Services Commission registry and claims information to improve the quality of data available in each file.

Looking for record linkage possibilities is a useful mental exercise when dealing with administrative databases. Perhaps the researcher should look first at what is desirable, and worry about what is practical later. This approach has led to several different linkages in our Manitoba work on common surgical procedures:

1. Linkage of hospital claims with primary data on anesthesia and its outcomes to produce a rich data set
2. Linkage of hospital claims with physician claims to verify fact of surgery and to add operation date to the hospital claims
3. Linkage of the enrollment file with vital statistics information to verify deaths and provide cause of death information

Although the linkage techniques that were used differed in each example, the linked files all proved helpful. Such linkages permit analysis at the individual level and dramatically increase the amount and quality of data.

Such data can be generated in other jurisdictions. If names and/or identifying numbers are not available on two potentially linkable files, investigators should look for four or five similar variables on the two data sets. Those may be all that are necessary to both link the files and use proven methods for assessing quality of the matches.[43,44,66]

Software

The preceding discussion has concentrated on conceptual building blocks for working with administrative data: research design, database quality and comprehensiveness, definition of outcomes, and casemix measurement. On the practical side, appropriate software represents one step toward making the approaches described here available to a larger audience. A system to facilitate small area analysis, longitudinal studies, record linkage, as examples, is needed to efficiently use existing databases. When a number of different analysts want to work with information formatted in various ways, easy to use software is particularly important.

In Canada the provincial health care bodies vary considerably in the amount of information collected and the format used for data management. Although items on the uniform hospital discharge data set seem available for each province, analysis is characteristically carried out at provincial rather than national levels. With considerable effort, Statistics Canada is able to put together a minimum hospital data set for the country as a whole. In similar fashion, the collection of United States Medicare data has been decentralized to the state level, but Health Care Financing Agency has imposed nation-wide standards for data submission to Washington. Software to improve their "inhouse" analytical capability might interest such groups as the provincial Colleges of Physicians and Surgeons in

Canada, peer review organizations (PROs) in the United States, insurers of various types, and hospital associations across North America.

In addition to the general capabilities outlined here, such a system should also be versatile, user-friendly, and reasonably economical of computer time. Speed of system development, ease of modification, and operation on a variety of machines are important factors. In the authors' experience, the widely adopted SAS language has proved ideal for development of a management information system for health analysts. SAS features flexibility in combining several variables, such as diagnoses and procedures, and good data subsetting capabilities for producing an abbreviated file containing selected claims and variables. SAS features facilitate working across several databases in the same run. Increasing computer power makes the greater running time associated with using such high-level languages of less concern.[19]

SAS' macroprocessor and accompanying macrolanguage were used to develop procedures to perform the functions outlined above. This macroprocessor "provides a way to store and retrieve SAS jobs that must be tailored to changing details." When appropriate, commands are common across the programs, and the syntax in the modules corresponds to that used by SAS. Regular SAS features are used to manipulate and analyze the data. In this way a coherent software system can be developed rapidly by building on existing fourth generation languages.

DISCUSSION

This chapter has reviewed approaches to the information-rich environment available to researchers, policy makers, and managers. Research on cost control and quality of care can have an obvious impact on the amount and distribution of resources for health care. Issues in identifying institutions with outcomes that should be carefully reviewed have been highlighted. The comparisons of the outcomes of different treatment alternatives are directly applicable to the emerging fields of clinical epidemiology and medical decision making.

Existing administrative databases are important for monitoring outcomes of many procedures, given both the North American "explosion in surgical utilization among the elderly"[65] and the great concern about health care costs. Specifying particular variables as predictors of postsurgical outcomes can help the physician decide on the appropriate treatment alternative. Thus the reporting of relatively high mortality after prostatectomies on nursing home patients resulted in a reduction of such operations by Maine urologists.[11]

Given the limited population entering most clinical trials, cohort studies using claims databases may be the major source of outcome data for operations performed on some age groups. For example, only claims data can provide ongoing information on mortality, readmissions, and "intervention-free" survival after coronary artery bypass graft surgery among the elderly. This procedure has grown rapidly among patients older than 65 years with some longitudinal series, but there has been no accompanying information from randomized clinical trials.[2,42]

What will it take to improve outcomes of surgery? Although the United States and Canadian experiences in cost control have differed, health care expenditures have risen in both countries since the early 1970s. Such increases have occurred in delivery of care in specific institutions[58,59] and at a systems level.[15,36] It is not cost of health care per se but cost in relation to quality of care and outcomes that is most important.[58] However, data relating specific cost increases to particular changes in quality of care are almost uniformly unavailable. Increases in direct hospital expenditures during the past decade should have improved the quality of care. More intensive monitoring of surgical patients, more aggressive postoperative care, and more highly trained nursing staff are all developments that have occurred across North America. The major rationale for these changes has been to improve quality. During the past 10 years, Manitoba also experienced a centralization of high-risk procedures and a limitation of the surgical privileges of nonspecialists.

However, research has shown little or no improvement in the outcomes associated with three common surgical procedures—hysterectomy, cholecystectomy, and prostatectomy—performed during a 10-year period in Manitoba.[40] Three surgical cohorts (all those undergoing surgery in 1972 to 1973, 1977 to 1978, and 1982 to 1983 were examined without finding significant decreases in the postoperative mortality, in the rate of readmission to hospital in the immediate postoperative period, of in the rate of readmission to hospital for adverse surgical outcomes in the 15 months after surgery. These data suggest "flat of the curve" medicine.[32] In the early 1970s, the organization and delivery of care for these three procedures was of such a quality that improving surgical outcomes proved difficult despite ever increasing expenditures on the hospital sector.

Careful monitoring of and feedback to institutions with poorer-than-expected outcomes seems likely to have a much greater impact on quality than the incremental system-wide increases in expenditures, which are the norm. Given reasonably high overall quality, achieving even small improvements are difficult. An emphasis on monitoring and feedback directs efforts toward the hospitals where improvement is more feasible. Where cost control is the issue, the techniques discussed here make it possible to focus on particular areas or particular hospitals rather then cutting across the board.

The maintenance, analysis, and improvement of existing databases represents a cost-effective way to better understand issues of access to and quality of surgical care. The technology and data are available; now funding to conduct the necessary research and the will to put findings into practice are necessary.

References

1. Abrams HB et al: Is there a role for surgery in the acute management of infective endocarditis? A decision analysis and medical data base approach, Med Decis Making 8:165, 1988.
2. Anderson GM and Lomas J: Monitoring the diffusion of technology: coronary artery bypass graft surgery in Ontario, Am J Public Health 78:251, 1988. (in press).
3. Barer M L et al: Aging and health care utilization: new evidence on old fallacies, Soc Sci Med 24:851, 1987.
4. Blumberg MS: Risk adjusting health care outcomes: a methodologic review, Med Care 43:351, 1986.
5. Brook RH and Lohr KN: Efficacy, effectiveness, variations, and quality: boundary-crossing research, Med Care 23:710, 1985.
6. Caper P: Variations in medical practice: implications for health policy, Health Affa 3:110, 1984.
7. Charlson ME et al: A new method of classifying prognostic comorbidity in longitudinal studies: development and validation, J Chronic Dis 40:373, 1987.
8. Cohen MM and Duncan PG: Physical status score and trends in anesthetic complications, J Clin Epidemiol 41:83, 1988.
9. Cohen MM et al: A survey of 112,000 anesthetics at one teaching hospital (1975-83), Can Anaesth Soc J 33:22, 1986.
10. Cretin S and Worthman LG: Alternative systems for case mix classification in health care financing (Rand R-3457-HCFA), Santa Monica, Calif, 1986, Rand Corporation.
11. Davis H: Was surgery needed? The Baltimore Sun, Apr 6, 1986.
12. Demlo LK and Campbell PM: Improving hospital discharge data: lessons from the National Hospital Discharge Survey, Med Care 19:1030, 1981.
13. Egdahl RH: Ways for surgeons to increase the efficiency of their use of hospitals, N Engl J Med 309:1184, 1983.
14. Eisenberg JM: Physician utilization: the state of research about physicians' practice patterns, Med Care 23:461, 1985.
15. Evans RG: Finding the levers, finding the courage: what have we learned about cost containment in North America? J Health Polit Policy Law 11:585, 1987.
16. Feinleib M: Data bases, data banks and data dredging: the agony and the ecstasy, J Chronic Dis 37:783, 1984.
17. Fetter RB et al: Case mix definition by diagnosis-related groups, Med Care 18:1 (supp), 1980.
18. Griffith JR et al: Measuring community hospital services in Michigan, Health Serv Res 16:135, 1981.
19. Harel EC and McLean ER: The effects of using a nonprocedural computer language on programmer productivity, MIS Quarterly 9:109, 1985.
20. Hornbrook MC: Techniques for assessing hospital case mix, Annu Rev Public Health 6:295, 1985.
21. Horwitz RI: The experimental paradigm and observational studies of cause-effect relationships in clinical medicine, J Chronic Dis 40:91, 1987.

22. Jencks SF and Dobson A: Strategies for reforming Medicare's physician payments: physician diagnosis-related groups and other approaches, N Engl J Med 312:1492, 1985.
23. Jencks SF and Dobson A: Refining case-mix adjustment: the research evidence, N Engl J Med 317:679, 1987.
24. Klingman D, Pine P, and Simon J: Outcomes of surgery among Medicaid recipients in Georgia and Michigan, 1981-1982, Presented at American Medical Review Research Center, Second Annual Research Symposium, Washington, DC, Sept. 10, 1987.
25. Luft HS: Regionalization in medical care, Am J Public Health 75:125, 1985.
26. Luft HS, Bunker JP, and Enthoven AC: Should operations be regionalized? The empirical relation between surgical volume and mortality. N Engl J Med 301:1364, 1979.
27. Luft HS and Hunt SS: Evaluating individual hospital quality through outcome statistics, JAMA 255:2780, 1986.
28. Reference deleted in proofs.
29. Maerki SC, Luft HS, and Hunt SS: Selecting categories of patients for regionalization: implications of the relationship between volume and outcome, Med Care 24:148, 1986.
30. Mossey JM and Roos LL: Using insurance claims to measure health status: the illness scale, J Chronic Dis 40:41S (suppl), 1987.
31. Mosteller F, Gilbert JP, and McPeek B: Reporting standards and research strategies for controlled trials, Controlled Clin Trials 1:37, 1980.
32. Neuhauser D: Cost-effective clinical decision-making: implications for the delivery of health services. In Bunker JP, Barnes BA, and Mosteller F, editors: Costs, risks, and benefits of surgery, New York, 1977, Oxford University Press, Inc.
33. Owens WD, Felts JA, and Spitznagel EL Jr: ASA physical classifications: a study of consistency of ratings, Anesthesiology 49:239, 1978.
34. Patricelli RE: Employers as managers of risk, cost, and quality, Health Aff 6:75, 1987.
35. Pauker SG and Kassirer JP: Decision analysis, N Engl J Med 316:250, 1987.
36. Reinhardt UE: Resource allocation in health care: the allocation of lifestyles to providers, Milbank Mem Fund Quart 65:153, 1987.
37. Roos LL: Alternative designs to study outcomes: the tonsillectomy case, Med Care 17:1069, 1979.
38. Roos LL, Nicol JP, and Cageorge SM: Using administrative data for longitudinal research: comparisons with primary data collection, J Chronic Dis 40:41, 1987.
39. Roos LL, Roos NP, and Henteleff PD: Assessing the impact of tonsillectomies, Med Care 16:502, 1978.
40. Roos LL, Roos NP, and Sharp SM: Monitoring adverse outcomes of surgery using administrative data, Health Care Finan Rev 7:5 (suppl), 1987.
41. Roos LL and Sharp SM: Becoming more efficient at outcomes research, Int J Tech Asses Health Care, 1988. (forthcoming.)
42. Roos LL and Sharp SM: Innovation, centralization, and growth: coronary artery bypass graft surgery in Manitoba, 1987. (submitted for publication.)
43. Roos LL, Sharp SM, and Wajda A: Assessing data quality: a computerized approach, Soc Sci Med, 1988. (forthcoming.)
44. Roos LL, Wajda A, and Nicol JP: The art and science of record linkage: methods that work with few identifiers, Comput Biol Med 16:45, 1986.
45. Roos LL et al: Using administrative data banks for research and evaluation: a case study, Eval Q 3:236, 1979.
46. Roos LL, et al: How good are the data? Reliability of one health care data bank, Med Care 20:266, 1982.
47. Roos LL et al: Using computers to identify complications after surgery, Am J Public Health 75:1288, 1985.
48. Roos LL et al: Centralization, certification, and monitoring: readmissions and complications after surgery, Med Care 24:1044, 1986.
49. Roos, NP: Hysterectomies in one Canadian province: a new look at risks and benefits, Am J Public Health 74:39, 1984.
50. Roos NP: What is the potential for moving adult surgery to the ambulatory setting? Can Med Assoc J 138:809, 1988.
51. Roos NP and Danzinger RG: Assessing surgical risks in a population: patient histories before and after cholecystectomy, Soc Sci Med 22:571, 1986.
52. Roos NP, and Lyttle D: Hip arthroplasty surgery in Manitoba: 1973-1978, Clin Orthop 199:248, 1985
53. Roos NP, and Ramsey E: A population-based study of prostatectomy: long term outcomes associated with differing surgical approaches, J Urol 137:1184, 1987.
54. Roos NP and Roos LL: High and low surgical rates: risk factors for area residents, Am J Public Health 71:591, 1981.
55. Roos NP et al: Variations in physicians' hospitalization practices: a population-based study in Manitoba, Canada Am J Public Health 76:45, 1986.
56. Roos NP et al: Using administrative data to predict important health outcomes: entry to hospital, nursing home and death, Med Care 26:221, 1988.
57. Schwartz WB: The inevitable failure of current cost-containment strategies: why they can provide only temporary relief, JAMA 257:220, 1987.
58. Scitovsky AA: Changes in the costs of treatment of selected illnesses, 1971-1981, Med Care 23:1345, 1985.
59. Showstack JA, Stone MH, and Schroeder SA: The role of changing clinical practices in the rising costs of hospital care, N Engl J Med 313:1201, 1985.

60. Showstack JA et al: Association of volume with outcome of coronary artery bypass graft surgery: scheduled vs. nonscheduled operations, JAMA 257:785, 1987.
61. Sloan FA, Perrin JM, and Valvona J: In-hospital mortality of surgical patients: is there an empiric basis for standard setting? Surgery 99:446, 1986.
62. Smith ME: Record linkage: organizing the facts together. In Bennett BM and Trute B, editors: Mental health information systems: problems and prospects, New York, 1984, The Edwin Mellen Press.
63. Stern RS and Epstein AM: Institutional responses to prospective payment based on diagnosis-related groups: implications for cost, quality, and access, N Engl J Med 312:621, 1985.
64. Thomas JW, Ashcraft MLS, and Zimmerman J: An evaluation of alternative severity of illness measures for use by university hospitals, Ann Arbor, Mich, 1986, Department of Health Services management and Policy, School of Public Health, University of Michigan.
64a. US Congress, Office of Technology Assessment, The quality of medical care: information for consumers, OTA-H-386, Washington, DC, June 1988, US Government Printing Office.
65. Valvona J and Sloan F: Rising rates of surgery among the elderly, Health Aff 4:108, 1985.
66. Wajda A and Roos LL: Simplifying record linkage: software and strategy, Comput Biol Med 17:239, 1987.
67. Wennberg JE: Commentary: on patient need, equity, supplier-induced demand and the need to assess the outcome of common medical practices, Med Care 23:512, 1985.
68. Wennberg JE: Which rate is right? N Engl J Med 310:310, 1986.
69. Wennberg JE: Commentary: using claims to measure health status, J Chronic Dis (suppl) 40:51S, 1987.
70. Wennberg JE and Fowler FJ: A test of consumer contribution to small area variations in health care delivery, J Maine Med Assoc 68:275, 1977.
71. Wennberg JE, Freeman J, and Culp WJ: Are hospital services rationed in New Haven or over-utilised in Boston? Lancet, May 23:1185, 1987.
72. Wennberg JE, McPherson K, and Caper P: Will payment based on diagnosis-related groups control hospital costs? N Engl J Med 311:295, 1984.
73. Wennberg JE et al: Changes in tonsillectomy rates associated with feedback and review, Pediatrics 59:821, 1977.
74. Wennberg JE et al: Use of claims data systems to evaluate health care outcomes: mortality and reoperation following prostatectomy, JAMA 257:933, 1987.
75. West R, Sherman GJ, and Downey W: A record linkage study of valproate and malformations in Saskatchewan, Can J Public Health 76:226, 1985.

WILLIAM R. DRUCKER

William R. Drucker is professor of surgery at the Uniformed Services University of the Health Sciences. Formerly he was Chairman of the Department of Surgery at the University of Rochester School of Medicine and Dentistry, Chairman of the Department of Surgery, University of Toronto, and Dean of the School of Medicine, University of Virginia. A graduate of Harvard College (1943) and The Johns Hopkins School of Medicine (1946), he received residency education in internal medicine and research at Johns Hopkins, Yale, and Case Western Reserve and residency education in surgery at the University Hospitals in Cleveland.

J. WILLIAM GAVETT

J. William Gavett, professor emeritus, holds dual appointments in the Simon Graduate School of Management and the Department of Preventive, Family and Rehabilitation Medicine at the University of Rochester School of Medicine and Dentistry. Dr. Gavett received a BSME degree from the University of Rochester in 1943, an MME degree from Cornell University in 1952, and a PhD from Cornell in 1956. He has served as consultant for industrial firms and health care organizations and has conducted research for the Small Business Administration, the Rochester Regional Medical Program, Rochester Regional Hospital Corporation, and Welfare Research, Inc.

16

The High-cost Surgical Patient

WILLIAM R. DRUCKER
J. WILLIAM GAVETT

In this chapter surgical patients whose hospital care has generated high costs will be considered relative to the causes leading to these costs and the strategies to reduce them. Attention will be directed to a category of high-cost patients designated as "ambiplex" to reflect ambiguity of the focus and complexity of the many problems that they harbor. The ambiplex patients were selected for special attention because they exemplify many of the managerial problems evident in high-cost hospitalized patients.

PHYSICIANS AND CLINICAL COSTS

A growing litany about cost containment has pervaded the health care literature for the past decade.[64,67,74,76] Suggestions and efforts to improve the economics of health care have varied. Considerable attention has been directed to relatively broad issues of reimbursement controls, consumer incentives, and organizational design.* There is increasing awareness that the success of these cost-containment efforts is limited.† The economic growth of the country is supplying only part of the additional resources that are needed to cover increases in health care costs. Hospital charges rose 19% in 1986 in contrast with a 1.9% rise in the consumer price index (CPI).[1] At the beginning of 1988 there was a surge in health insurance premiums, reflecting the failure to bring medical costs under control.[61,66]

As health care expenditures have continued to absorb an increased percentage of the gross national product, it is logical that efforts to contain costs should shift to the hospital where more than 40% of the total health dollar is spent. But until very recently, incentives to contain costs within hospitals have been either weak, nonexistent, or counterproductive.[12,23,36,40] This deficiency reflects in large measure the prevalent view that hospitals are the private preserve of physicians. Physician-directed activities within the hospital, exclusive of physician fees, are estimated to influence at least two thirds of total hospital expenditures. Consequently, physician managerial performance promises to be a fertile hunting ground for sharp-eyed cost cutters looking for ways to control hospital costs.[65]

Early questioning of physician management in hospitals demonstrated that laboratory tests frequently are overused.* After it became clear that relatively small financial gains accrued from the discriminative use of the laboratory, more direct regulatory measures were sought. Econo-

---

*References 24,25,27,31,49.
†References 2,3,5,44,45.

*References 16,24,37,38,73.

my-minded employer benefit plans and the government-sponsored Medicare program focused on the length of stay (LOS) of patients as a prime target for reducing costs.[53,62,77] The reactive cry from physicians about infringement on the quality of patient care has been ignored largely because the measures of quality required to validate physician concern are so imprecise. That is, the processes of clinical medicine that physicians control increasingly are being judged in economic terms. The very core of clinical medicine, the part that is under physician control, is being attacked for the economic benefits its modifications might reap.[76,81,83]

Although it can be expected that those footing the bill for health care will continue the impetus for cost containment, it is reasonable to expect that pressure will be placed on the medical profession. Reduction of LOS, use of intensive care units, efficient use of ancillary services, withholding medical procedures, allocation of decision rights to paraprofessionals, and hospital admission decisions all involve professional evaluations that only the physician can render.*

To gain better insight into how physicians influence hospital costs and to use this information for the development of strategies for physician-directed cost containment, studies were undertaken of hospitalized patients.[21,22,35] The hospitalization process in which a patient participates was considered to be the focal point of physician management and therefore a source for analysis. Recent literature suggested that attention to high-cost inpatients would limit the study group size and would provide a focus and leverage in the containment of costs, because these patients consume a disproportionate share of hospital resources.[50,71,72,84]

PRELUDE TO A STUDY OF HIGH-COST PATIENTS

A study of the inpatients in Strong Memorial Hospital (SMH), an institution owned and operated by the University of Rochester, was a collaborative effort among the faculty of the Simon Graduate Business School; the Department of Preventive, Rehabilitation, and Family Medicine; and the Department of Surgery of the University. The study was sponsored by the Rochester Hospital Experimental Payment Program (HEP), a cooperative program designed to contain the costs of the nine nonprofit hospitals in two counties of upstate New York. The intent of this study was to identify those factors under physician control that contribute to the high cost of patients and to suggest strategies based on these findings that might give clinicians the leverage to reduce the costs of hospital care. During the study a subset of patients who did not conform to conventional diagnostic, procedural, or service categories was found. They were designated ambiplex to embrace the complexity of their multiple independent illnesses lacking a well-focused disease problem and to emphasize the consequent ambiguity of their clinical description and therefore their management.

Background

Pareto's law is one of the economist's elementary descriptions of human activity: "in a play, only a few of the actors have most of the lines to say." That is, in a given activity a relatively small number of the actors contribute to a disproportionate share of the action.[63] Many examples of this can be found: only a small proportion of a bank's accounts (actors) contain most of the bank's dollar deposits (activity); only a small number of patients (actors) account for most of a hospital's annual billings (activity). In a recent note to the *New England Journal of Medicine,* the Hon. Henry A. Waxman, Chairman of the Subcommittee on Health and the Environment in Congress, observed that a tiny fraction of incompetent physicians (actors) are responsible for a large share of the paid malpractice claims (activity).[82]

This distribution is variously referred to as Pareto's law, named in honor of the noted Italian economist who recognized its universality, or the Lorenz curve, named after an economist who

---

*References 18,41,48,49,78,80.

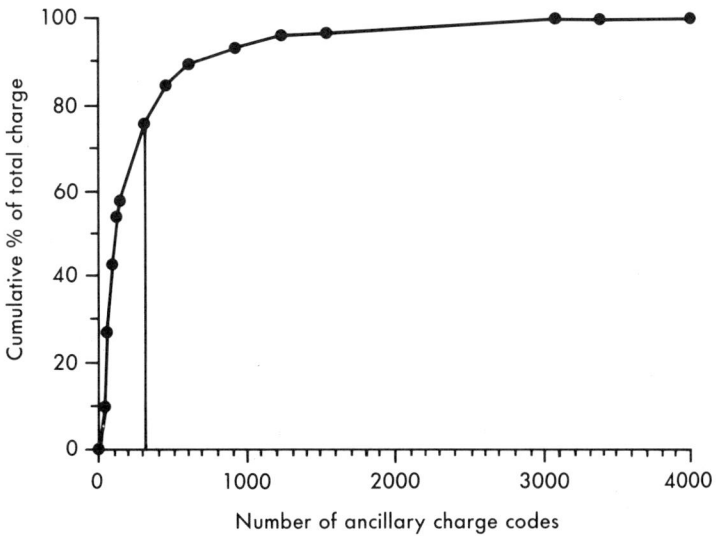

Figure 16-1. Use of ancillary hospital charges (Lorenz curve, illustrating Pareto's law).

popularized the applicability of Pareto's law to family incomes.[54] Subsequently, several "rules" of disproportionality have come into fashion, such as the 80/20 rule denoting that approximately 20% of the items account for 80% of an activity or the 50/10 rule indicating that 10% of the items account for one half of the resulting activity.

A quantitative descriptor of this relationship of disproportionality is shown in Figure 16-1. A teaching hospital catalogues 4000 ancillary procedures, such as drugs, tests, and x-rays examinations. These (actors) can be ranked in descending order of their annual dollar charges and then plotted against the cumulative dollar charges for all ancillary procedures (activity). This reveals that about 10% (400) of the ancillary procedures in the hospital are used with such frequency that they account for about 80% of the annual revenue from all procedures. Conversely, 90% (3600) of the procedures account for only 10% to 20% of total revenues.

The underlying rationale for describing an activity in terms of the Pareto phenomenon relates to the efficient management of the activity. It suggests that variable policies and controls should be applied to the classes relative to their activity value. Thus one directs more attention to the small number of prime actors (often referred to as class A items). The principle is appealing when the manager is faced with a large number of units (bank deposits, tax returns, hospital patients) to analyze, evaluate, or manage. The relatively small number of major actors facilitates focused management, presumably where the yield will be the highest. In contrast, the large number of minor actors (class C items) are candidates for generalized policies, plans, or designs that entertain economies of scale.

In spite of the prevalent recognition and use of this classification in the industrial and business world, it has only recently received attention in the health care field. In an isolated early study, Densen et al. in 1959 reported the use of this classification in a study of the intensive users of an HMO service.[17] Twelve percent of the HMO members generated 50% of the annual visits. More recent literature about high-cost inpatients indicates that about 10% to 15% of the acute patients in general hospitals account for as much of the annual hospital charges as the complimentary 85% to 90% of the inpatients, or 50% of the charges are accounted for by 10% of the patients (50-10 rule).[71,72,84]

Hospital Utilization Measures

Any study of the high-cost phenomenon will be influenced by the choice of the unit of activity (actor). To define the unit of activity it is necessary to review the time-oriented process of an individual's hospitalization. This process is seldom delineated or fully appreciated by economy-minded reviewers unfamiliar with the complexities of patient movement within the hospital and throughout a period of hospitalization.

A patient is admitted to the hospital for a single uninterrupted duration termed the length of stay (LOS). The hospital admission or discharge of a patient historically is the most prevalent unit of activity. During a single admission, however, a patient may be transferred among several geographically and administratively different clinical services or patient care units (PCUs), including intensive care units (ICUs). An encounter is a microunit of activity defining an uninterrupted duration of a patient's time on a given PCU. In a "macro" sense a given individual may experience more than a single hospital admission in a given period, such as a year. Under this circumstance the patient becomes the unit of activity. Several of these terms are illustrated in Figure 16-2, a flow diagram of a high-cost patient's activities during a single year.

Hospitalized patients receive a common battery of ancillary procedures (x-rays examinations, laboratory tests, and drugs, as examples.) In addition, a large number of special therapy procedures, also classified as ancillary procedures, are specific to some admissions. Thus, as noted in the discussion of Pareto's law, the hospital is a heavy user of standard procedures and a light user of many specialty and high technology procedures. Hospital accountants gifted with imagination have been able to group many costs under the rubric of ancillary charges.

In most of the early studies the surrogate for cost was hospital charges or billings.[29] Although charges may be an accurate measure of the cost to most reimbursing agencies, they do not represent true hospital marginal or average costs. If actual costs are used, one would expect a more pronounced ratio or a steeper Lorenz curve (Figure 16-1). Before the current use of prospective reimbursement methods, charges were partially leveled as a result of the common per diem: patients were charged a standard room rate regardless of the severity of their illnesses. Obviously this neglects the fact that resource consumption varies among individual patients.[30,32,33] In addition, the charges in the study represented hospital charges solely and ignored physician fees and outpatient charges.[34] These disregarded charges also serve to increase the differences between high- and low-cost patients. With these caveats in mind in comparing different classes of patients, charges still provide a useful relative measure of resource consumption.

Definition of High Cost

Depending on the purpose of a study, the cost of a patient's activity can be assigned to encounters, specific admissions, or the aggregate of multiple admissions over an extended time. Obviously the number of high-cost patients in a given institution increases as the time horizon is extended. Patients who are classified as low cost in a given year may become high cost in terms of cumulative activity over consecutive years.

Cost per unit is a continuous variable. Segregating patients into the dichotomy high cost and low cost is arbitrary and may appear to be capricious. Nevertheless, it is practical. It is difficult to adjust management or research attention on a continuous scale. It is much easier and it is satisfactory for the purposes of study to select the top 10% of the most costly patients or to select all patients whose cumulative charges across a given period exceed an arbitrarily chosen figure, such as $20,000 in one year.

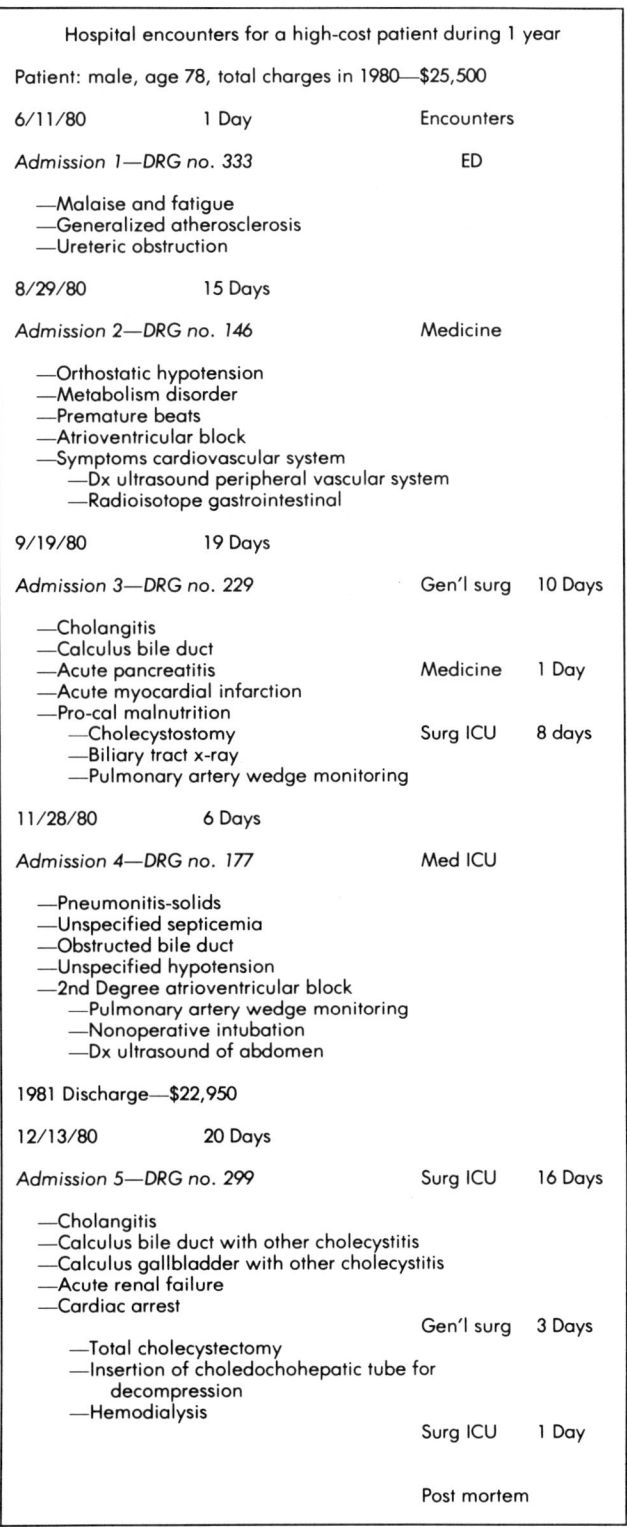

Figure 16-2. Admissions and encounters in 1980-1981 for a high-cost patient.

THE AMBIPLEX PATIENT STUDY

In 1983 an initial study of high-cost surgical patients was conducted at Strong Memorial Hospital.[22] This study employed a base of patient utilization data. The base contained detailed patient and billing information about all inpatient discharges on an annual basis. Specifically, the file contained patient demographics (age, sex, ethnic origin), room and ancillary charges, source of reimbursement (Medicare, Medicaid, Blue Cross, other), hospital days, discharge clinical service, discharge disposition, five levels of primary and secondary ICD-9-CM diagnostic codes, five levels of ICD-9-CM operating and diagnostic procedure codes, a diagnosis related group (DRG) code, and patient ancillary procedures including the procedure code (charge code), the date the procedure was applied, the charge, and the units delivered. In addition, room charges, ancillary procedure charges, and hospital days were recorded for each patient encountered on a clinical patient care unit (PCU) and in an intensive care unit (ICU).

For this study, computer-produced statistics were augmented with manual tabulations when computer and/or programming capabilities were temporarily inaccessible. Three units of analysis were used: patient, admission, and encounter. The prime unit of analysis was the patient's utilization statistics aggregated across 1 year. Although data for subsequent years became available in time, when this study was started, only data for 1980 were available and became the reference year for all future work. Charges were used throughout the study as a convenient surrogate of costs.[29]

The general purposes of this study were to reaffirm the disproportionality of hospital charges for a small number of patients and to make preliminary patient classifications that would be useful in focusing on the causes for high cost. From a population of 21,820 inpatients in the study year (1980), 3935 patients were identified as having at least one encounter with one or more of five general surgical PCUs including a surgical ICU. Within this population of surgical patients, 261 patients each had total 1980 SMH charges of $20,000 or more. These surgical patients, defined arbitrarily as high-cost, consumed a disproportionate share of hospital resources (Table 16-1).

In the initial phase of the research, a particular group of high-cost patients, labeled "complex," were discovered.[22] The next phase of research was directed to a study of the total population of high-cost patients in Strong Memorial Hospital, paying particular attention to these "complex patients."[35] It was hypothesized that these patients would present a special problem of management and opportunity for cost containment. This subset of high-cost complex patients did not easily fit into conventional diagnostic, procedural, or service categories. It was believed that they were not peculiar to surgery but present in the general hospital population. Therefore the 1980 hospital inpatient population was surveyed for their presence. Their designation was changed to ambiplex to embrace both the complexity of their multiple and often independent illnesses lacking a well-focused disease problem and the consequent ambiguity of their clinical description and management. Our initial study led to

Table 16-1. Utilization of general surgical resources by the 261 high-cost general surgical patients

100%	3935	General surgery patients
6.6%	261	Patients with charges ≥ 20,000
		These patients were responsible for:
32%		Total hospital charges for general surgery
32%		Total hospital days for general surgery
54%		Charges for just general surgical days
40%		All ICU days
30%		Ancillary charges

the belief that ambiplex patients would not necessarily be involved with high-cost technically complicated lifesaving procedures, such as coronary bypass surgery, transplantation surgery, and intensive care. Rather, they would be long-term or recurring occupants of the general medical and surgical services. They would have a disproportionate impact on hospital resources similar to other high-cost patients with focused illnesses. Finally, perhaps uniquely among the high-cost patients, these ambiplex patients might lead us to identify areas in which physicians, through changes in their managerial practices, could help bring costs under better control.

Definition of Ambiplex

Clinical studies classically focus on patients categorized by specific medical problems, diagnoses, operating procedures, or services, for example, cirrhosis of the liver, open heart surgery, trauma, renal, SICU. In contrast to these well-focused categorizations is the group of ambiplex patients. The criteria of ambiplex include a set of comorbidities that are not necessarily interrelated, multiple hospitalizations in terms of admissions, within-admission transfers (encounters) among different clinical services, and long hospitalizations. Patients are likely to be older. The several medical problems are largely independent, such that intervention to treat one problem simply shifts another to primacy. The prognosis for an overall satisfactory outcome is poor and the likelihood of death within a relatively short term is high. The hospital ancillary charges for this group of patients are also likely to be high. Thus the assignment of such patients to a focused problem or service set (diagnosis, DRG, ICU) may not be particularly meaningful. Ambiplex inpatients are a class by themselves, discernible primarily by an awareness of their existence.

An early hypothesis in the research was that ambiplex patients present a special leverage for cost containment. The general ambiguous nature of the diagnoses and/or therapies of these patients provides an ambience for potential indecision and variation in the choice of modalities of care. High cost might be attributed as much to the "search" for optimal modes of care in a nonemergent climate as to direct and noncontroversial medical interventions. In contrast, high-cost trauma patients might represent patients at the opposite end of the scale. The problems of trauma patients are seldom ambiguous: when a diagnosis is established, the modes of intervention usually are clear. Patients are likely to be younger: if death occurs, it is often early before extensive resources have been used. Except for rehabilitative services, the number of inpatient admissions per patient is small, although length of stay may be long. Care is intensive and emergent in the early stages after injury, tapering off to recuperative services as time ensues.[21]

Similarly, other "focused" patient problems contrast with the ambiguity of the ambiplex patients, such as open heart surgery, cancer, mental disorders, and renal disease, although there are some patients whose multiple problems intersect these categories and who become candidates for the ambiplex class.

The literature of hospital cost containment and clinical management does not specifically recognize this general class of patients. Complexity and ambiguity do not exist as commonly accepted and quantifiable variables. They are a construct, that is, defined in terms of other accepted and measurable variables. Although we have limited their characterization to hospital inpatient status, it is hypothesized that these patients are frequent users of other community health resources. Such patients are probably implicitly included in discussions and analyses of the broad class of chronic or long-term care elderly patients. Whether the explicit recognition of ambiplex patients is clinically and economically useful was the issue of this research. Beyond this definition there are a number of associated problems encountered in dealing with ambiplex patients. These are (1) the retrospective identification of such patients from a historical data base for purposes of research and analyses; (2) their prospective identification (prediction) from current admissions or a census for purposes of (a) resource management and (b) the anticipatory guidance for patients and their families; and (3) development of prognoses for both short- and long-term outcomes. Thus identification, prediction, and prognoses are different but not independent problems.

Methods

The patient rather than the single admission (discharge) was the unit of analysis. Also, again, patient charges (billings) were used as a surrogate of cost. Previous studies demonstrated that 20% of a patient's ancillary procedures usually account for 80% of the patient's ancillary charges.[22] Therefore detailed information about a given patient's ancillary usage was confined to those 20% of the procedures. Outpatient data and physician fees were not included in this study. High-cost patients were first defined in terms of aggregated charges greater than $20,000 across their 1980 SMH discharges. This yielded a study population of the 594 high-cost individuals of the total 1980 SMH population of 21,820 patients from which to search for the ambiplex patients.

The next step was to eliminate from the subset of 594 high-cost patients, those assumed to have relatively focused medical problems. A simple, bounding rule was used to segregate such patients into six arbitrarily defined groups with focused criteria, namely trauma, pediatric, psychiatric, cardiac (open heart), cancer, and renal (see box). Though crude, this method of step-by-step elimination identified sufficient ambiplex patients to provide the basis for the analyses of their clinical course and costs. The rationale for the bounding criteria selection was based on the initial assumption that there would be few ambiplex patients within the six groups with focused problems. A final class of patients left over after this assignment was referred to as the residual class, assumed to contain, among others, most of the ambiplex patients. After the initial segregation of patients into these seven classes by the computer, the classes were reviewed manually, and a small number of patients (4.7%) were reclassified based on the mix of the primary and four secondary diagnostic codes for each discharge.

The next step of this study was to purify the residual set of patients to ambiplex only. The selection was made by physician judgment according to the definition of ambiplex and by information in the clinical/financial file. The crit-

---

Criteria for Selecting Seven Groups of High-Cost Patients

1. Trauma — Any patient having a *primary* diagnostic ICD-9-CM code 900.00-959.90 in at least one of the patient's discharges if more than one discharge was involved.

2. Pediatrics — Any patient (not selected in group 1) having an age equal to or younger than 12 years.

3. Psychiatric — Any patient (not selected in groups 1 and 2) having a primary diagnostic ICD-9-CM code 290.00-319.00.

4. Cardiac — Any patient (not selected in groups 1 to 3 having a primary ICD-9-CM operation code 350.0-369.9. These were predominantly patients who had open heart surgery.

5. Cancer — Any patient (not selected in groups 1 to 4) having a primary diagnostic ICD-9-CM 140.00-239.90.

6. Renal — Any patient (not selected in groups 1 to 5) having a primary diagnostic ICD-9-CM code 585, 586, 584, 555.3.

7. Residual — All remaining patients.

ical data were the constellation of ICD-9-CM diagnostic and procedure codes available for all 1980 patient discharges. The primary and secondary diagnoses most frequently found in the ambiplex patients included diabetes mellitus (with or without complications), obesity, anemia, essential hypertension, hypertensive heart disease, atherosclerosis, coronary arteriosclerosis, heart failure, renal failure, chronic airway obstruction, and intestinal obstruction.

The final step in this study was random selection of a subset of 20 ambiplex patients from the set of 63 high-cost ambiplex patients identified within the group of residual patients. This study group was subjected to intensive clinical analysis. At least two physicians made an independent exhaustive review of each patient's hospital record and clinical/financial data including 1980 activity and any SMH activity in the years immediately subtending 1980. Each review was presented to the total group of four investigators (Drs. John Dickinson, William Drucker, J. William Gavett, and Margery McCrum) for assessment and integration into the final report. Demographic, emotional, social, clinical, and financial information were summarized by each of two reviewers and supplemented with detailed observations/inferences about clinical management. Completed summaries were discussed by the team to clarify discrepancies and assure completeness. Patients who had not died in SMH as of December 31, 1980 were traced to determine their survival status from 1981 to 1983. A composite description was then made for each subject. Observations from all 20 patients were collated into a taxonomy of management problems typical of ambiplex patients.

Results

594 High-cost patients. The Pareto phenomenon was observed again: patients with annual 1980 SMH charges of $20,000 or more accounted for only 2.7% of the total SMH patient population (Table 16-2); however, their charges and hospital days were about 24% and 20%, respectively, of the hospital's totals. The average daily census of high-cost patients was estimated to be about 20% of the hospital's average daily census. Almost 18% of these patients died in SMH in 1980 compared with 3.2% of the remaining population of patients; that is, 13% of the hospital's terminal patients were identified within the high-cost group.

Study group of 20 ambiplex patients. The 20 ambiplex patients extracted a disproportionate share of hospital resources (Table 16-3); the mean use of resources per patient was: $44,490, 105 days, 3.4 admissions, and daily intensity of $423. Nine (45%) died in 1980, and 14 (70%) died within the 4-year period (1980 to 1983). Only 3 of the 11 patients alive at the end of 1980 did not return to SMH at some time during the 3 subsequent years. It was recognized that some of these patients may have returned to hospitals other than SMH. Utilization of clinical services was as follows: more than half of their total days were on the medical service, including 10% of their days assigned to the medical intensive care unit (ICU); 28% were on the general surgical service, including 7% on the surgical ICU; and 18% of their days were on other clinical services (Table 16-4).

Contributors to high cost. The majority of these ambiplex patients received acceptable medical care in conventional terms. Nine factors, almost universally evident, were observed and judged to contribute to the higher cost and less than optimal care for these patients.

1. Lack of patient agent. The ambiplex patient in the hospital suffered from the lack of a comprehensive management; there was no identifiable central physician, or "patient agent", responsible for overseeing continuity of care. This judgment was based on the absence of a written plan for patient care, failure to document integrated patient assessment, apparent failure to recognize events of previous admissions, multiplicity of decision makers including an average of 10 residents and 6 specialists

Table 16-2. 1980 Summary data for 594 patients with annual charges ≥ $20,000 compared with the complement of the population of SMH patients

	High-cost Population	Remaining SMH Population
Total annual SMH charges per patient	$ ≥ 20,000	$ ≥ 20,000
Number of patients	594	21,300
Patients as percentage of all SMH patients	2.7%	97.3%
Total charges	$19,900,000	$62,467,000
Average charges per patient	$33,500	$2930
Charges as percentage of total hospital	24.1%	75.9%
Total hospital days	46,445	185,990
Average days per patient	78.2	8.7
Days as a percentage of total hospital	20%	80%
Total admissions	1232	23,090
Average admissions per patient	2.07	1.08
Average charges per day	$428	$336
Estimated daily census	120 (20%)	508 (80%)
Terminal in SMH in 1980	105 (17.7%)	684 (3.2%)

per patient without evidence of coordinated authority, delay by specialists in management of the patient until well after the first evidence of the relevant problem, and delays in patient discharge caused by hesitant decision making.

2. Lack of broad perspective of the patient's environment. The attending physicians and house officers frequently did not demonstrate a broad perspective in their assessments of the patients. They were noted to concentrate on a specific patient problem (clinical myopia) or they adopted an aggressive approach to remedying one or more of the patient's problems without consideration of the patient's total welfare.
3. Multiple encounters and decision rights. The organization of the hospital into traditional separate clinical services often necessitated patient transfer among specialized patient care units both between and during admissions. Placement of a patient within the hospital was dictated by the medical problem of momentary concern among his complex array of disorders rather than by a plan for preventive, comprehensive, or continuous care. Each new environment presented adaptation challenges, repetitious examination, and questioning with little attention to the past medical record.
4. Consultations. Multiple morbidities are inherent in ambiplexity. It was not surprising that many consultants were asked to see these patients. However, the high rate of consultation was rarely followed by incorporation of the consultants' recommen-

Table 16-3. Use of hospital resources by the study group of 20 ambiplex patients (compared with the total high-cost and remaining SMH populations)

	Ambiplex Study Group	High-cost Population	Remaining SMH Population
Number of patients	20	594	21,300
Total charges	$889,830	19,891,400	62,478,600
Average charges per patient	$44,490	$33,500	$2930
Range of charges	$20,709–$88,983	—	—
Total hospital days	2103	46,445	196,669
Average days per patient	105	78.2	8.7
Range of hospital days	48–303	—	—
Total admissions	68	1232	23,088
Average admissions per patient	3.4	2.07	1.08
Range of admissions	1–8	—	—
Average intensity $/day	$423	$428	$336
Terminal in SMH—1980	5 (25%)	105 (17.7%)	684 (3.2%)

Table 16-4. Clinical service utilization by 20 ambiplex patients in 1980

Service	Days	Percent
General medicine	936	44.5
General surgery	456	21.7
Gynecology	35	1.7
Neurology	296	14.1
Neurosurgery	8	0.4
Plastic surgery	11	0.5
Emergency	16	0.7
Medical ICU	209	9.9
Surgical ICU	136	6.5
TOTAL	2103	100.0

dations into a basic plan. Consequently, a house officer was left with a bombardment of suggestions from each consultant without an indication that a more senior physician was available to help sort out the overlap and potential danger of simultaneous study and therapy of multiple problems in the same patient.[47]

5. Profligate use of ancillary services. House officers had significant decision rights consistent with the delegation of responsibility as a prerequisite for the education of residents. Consequently, numerous tests and procedures were ordered for the patients without a well-organized plan. Often there was no evidence that results had any influence on subsequent planning. Many tests were judged to be repetitious or unnecessary. Stat (expedited) tests were commonplace and frequently without justification for the urgency or cost of the test.

6. Length of stay. The LOS of these patients was well beyond the norms for the general medical or surgical services in SMH.[4] To a certain extent this was traceable to the complexity of the medical problems that required care; it also reflected the lack of

both a well-organized care plan and a discharge plan for care in a more appropriate facility. However, securing placement in external facilities also was hampered by the complexity of the patients' illnesses and the unavailability of such facilities.

7. Poor communication. In the records of eight patients, there was strong evidence that lack of proper communications among interested parties led either to higher costs, compromised quality of care, or both. Environmental factors, particularly socioeconomic, usually were ignored in the formal record. Thorough and meaningful summary notes were missing. Useful notes by attending physicians were absent.[47] The medical record often was burdened by repetitious information from physicians, nurses, and social workers. Transfer notes were sparse and lacking a succinct summary of the reasons for transfer, the patient's course to date, or a list of the significant problems that were under study or therapy. Discharge summaries were nearly always inadequate.

8. Psychosocial and economic. Eight patients were judged to have psychosocial variables that contributed to hospitalization or to the exacerbation of their problems. In general, this information was obtained by social work interviews only.

9. Ethical/moral issues. Consideration of these issues almost never was evident in the medical record although conversation with the family or among the many physicians who participated in the care may have occurred. There was an almost uniform lack of consensus about DNR (do not resuscitate) status. Often the record suggested unwillingness of attending physicians to secure a DNR agreement from the family.[11]

DISCUSSION

The nature of this study precludes easy (valid) extrapolation of the results and conclusions to other populations. Judgment of the assessment of the management of these patients refers only to the experience of a single tertiary university hospital (SMH). The study raised many questions that beg further research. The increasing influence of prospective payment systems, the rise in the aged population, and the ever-developing lifesaving technology are just some of the factors emphasizing the need to identify and study the ambiplex patients as a special population contributing to the rising costs of medical care.

The 63 high-cost ambiplex patients represented only a small proportion of the hospital's annual patient population (0.2%) and only 2.7% of the annual charges. Although this does not appear significant, it is important to remember our definition of high cost. The rigidity of cost definition determines the number of ambiplex patients. Certainly, patients whose 1980 charges were $10,000 to $19,999 could be labeled high cost also. In addition, a group of ambiplex patients whose multiple admissions over a 4-year period (1980 to 1983) generated charges equal to or greater than $20,000 per patient were identified but not studied in detail. Their frequency in a 4-year span roughly equaled those who developed a high-cost status solely within a single year. Finally, we hypothesize that the problems of management associated with the ambiplex patient also will be present to some extent with other high-cost patients.[52]

Genesis of the Ambiplex Patient

Cursory review reveals that the ambiplex patient is not a newcomer to the hospital. Why then has the ambiplex patient not been characterized before? All too often the focus is on disease or procedure rather than on the patient. Retrospective analysis of hospitalized patients by physicians would not be expected to reveal the ambiplex patient because of orientation to a single disease process or to the response from specific intervention with drugs or surgery. Health systems planners also have overlooked the ambiplex patient because of their focus on admissions, discharges, or DRGs as units of analysis. The ambiplex phenomenon became apparent only when a study was focused on the long-term course of patients without regard to particular illnesses or a limited period of hospital care.

This group of patients does not represent a new disease process; rather, these patients can be regarded as products of the therapeutic effectiveness of modern medicine in delaying death. As such, their numbers may be expected to increase. In the past, certainly a quarter of a century ago, patients who developed any of the several disorders harbored by ambiplex patients would have died within a brief time at little or moderate financial expense to their families or society. Antibiotics, intensive care, an array of other potent new drugs and anesthetics, mechanical support for respiratory and cardiac functions, renal dialysis, replacement of diseased blood vessels and joints, and the trend for medical and surgical care to be based on physiologic concepts have contributed impressively to prolonging life and often improving its quality. Today, patients afflicted by multiple diseases are capable of leading reasonably productive lives. They enter the high-cost ambiplex category only when their tolerance for multiple comorbidities begins to deteriorate, necessitating a move from ambulatory to hospital care.

An alternative hypothesis explaining the genesis of ambiplex patients begins with a single chronic disease such as diabetes mellitus. Although patients with this disorders are not cured, modern therapy has greatly improved the quality of their lives and extended their life expectancy. The complications of the basic disease in time develop a relatively independent course with little relation to the vicissitudes of the disease that spawned them. Thus the vascular failure of a diabetic becomes in time a self-sustaining problem.

Drawing on this characterization, it is clear that ambiplex patients do not spring into being suddenly. Multiple disorders develop over time and become additive to challenge the patient's well-being. The ambiplex patient has always been a part of the acute hospital scene. More appropriately, the ambiplex is, in part, a constituent of the population of elderly, chronically ill, and often imminently terminal patients who are subjects of much current debate and dialogue relative to their care.[7-10,55] Even though not all ambiplex patients are elderly, focus is on this age group, both because of their relatively large numbers among the ambiplex set and because of the implications of advanced age in the decisions about their care. Therefore the results are highly relevant to the broader issue of geriatric care and its future development.

During the extended term of chronic illness, there are periodic acute and long-term hospital or institutional interventions, especially just before death. During the acute interventions, the care is a medical prerogative, and longer-term geriatric goals are subsidiary to the more immediate goals associated with medicine in a tertiary and teaching acute care hospital. The two may be incompatible as Gillick notes: "The goals of long-term care and of acute care may be irreconcilable.[36] The fundamental concern of long-term care is quality of life and restoration of function; for acute care the goals are treatment and cure of medical illness."[36,58] If, however, a health care plan is in operation from the start, it should be possible to harmonize the conflict between the goals of long-term and short-term care.

Hospital Economics

Because of the ambiguity and sometimes non-emergent character of the ambiplex patient's problem, such patients offer more flexibility in responding to current economic incentives. Patients whose high costs are concentrated in one or two admissions are clearly economic losers under the DRG payment system.[26,43,62,68] In contrast, the patient whose high cost is an aggregation of a large number of low cost admissions is a net income gainer under this system. One can envision the situation where the patient is transferred among organizations, within and without hospital settings, with each facility seeking to limit its contribution to the patient's care.[55]

Ambiplexity has been viewed in its acute inpatient stages at the point where costs are precipitous. In order to alter the course of hospital interventions, it is desirable to identify this patient in time for appropriate action. If high costs are associated with a concentrated hospitalization, a single admission, or a number of admissions clustered in a limited period, the problem of identification is not serious. Critical information includes the history, costs of previous admissions, and the potential for high cost based on criteria such as age, multiplicity and mix of problems, and socioeconomic ambience. Information can be neatly packaged through available computer-based real-time systems.

Prediction is defined as the anticipation of the early onset of the conditions that eventually will precipitate a high-cost event. Attainment of the desirable goal of early prediction probably will remain elusive until more experience has been obtained with this group of patients. But even with reliable predictions, it is not known what constitutes good long-term patient management. The management of ambiplex patients should be high on the agenda of those concerned with family medicine, primary, and long-term care.*

MANAGEMENT STRATEGIES
Recognition

The first management strategy for ambiplex patients is to create an awareness during clinical rounds of their importance as special inpatients. The immediate practical issue is to gain the participation of different clinical specialities, especially surgery and medicine, in discussions about factors contributing to the high cost of these patients.† In time it should be possible to construct a logical structure, such as multivariable analysis, that will predict the likelihood of a patient becoming ambiplex.

Reduce Hospitalization

Adopting preventive measures as a means of reducing the cost of a particular disease is not feasible in the instance of ambiplex patients because of their presumed genesis. Nevertheless, an identification of the potentially high-cost ambiplex patient should foster planning for management that will reduce the need for recurrent or lengthy hospitalization. A deficiency in the study is the lack of information about the management of ambiplex patients on an ambulatory basis and in other community institutions.[34] However, it is assumed that costs for ambulatory care are a relatively small fraction of those for hospital care. This early step toward reducing the overall cost of these pateints would be to keep them out of the hospital but at an appropriate level of care, such as a skilled nursing facility (SNF) or a health-related facility (HRF).

Need for a Patient Agent

The primary problem in the overall management of these patients is the lack of a physician who provides comprehensive care on a continuing basis. This position is referred to as the patient manager or, to borrow a term from the world of business, a patient agent.[20] Clearly, the physician who assumes responsibility for planning and directing the total care of the ambiplex patient must have a broad perspective of medical and social knowledge and technology. There must be an awareness of the patient's long-term clinical course and an understanding of psychosocial and economic factors that influence the patient in the nonhospital environment. Many primary physicians are qualified to function in this capacity, but our study indicated that they do not pursue their role as the patient agent when hospitalization becomes necessary.

---

*References 6,19,59,65,76,83.
†References 13, 15, 57, 60, 69.

Decision rights. In order to meet the responsibilities as the patient agent, this individual must be welcomed into the hospital and have authority over the total hospital care of the patient. If this agent is to assume this responsibility in the hospital, there must be clarification of the decision rights currently diffused across the various participating physicians (attending physician of record, house staff, specialist, consultants). This problem can be resolved, however, by recognition that decision making has four components: (1) initiation of optional courses or plans of action, (2) ratification of the plan, (3) implementation of the chosen plan, and (4) monitoring or evaluation of the outcomes (Jensen).[46] For instance, in an educational environment the patient manager, or agent, might assign the rights of initiation and implementation to house officers while retaining residual rights to ratification and monitoring.

Another fundamental responsibility of the patient agent is to monitor and intervene as necessary regardless of the patient's movement throughout the hospital. Ideally this continuity of care should continue after discharge. The agent should be involved personally in preparing a written discharge plan, in predischarged teaching sessions, and in the provision of ambulatory care.

Our study indicates that prospective payment systems will make management of the ambiplex patient an unrewarding task because of the potential for their high costs.[35] To the extent that hospitals are required to accept a certain number of ambiplex patients or that academic programs will benefit from this type of patient, there will be increased pressure to organize efficient and effective plans for their care. It is improbable that additional revenues will be forthcoming. Consequently, this new hospital specialist, the patient manager or agent, will need to share a slice of the reimbursement pie already expected to be reduced in total.

Thus the specific problems regarding the development of a patient agent are: (1) recognition that cost-effective and high quality care of ambiplex patients requires the leadership of a single physician who has the rights to plan and oversee the total care of the patient, (2), acceptance of this new actor by specialists and house officers and, (3) development of a program that rewards or penalizes all who participate in the care of these patients according to the success in achieving the goals of cost and quality control. The development of organization controls (rules of the game) that will promote this cooperative behavior is not a trivial endeavor. The magnitude of designing the organizational structure that will induce this cooperative behavior transcends the scope of this chapter.

Impact on Educational Practices

The managerial problems identified in the study of ambiplex patients suggest reordering of educational concepts and practices.* Predictably, difficulties will arise from the conflicting interests of education and patient care when an ambiplex patient is placed in a teaching hospital. Here again the issue of the assignment of decision rights is involved.

One precept of a sound residency program is the delegation of authority and responsibility for patient care to residents under the supervision of attending faculty. This study of 20 ambiplex patients clearly indicated adherence to this fundamental tenant of postgraduate medical education. On the other hand, the precise role of the attending faculty members was less evident, often to the apparent detriment of quality of patient care and hospital cost.

The process and extent of assigning decision rights to house staff must be reviewed. The four elements, initiation, ratification, implementation, and monitoring may be assigned in total or in part, depending on the nature of the decision and the maturity of the resident. In an ideal edu-

---
*References 22, 32, 47, 79, 81.

cation program, the right of decision initiation and implementation should continue to be assigned to these postgraduate students. At least with reference to ambiplex patients, however, the control of decisions through ratification and monitoring should be more strongly exercised by the principal physician. This should improve quality of care, contain costs, and enhance education.

Another major deficiency in the current programs of education is the myopic secular interest of established disciplines. It is expected that all residents acquire a core of general information and skills during their initial postgraduate year. Yet each discipline, such as medicine, psychiatry, or surgery, undertakes this task as a unique isolated responsibility. A multispecialty or interdepartmental program to provide this instruction for house officers would enhance the educational experience for all. Ambiplex patients, by definition having only transitory allegiance to a particular speciality, would be an ideal population for such an interdisciplinary program.

Beyond the focused problems of tests and procedures is the broader issue of the costs and benefits of hospitalization and associated clinical interventions. Attention to the ambiplex patient will require emphasis on the critical assessment of clinical costs and benefits for their diagnostic and therapeutic procedures.* As part of the periodic morbidity, mortality, and quality assurance conferences held on clinical services, there is a growing inclination to include assessments of the cost benefit of patient care practices. Many physicians feel inadequate for the task, however, by virtue of the unfamiliar vocabulary and the techniques of analysis. This suggests the desirability of enlarging the traditional closed shop clinical conference to include experts from other professions. The reticence of clinicians to utilize concepts that are foreign to them and that inherently will criticize their performance is matched by the lack of experts in managerial theory and practices as applied to clinical medicine. Financial clinical analysis is neither a fully developed nor familiar endeavor.*

Nevertheless, the saga of ambiplex patients demonstrates clearly the overwhelming need for this type of interdisciplinary conference as a means to improve the quality and to reduce the costs of their care.

Impact on Career Selection

Although it is difficult to obtain convincing data about the factors influencing the selection of careers within the broad field of clinical medicine, certain negative influences can be identified. When questioned about the factors governing their selection of a residency, students today express concern about a career that would involve responsibility for a large number of the "unrewarding" patients encountered during their clerkships. These patients were chronically ill, aged, possessed large number of unrelated disorders, had frequent or prolonged periods of hospital care, and often came from unfavorable socioeconomic backgrounds—the heretofore characterized ambiplex patient! Students' frustrations encountered by inefficient management, lack of improvement in the overall well-being of these patients despite episodic limited therapeutic triumphs, and the experience of receiving often conflicting advice from consulting specialists are specific factors contributing to student disinclination to pursue careers involving responsibility for significant numbers of these patients. The absence of a physician role model interested and skilled in the total management of ambiplex patients may represent a significant factor in the development of negative attitudes among young physicians regarding the care of these patients. Thus the ambiplex patient represents both a practical economic problem in need of solution as well as an overt challenge to the educational system. Finding more efficient and

---

*References 16, 24, 28, 37, 67, 73.

*References 3, 4, 8, 12, 18, 19, 23, 39, 64, 70, 78, 80.

effective ways of caring for the ambiplex patient should help resolve the disinclination of students to pursue a career that involves the need to care for these patients.

Patient Management Plan

One of the most important strategies will be to formulate a plan of management at the time of admission. This plan will change, of course, according to the patient's response to therapy and as information is obtained from tests and procedures during the course of hospitalization. The plan for the ambiplex patient differs only in the greater number of people involved in its formulation and the need to pay particular attention to the complete past medical record.

A determinant of the patient agent's success will be the degree to which the attending physicians and house officers abate the profligate use of resources by better planning and control. Elimination of unwarranted tests (repetitive and stat) and reduction of the overuse of otherwise appropriate procedures and tests is a result of the control exerted by the patient agent supported by a real-time on-line information system. Planned sequencing of tests and procedures must be conducted amid the bombardment of suggestions and requests from consulting specialists plus presumed and real legal pressures. Special care must be exercised, of course, to ensure that iatrogenic complications such as drug interactions and toxicity do not develop in these patients who have complex medical problems. This imposes on the patient agent yet another major demand—to be conversant with the pharmacologic parameters of each drug and of the patient's response to medications. Perhaps the problem of excess tests and procedures will be solved by advances in clinical decision making, but the ambiplex patient may be too unfocused for management by a fixed logical decision structure.

Moral and Ethical Considerations

Because of the moral, ethical, and social issues that must be addressed, the strengths and weaknesses of alternative plans must be identified. Members of the family will be expected to participate fully in this phase of planning. We can anticipate that a major contribution of the patient agent will be to advise the family against the current proclivity "to spare no expense" in providing all that modern medicine has to offer. Discussion will be guided by ethical and moral issues to achieve efficient humane care and, as prophylaxis against legal redress. We can only hope that in time the expectations of society will mature through experiences with the consequences and costs of excessive medical therapy.*

DNR (Do Not Resuscitate)

The prognosis of disease outcomes is a crucial element in the process of patient planning. All decisions regarding the various interventions will be guided by possibilities and probabilities of alternative outcomes, particularly the prognosis of mortality. The response to these prognostications are intimately guided by the current milieu of moral and ethical questions and resolutions. But resolutions are imperative to the management of the ambiplex patient and are manifested in the formulation of the DNR (do not resuscitate) policy. Indeed, setting DNR policy within a given hospital is a crucial step in the management of the ambiplex patient.[11]

Discharge Planning

Ideally the plan developed by the patient agent will be sufficiently comprehensive to include arrangements for placement and follow-up on discharge of the ambiplex patient from the hospital. Emphasis on finding a suitable out-of-hospital environment should help reduce the frequency of readmission to the hospital. Often the medical care of these patients does not require the high-cost resources of the modern "tertiary" hospital. Hospitalization may reflect a deficiency in the

---

*References 3, 7, 8, 10, 41, 49, 70, 78.

nonintegrated organization of the community health care system.

Medical Information System

An effective plan for management of the ambiplex patient requires an appropriate hospital information system (HIS). Perhaps it is the fault of the design of the currently available information system, the traditional attitude of the attending physician, or chance alone, but the study demonstrated the failure of the existing information system to support efficient and high quality care of these patients. There is an urgent need for an information system that will serve the following functions: (1) record an organized plan for care and study of these patients, (2) provide an accounting of charges subdivided into several categories, (3) profile physician performance relative to standards of quality and costs, (4) summarize real-time clinical information, (5) provide some index of the severity of illness or injury, and (6) communicate, for example, suggestions from consultants and observations of nurses and social service personnel.*

CONCLUSION

The "ambiplex" surgical patient is not a new discovery. He/she has always been an inhabitant of acute hospital wards. The frustration and minimal rewards associated with the inpatient management of these patients is manifested by their derisive classifications as "crocks, gomers, dwindlers." Their unique identity in studies of health costs has been obfuscated by failure to study the total patient over time. Previous studies have focused on the current malady of paramount concern for the patient. In this study an attempt was made to learn about them as a special class of patients that is overlooked when attention is confined to well-focused or specific diagnoses, procedures, admissions, or service statistics. They are individuals whose varied health problems are susceptible to more productive cost management and probably to a higher quality of care when they are viewed in their totality and across a time continuum.

It can be argued that the conscious recognition of the ambiplex patient will be a natural by-product of the current movement toward "case management" by both employers and providers. Traditionally this implies guiding the patient through an interinstitutional system usually by nonphysician professionals (social workers, nurses, case managers). In this chapter we suggest that strategies designed to provide more efficient and higher quality management of these patients should be focused on the clinical arena and physician decision rights. This concept presents special problems in regard to the identification and employment of a physician patient manager or agent. These include the partitioning of decision rights among residents, specialists, and paraprofessionals; the availability of sophisticated information systems; a willingness to address moral/ethical managerial issues; and communication with the nonhospital segments of the patient's life and progress.

The ambiplex patient represents both a practical economic problem in need of solution as well as an overt challenge to the educational system. Finding more efficient and effective ways of caring for the ambiplex patient should help resolve the disinclination of students to pursue a career that involves the need to care for these patients.

With the expanding core of technical knowledge, the average surgeon is hard pressed for time to absorb the new managerial/economic requirements of the task inherent in patient agency. There are no data to confirm that the benefits of a new role of patient agency will outweigh the added costs of maintaining that role. As with many studies of this kind, the conclusion is the injunction that more research is necessary. At least dialogue about experiences with this special kind of patient will be profitable. The strategies

---

*References 26, 42, 51, 56, 60, 69.

suggested for management of the ambiplex patient, however, are more than simple caveats. They are likely to be forced on the clinical arena by the kaleidoscope of changing rules of the game.

References

1. Bean E: Latest survey shows hospital charges increasing far more quickly than CPI, The Wall Street Journal, p 17, Jan 6, 1988.
2. Birnhaum H: The cost of catastrophic illness, Toronto, 1978, Lexington Books.
3. Bloom BS and Peterson OL: End result, costs and productivity of coronary care units, N Engl J Med 288:72, 1973.
4. Blumberg MS and Gentry DW: Routine hospital changes and intensity of care: a cross-section analysis of fifty states, Inquiry 15:58, 1978.
5. Bunis D: Doctors losing faith in HMO, Democrat and Chronicle, Rochester, NY, p 1, Jan 11, 1988.
6. Butler JA, Rosenbaum S, and Palfrey JS: Ensuring access to health care for children with disabilities, N Engl J Med 317:162, 1987.
7. Campion EW et al: Medical intensive care for the elderly: a study of current use, costs, and outcomes, JAMA 246:2052, 1981.
8. Campion EW et al: Prognosis, survival, and the expenditure of hospital resources for patients in an intensive care unit, N Engl J Med 305:667, 1981.
9. Chalmers TC and Stern AR: The staggering cost of prolonging life, Business Week Feb 23, 1982.
10. Chassin MR: Costs and outcomes of medical intensive care, Med Care 20:165, 1982.
11. Chernow B and Snyder R: Orders not to resuscitate: the DNR patient, Crit Care Med 12:922, 1984.
12. Civetta JM: The inverse relationship between cost and survival, J Surg Res 14:265, 1973.
13. Couch NP, Tilney NL, and Moore FD: The cost of misadventures in colonic surgery: a model for the analysis of adverse outcomes in standard procedures, Am J Surg 135:641, 1978.
14. Couch NP et al: The high cost of low-frequency events: the anatomy and economics of surgical mishaps, N Engl J Med 304:634, 1981.
15. Cullen DJ et al: Survival, hospitalization charges and follow-up results in critically ill patients, N Engl J Med 294:982, 1976.
16. Daniels M and Schroeder SA: Variation among physicians in the use of laboratory tests II. Med Care 15:482, 1977.
17. Densen PM, Shapiro S, and Einhorn M: Concerning high and low utilizers of service in a medical care plan, and the persistence of utilization levels over a three year period. Milbank Mem Fund Quart 37:218, 1959.
18. Detsky AS et al: Prognosis, survival, and utilization of hospital services for intensive care unit patients, N Engl J Med 305:667, 1981.
19. Diggs WW: Patient mix: the missing ingredients in understanding hospital costs, Hospital Topics 15:15, 1973.
20. Dranove D and White WD: Agency and the organization of health care delivery, Inquiry 24:405, 1987.
21. Drucker WR: The management of trauma: imperatives for hospital cost containment, Bull Am Coll Surg 69:12, 1984.
22. Drucker WR et al: Toward strategies for cost containment in surgical patients, Ann Surg 198:284, 1983.
23. Eisenberg JM and Rosoff AJ: Physician responsibility for the cost of unnecessary medical services, N Engl J Med 299:76, 1978.
24. Eisenberg JM et al: Computer-based audit to detect and correct overutilization of laboratory tests, Med Care 15:915, 1977.
25. Entoven AC: Health plan: the only practical solution to the soaring cost of medical care, Reading, Mass, 1980, Addison-Wesley Publishing Co, Inc.
26. Fetter RB: AUTOGRP patient classification scheme and diagnosis related groups (DRGs). HEW Pub No (HFCA) 03011 9-79, US Dept of Health, Education and Welfare.
27. Fetter RB et al: A system for cost and reimbursement control in hospitals, Yale J Biol Med 49:123, 1976.
28. Fetter RB et al: The application of diagnostic specific cost profiles to cost and reimbursement control in hospitals, J Med Syst 1:2, 1977.
29. Finkler SA: The distinction between cost and charges, Ann Intern Med 96:102, 1982.
30. Flood AB et al: The relationship between intensity and duration of medical services and outcomes for hospitalized patients, Med Care 17:1088, 1979.
31. Fuchs VR: A more effective, efficient and equitable system. West J Med 125:3, 1976.
32. Garber AM, Fuchs VR, and Silverman JF: Case mix, costs, and outcomes: differences between faculty and community service in a university hospital, N Engl J Med 310:19, 1984.
33. Garg ML et al: Evaluating inpatient costs: the staging mechanism, Med Care 16:3, 1978.
34. Gavett JW: Classification of home health patients by intensity of utilization of nursing service. Working paper, Department of Preventive Medicine and Community Health, University of Rochester, Oct 1975.

35. Gavett JW et al: A study of high cost inpatients in Strong Memorial Hospital, Final report to the Rochester Area Hospital's corporation. January 1985, p 83.
36. Gillick MR: Is the care of the chronically ill a medical perogative, N Engl J Med 310:190, 1984.
37. Griner PF et al: Use of laboratory tests in a teaching hospital: long term trends: reduction in use and relative costs, Ann Intern Med 90:243, 1979.
38. Griner PF and Liptzin B: Use of the laboratory in a teaching hospital, Ann Intern Med 75:2, 1971.
39. Herron D: Industrial engineering applications of ABC curves, AIIE Transactions 8:2, 1976.
40. Hillman AL: Financial incentives for physicians in HMOs: is there a conflict or interest, N Engl J Med 317:1743, 1987.
41. Hook EW III, Horton CA, and Schaberg DR: Failure of intensive care unit support to influence mortality from pneumococcal bacteremia, JAMA 249:1055, 1983.
42. Horn SD and Schumacher DN: An analysis of case mix complexity using information theory and diagnostic related grouping, Med Care 17:382, 1979.
43. Horn SD and Sharkey PD: Measuring severity of illness to predict patient resource use within DRGs, Inquiry 20: winter, 1983.
44. Iglehart JK: Second thoughts about HMOs for Medicare patients, N Engl J Med 316:1487, 1987.
45. James FE: Medical expenses resist controls and keep going one way: higher. The Wall Street Journal, p 41, July 29, 1987.
46. Jensen MC: Organization theory and methodology, The Accounting Review 58:2, 1983.
47. Jones KR: The influence of the attending physician on indirect graduate medical education costs, J Med Educ 59:789, 1984.
48. Knaus WA: Changing the cause of death, JAMA 249:1059, 1983.
49. Knaus WA, Draper EA, and Wagner DF: The use of intensive care: new research initiatives and their implications for national health policy. Milbank Mem Fund Quart, 61:561, 1983.
50. Kobrinski EJ and Matteson AL: Characteristics of high cost treatment in acute care facilities, Inquiry 18, Summer, 1981.
51. Krischer JR: Indexes of severity: underlying concepts, Health Serv Res 11:143, 1976.
52. Lairson DR, Forthofer RN, and Glasser JH: Catastrophic illness in an HMO, Inquiry 16:119, 1979.
53. Lind S: Transferring the terminally ill, N Engl J Med 311:1181, 1984.
54. Lorenz MC: Methods of measuring the concentration of wealth, Pub Am Statist Assoc 9, Sept, 1905.
55. Lubitz J and Prihoda R: Use and costs of medicare services in the last years of life, National Center for Health Statistics, DHHS Pub No (PHS) 84-1232, Public Health Service, Washington, DC, Dec 1983.
56. Luke RD: Dimensions in hospital case mix measurement, Inquiry 16, Spring, 1979.
57. Mason LB and Garcia AG: Hospital costs of surgical complications, Arch Surg 119:1065, 1984.
58. McCall N and Wai HS: An analysis of the use of Medicare services by the continuously enrolled aged, Med Care 21:567, 1983.
59. Morrow JS: Toward a more normative assessment of maldistribution: the Gini Index, Inquiry 14:3, 1977.
60. Munoz E et al: The identifier concept: clinical variables to manage costs for surgical patients, Hospital Health Serv Admin, Feb 1987.
61. New York Times: Health insurance boosts stun millions. In Times-Union, Rochester, NY, p 1, Jan 12, 1988.
62. Omenn GS and Conrad D: Implications of DRGs for clinicians, N Engl J Med 311:1314, 1984.
63. Pareto V: Cours d'Economic Politique 2:Lausanne, Switzerland, 1987, F Rouge, 1897.
64. Rassman WR: Why health care is a costly disgrace, Business Week, p 16, Jan 1981.
65. Reagan MD: Physicians as gatekeepers, N Engl J Med 317:1731, 1987.
66. Rundle R: Rapid increases in health insurance costs catch employers and insurers off guard, The Wall Street Journal, p 41, May 15, 1987.
67. Russell LB: The role of technology assessment in cost control. In McNeil BJ and Cravalho EG, eds: Critical issues in medical technology, Boston, 1982, Auburn House, Publishing Co.
68. Rutkow I: Rates of surgery in the United States: the decade of the 1970s, Surg Clin North Am 62:559, 1982.
69. Rutkow I: Surgical operations in the United States 1979-1984, Surgery 101:192, 1987.
70. Schneider KC and Dove HG: High users of VA emergency room facilities: are out-patients abusing the system or is the system abusing them, Inquiry 20:Spring, 1982.
71. Schroeder SA, Showstack JA, and Roberts HE: Frequency and clinical description of high-cost patients in 17 acute-care hospitals, N Engl J Med 300:1306, 1979.
72. Schroeder SA, Showstack JA, and Schwartz J: Survival of adult high cost patients: report of a follow-up study from nine acute-care hospitals, JAMA 10:245, 1981.
73. Schroeder SA et al: Use of laboratory tests and pharmaceuticals: variation among physicians and effect of cost audit, JAMA 225:969, 1973.

74. Schumacher DN et al: Hospital cost per case, Med Care 17:1037, 1979
75. Sorensen A, Saward E, and Stewart D: Hospital cost containment in Rochester: from maxicap to the hospital experimental payments program, Inquiry 19:327, 1982.
76. Starr P: The social transformation of American medicine, New York, 1982, Basic Books, Inc, Publishers.
77. Studnickl J: Differences in length of hospital stay for Medicaid and Blue Cross patients and the effect of intensity of services, Public Health Reports, Vol 94, No 8, Sept-Oct 1979.
78. Thibault GE et al: Medical intensive care: indications, interventions, and outcomes, N Engl J Med 302:938, 1980.
79. Thompson JD et al: One strategy for controlling costs in university teaching hospitals, J Med Educ 53, March, 1978.
80. Turnbull AD et al: The inverse relationship between cost and survival in the critically ill cancer patient, Crit Care Med 7:20, 1979.
81. Tyson WT and Merill JL: Health care institutions: survival in a changing environment, J med Educ 59:773, 1984.
82. Waxman HA: Medical malpractice and quality of care, N Engl J Med 317:943, 1987.
83. Winkenwerder W and Ball JR: Transformation of American health care, N Engl J Med 318:317, 1988.
84. Zook CJ and Moore FD: High-cost users of medical care, N Engl J Med 302:996, 1980.

FRANCIS D. MOORE

Francis D. Moore is a graduate of Harvard College (1935) and Harvard Medical School (1939). He had his initial residency training at the Massachusetts General Hospital. In 1948 he was appointed Moseley Professor of Surgery at Harvard and Chairman of the Department of Surgery of Harvard Medical School at the Peter Bent Brigham Hospital. At present he is Moseley Professor of Surgery, Emeritus, and a member of the editorial staff of *The New England Journal of Medicine*.

17

Commercial Constraints on Surgical Quality

FRANCIS D. MOORE

A professional is one who places the immediate interest of his patient or client above that of his own; the merchant places his own profit above the interest or welfare of his client. The tension between these two contrasting traditions of human behavior in our culture is responsible for much of the health of an open society. Providing goods and services in parallel, these two modes of behavior—professionalism and commercialism—have served us well since the root periods of Western culture in Egypt and Mesopotamia. Each is a counterbalance to the other.

Although those of both styles of service must acquire enough money to live comfortably, personal gain for the professional is based on service fees or salary. Corporate investment and joint profitability among stockholders with capital gains are intrinsic to the entrepreneurial role of merchants. The professional often practices alone and in any case deals directly with the patient or client. By contrast, merchants proliferate outlets: owners and stockholders; only a few lower level employees deal directly with the public.

When players in either social tradition—professionals and merchants—depart their accustomed roles, we become suspicious and distrustful of them. This is especially true if they maintain the facade of their accustomed social pattern as a screen for some other activity. When the professional—a physician for example—plays the role of selfless generous caregiver only to maximize his personal income with low-quality mass-produced services, we suddenly and irretrievably lose confidence. By the same token, when the merchant "gives away the store" for charity, no matter how worthy, we lose interest in owning stock in his company and in the quality of goods. This distrust has had a healthy effect because it has led to the establishment of charitable foundations by corporations, a step that leaves the corporation clearly the money earner, while the foundation seeks other ends (often of a professional nature) with some of the profits.

The physician's behavior as professional is increasingly at risk because of two current trends that arise from the commercial and entrepreneurial aspects of medicine. Although these distractions are not in any sense new, they are now assaulting the practitioner from every side with renewed and vicious impact. These two trends are intense competition for fiscal success in medical market outlets, and standardization of health practices. In simplest terms, an overemphasis on the fiscal success of highly competitive hospitals or clinics clearly jeopardizes medical care, much of which is expensive, nonprofitable, provided to the poor and uninsured, and with profits necessarily meager. At the same time, when every patient's problem is truly unique and a large percentage of patients show multidimensional departures or variations from the norm or the "expected" average manifestations of disease, standardization places at high risk the patient with an aberrant form of disease.

Fiscal competition and practice standardization both interfere with the latitude of judgment, the freedom to depart from the norm, and the willingness to fulfill the unprofitable need that are at the heart of Western traditions in medicine and medical care. The purpose here is to analyze these two factors that are adverse to the quality of care, as we enter the last decade of this century.

COMPETITION

A strong element of competition has always existed in the practice of medicine and in the life of hospitals. The young person in practice must of necessity compete with older more experienced colleagues; they, in turn, as they approach retirement, must learn to accept with equanimity the advent of a new younger generation who know many things they never learned. The small community hospital is always competing with the large urban center; at the same time, the urban center may lack the neighborliness or the convenience of the local hospital; the county and municipal tax-supported hospitals compete for patients and "status" with the private trustee-owned hospitals, and they in turn with the sectarian hospitals (Catholic, Lutheran, Jewish).

But even beyond this normal professional and institutional competition, the physician has survived professionally in a profit-oriented matrix beyond his control for at least 350 years, the entire period of medical care in this country. The profit-making aspects of medicine have been particularly notable in the development and sale of drugs and equipment. Remarkable drug monopolies (ether, insulin, and the many new synthetic drugs) have increased the cost of medicine while lining the pockets of corporations and stockholders with billions of dollars, usually under the wing of the patent laws. Equipment essential to the practice of medicine (such as x-ray or computed tomography apparatus, laboratory analytic equipment or surgical equipment) has been sold to hospitals, often exploiting the technical naivete of the purchasers. In both instances (drugs and equipment) we have tried to assuage our dissatisfaction with the merchant invasion of professional life by relying on "market forces." By this token, he who sells the false mousetrap will soon come to fiscal grief. At this late date one can ask how often market forces operate in medical care. The answer seems to be: rarely and unreliably.

In the past decade, several factors have greatly heightened this competitive environment in medicine.

Consumer Choice Pricing

The emergence and strong advocacy of competitive "consumer choice" pricing of health insurance plans and HMOs are allegedly consumer-oriented concepts. Advanced and strongly pushed by Enthoven,[3,4,5] consumer choice pricing places pricing above all other criteria of accessibility in the purchase of a health plan, either by patients or collective patients, such as employees, or those who collectively finance patient aggregates, that is, employers. It is entirely based on a concept of market forces: plans that fail to attract customers by their low prices will fail. The hazards here are too numerous and obvious to bear much further discussion. The main hazard is that every patient and employer understands price but rarely if ever understands the medical and quality implications (or limited coverage) of a cheap product. This is in contrast to the purchase of an automobile or refrigerator where even the average consumer has a very good idea of what constitutes quality, and if quality is not there, the family may collect on the warranty or simply buy a different brand next time. In medical care there is no warranty on which to collect. If you have not had cardiac catheterization after your acute myocardial infarction because it is too expensive for your "plan," and thus have missed the chance for angioplasty, bypass, or enzyme infusion, not only has the chance for merciful pain relief been lost, but also possibly your life. The most vicious aspect of the Enthoven concept is that it maximizes the commercial, adversarial, and often misleading merchant impulses of every insurance company or HMO: the incentive is to reduce price and thus reduce cost (and thus services) so as to widen the market; in reducing services and coverages, the incentive is to do it in such a way that the customer is unaware of it, by "fine print." In point of fact, widening of the market and increased sales have nothing whatsoever to do with the quality of medical care.

Emergence of For-profit Hospitals

The possible hazard of the investor-owned for-profit (IOFP) hospital to patient welfare has been extensively aired in the literature[7,8,15-18]. In recent examples, for-profit hospital chains continued to harbor incompetent physicians despite multiple suits against them and their borderline practices, simply because they brought in large numbers of patients. Investor-owned for-profit hospitals must make money somehow, and one way to do it is to reduce the cost of physicians' and nurses' services and maximize the use of profitable ancillaries. Stories of the work of physicians being compromised by pressures from hospital directors are still in the anecdotal stage; there is a need for carefully designed studies on this. The cardiac surgeon is told not to take on high-risk patients because mortality will rise and the hospital might lose money. In fact, for many patients it is the very willingness of a physician or hospital to take on difficult responsibility even though it is at some risk that is the touchstone of a precious quality factor in U.S. medicine.

Need for Profit by Nonprofit Hospitals

The need for nonprofit hospitals to make a profit has become evident. Here, the operative platitude is "philanthropy can no longer make up the deficit." Cross-subsidization (by which expensive private facilities help pay for the deficits of care for the indigent) has also become illegal and ethically unacceptable. For this reason many large trustee-owned and university teaching hospitals and some tax-supported hospitals are applying the same sort of pressures to their staff found in the for-profit hospitals. They state, "We make no profit, but we must operate in the black." There is an apparent injustice here, since the for-profit hospitals have to pay taxes on more accounting components than do the nonprofits. And yet this seeming injustice is offset by the nonprofits taking on nonprofitable care entities (stroke, paraplegia, severe burns, long term retardation) and welfare, uninsured, or no-pay patients to an extent far greater than the IOFP. In turn, a third category of hospitals, those financed by taxes and including municipal, city, county, and state hospitals (as well as the state university hospitals), are often subjected to "dumping" by both the other categories (IOFP and trustee-owned) because of the adverse effect of profitless patients on annual balance sheets.[11]

Tensions Established by DRG Reimbursed System

When the placement of a disease entity in a diagnostic category is the sole criterion of remuneration, we are dealing with a form of competition that is not based on pricing alone, nor is it structural; it is instead based solely on classification and nomenclature. The DRG system must acquire a severity index or corrector if it is to be used as the primary basis for remuneration in a competitive environment. When a physician or hospital is penalized for giving appropriate care to unusual patients, quality is threatened.

Hardball Marketing of Insurance Policies

Aggressive marketing of insurance policies is an aspect of the "consumer's choice" concept mentioned above. Clearly, an insurance company can somehow arrange to sell coverage to large numbers of employees (or to the employers) at lower cost. This lower cost always means less access, less coverage, or higher deductibles—there is no "free lunch." The difficulty is exacerbated when this insurance policy is sold to individuals rather than group purchasers. This is the case with some types of disability insurance, some types of "over the limit" Medicare underwriting, dental insurance, and some nursing home coverages. Here the individual is asked to make a quality choice that requires delicate medical judgment, wholly on the basis of a bluntly profit-oriented pricing structure. Even the most sophisticated of purchasers claim, with a complaining voice, "How do I know which is best for my family?" The general public is at a terrible disadvantage. They are consumers who are not too anxious to choose.

Advertising and Selling of HMOs

In Massachusetts, where one of the larger university-based HMOs (Harvard Community Health Plan) has pursued a steady growth for the last quarter century and is now investing in investor-owned for-profit (IOFP) medical enterprises of "managed care," the new marketing of HMOs is particularly offensive. The Madison Avenue approach enters with a statement that this company's policy will "buy you more". More what? It is reminiscent of the old joke about the advertising of soap as "99 and 44/100% pure"...what? Poisoning the delicate decision making that parents should make for the total coverage of their family by placing "cure for the blues" advertising is offensive. Institutions that do this advertising should be taken promptly to court for misleading advertising practices—misleading both in form and content.

Advertising must place a premium on some epiphenomenon of the item being sold. This is the essence of advertising. In advertising cigarettes a beautiful woman is shown smoking; in advertising an automobile it is shown proceeding at 120 miles an hour on a large highway or ascending a series of bumpy rocks on a mountain; even for shoe polish a beautiful woman is shown accompanying the man with the high polish (of his shoes). The advertiser has in essence chosen a property of the product that he wishes to emphasize, an epiphenomenon, quite without respect to its more important features.

It is this aspect of medical advertising that is so unhealthy. Two of the prime health concerns of young families are night calls for critically ill children and dental care. Some insurance and HMO contracts cover these needs, others do not. One never sees any mention of either of them in the advertising. One would have thought that cautious and judicious hospital administrators in the teaching hospitals would have avoided this trap. The situation is quite the contrary. A prominent teaching hospital in the Harvard family has recently published the picture of the naked back of a man, indicating that "this is the way we they take care of renal stones." There are no scars. The implication is that lithotripsy was used, and they have it while their competition do not have it (yet). Nowhere in the advertisement is there a statement to the effect that this is actually not the back of a patient with renal stones (which in point of fact it is not). A teaching hospital is thus advancing a baldfaced medical lie. But more important, the effectiveness of lithotripsy is not to be gauged by the welfare of a single patient but rather by some sort of stochastic likelihood based on numbers of cases, that is, by the probabilistic analysis of an aggregate of cases, not by a single testimonial! As Cicero said in desperation, "Quo usque?"

Publication of Crude Mortality Statistics

The government has led the charge for a false criterion of quality by publishing crude mortality statistics. There are certain statistical aspects of surgical care that indeed could be published that would give some idea of quality. Examples would include length of stay, complications in relation to comorbidities, and, if mortality is to be used, mortality corrected for a severity index. The crude mortality number alone means nothing. In general, the higher quality institutions often have higher mortalities because they are willing to take on the high-risk patients. Some years ago the highest mortality for hysterectomy in the state of Massachusetts was exhibited by a gynecologic service that was generally regarded as one of the best in the world. This occurred because very high risk women with carcinomas of the endometrium who were also suffering from diabetes and pernicious anemia were sent to that institution for care.

Were it not for the competitive environment,

there would be no urge to publish such simplistic mortality statistics. If the government in a sudden and unaccustomed fit of "consumerism" feels it is wise for consumers to distinguish between "good" and "bad" hospitals in their community, assuredly they should publish some data more demanding of skill and statistical expertise than a single uncorrected mortality.

STANDARDIZATION

For the administrators of health care, be they insurance executives, hospital superintendents, or the chief executive officers of health maintenance organizations, nothing is more puzzling and frustrating than the seemingly endless chaos of cases, and nothing is more gratifying than standardization.

The manifestations of disease are extremely variable. The ability of physicians to adapt to this variability is crucial to their success in delivering high quality care. For the administrator, however, this variability defies his sense of order, of accounting, and of predictability. A much simpler approach would be to force all of medical care into a series of parallel molds where, given a diagnosis, a certain treatment follows, a certain charge is entered, no aberration is tolerated, and the computer can sail on with a very simple helmsmanship program.

Concepts of standardization in medicine also have a statistical origin in the analysis of outcomes referred to as "the clinical literature." It is a natural human tendency to seek a "best way" and when it is found by defining homogeneous patient aggregates, some degree of standardization results.

Thus efforts to find homogeneity and to standardize medical care are based both on commercial enterprises and clinical research. The hazard lies not in seeking common denominators but in overemphasis on standardizing procedures (study, tests, operations, length of stay) for large diagnostic categories. The hazard is evident when standardization unduly constrains the intrinsic variability in treatment required by the naturally variable phenomena of disease.

Although such tendency to real or imagined standardization of health care has many roots, it became accentuated in the 1960s and early 1970s when the Medicare agencies tried to standardize care by a series of consensus panels and paper conferences whereby the "indications for operation X" could be listed concisely. Departures (regardless of patient variability) could then be disallowed for payment or reimbursement.

In 1979 the studies of Lewis on the state of Kansas emerged into this climate showing that there was remarkable variability between small adjacent geographic areas in the frequency of certain operations.[9] This beacon was immediately taken up by Wennberg and Gittelsohn.[21] Since that time they have sprouted a huge literature on "small area variations".[19,22,23] This literature assumes that all variability is a result of "practice style." This is clearly stated in the articles. It is a statement that could not be made without the logical assumption that all diseases are constant in incidence and phenomenology, that complaint frequencies are absolutely uniform throughout populations, and that the only variable is physician-generated.

Critiques of the Wennberg thinking and method have been published and will not be reviewed here in detail.* The most important difficulty is that disease is definitely nonrandom in distribution, showing variability according to age, sex, ethnic group, occupation, and economic status, as well as education. Also, the small area variation (SAV) method looks solely at a single procedure, and it examines procedure frequencies without reference to the use of competing procedures or alternate treatment options. Finally, the small area variation literature has confined its study to a single year and in many instances to just a few months extrapolated to a year.

Beyond the standardization impulse provided by government consensus panels and SAV literature, the DRG system itself must be regarded as a bias towards excessive standardization.

To understand this, one must trace back the

---
*References 1,2,6, 10,12,13,14,20.

origins of the DRG system. This was developed by a group of scholars in the nursing faculty at Yale who were seeking to aggregate the tens of thousands of diagnoses in the ICD-9-CM classification and the thousands of procedures into sensible clinical groupings. These were done in part according to length of stay and resource utilization, in part by biological affinity, for example, congestive heart failure and valvular disease, and in part by procedural commonality, such as gynecologic disorders potentially treated by hysterectomy.

The method was then seized upon as a fiscal criterion establishing acceptable limitations for resource utilization and length of stay. According to this system some 470 individual diagnostic related groups were established among 45 major diagnostic categories (MDC).

The method itself was a praiseworthy first step (now with modifications a second or third step) toward sensible aggregation and simplification of medical phenomenology. But it is often quite blind. For example, there is no DRG for carcinoma of the endometrium; there is no way of differentiating a traumatic from a spontaneous separation of the retina; the assignment of a cause to congestive heart failure can only be done by listing comorbidities; and there is no procedural DRG for new things coming on the scene, such as the infusion of enzymes or thrombolytic agents for coronary artery disease.

But for the purpose of this discussion, the worst failing of the DRG is the forcing of physicians into a behavioral mold, treating all loosely aggregated "similar" cases as identical without any severity coefficient. From the very start, the proviso has always been specific; when the welfare of an individual patient was put at risk by premature discharge, for example, the physician could object to the hospital administrator and seek a waiver. Already beset by a tremendous new overlay of paperwork as a result of the tendencies to competition and standardization that form the subject of this paper, we now are asking the busy physician to make a call to the hospital administrator (who rarely can be reached on the telephone anyway) to seek a waiver for sending Mrs. Jones home on the same day specified by the DRG when she in point of fact is very elderly and has no one to look after her at home. This is an obvious example of an unjustified effort at standardization that limits the choices, the decision making, and the latitude of professional judgment of the physician.

THE NEW PROFESSIONS OF MEDICINE

A large new cadre of people has been injected into the policy- and decision-making aspects of medicine in the United States. This dates back at least to the enactment of the Medicare legislation. These are the "regulators." Some achieve regulation through Washington bureaus and offices, others through the adminstrative offices of hospital superintendents, and still others ply their trade as executives of HMOs or insurance companies. The sheer magnitude of this profession is awe inspiring. They number in the hundreds of thousands and probably outnumber the physicians whose work they seek to regulate.

Efforts to promote competition and foster standardization come largely from this segment of medicine in this country: the regulators, the policy makers, the policy analysts, the entrepreneurs, the "medi-business" executives, and the legislators.

If we are to look to the next century as one of maintaining and increasing the high quality of Western medicine in general and U.S. medicine in particular, we must begin to demand a new standard of this new group as professionals.

To do this, they must have an education that includes firsthand contact with the care of the sick. Many people plying their trade as hospital directors, Medicare executives, or HMO executives have never seen a baby born, nor have they seen a patient die; they have never talked to the distressed family of a retarded newborn, nor have they discussed with a family the prognosis of a malignancy found at operation. They have been so far removed from the realities of medical care that their only recourse is to ignore such realities or to base their ideas on their own personal experience, an experience that is highly random and often zero.

One senses this narrowness of view in talking to foundation executives who, for example, anxious to emphasize their humanistic tendency, will relate that they "saw a woman injured on the street and no one could get an ambulance." Thus they have put huge amounts of money into trying to improve the ambulance service. Although this may be an entirely praiseworthy undertaking, it is clearly based on a random one-hit episode and does not recognize the many needs of the rest of the emergency medical situation in that city, such as head-injury triage, a burn center, facilities for organ donation, and a host of other unmet needs in most cities. Often, narrow funding objectives of foundations are based on executive ignorance of the realities of medicine.

We must devote resources to an improved education of those who are destined to make careers as the regulators or financiers of our medical care system. It is entirely unrealistic to expect physicians to engage to a greater extent in this regulatory or legislative undertaking. One hears the complaint, "If only physicians would get involved themselves." Considering that most physicians work long hours and are chronically behind with paperwork, it is unrealistic to expect the physician to be distracted into becoming a regulator.

Instead, we must help organize postgraduate curricula in health policy so that we will raise a new generation of regulators who will perceive the adverse effect of excessive fiscal competition and unrealistic clinical standardization on the quality of care, and seek, themselves, to soften or mollify the impact of these laws, guidelines, regulations, and trends so that physicians may continue to give the highest quality of patient care.

References

1. Brook RH et al: Geographic variations in the use of services: do they have any clinical significance? Health Aff 3:63, 1984.
2. Caper P and Spitzer M: In defense of small area analysis, Health Aff 4:115, 1985.
3. Enthoven A: Consumer-choice health plan, N Engl J Med 298:650 and 709 (Parts I and II), 1978.
4. Ginzberg E: The grand illusion of competition in health care, JAMA 249:1857, 1983.
5. Ginzberg E: The monetorization of health care, N Engl J Med 310:1162, 1984.
6. Gittelsohn A and Wennberg J: The authors respond, J Maine Med Assoc 68:53, 1977.
7. Kleinfield, NR: Operating for profit hospital corporation: the private sector's surge into medical care: the chains keep growing, The New York Times, May 29, 1983.
8. Lewin LS, Derson RA, and Margulis R: Investor-owneds and non-profits differ in economic performance, Hospitals 55:52, 1981.
9. Lewis CE: Variations in the incidence of surgery, N Engl J Med 281:880, 1969.
10. Moore FD: Small area variations in health care delivery: a critique, J Maine Med Assoc 68:49, 1977.
11. Moore FD: Who should profit from the care of your illness? Harvard Magazine, Nov-Dec, 1985, p 45.
12. Moore FD: Commentary: Small area variations studies: illuminating or misleading? Health Aff 4:96, 1985.
13. Moore FD: Letter to Editor: Variations in the use of medical and surgical services, N Engl J Med 315:649, 1986.
14. Moore FD and Pratt LW: Tonsillectomy in Maine: regulation versus education as modulators of medical care, Ann Surg 194:232, 1981.
15. Pattison RV and Katz HM: Investor-owned and not-for-profit hospitals: a comparison based on California data, N Engl J Med 309:347, 1983.
16. Relman AS: The new medical industrial complex, N Engl J Med 303:963, 1980.
17. Relman AS: Investor-owned hospitals and health care costs, N Engl J Med 309:370, 1983.
18. Sloan FA and Vracu RA: Investor-owned and not-for-profit hospitals: addressing some issues, Health Aff 2:25, 1983.
19. Wennberg JE: Dealing with medical practice variations: a proposal for action, Health Aff 3:6, 1984.
20. Wennberg JE: Reply "To the Editor", N Engl J Med 315:650, 1986.
21. Wennberg J and Gittelsohn A: Small area variations in health care delivery, Science 182:1102, 1973.
22. Wennberg J and Gittelsohn A: Health care delivery in Maine. I. Patterns of use of common surgical procedures, J Maine Med Assoc 66:123, 1975.
23. Wennberg JE, Gittelsohn A, and Shapiro N: Health care delivery in Maine. III. Evaluating the level of hospital performance: J Maine Med Assoc 66:11, 1975.

PAUL A. EBERT

Paul A. Ebert is Director of the American College of Surgeons. Born in Columbus, Ohio, Dr. Ebert received his BS degree from Ohio State University (1954) and his MD degree from the same institution (1958). He was an intern in surgery at the Johns Hopkins Hospital, followed by a year at the hospital as an assistant resident surgeon. From July 1960 to June 1962, Dr. Ebert served at the National Heart Institute, returning to Johns Hopkins Hospital in July 1962 until June 1966. He subsequently was on the surgical faculty at Duke University Medical Center, where he remained until January 1971. In that year Dr. Ebert was appointed Chairman of the Department of Surgery and Johnson and Johnson Professor of Surgery at Cornell University Medical College. He assumed the position of Professor and Chairman of the Department of Surgery at the University of California, San Francisco Medical Center in 1975 before becoming the eighth director of the College in 1986.

18

Implications of Federal Legislation for Surgical Practice

PAUL A. EBERT

During the past 5 years both federal and state governments continue to be more active in policies of health care. With an increasing aging population and a greater need for health services, the main procurer of these services has become the Medicare program. Obviously in areas such as cataract surgery, the Medicare program is almost the sole purchaser of such services. As the volume of services purchased by Medicare increases, the strain on already diminishing funds has caused panic in the finance committees of the House and Senate as they face the reality that the system may, in fact, be in negative balance in the coming years. Thus health services under Medicare have essentially become a cost-driven system in which the government recognizes that it must purchase more service for essentially the same or even a lower price. This recognition probably has led to the most radical changes in the health care system in the past 5 years. It is likely that more radical and sometimes unpredicted alterations can be anticipated in the near future.

DRG REIMBURSEMENT SYSTEM

The Social Security amendments of 1983, which authorize the diagnostic related group pricing for hospital services, must be regarded as some of the initial major changes in financing of health care. The so-called DRG reimbursement system was essentially unanticipated by the health providers and has had a major effect in the delivery of services. The concept that a specific DRG inpatient service would be paid at a fixed rate has decreased hospital stays, eliminated many admissions, and moved many services to the outpatient arena. These changes have affected surgical practice by necessitating a more efficient outpatient workup, by not allowing patients for many diagnoses to be admitted before the day of operation, and by reducing the total length of stay. Shortened postoperative hospital stays have caused increased pressure on rehabilitation services whether provided by nursing homes, specific centers, or visiting therapists and home nurse programs. The initial experience of the DRG program provided little financial difficulty to hospitals. But as readjustments of the specific rates per diagnosis have been made, more hospitals are finding it difficult to stay financially solvent with the reimbursement methods. Hospital occupancy has decreased, and it is anticipated that, during the next 5 years, 10% of hospitals in the United States will close. This legislative activity has increased quality assurance programs and physician review mechanisms in hospitals to guarantee no overuse of facilities. Obviously this has had a major effect on surgical services, because a large proportion of hospital admissions are still for major operative procedures.

The issue of quality care remains important within the profession but seems to generate less interest at the federal level. Since inception of the DRG program, there are increasing data that patients may not be receiving optimum care when faced with premature discharges related to hospital reimbursement. The influence on surgical practice has been immense as many procedures considered to be routine inpatient operations have been relocated to the outpatient or ambulatory surgical center. The large increase in ambulatory services was noted as one of the major goals of the federal legislation, and at this time ambulatory services have remained somewhat immune from federal financial restrictions. In some ways this overemphasis on outpatient surgery has enticed some surgeons to perform major operations that have greater potential for patient harm in the ambulatory setting only because service is reimbursed at a higher level and with less involvement from physician review organizations.

Ambulatory surgery centers in 1988 must start collecting the 20% Part B copayment from patients on physicians' services. This will reduce a key competitive advantage over hospital outpatient facilities. This type of geographic payment enticement seems unfair, since it favors surgical offices that are equipped for minor surgical procedures. This may entice surgeons to increase office expenditures and again promote performance of procedures in office settings that may have been more safely performed in hospital outpatient or ambulatory care centers.

In the spring of 1987 a DRG process was proposed for physician reimbursement of anesthesiologists, pathologists, and radiologists because the majority of their activity is hospital based. It was suggested that, because these individuals rarely do primary or direct patient management but simply assist as consultants, it would be logical to tie their cost into the basic DRG process of the hospital. Obviously this would represent a philosophic change in the practice of medicine and has been strongly opposed by the entire profession. However, one would believe that it is unlikely that this is the last time that this suggestion will be presented.

SURGICAL MANPOWER
Financing of Graduate Medical Education

After completion of the GMENAC report, there has been little discussion at the federal level regarding implementation of manpower recommendations from that report. There has been considerable discussion in the committees of the House of Representatives regarding who should pay for graduate medical education. The scenario has vacillated between (1) if residents are truly students, shouldn't they pay for their own education, and (2) graduate medical education is a national resource and thus should be supported by the federal government. In 1986 a vigorous attempt was made by the House of Representatives to implement some of the GMENAC recommendations by increasing support for general practitioners and family practitioners to provide more primary care, especially in rural and some underserved urban areas. The outcome was that legislation was passed that financing for graduate medical education would support residents to primary board certification. Thus surgeons in residency training, such as pediatric and thoracic or in fellowships for added qualifications would not be financed by Medicare, since these surgeons had already completed a primary board residency requirement such as the American Board of Surgery. As yet, this has not altered the graduate medical training because other means of financing this relatively small number of individuals has been accomplished by their respective institutions. There has been considerable discussion to limit support of graduate medical education to a specific number of years after medical school. The common number seems to be either two or three. This obviously could have significant effect on residency training in specialties that require more time. Little was said in congressional discussion during 1987, and thus surgical residency training remains essentially as for the previous year.

Training of Specialists

During the past 5 years there has been more interest in several states regarding the number of specialists to be trained in those states. Thus it is difficult to assume that only federal legislation may affect graduate medical education. The states of New York and California are showing considerable interest in the number of generalists versus specialists to be trained. Residency programs in these states have incurred reduction in some specialty programs of surgery during the past 3 years. These states, as well, have pending legislation that may reduce the number of hours that a resident would be on call. This innovation attempts to protect a resident from being overcommitted and reflects the assumption that the rested individual is more apt to make correct clinical decisions.

Although little data have been presented regarding errors in clinical decision making related to time awake or on call, the assumption seems to be accepted. Thus the question of continuity of care—the person present at operation is the most informed regarding potential postoperative complications and postoperative care is best delivered by the operating surgeons—may be disregarded by attempts to regulate specific time periods that a resident and possibly even the attending surgeon may be able to respond to the patients' needs. This could obviously have a striking impact on future surgical practice.

In 1986 Congress appointed a commission on graduate medical education to study manpower needs and distribution in various specialties. This commission has a limited budget and is unlikely to be able to perform a major manpower study similar to GMENAC. Regarding surgical trainees, it is clear that there has been little significant change in the total number of surgeons in residency programs in the past decade. Some may argue that there are too many or too few. The absolute figures are relatively stable, and compared with a large increase in medical students over the same time, there has not been a proportional increase in surgical specialists. It is anticipated that the commission on graduate medical education will be able to continually advise the House subcommittees on the physician manpower status in the United States.

PHYSICIAN REIMBURSEMENT

The American Hospital Association has described 1988 as potentially the "year of the physician." This is not necessarily complimentary, but certainly federal legislative changes in 1988 regarding physician reimbursement may have a more direct effect on surgeons than any previous legislation. It is clear that Congress has been interested in physician reimbursement for some years but has failed to take any serious action in this area. The pattern for physician reimbursement payment reform began in 1983 legislation when Congress suggested to Health Care Financing Administration that the DRG system should be evaluated as a method for paying physicians. It actually resulted in HCFA contracting through the AMA for a resource based relative value scale to be developed to compare physicians' worth for reimbursement purposes. Thus the contract to the Harvard School of Public Health under Dr. Chiau-Wen Hsaio was implemented. The impact on surgeons from this relative value comparison is likely to result in reduced payment per service for the majority of surgical procedures. The actual impact on surgical practice can only be anticipated at this time.

The Budget Reconciliation Act of 1988 authorized the Secretary of HHS to develop a fee schedule for radiology services provided by board-certified and board-eligible radiologists. This is a particular interest because the results of the resource-based relative value scale were to be reported within 6 months of the date of this enactment. Thus one could anticipate that if a fee schedule was developed for radiology, it may be forthcoming for other specific specialties.

Congress in 1986 actually decided that a procedure, the cataract operation, was overpriced and the Medicare reimbursement for this procedure was reduced. It is obvious that Medicare is looking at the more frequently used procedures for which they are responsible for payment. Thus in 1987 Congress recommended that nine surgical procedures were overpriced and should be reduced between 10% and 15%. The Budget Reconciliation Act of 1988 actually increased this number of procedures to 15. This represents simple budget reductions based on what many would say are somewhat arbitrary methods of determining overpricing. The recommendation regarding overpricing came from the Commission for Physician Payment Reform that was developed in 1986 by Congress.

This commission was charged with determining changes in the reimbursement system for physicians. Obviously there are only two methods by which the federal government has been able to reduce costs. One is reduction of the price of a procedure, and the other is to reduce the volume. As yet, no attempt has been made to reduce volume of service but only to reduce the price of each procedure. It is obvious that most surgical procedures cannot be repeated, and with fairly strict PRO regulation in effect, the likelihood of a reduction of price of an item resulting in an increase of volume is unlikely. However, for simple office visits or other less rigidly defined medical practice, the question has been raised as to whether constant price reducing per unit will result in an increased volume of the practice of medicine in order to maintain a somewhat constant income. Obviously none of these legislative enactments directly affect the physician in dealing with his patient. The indirect consequences are difficult to anticipate or determine. It is obvious that the physician review organizations will receive continued support by Congress and likely will become more active in the coming years. Thus the feeling of more external review of an individual's practice activity should be anticipated. The PRO per se will focus mainly on length of stay, indications for operations, and overuse of hospital services. However, the implication of the legislative initiatives are to ultimately review outcome. One has already seen this in HCFA's 1986 release of mortality figures for coronary artery bypass surgery. These numbers are simple raw mortality figures for each hospital with no attempt to equate severity of illness or type of patients among hospitals. The 1987 release of hospital mortality figures encompassed a wider range of disease entities, but again no severity of illness index was attached to the mortality figures, and the actual interpretation of this type of data remains obscure. A major concern is whether hospitals and physicians will begin to limit services in many of these higher-risk areas simply because they are fearful of what future implications of mortality data released may bring. It is hard to see how standard of care or the ability to select a particular physician or hospital is enhanced by this particular practice.

Many seriously question whether this type of data has any particular value. HCFA states that this is an attempt to enable individual patients to make informed selections based on outcomes as such data are released regarding specific hospitals and probably in the future, individual surgeons. It is likely that this outcome information will be extended to other operative procedures and involve a more standardized form of practice among surgeons performing the same procedures. Thus indications and outcomes for an operative procedure will more likely be similar in the future. Also, the entire practice pattern of each surgeon is likely to be more similar, and it is hoped it will result in improved quality of care. It may, however, result in a less creative atmosphere in medicine because divergence from the accepted line of practice may be unrewarding. We hope that this more rigid approach to standardizing practice will not inhibit creativity and will allow progress in surgical therapy.

Although legislation clearly states that the Medicare and Medicaid systems would prefer some type of capitated health plan, as yet it has not been possible for implementation of these programs. As HMOs have developed more financial difficulties in the past few years, there has been a reluctance at the federal level to seriously encourage a capitated system for all Medicare/Medicaid patients. This is, however, still a dominant feature in the long-term plans of the current HHS administration.

CONCLUSION

Although these comments are not totally comprehensive of the legislative activities of the past 5 years, they do, I believe, represent the issues that are most likely to affect the immediate future of surgical practice and the education of surgeons. If one anticipates the future based on the past 5 years, one sees a much more active congressional effort related to health care of the indigent and elderly. We must all recognize that the main force behind the congressional concern for health care is expense, and today this clearly is a cost-driven system, and thus future legislative actions will most likely also be driven by cost. It is hoped that new legislation will have minimal effect on the quality of care, but we all must realize that the health care budget can be restricted only so much before a reduction in quality of care is inevitable.

PART FOUR

Legal and Ethical Issues in Surgery

19. CLINICAL SURGICAL DECISION MAKING
    John R. Clarke
20. UNNECESSARY SURGERY
    Ira M. Rutkow
21. SURGICAL EDUCATION AND CERTIFICATION REQUIREMENTS
    Ward O. Griffen, Jr.
22. THE MALPRACTICE CRISIS AND THE SURGEON
    Barry M. Manuel
23. THE SURGEON IN COURT
    Sal Fiscina

JOHN R. CLARKE

John R. Clarke is Professor of Surgery at the Medical College of Pennsylvania. He received his MD from the University of Pennsylvania in 1968 and completed his surgical internship at Presbyterian St. Luke's Hospital in Chicago, now the Rush Medical College. After 2 years as an emergency medicine physician in the military service, he finished his general surgical training at St. Joseph Mercy Hospital in Ann Arbor, Mich. Dr. Clarke undertook a trauma research fellowship at Boston City Hospital from 1975 to 1976 and subsequently joined the faculty at the Medical College of Pennsylvania. During the past 12 years he has served as Chief of the Trauma Service and now Director of the Regional Trauma Center. Dr. Clarke is on the Editorial Board of the journal *Medical Decision Making*.

19

Clinical Surgical Decision Making

JOHN R. CLARKE

WHAT IS SURGICAL JUDGMENT?

Surgeons, like all humans, make decisions every day. Judgment can be considered the ability to make those decisions correctly with incomplete, uncertain, or conflicting information.[25] The ability to make correct decisions about a patient's diagnosis, prognosis, or treatment is called clinical judgment. For this discussion, we shall define surgical judgment as a very specific form of clinical judgment, comprising decisions (1) to operate or not and (2) what operation to do.

Surgical decisions form a distinct class of decisions in another sense, too. Students of decision making are fascinated by surgical decisions because of their special characteristics. Unlike many other kinds of decisions, surgical decisions are generally irrevocable, frequently unavoidable, often urgent, and commonly associated with the possibility of significant loss.

Clinical decision making in general and surgical decision making specifically are forms of human decision making. In order to understand surgical decision making, we need to review some of the fundamental concepts of human decision making, particularly the combination of heuristics and logic.

DECISION MAKING AS LOGICAL DEDUCTION

Humans have limited short-term memory. The average person can retain only about six new and independent pieces of information in working memory without resorting to long-term memory.[31,37] When people are faced with a complex problem that involves many facts, such as making a medical diagnosis, they will consolidate a set of individual facts into a single concept to stay within the limits of working memory. Thus an otherwise healthy 12-year-old boy with pain in the right lower quadrant of the abdomen (five facts) becomes possible appendicitis (one concept).

Elstein and his colleagues examined the process of medical diagnosis.[16] They confirmed that physicians consolidate the initial information elicited from a patient into hypotheses, or working diagnoses, and use subsequent information to confirm or reject the hypotheses. The process of constructing hypotheses to explain a limited set of facts and then testing them with subsequent facts is called the hypothetico-deductive model of decision making. It follows naturally from the constraints of being limited to half a dozen pieces of information in working memory.

Artificial intelligence is a discipline of computer programming that attempts to make computers produce conclusions by manipulating information the same way people do.[3] One of the fundamentals of artificial intelligence is that information is manipulated by the principles of logic. In fact, artificial intelligence has been described as programming by logic. Programs using the techniques of artificial intelligence have been much more successful in reproducing the expertise of clinicians than programs using traditional programming techniques.

Buchanan and Shortliffe demonstrated that successful medical diagnostic and therapeutic programs could be made by rephrasing clinical principles as logical statements and then manipulating those statements using the rules of logical inference.[5] Clinical principles are written as conditional statements called decision rules: If the patient has a ruptured abdominal aortic aneurysm and the patient is treated without an operation, then the patient will die. Elementary logic requires that such conditional statements are absolutely true.

However, few of the principles people use to make decisions are absolutely true. Much more typical is the conditional statement: if the patient has appendicitis, then he or she will have an elevated white blood cell count. This rule is usually, but not always, true. Buchanan and Shortliffe had to program their computer to accommodate this uncertainty, that is, to infer using the less structured rules of probabilistic logic in order to produce decisions that matched those decisions of experienced clinicians. Real information is uncertain. Actual decision making requires that people account for uncertainty in their inferences.

Although Buchanan and Shortliffe used explicit rules of probabilistic inference for their computer programs, people use less exact methods. Based on extensive work, Kahneman and Tversky propose that humans use heuristic rules to draw conclusions from uncertain information.[24,39] They have been able to explain some of these heuristic methods of reasoning, particularly heuristics based on availability, representativeness, and adjustment from an anchor. Another characteristic of human decision making is an aversion to risk.[38,40] The strength of these heuristic ways of processing information is that they are simple. The weakness is that they make us susceptible to predictable biases.[23]

HUMAN REASONING: HEURISTICS AND BIASES

One heuristic that people use when reasoning is the availability heuristic. We tend to use the information that is available rather than the information we need. More precisely, when processing uncertain information, we assess higher probabilities to information that can be easily checked than to information that is difficult to find. Generally, available information is more relevant; that is why it was collected. But occasionally this can lead to an availability bias. Most people would say that the number of words with R as their first letter is larger than the number of words with R as their third letter, even though the opposite is true, because it is easier to think of words that start with R. Most patients with appendicitis are between 10 and 29 years, a fact well known, but patients with nonspecific abdominal pain have virtually the same age distribution, a fact not well known.

Another heuristic is the representative heuristic. The more that one thing resembles another, the more probable a relationship between the two. If a patient has all the findings associated with appendicitis, we reason that it must represent an example of appendicitis. Although this heuristic makes sense, it can occasionally result in erroneous processing of uncertain information.

One of these errors is ignoring the base rate.[2] A patient enters the emergency department with pain in the right lower quadrant of the abdomen. You think the patient has appendicitis. The resident has just been reading about the rare disease acute intermittent porphyria and points out that the patient's abdominal signs and symptoms, although not inconsistent with appendicitis, match the description of porphyria perfectly. He concludes that porphyria is the more likely diagnosis because the signs and symptoms match porphyria more closely than appendicitis. You point out, correctly, that appendicitis is still more likely only because appendicitis was much more likely before any signs or symptoms were considered.

When features that represent a match with the prototype also have relationships among themselves, people get the illusion of validity. If anorexia, nausea, and vomiting are considered independent elements of a match, the match may seem closer than if they are considered different manifestations of the one problem, disturbance of gastrointestinal function.

Another error is the failure to consider the variability of small samples. Most people would say that it is equally likely (or unlikely) that boy babies will outnumber girl babies by a ratio of 3:2 at the Nantucket Cottage Hospital (50 births per year) as at the Medical College of Pennsylvania (1500 births per year). One has only to consider a hospital with 5 births per year to realize that smaller series are expected to be more variable. As another example, a report of two cases with one fatal outcome does not extrapolate to a death rate of 50%. Another form of this error is the failure to consider regression to the mean. The percentage of diseased appendixes that are perforated before removal is about 20% nationally. You note with some satisfaction that your percentage in your first 25 cases is 8%, obviously because of your superior judgment. However, after 100 cases your percentage has crept up to 16%. Disappointed? You shouldn't be. The larger the series, the more likely the proportion of events will approximate the mean of the entire population, all other factors being equal.

The gambler's fallacy is the erroneous belief that any reasonable segment in a series of independent events must reflect the correct probabilities of those events. Having flipped a fair coin four times and obtained heads each time, people will expect tails to be more likely than heads in the next four flips. In fact, the probabilities will remain the same. They are not affected by the unrelated independent events that preceded it, nor will they affect the unrelated independent events that follow.

The third heuristic we will examine is the anchor-and-adjust heuristic. To make optimal decisions with uncertain information, people must accurately estimate the level of uncertainty. A common way to estimate the probability of an event is to estimate a starting point (the anchor) and then make an appropriate adjustment. For example, we know the death rate for an operation and the characteristics of a typical patient having the procedure. If our patient is younger and healthier, we lower the average death rate in making decisions about our patient.

However, people are poor at estimating probabilities, including the anchors. People tend to overestimate the probabilities of infrequent events and underestimate the probabilities of frequent ones. We also overestimate the probability that two independent events will occur together and underestimate the probability that either one or the other will occur. As you will see, this may improve with feedback.

Another characteristic of human decision making is aversion to risk or uncertainty. Although this trait varies with both the person and the task, most people try to avoid risk or uncertainty in the probability of the outcome of their decisions. They are described as being risk-averse. For instance, most people will accept a sure thing over a double-or-nothing bet. Aversion to risk is obviously a sensible concept, but it can result in biases.

Aversion to uncertainty creates conservatism, leading to conservative adjustments to probabilities. People tend not to change probabilities as much as they should from the anchor.

Regret or value-induced bias is the distortion of the expected outcome of an event because of uncertainty about the consequences.[12,22,30,43] Thus people behave as if the probability of an event is higher when the consequences of being in that state may be severe.

For physicians at least, Scheff proposes that there is a bias favoring errors of commission over errors of omission.[36] Although not mentioned by Scheff, this bias may be motivated by the desire at least of the physician to reduce uncertainty.

Framing is a psychologic phenomenon associated with risk aversion and resulting in biases.[40] Framing is the influence of the method in which the information is presented. When asked to chose between an operation with a 95% survival rate and one with a 5% death rate, a significant majority of people will predictably choose the first even though they know the two are equivalent.

Other psychologic processes and biases, not associated with heuristics, also can affect human decision making.[12,14] People have selective memories. We ignore negative or disconfirming evidence. The ego bias produces the finding that people overestimate probabilities associated with their own performance. With the hindsight bias, estimates of probabilities for the actual outcomes are higher if the results are already known at the time the estimates are given.[1] This, of course, is one of the more obvious biases.

PHYSICIAN ERRORS

Unfortunately, physicians are no less susceptible to biases when reasoning than anyone else. Arkes demonstrated the hindsight bias on physicians.[1] Berwick tested understanding of statistical concepts in physicians and replicated the failure to consider the variability of small samples, the failure to consider regression to the mean, and errors in estimating conjoint ("and") and disjoint ("or") probabilities.[4] Wallsten confirmed that physicians fail to consider the base rate, and they exhibit value-induced bias.[43] Detmer studied surgeons and noted insensitivity to sample size, the gambler's fallacy, ego bias, and hindsight bias.[14] Rutkow demonstrated inconsistency in surgeons' decisions.[34]

Voytovich has studied physicians' diagnostic errors and classifies them as four types.[42] The first and most obvious error is to be flat-out wrong. This error is an incorrect synthesis of information caused by a deficit of knowledge about the subject. A second, related error is the inability to arrive at a conclusion when the necessary information is available. This error is an incomplete synthesis of information, again because of a deficit of knowledge. The third error is to ignore inconsistent or contradictory information. This error is one of the errors of human information processing that we have discussed already. The fourth error, and the only one that is as prevalent in mature clinicians as novices, is what he calls premature closure, but what is commonly called jumping to conclusions. This error occurs when physicians reach conclusions although the alternative hypotheses have not been realistically excluded. Voytovich does not elaborate extensively on the relationship between premature closure (jumping to conclusions) and the errors in human information processing that are mentioned above, but several are likely to contribute, such as the illusion of validity and the overestimation of probabilities that two independent events will occur together.

We have illustrated that the human methods of decision making have, as side effects, predictable errors that can be reproduced in studies of clinical decision making by physicians and even surgeons specifically. Of course we can't realistically expect surgeons to be better decision makers than any other people in critical positions. Nevertheless, if we examine surgical decisions, that is, the decision to operate or not and what operation to do, we may be able to see where improvements can be made and where results are beyond the control of the individual surgeon.

ARE SURGEONS RATIONAL DECISION MAKERS?

We must accept that surgeons have no more immunity to biases in human reasoning than other rational thinkers, such as statisticians and business executives. For the rest of the discussion, let us set aside the universal psychologic processes and look specifically at surgical judgment. Let us examine other evidence for or against surgeons as rational decision makers. Operative rates do vary among surgeons, and these variations seem to reflect different treatment practices among the physicians.[19,20,35,45]

The U.S. government through the Health Care Financing Administration (HCFA) has posted in the public record crude death rates for Medicare patients by hospital for a variety of diagnoses and procedures.[15] These death rates sometimes vary widely from hospital to hospital much to the consternation of some hospital administrators and medical staffs. The simplistic conclusion is that these variations are the result of differences in the technical and/or cognitive skills of the practitioners. Other obvious causes are differences in the severity of the patients' illnesses and variations resulting from small sample sizes.[15] Other factors that cannot be ignored are the effect of the patients' preferences on the treatment selected and simple random variation. It is undoubtably premature to try to make conclusions about decision-making skills from these data.

Surgical second opinion programs provide the current "gold standard" for surgical decision making. However, it would be incorrect to extrapolate error rates for surgical decision making from the results of surgical second opinion programs. There is a fundamental flaw in the proposition that the results of surgical second opinion programs identify errors in surgical judgment and prevent unnecessary surgery. An alternative explanation is that the results are the predictable consequences of differences in physicians' treatment practices.

Two extremely informative studies about surgical decision making were done by Rutkow.[34,35] He sent patient management problems to randomly selected, board-certified surgeons and asked them to decide whether they would advise operation. Some of the vignettes described problems in definite need of surgery as case controls. Others problems required more judgment, presumably because the differences in the expected outcomes of the choices were less.

Among the control cases, from 95% to 100% of the surgeons chose the desired responses, suggesting an error rate of 5% or less, which is what would be expected. Among the 19 test cases, 7 had majorities of 80% to 89%, 3 from 70% to 79%, 4 from 60% to 69%, and 4 from 50% to 59%. He deduced marked patterns of disagreement among surgeons for patient management problems requiring judgment, possibly representing only reasonable differences in clinical practice.

Two years later he sent the same problems to the same surgeons. The percentage of recommendations for and against surgery were not substantially different, but the people making them had changed. Nine test cases had no more than 2% change in the percentage of recommendations for or against surgery between the two studies. In four of the nine, 20% to 29% of surgeons changed their recommendations; in two, 30% to 39% of surgeons changed; and in one, more than 40% changed. The study strongly suggests that surgeons are inconsistent from case to case.

Work at the Medical College of Pennsylvania confirmed Rutkow's observation that there was disagreement among surgeons giving advice for patient management problems and reenforced the premise that some of the disagreement represented reasoned differences in clinical practice.[9] As an example, for a vignette describing a patient who may or may not have had appendicitis, 44 surgeons were evenly divided between recommending appendectomy and recommending observation. After errors in their decision-making processes were corrected, they were divided 59% to 41% in favor of appendectomy.[8,9]

We compared general surgeons' opinions with decisions derived mathematically using decision analysis.[8] For six patient management problems, we solicited the surgeons' opinions in addition to their estimates of the probabilities and impact of each possible outcome. We then used each surgeons' estimates to solve the problems mathematically. In 92% of 236 individual examples, the surgeons' opinions were rational in that they were consistent with the results of the analyses done using their own estimates for the components of the decisions.

Much of the disagreement among surgeons can be attributed to different methods of treating patients based on training or experience or potentially on different preferences exercised by patients. Surgeons are rational in that they are consistent when making a decision for an individual problem between their opinions and the information on which the opinions are based. Surgeons do make the expected errors in processing that information. Most notably, although consistent within a single patient care situation, they are inconsistent between cases. This inconsistency will be explored in more detail.

ARE SECOND OPINIONS BETTER THAN FIRST OPINIONS?

In keeping with our emphasis on clinical decision making, let us look at the use of other decision makers to confirm surgeons' decisions. The results of surgical second opinion programs suggest that errors in decision making are seen with peer or expert review and by extension, that unnecessary surgery exists when these errors are not detected. Certainly errors occur. However, as we have seen from Rutkow's work, there also can be legitimate disagreement among surgeons about the best treatment. Let us explore what should happen when we check imperfect decision makers with disparately opinionated decision makers using a method that is systematically biased to check only the decision to operate.

For simplicity we will establish some logical constraints. Second opinions will imply that the surgeon giving the first opinion is qualified to do so and that the surgeon giving the second opinion is equally qualified, that is, the surgical second opinion program is a peer review process. Therefore, we will also assume that the second or even third doctor seen is just as likely to make a mistake or to advise the minority position in a scientific controversy as the first. The third doctor will be used if the second disagrees with the first. We will limit the second opinion to two options: agree or disagree. We will also assume that, either because of differences in training or experience or because of errors in decision making, some but not all of the surgeons will recommend operation, and the remainder will not.

Now let us implement a conventional surgical second opinion program as originally described by McCarthy.[29] You get an opinion from one of the qualified surgeons about whether you need an operation. If he or she advises against the operation, you accept that advice. If he or she advises in favor of the operation, you get a second opinion from another qualified surgeon. If the second surgeon agrees with the first, the decision to operate is considered confirmed. If the second surgeon disagrees, you see a third qualified surgeon to get a majority opinion.

The probability that an operation will be the final recommendation from this process can be calculated knowing only the proportion of qualified surgeons who would favor operation (probability = $2 \times \text{proportion}^2 - \text{proportion}^3$).[9] The probability that an operation will be the final recommendation will always be less than the proportion of surgeons who recommend the operation, whether or not operating is the correct decision. Therefore, this difference does not axiomatically represent errors in decision making or unnecessary surgery. Rather, it is the inevitable and obvious result of reviewing only decisions to operate. If the surgical second opinion program reviewed only decisions to not operate, the number of operative recommendations would increase, and people might be debating the possibility that patients are being deprived of necessary surgery!

If the majority of surgeons would operate, and operation is in fact the correct choice, the conventional surgical second opinion program will actually increase errors. For instance, if 80% of all surgeons would operate, only 77% of patients would get confirmed recommendations for operation from a conventional surgical second opinion program. If the surgeon giving the second opinion has more expertise, thereby changing the process to an expert review, more errors would probably be identified, but the process still would be biased by reviewing only recommendations for operations. The bias would also have an effect if the choice involved more than two options.

Surgical second opinions do have a place in clinical medicine. For the patients there is more dialogue about the decisions they must ultimately make. For the payer there is possibly a sentinel effect.[17] However, surgical second opinion programs measure agreement among physicians, not the correctness of their decisions. For conventional surgical second opinion programs, nonconfirmation is a statistical inevitability even when the majority of qualified surgeons advise operating. As we will see, several models of decision making have the potential to control some of the errors in the human decision-making method.

DECISIONS AS TRADEOFFS

Judgment has already been defined as the ability to make correct decisions when information and outcomes are uncertain. We have also determined that real problems usually require that we account for uncertainty by including probability in our reasoning. We have illustrated that people make errors when making decisions by probabilistic reasoning or under conditions of uncertainty.

In the 1940s von Neumann and Morgenstern developed mathematical methods for defining the best strategies for situations in which outcomes could not be predicted with certainty.[41] Later Raiffa extended the method and popularized the currently used method of analyzing decisions using decision trees.[27,33] Ledley and Lusted were the first to suggest that these analytical methods could be applied to medicine.[26] Lusted subsequently explored the prospect in depth.[28] Gorry began a tradition at Tufts of using formal decision analysis to characterize clinical problems.[21] Bunker was the first to extensively apply the method to surgical problems.[6]

Deciding between two or more options usually involves choosing between tradeoffs. Some decisions involve tradeoffs that are relatively certain; that is, each choice has advantages and disadvantages that are obvious to the decision maker. The decision maker chooses the option with the best net advantage. Decisions about which apartment to rent or which car to buy are examples of tradeoffs in which the results of the decisions are relatively certain.

Medical decisions more likely would be considered decisions made in the face of uncertainty. At the time a physician makes a decision, he or she does not know whether the choice will result in a good outcome or a bad one. The outcome of the decision will become known only some time after the decision is made. Not only must medical decision makers consider the desirability of each outcome but they must consider the probabilities that they will get a desirable outcome or an undesired one with each of the options. They must consider tradeoffs between the desirability of each outcome and the probability that it will occur. Decision analysts call these decisions under risk.[27]

Decision analysis is a formal process of representing and analyzing decisions in which the outcomes are uncertain. The decisions are represented in the form of decision trees. We will include only the most basic elements of decision analysis in this discussion. The specifics of the technique are nicely covered in a medically oriented textbook by Weinstein.[44]

A decision implies a choice between at least two options. This decision point is called a decision node and conventionally is represented by a square. (Think of it as a ballot box.) From this decision node emanate the options (Figure 19-1). For this simple example of surgical decision making, we will consider the options to treat with an operation and to treat with medication.

Each option can result in a spectrum of outcomes. Because the outcome that will occur is not known at the time the decision is made, it is considered an uncertain event to be determined

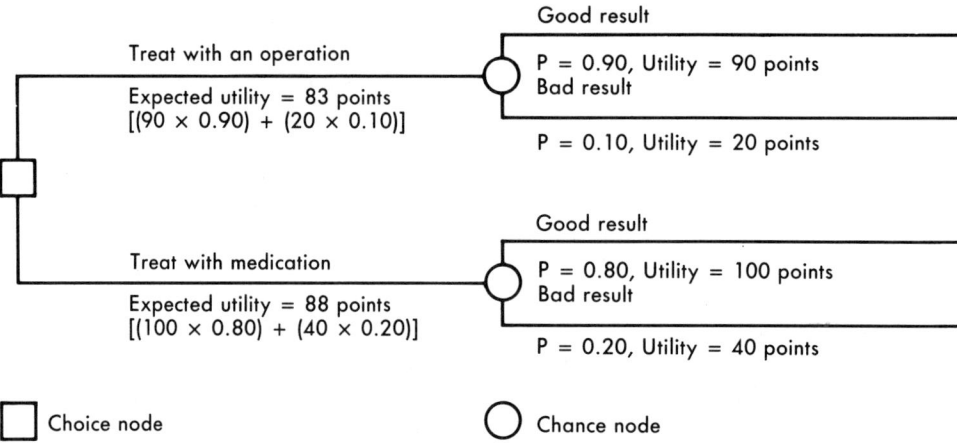

Figure 19-1. A simple surgical decision represented as a decision tree. The square represents a decision node; the circle represents a chance node. The decision has been solved by calculating the expected utilities for the two alternatives from the probabilities and utilities of all the outcomes.

in the future. The point at which the actual outcome will be determined is called the chance node. It is conventionally represented by a circle. (Think of it as a wheel of fortune.) In this example we will consider two possible outcomes for each option, a good result and a bad result.

Having defined all the outcomes that are associated with each option, we can assign each outcome a probability that it will occur if that option is chosen. These probabilities can be estimated subjectively, with the errors that we know are inherent in that process, or they can be derived statistically. For this example, we will consider that surgical treatment yields good results for 90% of patients and medical treatment yields good results for 80% of patients.

Assuming that an outcome does occur, it can be assessed a value by the patient. These measures of outcome are not strictly mathematical quantities, such as days sick or dollars spent. They also incorporate the patients' psychologic attitudes toward the outcomes, such as the impact of aversion to risk. This adjustment of the objective measures is done by a series of theoretic tradeoff decisions. Decision analysts call these outcome measures utilities. For example, the average person would choose a guaranteed $5 rather than a 50-50 chance of $10 or nothing, even though the two choices have the same mathematical value. The person may be ambivalent between a guaranteed $4 and a 50-50 chance of $10 or nothing. The utility of this $10 lottery would be equivalent to $4, with the $1 difference an indication of the person's attitude toward the risk inherent in the uncertain outcome.

In the example we will arbitrarily consider that a good result with medical treatment has a utility of 100 points on a relative scale; a good result with surgery, 90 points; a bad result with medical treatment, 40 points; and a bad result with surgery, 20 points. We now have outlined the tradeoff. The option of operative treatment is more likely to produce a good outcome than the option of medical treatment, but the outcomes of surgical treatment, good and bad, have less utility to the patient than the outcomes of medical treatment. Should the physician recommend surgery, which is more likely to be successful, or medical treatment, which will give a better result if it is successful? Considering both the probability and the utility of good and bad outcomes with each option, medical treatment will produce, on the average, a superior result. (An 80% chance of 100 points plus a 20% chance of 40 points is greater than a 90% chance of 90 points plus a 10% chance of 20 points. These average payoffs are called expected utilities.)

Notice that such an analytic approach makes the tradeoffs explicit. One can calculate the number of people who will get good results and bad results and the cost/benefit ratio of the alternative strategies.

As any surgeon knows, surgical judgment involves making tradeoffs under conditions of uncertainty or risk. A question was posed in the Department of Surgery at the Medical College of Pennsylvania. Do surgical decisions fit the decision analyst's tradeoff model or at least, can they? At that time (1978) no systematic investigation of how surgeons made decisions had been published. We started such an investigation.

We interviewed 37 randomly selected, board-certified surgeons in all the surgical specialties, including oral surgery and ophthalmology, in Philadelphia to generate hypotheses.[8] Based on these interviews, we constructed a model of the surgeons' decision-making process. This model was not intended to represent how these surgeons actually made their decisions, but to capture the elements of their decision making in a model consistent with the decision analyst's tradeoff model.

The hypotheses and the model were then validated two ways. We queried 155 randomly selected, board-certified surgical specialists of all types in Pennsylvania, representing about 5% of all the surgical specialists in the state. This query was done using a mailed questionnaire. We also interviewed 21 surgical specialists of all types at university hospitals in Philadelphia as they made decisions about 103 actual patients.

The results confirmed that surgical decisions could be represented by decision trees and solved by decision analysis. Surgical decisions, that is, the decisions to operate or not and what operation to do, consisted of one or at most two decision points per patient. Although the specific tradeoffs in the decisions varied among disciplines, the structures of the decision trees could be classified into very few types.

Most decisions consisted of the simple tradeoffs outlined here between two treatment options, each with the potential for good or bad results. One treatment option was always an operation, of course. The alternative was either no treatment, medical treatment, radiation therapy, another operation, or the same operation at a later time.

Another type of decision was more complex. It was called the decision about prophylactic surgery (Figure 19-2). This decision structure could be used to describe the decisions about operating for a variety of conditions such as possible appendicitis, asymptomatic gallstones, and inguinal hernias. The decision is whether to operate on a patient with a simple problem to prevent complications or to wait. By waiting, the patient may avoid surgery by not developing the feared complication. The other side of the tradeoff is that he or she may get the anticipated complication and be worse off.

When we looked at how surgeons made decisions, they could be described as using a form of the anchor-and-adjust heuristic. When presented with a problem, they drew upon a standard solution. This protocol was usually one that they had learned from their training or experience to be generally useful to solve the problem.

They then estimated whether the particular patient was representative of the patients associated with the protocol. If so, they applied the rule. If not, they adjusted the probabilities and outcome measurements to fit the particular patient and solved the specific tradeoff problem for that individual.

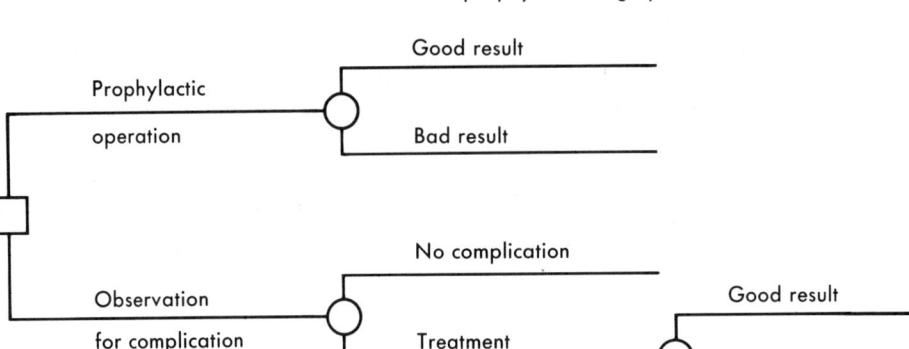

Figure 19-2. A more complex surgical decision representing the tradeoffs between operating prophylactically to avoid complications and operating only on those who develop the complications.

Sometimes they even went one step further. If the best of the tradeoffs was not good, they considered more aggressive, but riskier, treatment that offered opportunity for a better outcome but with more risk. For example, if a patient has severe coronary artery disease, surgery may carry a prohibitive risk. The risk of a heart attack from the stress of surgery can be reduced by supporting the patient with an intraaortic balloon pump, but the device carries its own risk of complications. Thus the surgeon occasionally created an additional tradeoff that needed resolution.

In one half of the actual decisions discussed, the most important component of the decision to the surgeon was the adjustment of the probabilities and patient's utilities. When done subjectively, as it usually is by surgeons, probability revision is vulnerable of course to some of the biases mentioned above. Accurate probabilities derived objectively with statistical methods are preferable. Because utilities measure the patients' attitudes and value system, two patients facing the same tradeoffs and having the same probabilities of good and bad results can have different preferences for treatment because they have different utilities.

Assessments of patients' utilities are the weakest part of the analytic concept. Utilities are inherently subjective, measuring the attitudes and values of individual people. They are expected to reflect the pyschologic processes mentioned early in this chapter, particularly aversion to risk. Unfortunately, they are also subject to biases in the measurement, such as those caused by regret and framing. Because there are no objective standards, it is difficult to tell whether a peculiar measurement is the result of a different value system or an erroneous measure of a conventional value system.

Bunker had demonstrated how decision analysis could be applied to surgical decisions.[6] Overall we felt that the decision analyst's tradeoff model could appropriately represent surgical decisions. Although surgeons had reduced the decisions for many common problems to standard protocols, there seemed to be an underlying tradeoff structure inherent in the solutions. It was still unclear whether the human biases in assessing the components of a decision-tree model would overwhelm the analytic process.

The potential for the analytic decision-tree tradeoff model to replicate surgical judgment was tested further. Six challenging general surgical patient management problems with analytic solutions that could be defended from the literature were presented to 50 board-certified general surgeons in the Philadelphia area who would be regarded as expert by any surgical second opinion program.[8] For validation one of the cases was a replication of one of Rutkow's cases.[34,35] Each surgeon was asked first to recommend treatment for each patient problem. Then each was asked to give subjective estimates of the probabilities and patient utilities necessary to solve the tradeoffs using a decision tree.

Using the predetermined analytic solution as the correct response, mathematical solutions of the decision trees using the surgeon's own subjective estimates were slightly but significantly more accurate than the surgeons' initial recommendations. In a subsequent theoretic challenge, the mathematical solutions also proved to be more accurate than surgical second opinion programs.[9] The problems were, for the most part, difficult and complex. The analytic tradeoff model proved to be a valid model of surgical judgment, producing better recommendations than the human process or surgical second opinion programs even with the inherent biases of subjective estimates.

Why did the mathematical model outperform the surgeons whose data were used in the model? Models of decision making often outperform the person whose decision-making process is being modeled, even when the model is imperfect.[11] The phenomenon is termed bootstrapping by experimental pyschologists.[23] Bootstrapping is probably the result of the ability of the analytic model to control some of the errors in human reasoning, particularly inconsistency.

The theoretic advantages of the analytic decision-tree tradeoff model include systematic consideration of all elements of the decision, accurate manipulation of the probabilities and utilities, and consistency in identifying the best answer. We are forced to consider relevant information that is not easily available. We must confront negative information and give appropriate consideration to all possible outcomes. We can avoid errors in estimating the products of sequential probabilities. We can accurately incorporate objectively derived probabilities of particular outcomes. We can control value-induced biases by independently considering the probabilities and utilities of bad outcomes.

CONSISTENCY—MAN VERSUS MACHINE

We previously described Rutkow's work showing that inconsistency was a major source of error in surgical decision making. The finding that surgeons are inconsistent from case to case is no surprise. Inconsistency is characteristic of human reasoning and a major source of error with human information processing.[23] We will demonstrate possible reasons in a moment.

Teleologically, inconsistency is probably an advantage to a species in a competitive environment. Rational beings that always did things in the optimal way would not fare well in the Darwinian jungle. You are trying to outsmart your competitors. Therefore, you instinctively mix your strategies. To optimize your results when competing against other people, inconsistency is important. In the children's game "Rock, Scissors, Paper" you shoot each with equal frequency. If you always threw "Rock," your opponents would always throw "Paper."

The use of an analytic method of decision making implies consistency, that is, you will always give the same advice for the same circumstances. It can be shown that to optimize your results when competing against chance, consistent selection of the most likely outcome is the optimal strategy. Clinicians may argue that such a policy doesn't provide a role for clinical intuition. Let us see.

Consider a patient with a set of findings that indicates that the probability of appendicitis is 0.80. Specifically you search for all the patients in the abdominal pain registry who have exactly the same set of findings as your patient. There are 100, and 80 of them had appendicitis. The analysis implies that you should diagnose the patient as having appendicitis. However, you say that the results also indicate that one patient in five did not have appendicitis and you, an experienced clinician, think this is the one.

If you base your clinical prediction only on the information in the database, your optimal strategy is to always diagnose appendicitis. Most people will use a mixed strategy, alternating predictions in the same ratio as the probability (in this case appendicitis 4 times in 5).[18] However, the mixed strategy or any other strategy is likely to give fewer correct predictions than always guessing appendicitis (which will be correct four times in five or 80% of the time). Although there is a 1 in 25 chance of matching with nonappendicitis by skipping around, there is only a 16 in 25 chance of matching with appendicitis. Skipping around will result in correct predictions only 17 times out of 25 or 68% of the time. Skipping around would be a rational strategy if the appendix were an adversary that would get inflamed or not depending on whether it thought you were going to operate or not. It is not the rational strategy when the appendix is inflamed whether or not you intend to operate.

If you, the expert diagnostician, base your clinical prediction on information that is not in the database, your estimated probability may be legitimately different. For instance, the patient has normal coloring, neither pale nor flushed. As an expert clinician, you estimate quite accurately that the odds of appendicitis based on this observation alone are 7 in favor and 8 against. Your estimated probability of appendicitis is now less (0.78, to be precise). Yet because appendicitis is still more likely than not, the best strategy is still to predict appendicitis. On the other hand, the patient has had a hysterectomy. She does not know whether she had an incidental appendectomy, and there is no way to find out. You estimate that because it is likely that the appendix has been removed, the probability of appendicitis must be less than 0.50. Now your best strategy is to predict that the patient does not have appendicitis.

Note that in all of these examples, the strategy to consistently choose the more likely disease is superior to any strategy involving going against the odds. The only reason for not choosing the more probable diagnosis is if further objective or subjective analysis drops the estimated probability below 0.50 and makes it the least probable diagnosis.

The same principles make the same strategy optimal when probabilities are multiplied by the patients utilities to produce the average payoff or expected utility for each choice. Again, the optimal strategy is to always select the strategy with the best expected utility. No mixed strategy of operating and not operating in any ratio can produce better results.

Consistency counts more than intuition. Consistency is necessary to make the best decisions for the largest number of patients during an extended clinical experience. If we are making many decisions, the long-term results from consistency will overwhelm any short-term gains from intuition. Consistency minimizes errors in reasoning beyond those caused by bias.

Methods for maintaining consistency include the use of protocols, algorithms, decision rules, and analytic models either in written form or computerized. As mentioned previously in the discussion of bootstrapping, a model using such techniques to minimize inconsistency will make more correct decisions than the person whose reasoning was formalized, even imperfectly.[11]

METHODS OF IMPROVING SURGICAL JUDGMENT

This review suggests that surgical judgment can be improved if biases in the heuristic methods of human reasoning are corrected and inconsistency is controlled. Current methods to improve surgical judgment include second opinions and various forms of critique with feedback, such as mortality and morbidity conferences, quality assurance programs, and malpractice suits.[13,17,29,45] Potential methods include decision models and education.

Let us return to the 6 patient management problems reviewed by 50 general surgeons and look at some potential methods to improve the decisions. These were theoretic cases, but as such they do permit comparisons that would not be possible with actual patient care situations.

The net improvement in the number of correct decisions was calculated and compared for five strategies to improve surgical judgment[8,9] (Table 19-1). One method that has already been discussed at length is a conventional surgical second opinion program. In this particular group of six, this strategy resulted in a decreased number of correct decisions. Consultations on all cases, not just the decisions to operate, led to a slight improvement.

As part of our original study, we returned the following feedback to each surgeon who provided complete information: the surgeon's decision for each problem, the majority opinion of the 50 surgeons, the results of the decision analysis using the information the surgeon had provided, and the analytically correct answer.[8] We asked each surgeon if he or she wanted to change any of his or her recommendations. Eighty percent responded; there were five changes. This critique with feedback reduced the number of errors 5%, from 97 to 92.

The mathematical solutions of the decision trees using the surgeon's own subjective estimates gave an estimate of the effect of correcting for errors in the way humans make decisions, such as ignoring negative or disconfirming information, inaccurately manipulating the probabilities and utilities, and inconsistency. When information was analyzed mathematically rather than in the surgeons' heads, the number of errors was reduced 12%. Adding accurate information to accurate analysis doubled the improvement. Because no hypothesis was presented, no statistical test will be done. Remember that the comparisons, although interesting, are theoretic.

We have already demonstrated the limited potential for second opinions to improve surgical judgment. Our experience with feedback is too limited to draw conclusions, but both Wennberg and Detmer among others report changes in operative rates with feedback.[13,45] As described, the effect appears to be an educational one influencing future decisions rather than an immediate one affecting the actual cases in which errors were made.

Both the work that we have described and a related study of surgical residents have suggested the importance of good information to process as well as good processing of information.[7,8] We postulated that both knowledge and decision-making skills were important for sound surgical

Table 19-1. The effect of different forms of critique on the overall accuracy of recommendations to operate

Case	N	Surgical Second Opinion Program	Routine Consultations	Feedback	Correction of Errors in Decision Making	Correction of Errors in Decision Making and Knowledge
1	40	− 1	+2	+1	+ 2	+ 2
2	37	+ 4	+5	+1	+ 1	− 1
3	44	− 8	0	+1	+ 2	+ 4
4	39	+ 3	−2	+1	+ 1	+ 1
5	32	− 3	+2	+1	+ 1	+13
6	44	− 6	−5	0	+ 5	+ 4
TOTAL	236	−11	+2	+5	+12	+23

judgment. In our six theoretic cases, the accuracy of the recommendations was proportional to the accuracy of the information used and the amount of accurate information used. It is no surprise that knowledge of the subject is considered important for good decision making. Now there is evidence that knowledge about the reasoning process is also helpful.[32]

However, because of consistency, models of the decisions should provide the most accurate recommendations. Protocols and algorithms have been useful, particularly those taught in the Advanced Cardiac Life Support (ACLS) and Advanced Trauma Life Support (ATLS) courses. For practical reasons, protocols and algorithms are limited to prototypic examples. When the clinical situation permits, idiosyncracies of individual patients can be considered with artificial intelligence medical expert systems that can mimic physicians' reasoning and with decision trees that analyze the patients' tradeoffs.

We have demonstrated more accurate decisions among experienced practitioners with decision analysis. Our studies suggest that methods incorporating accurate numbers derived from information bases should be superior to those just accurately manipulating physicians' estimates, which are themselves subject to the errors of human judgment. We also have demonstrated more accurate decisions among residents with artificial intelligence expert systems that incorporate our clinical protocols.[10]

IMPLICATIONS
Efficiency in Deduction

When we are presented with information, we can juggle just a few facts before we must join them into a hypothesis. To maximize efficiency, the most relevent facts should be presented first. Therefore, it is important that the decision maker understand which are the most powerful discriminators for any clinical conundrum. This is true not only for choosing questions during the history-taking session, but most important, for choosing tests that will be expensive, time consuming, and risky. Information about the false positive and false negative rates associated with various findings of specific diseases is important. With proper application of this information, physicians can minimize the efficiency of their diagnostic workups.

First Opinions

Surgeons do make rational recommendations. To minimize errors and maximize understanding by the patients, they should present both the pros and cons of both the preferred and alternative options. The surgeon should estimate for the patient the likelihood that any particular outcome will occur and listen to the patient's attitude about that outcome. The surgeon must be careful to avoid biasing the interaction by the way the information is presented (the framing effect). A patient who has a recommendation from a surgeon, who understands that the decision reached is the best of several possible tradeoffs, and who understands the nature of each tradeoff is as well informed as any patient could be after a discussion with a physician.

Consideration of Patients' Wishes

People, including both physicians and patients, are generally averse to risk. Different individuals have different experiences, value systems, and attitudes. Decisions must incorporate these considerations into the decision-making process. There is general agreement among decision makers that the utility measurement should be the patient's, not the doctor's. Therefore, two patients, with the same problem, the same options, the same possible outcomes, and even the same probabilities for each one of those outcomes being the end result, may have different correct solutions if the patients have different preferences. Protocols and policies should take those preferences into account.

Unnecessary Surgery

Unnecessary surgery is not axiomatically surgery that has not been confirmed. In particular, we have demonstrated that nonconfirmation is an inevitable consequence of conventional surgical second opinion programs, which review only decisions to operate. This method of confirmation is biased against finding offsetting instances in which surgery has been overlooked. Variations in operative rates, representing different experiences, are an alternative explanation for the results of surgical second opinion programs.

Any investigation of unnecessary surgery must accommodate two concepts. One is that, because of different training and experiences, surgeons vary in their opinions of which possible solutions are the best. The second is that, just as different options may be optimal in the hands of different surgeons, different options may be optimal in the minds of different patients because of their value systems.

Sources of Variation in the Results of Treatment

When operative death and complication rates for surgeons and operations vary from the norm, either up or down, the obvious thought is that there is a difference in performance. The surgeon or surgeons involved may have better or worse judgment skills or technical expertise or they may not. The differences may also represent differences in the scope of the patients' illnesses or even differences in the preferences of patients with the same illness for various outcomes. For instance, if patients in New York are willing to accept a 2% higher operative risk to relieve angina than patients in Florida, the operative death rate in New York may be higher than in Florida. Different rates and subsequent changes in rates may even represent just random variation, the variability of small samples, or regression to the mean.

Predictable Bad Outcomes

The analytic model makes the tradeoffs in a decision explicit. Let us return to the decision in Figure 19-1. The proper recommendation is medical treatment. Yet that choice will predictably result in 20% of the patients having bad outcomes. Those bad outcomes are not the results of bad judgment but of the reality that the potential for gain comes with a predictable risk for loss.

If the analysis was done properly, the patient preferred the gamble associated with the medical treatment more than the gamble associated with operative therapy. His preference indicated his willingness to accept this risk between a good outcome and a bad outcome, considering the alternative. Deciding between the alternatives involved consideration of both the probabilities and utilities of all the outcomes. The measurement of utilities captured the patient's attitudes about uncertainty, risk, regret, and excessive concern about particular dreaded events.

By bringing the patient into the decision so that he understands what the tradeoffs are and gives his preferences, the outcome of the preferred gamble should be more tolerable. The analytic model also makes exposure to any bad outcome more defensible. The predictability and the relative importance of each bad outcome are clearly stated and can be compared. Of course if the patient loses the gamble and gets the bad result, he is likely to exhibit hindsight bias: "If only I had known how great the risks were, I never would have agreed."

The Importance of Information

Knowledge is an important foundation for any decision. You can make reasonable decisions using a good understanding of the subject and everyday human reasoning. You cannot make good decisions if you don't know the subject, no matter how good you are at reasoning. Unfortunately, much of the information available is not what we need to make decisions, and much of the information we need is not available. Computerized databases and information systems may correct these deficiencies if the information that is collected is what is needed.

Feedback

Feedback improves patient care through education of the physician. Providing physicians with accurate counts of outcomes and the factors that influence them should improve their ability to estimate probabilities and decrease the effect of selective recall and some of the biases we have discussed. The process of feedback provides a sentinel effect. The results provide an awareness of the individual's competitive position. Both are usually motivators to improve results.

Following Protocols

Inconsistency is one of the major causes of poor decisions. People try to outguess the probabilities with deleterious results. The gains from intuition are overwhelmed by the losses for inconsistency. Because of consistency, models of decisions can outperform the human decision maker who was the basis for the model. Protocols, algorithms, mathematical models, decision trees, computer programs, computers, and artificial intelligence expert systems have the potential to improve decision making, provided they are sophisticated enough to represent the solutions accurately.

My opinion is that the best way to improve clinical judgment is to maintain consistency with sophisticated protocols that are complex enough that they fit all the patients' problems without requiring simplifications in the description of the patients in order to fit the protocols. The use of such protocols would require the assistance of computerized artificial intelligence expert systems. Because such systems must reason probabilistically, they would have to incorporate the principles of decision analysis to evaluate probabilities that decision rules are true and to determine thresholds for applying the rules.

References

1. Arkes HR et al: The hindsight bias among physicians weighting the likelihood of diagnoses, J Appl Psychol 66:252, 1981.
2. Bar-Hillel M: The base-rate fallacy in probability judgment, Acta Psychol 44:221, 1980.
3. Barr A and Feigenbaum E: Handbook of artificial intelligence, vol 2, Reading, Mass, 1981, Addison-Wesley Publishing Co, Inc.
4. Berwick DM, Fineberg HV, and Weinstein MC: When doctors meet numbers, Am J Med 71:991, 1981.
5. Buchanan B and Shortliffe E: Rule-based expert systems, Reading, Mass, 1984, Addison-Wesley Publishing Co, Inc.
6. Bunker JP, Barnes BA, and Mosteller F: Costs, risks, and benefits of surgery, New York, 1977, Oxford University Press, Inc.
7. Clarke JR: The role of decision skills and medical knowledge in the clinical judgment of surgical residents, Surgery 92:153, 1982.
8. Clarke JR: Surgical judgment using decision sciences, New York, 1984, Praeger Publishers.
9. Clarke JR: A comparison of decision analysis and second opinions for surgical decisions, Arch Surg 120:844, 1985.
10. Clarke JR, Cebula DP, and Webber BL: Artificial intelligence: a computerized decision aid for trauma, J Trauma 27:818, 1987.
11. Dawes RM: The robust beauty of improper linear models, American Psychol 341:571, 1979.
12. Dawson NV and Arkes HR: Systematic errors in medical decision making: judgment limitations, J Gen Intern Med 2:183, 1987.
13. Detmer DE and Frisch C: Improved results in acute appendicitis care following areawide review, Med Decis Making 4:217, 1984.
14. Detmer DE, Fryback DG, and Gassner K: Heuristics and biases in medical decision-making, J Med Educ 53:682, 1978.
15. Eastaugh S: Financing health care: economic efficiency and equity, Dover, Mass, 1987, Auburn House Publishing Co.
16. Elstein AS, Shulman LS, and Sprafka SA: Medical problem solving, Cambridge, Mass, 1978, Harvard University Press.
17. Finkel ML, McCarthy EG, and Ruchlin HS: The current status of surgical second opinion programs, Surg Clin North Am 62:705, 1982.
18. Gardner RA: Multiple-choice decision behavior, Am Psychol 71:710, 1958.
19. Gittelsohn AM and Wennberg JE: On the risk of organ loss, J Chronic Dis 29:527, 1976.
20. Gittelsohn AM and Wennberg JE: On the incidence of tonsillectomy and other common surgical procedures. In Bunker JP, Barnes BA, and Mosteller F, editors: Costs, risks, and benefits of surgery, New York, 1977, Oxford University Press, Inc.
21. Gorry GA et al: Decision analysis as the basis for computer-aided management of acute renal failure, Am J Med 55:473, 1973.
22. Hershey JC and Baron J: Clinical reasoning and cognitive processes, Med Decis Making 7:203, 1987.
23. Hogarth RM: Judgement and choice, Chichester, Eng, 1980, John Wiley & Sons, Inc.
24. Kahneman D, Slovic P, and Tversky A: Judgment under uncertainty: heuristics and biases, New York, 1982, Cambridge University Press.

25. Knafl K and Burkett G: Professional socialization in a surgical specialty: acquiring medical judgment, Soc Sci Med 9:397, 1975.
26. Ledley RS and Lusted LB: Reasoning foundations of medical diagnosis, Science 130:9, 1959.
27. Luce RD and Raiffa H: Games and decisions, New York, 1957, John Wiley and Sons, Inc.
28. Lusted LB: Introduction to medical decision making, Springfield, Ill, 1968, Charles C. Thomas, Publisher.
29. McCarthy EG and Widmer GW: Effects of screening by consultants on recommended elective surgical procedures, N Engl J Med 291:1331, 1974.
30. McGuire WJ: A syllogistic analysis of cognitive relationships. In Rosenberg MJ et al, editors: Attitude organization and change, New Haven, Conn, 1960, Yale University Press.
31. Miller GA: The magical number seven, plus or minus two: some limits on our capacity for processing information. Psychol Rev 63:81, 1956.
32. Nisbett RE et al: Teaching reasoning. Science 238:625, 1987.
33. Raiffa H: Decision analysis: introductory lectures on choices under uncertainty, Reading, Mass, 1968, Addison-Wesley Publishing Co, Inc.
34. Rutkow IM: Surgical decision making: the reproducibility of clinical judgment, Arch Surg 117:337, 1982.
35. Rutkow IM, Gittelsohn AM, and Zuidema GD: Surgical decision making: the reliability of clinical judgment, Ann Surg 190:409, 1979.
36. Scheff TJ: Decision rules, types of error, and their consequences in medical diagnosis, Behav Sci 8:97, 1963.
37. Simon HA: How big is a chunk? Science 183:482, 1974.
38. Slovic P and Lichtenstein S: The relative importance of probability and payoffs in risk taking, J Exp Psychol 78:Part 2, 1968.
39. Tversky A and Kahneman D: Judgment under uncertainty: heuristics and biases, Science 185:1124, 1974.
40. Tversky A and Kahneman D: The framing of decisions and the psychology of choice, Science 211:453, 1981.
41. von Neumann J and Morgenstern O: Theory of games and economic behavior, Princeton, NJ, 1944, Princeton University Press.
42. Voytovich AE, Rippey RM, and Suffredini A: Premature conclusions in diagnostic reasoning, J Med Educ 60:302, 1985.
43. Wallsten TS: Physician and medical student bias in evaluating diagnostic information, Med Decis Making 1:145, 1981.
44. Weinstein MC et al: Clinical decision analysis, Philadelphia, 1980, W.B. Saunders Co.
45. Wennberg JE et al: Changes in tonsillectomy rates associated with feedback and review, Pediatrics 59:821, 1977.

20

Unnecessary Surgery

IRA M. RUTKOW

What unnecessary surgery is and whether it exists are questions fundamental to the delivery of surgical health care. Although recent socioeconomic changes have thrust the term unnecessary surgery before the public, the concern has been present since the dawn of recorded history. Certainly the discovery of prehistoric skulls, on which trephination had been performed to release evil spirits, would attest to the presence of questionable surgery.

Unnecessary surgery has become a shibboleth for many of the problems with modern United States medicine.* The vociferousness of some consumer groups and government officials, for example, in discussing unnecessary surgery has led to the implication that such operations are one reason for the rapid rise in cost of health care. This chapter discusses the concept of unnecessary surgery regarding what it is and what it is not.

HISTORICAL PERSPECTIVE

Although the debate over unnecessary surgery seems of recent origin, it has been discussed and written about for centuries. As far back as 1775 John Jones in his classic work *Plain Concise Practical Remarks On The Treatment Of Wounds And Fractures*, the first surgical textbook written by a physician of the United States, stated[61]:

> As every operation is necessarily attended with a certain degree of bodily pain, as well as terrible apprehension to the patient's mind, a good surgeon will be in the first place, well assured of the necessity of an operation, before he proceeds to perform it; and secondly he ought to consider, whether the patient will in all probability be the better for it, or whether he may not be the worse.

In 1908 Ernest W. Hey Groves, a surgeon to the Bristol General Hospital in England, called for a uniform registration of operation results to monitor surgical procedures.[53] He suggested six ways to improve surgical outcomes and avoid unnecessary surgery. Among them were the establishment of a central authority, an organizing committee, a standard nomenclature of operations and diseases, and the recording of facts and statistics relative to the performance of all operations. As he wrote:

> In this way the profession would be afforded each year an absolutely authoritative and impartial report of the results of all the major operations performed in the United Kingdom. From this could be derived the most valuable knowledge as to the prognosis after operations, the increase or decrease of various diseases, and the different operations performed for their relief. And the improvement in results could be noted in each

---

*References 19,22,50,85,95,101,106,110,112,114,126,141.

procedure by the comparison of one year's results with another.

Hospital Studies

About the same time in the United States, the Clinical Congress of Surgeons of North America (forerunner of the American College of Surgeons) was grappling with ways to better measure the efficacy and efficiency of hospitals and the care they rendered to surgical patients. As Jones had stated about United States institutions more than a century and a quarter earlier[61]:

> Among the variety of public errors and abuses, to be met with in human affairs, there is not one perhaps which more loudly calls for a speedy and effectual reformation, than the misapplied benevolence of hospitals for the sick and wounded.

The modern movement to improve hospitals and their clinical care was headed by that great skeptic of all things surgical, Ernest Amory Codman.[20] It was he who, during the first decade of the twentieth century, developed and promulgated the "end-result plan" of tracking hospital patients long enough to determine effectiveness of treatments so that competence of hospital physicians, surgeons, and staff could be evaluated. Codman was appointed chairman of the Clinical Congress' Committee on Hospital Standardization, which initiated and crusaded for improvement and standardization of hospital treatment nationally. In an address before the Philadelphia County Medical Society (May 14, 1913) Codman defined standardization as[20]

> ... a general movement toward improving the quality of the products for which hospital funds are expended. As a rule standards are raised by stimulating the best—not by whipping up the laggards.

He went on to further state:

> We must formulate some method of hospital report showing as nearly as possible what are the results of the treatment obtained at different institutions. This report must be made out and published by each hospital in a uniform manner, so that comparison will be possible. With such a report as a starting point, those interested can begin to ask questions as to management and efficiency.

Other surgeons were trumpeting the same call. Robert L. Dickinson, a gynecologic surgeon from Brooklyn, stated before the American Medical Association's 65th annual session in 1914[30]:

> It is not easy to adjust our point of view to the idea that the actions of all of us are to be checked up and compared with certain standards while our breaks are calmly tallied and bulletined and our results are openly scheduled. As it is at present a visiting or associate surgeon may be a striking success in diagnosis or technic but in other points like after-care or progress or humanity be grievously defective. Who may tell how the balance is to be struck under present methods?

Horace G. Wetherill, a surgeon from Denver, in a 1914 speech before the Western Surgical Association declared[139]:

> The promotion of hospital efficiency and standardization, the elevation of hospital morals, and the exclusion of the unfit and the incompetent from hospital practice has now become a matter of paramount necessity because of the importance of the hospital in the present scheme of medical education.

It was John G. Bowman in 1920, as first director of the American College of Surgeons, who enunciated the concept of the "minimum standard".[13] In this way it would be possible to know

> ... if any unnecessary surgical operations are performed in the hospital; or if incompetent surgical operations are performed; or if lax, lazy, or incomplete diagnoses are made.

In a 1922 editorial "The Unnecessary Operation", William Haggard, a future president of the American College of Surgeons, wrote[54]:

> There yet remain well-meaning men who lack discrimination and experience and make the er-

ror of attempting to extend operative relief to . . . individuals upon insufficient clinical data and inadequate pathological criteria. There are regrettably some unconscionable pothunters who will operate on anybody that will hold still. Every hospital should eliminate that kind of man.

Hospital Accreditation

As an outgrowth of its interest in the standardization of hospitals, the American College of Surgeons established a permanent committee to deal with accreditation, survey, inspection, and reporting.[125] Beneficial results soon became obvious, and hospitals struggled to upgrade conditions. The expansion of the hospital inspection program eventually became too large a financial burden for the College to maintain without external assistance. In addition, the American Hospital Association had become a strong organization in its own right and wished to participate more actively in the accreditation of its member hospitals. In 1951 Evarts Graham proposed to the Board of Regents of the College that an independent commission of hospital accreditation be set up and financed by contributions from participating organizations. This ultimately led to the formation of the Joint Commission on the Accreditation of Hospitals.

Consumer Movement

With the advent of a strong consumers' movement in the United States, increasing numbers of articles have appeared in the lay press, government publications, and scientific journals alluding to certain common surgical procedures performed without proper clinical and pathologic justification. As arguments continued through the past 30 years, there have been a number of events that were most prominent in bringing the entire problem of unnecessary surgery to public scrutiny.

The first was twin studies conducted in 1962 and 1964 regarding the quality and costs of medical and hospital care secured by a sample of teamster families in the New York area.[128] The group was surveyed regarding various types of surgery they had undergone. It was found that one third of hysterectomies had been performed "unnecessarily" and that questions regarding advisability could be raised for another 10%. Serious concerns were raised about the necessity of more than half of the cesarean sections.

At the end of the 1960s an article by Lewis in which he analyzed records of the Blue Cross Association of the state of Kansas showed a threefold to fourfold variation in that state's regional rates for the performance of six common elective procedures.[68] Lewis went so far as to conclude that a surgical variation of Parkinson's law existed:

> . . . patient admissions for surgery expand to fill beds, operating suites and total surgical manpower.

The following year Bunker, in a still frequently quoted paper, compared operations and surgeons in the United States with those in England and Wales.[15] He noted that per capita the United States had twice as many surgeons as England and Wales and twice the number of operations performed per population. It was the preceeding two papers that helped propagate the concept that surgeons coming to a community perform surgery according to their own financial requirements. Therefore it could be construed that a portion of surgery in the United States is completed solely for remunerative purposes, which would deem it unnecessary.

These findings from medical literature were soon heralded by the insurance industry. Herbert S. Denenberg, Pennsylvania's Insurance Commissioner published a shoppers' guide to surgery.[26] In it he outlined 14 steps individuals could take to make certain they were not operated on unnecessarily or by incompetent surgeons.

In December 1974 McCarthy and Widner published their controversial surgical second opinion study, which showed that presurgical screening programs had a substantial benefit for cost reduction in an insured population.[79] This led to the federal government's notion that differences in surgical opinion are directly translatable into the amount of unnecessary surgery performed in the United States.

Representative John E. Moss' 1976 report *Cost and Quality of Health Care: Unnecessary Surgery* provoked a huge storm of criticism regarding surgical health care in the United States.[21,127] As he stated in his letter of transmittal to Representative Harley O. Staggers:

> The report concludes that second consultations before surgery can cut down on unnecessary surgical procedures . . . surgical payments by the fee-for-service mechanism encourages surgery in questionable situations . . . unnecessary surgery has deleterious effects upon the American public . . . there were approximately 2.4 million unnecessary surgeries performed in 1974 at a cost to the American public of almost $4 billion, and . . . these unnecessary surgeries led to 11,900 deaths last year.

In the same month (January, 1976) a five-part series of front page articles in *The New York Times* featured sensational accusations of both unnecessary and incompetent surgery. Jane Brody wrote[14]:

> . . . at least some surgeons "make work" for themselves by doing operations that are unnecessary.

In 1977 Bunker et al. edited a monograph devoted to the costs, risks, and benefits of surgery.[16] This work dealt extensively with socioeconomic principles and the delivery of surgical health care. The authors presented data that discussed the concept of unnecessary surgery relative to several specific operations.

Public Policy

During the early 1980s Rutkow edited the first book on formation of public policy specifically applied to surgery in the United States.[105] About the same time the question of a large surplus of surgeons in this country was raised for discussion in all levels of society. Implicit in this debate was the belief that "underemployed" surgeons would contribute further to problems of unnecessary surgery.

By the late 1980s public support for surgeons and the quality of their surgical health care had markedly declined. It is almost as if an adversarial relationship is established when a patient enters a surgeon's office. Consumerism, increasing health care costs, and the assumption that a significant amount of unnecessary surgery exists have led to the rapidly changing environment in which surgical decision making is carried out.

DEFINITION

In addressing the question of unnecessary surgery, it is of major importance that a workable definition be established. We need to know by whose terms and by what criteria a surgical procedure is being termed unnecessary.

Idealistically, the definition can be approached from two sides, that of the surgeon and the medical profession and that of the attorney and the legal profession. It is defined more pragmatically, however, by the final arbiter of all surgical procedures, the patient.

Medical Profession

The medical profession has had great difficulty defining unnecessary surgery. In 1953 Charles Letourneau, secretary of the Council on Professional Practice of the American Hospital Association stated[67]:

> . . . it is—a felony—for a surgeon to represent fraudulently to a patient that his physical condition requires a surgical operation and then to operate on him after obtaining his consent. In the first place the surgeon is guilty of a criminal assault on the patient, for consent obtained by fraud is no consent at all, and, if his sole intention in performing the operation is to obtain money from the patient, the crime then resembles theft with violence, known technically as robbery.

In 1954 Greer Williams, an official of the

American College of Surgeons, writing in the lay press stated[140]:

> Unjustified surgery—or unnecessary surgery . . . may be defined as an operation which is not supported by careful clinical reasoning and judgment, and not confirmed in diagnosis by any disease actually found.

George Crile feels it would be easier to supervise the quality of surgery if operations were judged not as being necessary or unnecessary but as appropriate or inappropriate.[23,24] He describes three classes of inappropriate operations: (1) operations that are inappropriate for the disease; (2) operations that are inappropriate for the individual patient; and (3) operations that are appropriate for the disease and the patient but are performed by a surgeon not appropriately trained to do them.

A frequently cited categorization of operations that might be termed unnecessary comes from the Study On Surgical Services for the United States.[4,143] In this multivolume report six categories of operations deemed unnecessary depending on their individual clinical frame of reference were outlined. They are (1) operations in which no pathologic tissue is removed, (2) operations in which indications are a matter of judgment, (3) operations to alleviate endurable or tolerable symptoms, (4) discretionary operations for asymptomatic, nonpathologic, or nonthreatening disorders, (5) operations now outdated, obsolete, or discredited, and (6) operations for which there is little justification by clinical, x-ray, or laboratory study.

There is little disagreement that operations in the latter two categories can be labeled as truly unnecessary, but those to alleviate endurable or tolerable symptoms and discretionary procedures enter the gray area of comfort surgery. Who is to say whether these are unwarranted?

The Board of Regents of the American College of Surgeons pronounced that unnecessary surgery[1,3]:

> . . . is a catchphrase that cannot be readily defined. However, the term has been widely used in conjunction with faulty statistics to suggest that unnecessary operations are being performed in huge numbers. It has also been implied that such operations make a major contribution to the rising costs of health care in this country. Both these notions are false, but they have been stated so often by congressional spokesmen, government officials, and the media that they have become a fixture in the collection of myths about medical care in the United States.

Legal Profession

The legal profession confronts the problem of unnecessary surgery on a more basic level than the physician. For the attorney a static definition must be delineated because rulings are needed in the courtroom. In a series of three articles on unnecessary surgery, Holder, an attorney on the staff of the Office of the General Counsel of the American Medical Association, writes[56-58]:

> . . .for purposes of determining liability, 'unnecessary' includes more than its dictionary definition. Unnecessary surgery would include those operations which not only turn out at or after the operation to have been not necessary but in which the decision to operate was erroneous based on the symptoms which existed at the time the decision was made. The negligence in these cases therefore appears to be predicated on negligence in diagnosis, not in the performance of the surgery itself. . . . Hindsight is better than foresight in surgery as in other areas of life. Courts do not expect surgeons to be wizards or soothsayers and as long as the original diagnosis is made with skill and care and attention, no liability will be imposed.

Ficarra, in his book *Surgical And Allied Malpractice* states[44]:

> Unnecessary surgery is a self-explanatory term. It means performing an operation which is not necessary or the removing of a normal organ with knowledge aforethought that no disease really existed.

Louisell and Williams, in *Medical Malpractice,* carry the legal definition one step further and write[73]:

> Although classification of surgery as 'necessary' or 'unnecessary' is largely a matter of medical judgment to be exercised under the facts of each case, there are nevertheless specific criteria which have been refined—and undoubtedly will be further refined—for the purpose of identifying surgical procedures which are performed without reasonable indications. Foremost among such surgical procedures are various gynecologic operations.

Other observers of the discussions about unnecessary surgery have provided interesting viewpoints. Annas states[5]:

> Continued debate about unnecessary surgery serves only to cloud the real issues. The term has become little more than a political slogan. The real issues of quality control, including certification, monitoring, and discipline of negligent surgeons, cost control, and patient access to information should be addressed directly.

Pauly has argued[91]

> ...that much of the confusion results from a failure of most medical or public health experts to state clearly what is meant by 'unnecessary surgery.' The problem is not, however, that the experts know what unnecessary surgery is, and have been unable or unwilling to communicate it, but, rather, that medicine as a discipline cannot generate either the conceptual apparatus or the complete information set needed to arrive at a general definition.

In a recent article Schacht and Pemberton write[113]:

> As the debate now stands, the grounds remain problematical for accepting any of a range of expert opinions over the views of consumers or indeed, for accepting the views of one expert over another. Judgements about the necessity (or otherwise) of particular instances of surgery are always, at least in principle, open to debate. Consequently, those who would claim that X is (or is not) an instance of unnecessary surgery should expose their assumptions, arguments, and evidence to critical scrutiny in a "public" forum... this could well be done in the context of an audit by a review committee.

Patient Perspective

For the patient the ultimate definition of unnecessary surgery depends on how well the surgical procedure alleviated the disease process. A procedure that is indicated clearly in the mind of the physician but does not help control the patient's suffering conceivably can be thought of as unnecessary by the patient. For instance, a cholecystectomy that fails to alleviate abdominal distress, although clinically indicated by the presence of cholelithiasis, nonetheless might be considered unjustifiable by the patient if his or her symptoms remain.

An unnecessary operation may seem very necessary beforehand, and the risks of not performing it far outweigh those of surgical intervention. Yet in retrospect it might be considered unnecessary by the expert witness. The problem remains that medicine is a semiexact scientific discipline. It would be nice to always have the advantage of hindsight; unfortunately, this is not possible.

The preceding attempts to define unnecessary surgery should not be misconstrued as recommendations but, rather, should be considered illustrations of the current problem. The debate about unnecessary surgery will not be settled until there is agreement on a clearer definition of the term. This will require that the indications for procedures be drawn with more precision than they are now. For the present there remains no generally acceptable means of assessing what percentage of operations is unnecessary.

MONITORING SURGICAL PROCEDURES
Hospital Tissue Committees

One of the early ways in which hospitals and their staffs attempted to monitor so-called unwarranted surgical procedures was through the use of the hospital tissue committee. This methodology is the forerunner of today's concepts of quality assurance and utilization review. Myers, in discussing tissue committees, noted the limitations placed on them by only examining the pathologic specimen[86]:

> The present misconception concerning the relationship of normal tissue rates to the justification of surgery stems from the now disproved theories of pioneers in hospital standardization who stated that the incidence of removal of normal tissue was an indication of unnecessary surgery and should not exceed ten percent . . . a normal tissue rate is not the sole criterion of the justification for surgery. This can be determined not only by the physician's evaluation of the clinical indications for surgery in each case.

It always intrigued me that as a general surgical resident I was constantly taught that 10% to 20% of exploratory laparotomies for presumed appendicitis should show normal pathology. The rationale for this was that a lower percentage indicated an overly cautious surgeon who did not operate in the early stages of the disease. If the percentage was higher, it meant the surgeon was too aggressive, and unnecessary laparotomies were performed. I would think that the percentage of negative laparotomies for presumed appendicitis should be as close to zero as possible. At the same time, there should be an effort to reduce morbidity from perforated appendicitis. It seems a foolish assumption to aim for anything less than perfect diagnostic evaluation. This is an impossible task, but why start the examination process under the ludicrous assumption that the surgeon will be wrong one of five times and view this as perfectly acceptable.

Among the first studies to demonstrate the effectiveness of hospital tissue committees in raising surgical standards was one completed by Weinert and Brill in 1952.[135] They showed that the percentage of appendectomies censured fell from 25% to 10% after the formation of their hospital's tissue committee. As a result there were fewer unnecessary emergency surgical operations at their hospital.

Henley et al. showed that with formation of a tissue committee, improvements were noted in the thoroughness of physical examination, frequency of consultation, quality of operation, and preoperative and postoperative care.[55] In 1958 Verda and Platt demonstrated that after implementation of a tissue committee, there was a 60% decrease in the number of appendectomies, although surgical admission rates remained constant.[132] Concurrently there was an increase of common bile duct explorations from 9% to 32% and an increase in operative chlangiograms from none to 17%. In another review of tissue committees, there was a decrease in noninflamed appendices noted on pathologic examination from 36% to 16% over 3 years.[118]

A study from Saskatchewan showed how the utilization of a combined physician-consumer-based tissue committee to monitor hysterectomies contributed to a decrease in the average proportion of unjustified hysterectomies from 24% to 8% over 5 years.[35] Overall, the absolute number of hysterectomies in the province dropped by 33% during the study. Wennberg et al. have demonstrated that the feedback of population-based data on the incidence of tonsillectomy and/or adenoidectomy to surgeons with the highest rates of performance resulted in significant decreases in their future tonsillectomy rates.[138]

Hospital Utilization Studies

In addition to tissue committee monitoring, both retrospective chart reviews and hospital utilization studies have been performed to analyze unnecessary surgical rates. The earliest such review was by Miller in 1946.[83] Although it was poorly controlled with no statistical analysis and a small operative group, he showed that 17% of women who underwent hysterectomy had no preoperative complaints, 19% manifested no pathologic findings on pelvic examination, and 31% had no abnormal histopathology on removal of the organ. Overall, one of six patients had no symptoms, no suspected disease on pelvic examination, and no microscopic evidence of disease. In the early 1950s Doyle published two reports that showed 48% of ovariectomies and 39% of hysterectomies to be unnecessary.[31,32]

Lembcke measured the quality of medical care through vital statistics based on hospital service areas.[66] He noted that considerably more appendectomies were performed than appeared indicated. Excesses of 25% to 100% were described. Interestingly, for areas with a low incidence of surgical operations for appendicitis, there was no evidence that it was associated with high death rates from misdiagnosed appendicitis.

The two Trussell et al. reports from the mid-1960s studied the quantity, quality, and costs of medical and hospital care received by a sample of teamsters' families in the New York City area.[128] More than 30% of hysterectomies were judged to be unnecessary, and 33% of the general surgical admissions were believed to be unnecessary. These studies have been justifiably criticized in that only one gynecologist was utilized as the chart reviewer for all of the hysterectomy cases. His indications for operation have been considered much too specific, because he believed that it was essential for a woman to have a dilation and curettage followed by an observation period of at least 1 week before a hysterectomy could be performed. If this sequence was not followed, the hysterectomy was labeled as "unwarranted."

Morton et al. evaluated the utilization of surgical beds in 1968.[84] Three reviewers agreed with the appropriateness of 85% of the elective admissions and 67% of the emergency surgical admissions. However, there was agreement in only 41% of the urgent admissions.

In response to the two Trussell et al. reports, committees were established by the New York State Medical Society to study cholecystectomies and hysterectomies.[87,88] Quality of care was assessed, leaving cost as another issue. Only 2% of the cholecystectomies and 3% of the hysterectomies were judged to have received inadequate or unacceptable care. It was also noted that the quality of care was higher in the voluntary and city hospitals than in the proprietary hospitals.

In a similar investigation, the Ohio chapter of the American College of Surgeons judged the necessity of 28,621 cholecystectomies performed from 1962 to 1966.[6] They found an overall mortality of 1.8%, with acute cholecystitis present in 15% of cases. Overall, cholelithiasis was noted in 93% of the gallbladders.

Peer Review

Fine and Morehead studied peer review of hysterectomy, appendectomy, and prostatectomy in New York City hospitals.[45] Case records were reviewed by board-certified surgical specialists. The findings showed that 86% and 91% of the appendectomy and prostatectomy admissions, respectively, were judged satisfactory. However, more than 50% of the hysterectomy admissions were considered unsatisfactory. As a conclusion, the authors stated that although the quality of professional care in other hospitals is not less competent in certain categories, the teaching hospital was clearly superior overall.

A study of pediatric surgical inpatient care reported in 1972 showed that 11% of all surgical admissions were considered to be unnecessary, and 16% of all surgical patients were deemed to have questionable management.[33] Of pediatric urologic patients, 67% were considered to have undergone improper therapy. A follow-up to this study demonstrated little change in the percentage of unnecessary surgical admissions and improper patient management except for urology, which had decreased to 53% improper therapy.[34]

Retrospective Chart Reviews

Two studies from the mid-1970s conducted by Emerson utilized chart review in an effort to determine whether unnecessary surgery was present.[41,42] He reported that less than 1% of cholecystectomies were unnecessary, with similarly low percentages noted for hysterectomies, meniscectomies, tonsillectomies, and appendectomies. In these studies the concept of "pre-set criteria" was introduced as the basis on which to study the incidence of unjustified surgery. Retrospective reviews were done by measuring the indications for surgery against preestablished criteria of the Joint Commission on the Accreditation of Hospitals, Performance Evaluation Procedure Medical Care Audit, and the Quality Criteria Predictors of Hospital Care of the Medical Society of the State of New York. These criteria are extremely broad, and they include a wide spectrum of indications. This was reflected in the low rate of unjustified procedures that was found. Whether this is a true accounting of unnecessary surgery depends on how willing one is to accept the operative indications that Emerson utilized.

LoGerfo et al. were able to document only 32% of children undergoing tonsillectomy to have met commonly promulgated indications for surgery.[71] It was concluded that a major reduction in the frequency of this procedure would be brought about by development of an audit strategy that assumed the indications stated by the surgeon met commonly recommended guidelines.

Pantell and Irwin studied the incidence of appendectomies during a physician boycott in 1975 and noted no appreciable change in the number of appendectomies performed during the boycott month when compared with a 6-month baseline period.[89] Similarly, no differences were noted in the percentage of affected appendices that had become perforated. These findings suggest that if unwarranted appendectomies were being performed before the boycott, the number must have been small.

In one of the few papers published by a Professional Standards Review Organization concerning surgical procedures, the Colorado Foundation for Medical Care studied 13 surgical operations to determine if they were performed in accordance with appropriate indications.[40] Of the 4850 cases, 97% either met indications for these procedures or were justified by physician review.

Criteria for chart review. Chart review by preestablished criteria is an attractive measure, because the methodology itself entails the formulation of guidelines and definitions of what is to be considered necessary. However, a number of criticisms have become apparent as more of these studies are published. Variations in the "tightness" of the criteria and in the stringency with which they are applied can result in different findings. Unless the indications are clear-cut, it is difficult to judge a chart adequately. Second, the background of the chart reviewer should be within the specialty of the procedure under review. Often this is not the case. For instance, the 1972 and 1975 reports on pediatric surgical inpatient care were completed without input from either a general surgeon or a pediatric surgeon.[33, 34] Instead, the patient reviews were performed by an internist or by a pediatrician who consulted the surgical literature for appropriate guidelines.

Criticism. In addition to the previously listed criticisms concerning studies of hospital utilization, a number of reports have investigated the entire area of peer evaluation and have demonstrated flaws that exist in attempting to achieve a consensus with regard to chart review. As early as 1957 Rosenfeld showed only 33% agreement among surgical specialists in their rating of surgical care according to chart review.[100]

DeRouville in 1971 found that in peer-judgment review, raters tended to change their self-imposed criteria for judging quality of care.[28] An audit was performed by 20 board-certified or board-qualified general surgeons who were in active clinical practice. There was a consistent trend toward more "unsatisfactory" reviews as the study progressed. it was one judge's opinion that in later reviews the surgeons unwittingly began to apply new criteria, and this was tied in directly with an increased compensation for previous leniency in ratings. As part of the same study, a second review of 50 cases that previously had been judged to be 4% unsatisfactory revealed a 26% unsatisfactory rating. It became apparent that there was a substantial degree of intraobserver and interobserver variation. The conclusion was that a review mechanism that relies on pure peer judgment by multiple assessors is a highly unsatisfactory tool for measuring the quality of medical care and for determining unwarranted surgery within a large population of cases. Therefore, to initiate a widespread state or national program of systematic review based on a method of peer chart judgment would not be desirable.

Richardson in 1972 showed that when surgeons were asked to separately review the hospital records of patients who had undergone surgical procedures, their judgments were far from uniform.[96] Eight of the surgical judges believed that 1 or 2 of 10 charts were unsatisfactory, 6 of the reviewers considered 2 or 3 of the charts to be unsatisfactory, 5 of the surgeons judged 3 or 4 of the charts as poor, 1 surgeon considered 4 or 5 of the charts as unsatisfactory, and the final reviewer judged 7 or 8 of the 10 charts as being unsatisfactory. Statistical analysis demonstrated that 21 surgical and 28 gynecologic reviewers would be required to produce a composite judgment of the quality of care of a single patient with a 95% confidence level. Clearly, it would be logistically impossible to provide such levels of surgical decision making for every patient in this country.

Rutkow reported three randomized mail surveys of surgical specialists (both national and international) that attempted to determine variations in clinical decision making for seven elective surgical operations.[103,104,108,109] A marked divergence of opinion concerning the need for surgery was evident. It remains an open question whether the magnitude of interobserver and intraobserver variation shown in these reports can be related to concerns about unnecessary surgery.

Geographic Variation

Although the preceeding tissue committee reports and peer review and chart evaluations are open to criticism, there are other types of investigations that purport to show a question of unnecessary surgery in the United States. Unexplained variations in surgical rates across geographic areas have been documented during the past 50 years.[130] These differences have been studied internationally, nationally, regionally, and locally. In 1965 Logan and Eimerl demonstrated wide variations in surgical rates between Canada, England, Sweden, and the United States for removal of hemorrhoids, tonsils, uteri, gallbladders, prostates, and varicose veins.[69] Vayda showed that surgical rates in Canada were 1.8 times greater for men and 1.6 times greater for women than in England and Wales. Bunker's classic study noted that per capita the Untied States had twice as many surgeons as England and Wales and twice the number of operations performed per population.[129] A more recent report by Vayda and Rutkow showed that surgical rates in the United States were 43% greater than in Canada and 125% greater than in England and Wales in 1976.[131]

Variations at the regional and local level have been well documented. Analysis of the records of the Blue Cross Association in Kansas showed a threefold to fourfold variation in state regional rates for the performance of six common elective surgical procedures.[68] In Massachusetts a fourfold variation in the tonsillectomy rate from one community to the next was noted.[7] Wennberg and Gittelsohn have reported extreme variations, as much as 1000%, in the patterns of use of nine common surgical procedures in Vermont and Maine.[136,137] In Wisconsin, Detmer and Tyson analyzed population-based surgical rates for primary appendectomy, cholecystectomy, herniorrhaphy, and tonsillectomy. Variations of as much as 800% in the rates of the procedures were found, even within large planning districts.[29]

McPherson et al. have examined small-area variations in the use of common surgical procedures among New England, England, and Norway.[80, 81] The degree of variation generally appeared to be more characteristic of the procedure than of the country in which it was performed.

Assessing Surgical Rates

It is probably not unreasonable to assume that a multitude of factors contribute to variations in surgical rates. Such differences in themselves, however, cannot be taken to mean that unnecessary surgery is performed in those countries with higher rates. Because there are currently no guidelines for determining which of the surgical rates are the most appropriate, could not, in fact, the higher rates represent the meeting of previously unmet needs for surgery? Conversely, it can be argued that because areas with lower rates of surgery do not appear to have significantly higher mortality than the areas with higher surgical rates, the higher rates represent unneeded surgery? However, the mortality argument can be countered because so few of the operations are a matter of life or death. Roos et al. reviewed this question of varying surgical rates and its relation to quality of care.[98, 99] They concluded that the complexity of physician practice patterns challenges the simplistic assumption that high elective surgical rates indicate lowered standards of practice.

"Population at risk" factor. Gittlesohn and Wennberg have proposed the important concept of "population at risk of organ loss" as a major factor in determining true surgical rates.[52] This principle simply reflects that once a person has undergone an operation for removal of an organ, he or she can no longer be considered at risk for a similar procedure. Consequently, they should not be considered in the population at further risk. This becomes important when it is realized that Walker and Jick showed that the estimated fraction of the United States' women with uterus intact by age 60 was only 64%.[133] Similar conclusions were reached by Koepsell et al.[64] Additional estimations should be performed for a wide range of the other most common operations currently performed, such as cataract extraction, herniorrhaphy, and prostatectomy.

Two investigations were completed to understand future rates of total hip arthroplasty and cardiac surgery. It was estimated that there was a true requirement of more than 100,000 total hip arthroplasties needed per year in this country.[82] This is well above current figures, and in 1982 it was estimated that direct medical costs for this operation alone would exceed 1 billion dollars annually. Conversely, it was found that further growth in the number of cardiac centers in the United States should be avoided because rates of operation will level off.[63]

Payment schemes. Another frequently cited indicator of unnecessary surgery is the difference in surgical rates among similar populations when they receive surgical care under varied payment schemes. In one of the earliest studies to investigate this issue, Densen et al. analyzed two populations receiving surgical care through fee-for-service solo practice or on a prepaid basis.[27] When the data were classified into admissions that involved surgery and those without surgery, the biggest difference between the two plans occurred among female surgical patients. The prepaid group's admission rates were lower at all age groups.

Six years later Perott also demonstrated that prepaid health plans had lower surgical rates than did the fee-for-service mode.[94] He considered the hospital experience of federal employees covered under different insurance plans. In comparing the rates of hospitalization for surgery, the data showed a tonsillectomy rate for the government Blue Shield plan more than 2½ times that of the prepaid group practice plan; for various types of gynecologic surgery it was 1½ times that of the group practice; and an appendectomy rate was twice that of the prepaid enrollees. For all surgical procedures, the Blue Shield insured employees had a rate of 7000 per 100,000 covered persons, while the prepaid practice had a rate of 3900.

Gaus et al. compared a health maintenance organization's performance with that of a fee-for-service system for Medicaid patients.[49] The prepaid group had a surgical admission rate of 24,000 per 100,000 population, while the fee-for-service rate was 82,000 per 100,000 population.

Wilson and Longmire found that the method of surgeon payment influenced several important aspects of surgical care.[142] In appendicitis, there was a trend of fee-for-service physicians to undertake earlier surgical exploration, which resulted in fewer secondary complications. Operative workloads were highest for surgeons receiving a salary plus a percentage in fee-for-service group practice.

LoGerfo et al. assessed the care received by persons enrolled in either a large prepaid group practice or in a prepaid independent practice setting in which surgeons were reimbursed on a fee-for-service basis.[70,72] It was found that for quite similar low-income enrollee groups with full prepaid benefits, the frequency of appendectomy, tonsillectomy, cholecystectomy, and hysterectomy was much higher under the plan in which physicians were reimbursed on a fee-for-service basis.

Although the majority of studies support the hypothesis that enrollees in prepaid insurance plans have lower surgical utilization rates than do member in fee-for-service systems, there are some investigations that refute these findings. Perkoff et al. found prepaid enrollees to use the same or more surgical care than did fee-for-service members.[92,93] Similarly, Scitovsky and McCall demonstrated that surgical admission rates were higher for a fee-for-service group plan when contrasted to a prepaid Kaiser plan.[116] However, when surgical procedures performed in the hospital on a nonadmission basis are added to surgical admissions, the surgical rates under the two plans became almost identical.

In a recent study, Robinson et al. showed that competitive pressures encourage hospitals to accommodate surgical patient and physician preferences for longer lengths of stay.[97] Increases in length of stay were identified for total hip replacement, prostatectomy, hysterectomy, cholecystectomy, herniorrhaphy, appendectomy, and coronary artery bypass surgery. It was concluded that there is a strong association between the number of hospital competitors in the local market and the average length of stay in United States hospitals.

Although one possible explanation for the lower surgical rates observed in prepaid group practices is that the absence of a financial incentive for overutilization reduces the amount of unnecessary surgery performed, a counter explanation can be offered: the prepaid system might be denying some patients surgery that is appropriate. Competitive pressures have begun to have enormous impact on utilization of surgical services, and these differences will need further investigation. Either way, the use of such variation data alone as a definite indicator of unnecessary surgery is precluded by the absence of a definition of what the appropriate or correct rates of surgery are.

Second opinion programs. The final set of data that many individuals have utilized to confirm the presence of unnecessary surgery is in reference to surgical second opinion programs. These presurgical screening programs, first reported by McCarthy and Widmer in 1974, rely on a board-certified surgeon's evaluation of the necessity for elective surgery after the patient initially has been recommended to undergo an operation.[79]

There has been a tremendous proliferation of such programs throughout the country. The findings have been both controversial and contradictory.[51,78,90] The data from McCarthy's group have shown an overall nonconfirmation rate of approximately 18%. Perhaps the most startling of their findings is that more than 10% of the patients who were confirmed for operation by two surgeons elected not to undergo the procedure. It is not known what effect this delay has on the economic aspects of the patients' future surgical health care.

From the standpoint of unnecessary surgery, the most difficult problem with surgical second opinion programs is the general feeling that nonconfirmation rates can be used as a measure of unwarranted surgery. It was the original McCarthy figure of 18% that the Moss subcommittee used to calculate the number of unnecessary operations (2,380,000) in the United States for 1974.[21] However, a critical analysis of this report and the misapplication of nonconfirmation rates reveal inevitable inaccuracies, statistical manipulations, and inappropriate extrapolations. McCarthy is the first to admit that the results from surgical second opinion programs cannot be used to justify any estimation of unnecessary surgery. At best, the figures represent the concept of "deferred surgery."

The fact that one surgeon believes a given patient needs surgery and a second surgeon believes the opposite or that the procedure should be deferred for now does not indicate that the second opinion was correct and that the first was incorrect. It would be foolish to equate a recommendation for operation that is not confirmed with one that is definitely unjustified or unwarranted.

Recent attempts to monitor the delivery of surgical health care and unnecessary surgery involves the establishment of professional review organizations.[124] To date there have been few published results of their audits in peer-reviewed journals. For this reason the validity of this method to study unnecessary surgery remains unknown.

Cost/Benefit Analysis

The debate about unnecessary surgery has direct ties to the fundamental goal of all medical care, that is, to improve the quality of life. It is also evident that this precept must now be accomplished within the parameters of a cost-effective health care delivery system. One way in which cost containment had been applied to the question of unnecessary surgery was the extensive use of cost/benefit analysis.[8-10] Cost/benefit analysis was originally a systematic method of setting out the relevant factors for choosing among alternative public works projects. With the burgeoning cost of medical care, the concept of cost/benefit analysis was extended to the health delivery field.[134] Surgical therapy, because of its discreteness, accomplishments, and cost, is particularly suited for such analysis.

The basic rule is that a surgical operation should be supported if benefits exceed the costs. Therefore a complete analysis attempts to identify all benefits and costs in economic or dollar terms. The best example of cost/benefit analyses applied to surgical therapy is the 1977 monograph by Bunker et al., *Costs, Risks, And Benefits Of Surgery*.[16] This elaborate text is comprehensive in scope and provides a thorough discussion of the entire subject. Among the operations that were assessed are inguinal herniorrhaphy, cholecystectomy, hysterectomy, appendectomy, mastectomy, and coronary artery bypass.

Unfortunately, the concept of cost/benefit analysis as applied to the delivery of surgical health care has serious limitations. For instance, in health-related statistics, the more precise data usually are available only for the immediate and past hospitalization experience as opposed to future events. Estimates of long-term changes in cost involve many unpredictable factors, and long-range planning becomes difficult. Further, separate costs and benefits are often so numerous that it is difficult to take them all into account. Benefits mean more than just survival or a decrease in morbidity but include quality of life and other unmeasurable effects. The relevant cost figures extend far beyond the direct fees of hospitals and physicians. These perplexities make utilization of cost/benefit analysis in the debate about unnecessary surgery a complicated task. Perhaps that is why so few investigations continue into cost/benefit analysis as it relates to surgery.

Socioeconomic Factors

Socioeconomic status is an important variable that affects medical care. It has been shown that poor people often carry a burden of ill health far greater than those living in better circumstances. However, there is no reason to suppose that certain pathologic conditions in need of surgical intervention, such as appendicitis, cholecystitis, prostatism, and cataract formation, should have a predilection for individuals at a particular socioeconomic level. Unfortunately, certain critics of surgery in the United States say that it is the lower socioeconomic classes who suffer most from unnecessary surgery. Several studies discuss this issue.

Bunker and Brown assessed the alleged overuse of surgical services in the United States, which is often attributed to lack of consumer education.[17] Assuming that physicians are the most educated group about medical problems, these authors examined the use of surgical services by physicians and their families and compared it with lawyers, ministers, and businessmen. It was found that surgical rates for physicians and their families were as high or higher than other groups. Overall, surgical rates for the four groups were estimated to be 30% higher than those for the country as a whole. It was concluded that as the public became better informed about surgical services, the demand for surgery would increase.

Bombardier et al. showed the opposite correlation with education.[11] In addition, they noted a large increase in utilization of surgery among economically disadvantaged groups, the aged, lower-educated groups, and nonwhites during the 1960s. Scott and Mackie, in a similar report, noted many frequently performed surgical procedures to have the same rate of operation for all socioeconomic levels.[117] Horne and Beck investigated the utilization of health services leading to cholecystectomy and noted that presurgical and surgical decisions were influenced by extramedical factors.[59] Among these were the social condition of the patient and the overall availability of health resources.

An analysis of the race and economic status of surgical patients and who performed their surgery concluded that blacks were more likely than whites to be under the care of surgeons in training.[38] Unfortunately, the only surgical operations analyzed in this report were inguinal herniorrhaphy and cholecystectomy. Whether this finding would be present for more complicated operations, for example, coronary artery bypass, was not studied.

That poor people may be more apt to have as their primary surgeon an individual in training was not a new or unexpected finding. The important question is whether patients taken care of by resident surgeons have better or worse outcomes than those under treatment by staff physicians. Kurtz and Wise have investigated this question and have shown that performance of gallbladder surgery by a surgeon in training with appropriate supervision did not have an adverse effect on the outcome of that surgery.[65]

In an interesting sociologic treatise on surgeons in training, Bosk in his book *Forgive And Remember: Managing Medical Failure* explored the way surgeons recognize, categorize, and punish surgical errors.[12] In doing so, he analyzes social control within the surgical community. Most significantly, he found that errors of judgment and skill that harm patients were considered less serious by a surgeon's peers than forms of uncooperative behavior that indicate that a surgeon in training does not acknowledge the standards and authority of his superordinates.

RECOMMENDATIONS

Egdahl has provided an extensive essay on the way in which surgeons can increase the efficiency of their use of hospitals.[39] In this way unnecessary surgery can be decreased. A large portion of this efficiency involves postsurgical care. Schoonhoven et al. have rated the complexity and uncertainty of surgical procedures and postsurgical care as to provide a means to better anticipate staffing needs on surgical floors.[115]

Cost of elective surgery and utilization of ancillary services are major problems when dealing with unnecessary surgery. Schwartz et al. investigated the effect of a 30% reduction in physician fees on Medicaid surgery rates in Massachusetts.[120] Although arguments could be made as to whether rates should increase or decrease, in the final analysis there was little change in any operative rates. It would appear that if unnecessary surgery was practiced financial remuneration did not appear to play as prominent a role as some individuals believe.[2]

In the final analysis, any discussion concerning unnecessary surgery must revert to the surgeon. Fuchs makes the point that surgeons induce their own demand for surgery.[48] In a paper from 1978 he presents a multiequation, multivariate analysis of differences in the supply of surgeons and the demand for operations across geographical areas of the United States in 1963 and 1970. His results support the hypothesis that surgeons shift the demand for operations. Thus, all things being equal a 10% increase in the surgeon/population ratio results in about a 3% increase in per capita utilization. Moreover, differences in supply seem to have an unlikely effect on fees, in that they are raised when the surgeon/population ratio increases.

These findings were reemphasized by Cromwell and Mitchell.[25] Their results provide definite support for the notion of competitive market failure when surgical health care delivery is involved. However, their shift elasticities were not as large as Fuchs' findings.

The presence of a physician-induced demand for surgery runs counter to what Rutkow has demonstrated utilizing data from the National Center for Health Statistics.[102,107,111] He has shown a decrease in age/sex standardized operative rates since the mid-1970s. This comes at a time when the supply of surgeons has dramatically increased. If there is a surgeon-induced demand for operations, it is not apparent in Rutkow's macrodatabase, which extends from 1970 to 1985.

One of the more interesting aspects of the debate about unnecessary surgery concerns the relationship between operative volume and mortality.* There have been many investigations of this question, and the concept of regionalization of health care has been touted as the answer. In 1979 Luft et al. found that the mortality of open heart surgery, vascular surgery, and transurethral resection of the prostate decreased with increasing numbers of operations performed.[75] Hospitals in which 200 or more of these procedures were done annually had death rates 25% to 41% lower than hospitals with smaller surgical volumes. Some procedures, such as cholecystectomy and vagotomy, demonstrated no relation between volume and mortality. These findings have been reemphasized in another investigation that analyzed surgical volume and incidence of postoperative wound infection. Farber et al. found a highly significant inverse relation between the frequency of operation and the infection rate for appendectomy, herniorrhaphy, cholecystectomy, colon resection, and abdominal hysterectomy.[43] Although the data clearly demonstrated higher morbidity in hospitals performing relatively little surgery, there were several possible explanations. As a result, no conclusions for surgical health care policy were drawn.

In concluding this discussion of unnecessary surgery, it becomes obvious that many questions remain unanswered. Numerous studies have been published that attempt to describe the amount of unnecessary surgery currently performed, but all are subject to major criticisms. The lack of a precise definition of what unnecessary surgery truly is continues to be the most

---

*References 18, 36, 37, 46, 47, 60, 62, 74, 76, 77, 119, 121-123.

imposing obstacle in the entire discussion.

Is the likelihood that an operation will lead to a more comfortable, useful, and rewarding life sufficient reason to justify accepting risks of death of 1 in a 1000, 1 in a 100 or 1 in 10? Will it ever be possible to achieve a consensus on what constitutes unnecessary surgery?

The most accurate statement of the problem appears to be that unnecessary surgery exists but to what extent remains uncertain. Both the patient and surgeon deserve the facts, but until further research on surgical health care delivery and unnecessary surgery can be carried out, the many questions that surround this controversial subject will remain unanswered.

References

1. American College of Surgeons: Statement of unnecessary surgery, Bull Am Coll Surg 63:8, 1978.
2. American College of Surgeons: Effects of withholding elective operations on surgical utilization rates, Bull Am Coll Surg 64:27, 1979.
3. American College of Surgeons: Statement on unnecessary surgery, American College of Surgeons' Reports, August, 1983.
4. American College of Surgeons—American Surgical Association: The study on surgical services for the United States, Chicago, 1975.
5. Annas GS: The extravagant, wasteful and superfluous debate about unnecessary surgery, Hastings Cent Rep 9:13, 1979.
6. Arnold DJ: 28,621 cholecystectomies in Ohio, Am J Surg 119:714, 1970.
7. Baldwin AD: Tonsillectomy and adenoidectomy in Massachusetts, N Engl J Med 285:1537, 1971.
8. Barnes BA: Cost-benefit analysis of surgery: current accomplishments and limitations, Am J Surg 133:438, 1977.
9. Barnes BA: Evaluation of surgical therapy by cost-benefit analysis, Surgery 82:21, 1977.
10. Barnes BA: Cost-benefit and cost-effective analysis in surgery, Surg Clin North Am 62:737, 1982.
11. Bombardier C et al: Socioeconomic factors affecting the utilization of surgical operations, N Engl J Med 297:699, 1977.
12. Bosk CL: Forgive and remember: managing medical failure, Chicago, 1979, University of Chicago.
13. Bowman JG: Hospital standardization, Bull Am Coll Surg, 1920.
14. Brody JE: Incompetent surgery is found not isolated, The New York Times, Jan 27, 1976.
15. Bunker JP: Surgical manpower: a comparison of operations and surgeons in the United States and in England and Wales, N Engl J Med 282:135, 1970.
16. Bunker JP, Barnes B, and Mosteller F, editors: Cost, risks and benefits of surgery, New York, 1977, Oxford University Press, Inc.
17. Bunker JP and Brown BW: The physician-patient as an informed consumer of surgical services, N Engl J Med 290:1051, 1974.
18. Bunker JP, Luft HS, and Enthoven A: Should surgery be regionalized? Surg Clin North Am 62:657, 1982.
19. Carey L: Unnecessary surgery: has the controversy been blown out of true perspective? Med Opinion 6:18, 1977.
20. Codman EA: The product of a hospital, Surg Gynecol Obstet 18:491, 1914.
21. Cost and quality of health care: unnecessary surgery, Report by the Subcommittee on Oversight and Investigations of the Committee on Interstate and Foreign Commerce, Washington, DC, 1976.
22. Coyne PS: May I cut in? Unnecessary surgery in America. Private Practice 7:12, 1975.
23. Crile G: The surgeon's dilemma; the built-in conflict in medical fees, Harper's Magazine, May 1975.
24. Crile G: Surgeons are the best judges of surgery, Mod Med, Aug 1, 1976.
25. Cromwell J and Mitchell JB: Physician-induced demand for surgery, J Health Econ 5:293, 1986.
26. Denenberg HS: A shopper's guide to surgery, Conn Med 37:321, 1973.
27. Densen PM et al: Prepaid medical care and hospital utilization in a dual choice situation, Am J Public Health 50:170, 1960.
28. deRouville WH: Peer review in biliary tract surgery, NY State J Med 71:1544, 1971.
29. Detmer DE and Tyson TJ: Regional differences in surgical care based upon uniform physician and hospital discharge abstract data, Ann Surg 187:166, 1978.
30. Dickinson RL: Standardization of surgery: an attack on the problem, JAMA 63:763, 1914.
31. Doyle JV: Unnecessary ovariectomies, JAMA 148:1105, 1952.
32. Doyle JV: Unnecessary hysterectomies, JAMA 151:360, 1953.
33. Duff RS, et al: Use of utilization review to assess the quality of pediatric inpatient care, Pediatrics 49:169, 1972.
34. Duff RS et al: A review of pediatric inpatient care, Am J Dis Child 129:1422, 1975.
35. Dyck FJ et al: Effect of surveillance on the number of hysterectomies in the province of Saskatchewan, N Engl J Med 296:1326, 1977.

36. Eastaugh SR: Cost of elective surgery and utilization of ancillary services in teaching hospitals, Health Serv Res 14:290, 1979.
37. Eastaugh SR: Organizational determinants of surgical lengths of stay, Inquiry 17:85, 1980.
38. Egbert LD and Rothman IL: Relation between the race and economic status of patients and who performs their surgery, N Engl J Med 297:90, 1977.
39. Egdahl R: Ways for surgeons to increase the efficiency of their use of hospitals, N Engl J Med 309:1184, 1983.
40. Elliot RV, Kahn KA, and Kaye R: Physicians measure up: a study of 13 surgical procedures, JAMA 245:595, 1981.
41. Emerson R: Unjustified surgery, fact or myth? NY State J Med 76:454, 1976.
42. Emerson R and Creedon JJ: Unjustified surgery dilemma: second opinion versus present criteria, NY State J Med 77:779, 1977.
43. Farber BF, Kaiser DL, and Wenzel RP: Relation between surgical volume and incidence of postoperative wound infection, N Engl J Med 305:200, 1981.
44. Ficarra BJ: Surgical and allied malpractice, Springfield, Ill, 1968, Charles C Thomas, Publisher.
45. Fine J and Morehead MA: Study of peer review of inhospital patient care, NY State J Med 71:804, 1971.
46. Flood AB, Scott WR, and Ewy D: Does practice make perfect? I. The relation between hospital volume and outcomes for selected diagnostic categories, Med Care 22:98, 1984.
47. Flood AB, Scott WR, and Ewy D: Does practice make perfect? II. The relation between volumes and outcomes and other hospital characteristics, Med Care 22:115, 1984.
48. Fuchs VR: The supply of surgeons and the demand for operations, J Human Resources 13(supplement):36, 1978.
49. Gaus CR, Cooper BS, and Hirschman C: Contrasts in HMO and fee-for-service performance, Soc Secur Bull 39:3, 1976.
50. Gertman PM and Mitchell JB: Surgical care: a policy focus of the 1980s, Med Care 18:881, 1980.
51. Gertman PM et al: Second opinions for elective surgery: the mandatory Medicaid program in Massachusetts, N Engl J Med 302:1169, 1980.
52. Gittelsohn AM and Wennberg J: On the risk of organ loss, J chronic Dis 29:527, 1976.
53. Groves EWH: Surgical statistics: a plea for uniform registration of operation results, Br Med J 2:1008, 1908.
54. Haggard WD: The unnecessary operation, Surg Gynecol Obstet 35:820, 1922.
55. Henley PG, Duzan KR, and Robins RB: Use and abuses of the tissue committee, JAMA 168:2243, 1958.
56. Holder AR: Unnecessary surgery, JAMA 213:1755, 1970.
57. Holder AR: Recent decisions on unnecessary surgery, JAMA 22:1593, 1972.
58. Holder AR: Unnecessary surgery, JAMA 232:1059, 1975.
59. Horne JM and Beck RG: Temporal patterns in the use of health services leading to cholecystectomy, Med Care 16:1006, 1978.
60. Hughes RG, Hunt SS, and Luft HS: The effects of low surgeon volume on hospital quality, Med Care 25:489, 1987.
61. Jones J: Plain concise practical remarks on the treatment of wounds and fractures, New York: John Holt, 1775.
62. Kelly JV and Hellinger FJ: Physician and hospital factors associated with mortality of surgical patients, Med Care 24:785, 1986.
63. Kennedy RH et al: Cardiac catheterization and cardiac surgical facilities, N Engl J Med 307:986, 1982.
64. Koepsell TD et al: Prevalence of prior hysterectomy in the Seattle-Tacoma area, Am J Public Health 70:40, 1980.
65. Kurtz LM and Wise L: A study of the impact of resident participation on the results of surgery for cholecystitis, Surgery 86:530, 1979.
66. Lembcke PA: Comparative study of appendectomy rates, Am J Public Health 42:276, 1952.
67. Letourneau CU: The legal and moral aspects of ''unnecessary surgery,'' Hospitals 27:82, 1953.
68. Lewis CE: Variations in the incidence of surgery, N Engl J Med 281:880, 1969.
69. Logan RFL and Eimerl T: Case loads in hospital and general practice in several countries, Milbank Mem Fund Quart 43:302, 1965.
70. LoGerfo JP: Organizational and financial influences on patterns of surgical care, Surg Clin North Am 62:677, 1982.
71. LoGerfo JP et al: Tonsillectomies, adenoidectomies, audits: have surgical indications been met? Med Care 16:950, 1978.
72. LoGerfo JP et al: Rates of surgical care in prepaid group practices and the independent setting: what are the reasons for the differences? Med Care 17:1, 1979.
73. Louisell DW and Williams H: Medical malpractice, New York, 1976, Matthew Bender & Co, Inc.
74. Luft HS: The relation between surgical volume and mortality: an exploration of causal factors and alternative models, Med Care 18:940, 1980.

75. Luft HS, Bunker JP, and Enthoven AC: Should operations be regionalized? The empirical relation between surgical volume and mortality, N Engl J Med 301:1364, 1979.
76. Luft HS, Hunt SS, and Maerki SC: The volume-outcome relationship: practice-makes perfect or selective-referral patterns? Health Serv Res 22:157, 1987.
77. Maerki SC, Luft HS, and Hunt SS: Selecting categories of patients for regionalization: implications of the relationship between volume and outcome, Med Care 24:148, 1986.
78. McCarthy EG and Finkel M: Second opinion elective surgery programs: outcome status over time, Med Care 16:984, 1978.
79. McCarthy EG and Widmer GW: Effects of screening by consultants on recommended elective surgical procedures, N Engl J Med 291:1331, 1974.
80. McPherson K et al: Regional variations in the use of common surgical procedures: within and between England and Wales, Canada and the United States of America, Soc Sci Med 15A:273, 1981.
81. McPherson K et al: Small-area variations in the use of common surgical procedures: an international comparison of New England, England, and Norway, N Engl J Med 307:1310, 1982.
82. Melton LJ et al: Rates of total hip arthroplasty, N Engl J Med 307:1242, 1982.
83. Miller NF: Hysterectomy: therapeutic necessity or surgical racket? Am J Obstet Gynecol 51:804, 1946.
84. Morton JH, William JS, and Kutner FR: Evaluation of surgical bed utilization, Arch Surg 97:395, 1968.
85. Mosteller F: Dilemmas in the concept of unnecessary surgery, J Surg Res 25:185, 1978.
86. Myers RS and Stephenson GW: Evaluation form for tissue committees, JAMA 156:1577, 1954.
87. New York State Medical Society: Report of the cholecystectomy subcommittee of the quality care committee, NY State J Med 26:17, 1970.
88. New York State Medical Society: report of the hysterectomy subcommittee of the quality care committee, NY State J Med 28:17, 1972.
89. Pantell RH and Irwin CE: Appendectomies during physicians' boycott: analysis of surgical care, JAMA 242:1627, 1979.
90. Paris M, Salsberg E, and Berenson L: An analysis of nonconfirmation rates: experiences of a surgical second opinion program, JAMA 242:2424, 1979.
91. Pauly MV: What is unnecessary surgery? Milbank Mem Fund Quart 57:95, 1979.
92. Perkoff GT, Kahl L, and Mackie A: Medical care utilization in an experimental prepaid group practice model in a university medical center, Med Care 12:471, 1974.
93. Perkoff GT et al: Lack of effect of an experimental prepaid group practice on utilization of surgical care, Surgery 77:619, 1975.
94. Perott GS: Federal employees health benefits program: utilization of hospital services, Am J Public Health 56:57, 1966.
95. Pfeutze KD: "Unnecessary surgery": scientifically erroneous testimony in Moss subcommittee hearing, NY State J Med 76:2198, 1976.
96. Richardson FM: Peer review of medical care, Med Care 10:29, 1972.
97. Robinson JC et al: Hospital competition and surgical length of stay, JAMA 259:696, 1988.
98. Roos NP: Who should do surgery? Tonsillectomy-adenoidectomy in one Canadian province, Inquiry 16:73, 1979.
99. Roos NP, Roos LL, and Henteleff PD: Elective surgical rates: do high rates mean lower standards? N Engl J Med 297:360, 1977.
100. Rosenfeld LS: Quality of medical care in hospital, Am J Public Health 47:856, 1957.
101. Rutkow IM: Delivery of surgical health care in the United States, Arch Surg 116:963, 1981.
102. Rutkow IM: Rates of surgery in the United States: the decade of the 1970s, Surg Clin North Am 62:559, 1982.
103. Rutkow IM: The reliability and reproducibility of the surgical decision-making process, Surg Clin North Am 62:721, 1982.
104. Rutkow IM: Surgical decision making; the reproducibility of clinical judgment, Arch Surg 117:337, 1982.
105. Rutkow IM, editor: Surgical health care delivery, Philadelphia, 1982, WB Saunders Co.
106. Rutkow IM: Unnecessary surgery: what is it? Surg Clin North Am 62:613, 1982.
107. Rutkow IM: Surgical operations in the United States, 1979 to 1984, Surgery 101:192, 1987.
108. Rutkow IM, Gittelsohn AM, and Zuidema GD: Surgical decision making: the reliability of clinical judgment, Ann Surg 190:409, 1979.
109. Rutkow IM and Starfield BH: Surgical decision making and operative rates, Arch Surg 119:899, 1984.
110. Rutkow IM and Zuidema GD: "Unnecessary surgery": an update, Surgery 84:671, 1978.
111. Rutkow IM and Zuidema GD: Surgical rates in the United States: 1966-1978, Surgery 89:151, 1981.
112. Sammons JH: Statement by the American Medical Association on unnecessary surgery, J Med Assoc GA 66:633, 1977.
113. Schacht PJ and Pemberton A: What is unnecessary surgery? Who shall decide? Issues of consumer sovereignty, conflict and self-regulation, Soc Sci Med 20:199, 1985.

114. Schlike CP: Doctor, is this operation necessary? Am J Surg 134:3, 1977.
115. Schoonhoven CB et al: Measuring the complexity and uncertainty of surgery and postsurgical care, Med Care 18:893, 1980.
116. Scitovsky AA and McCall N: Use of hospital services under two prepaid plans, Med Care 18:30, 1980.
117. Scott HD and Mackie A: Decisions to hospitalize and operate: a socioeconomic perspective in an urban state, Surgery 77:311, 1975.
118. Sharpe HR: The effect of a tissue committee on appendectomy in a general hospital, Wis Med J 59:135, 1960.
119. Showstack JA et al: Association of volume with outcome of coronary artery bypass graft surgery: scheduled vs nonscheduled operations, JAMA 257:785, 1987.
120. Shwartz M et al: The effect of a 30% reduction in physician fees on Medicaid surgery rates in Massachusetts, Am J Public Health 71:370, 1981.
121. Sloan FA, Perrin JM, and Valvona J: Teaching hospitals' growing surgical caseload, JAMA 254:376, 1985.
122. Sloan FA, Perrin JM, and Valvona J: In-hospital mortality of surgical patients: is there an empirical basis for standard-setting? Surgery 99:446, 1986.
123. Sloan FA, Valvona J, and Perrin JM: Diffusion of surgical technology, J Health Econ 5:31, 1986.
124. Stephens SK and Cleeman JI: Review of surgery: staff paper prepared for the national professional standards review council, J Maine Med Assoc 68:462, 1977.
125. Stephenson GW: The college's role in hospital standardization, Bull Am Coll Surg 66:323, 1981.
126. Stroman DF: The quick knife: unnecessary surgery, USA, Port Washington, 1979, Kennikat Press.
127. Surgical performance: necessity and quality: Report by the Subcommittee on Oversight and Investigations of the Committee on Interstate and Foreign commerce, Washington, DC, 1978.
128. Trussell RE, Morehead MA, and Ehrlich J: The quantity, quality and costs of medical and hospital care secured by a sample of teamster families in the New York area, New York, 1972, 1974, Columbia University School of Public Health and Administrative Medicine.
129. Vayda E: A comparison of surgical rates in Canada and in England and Wales, N Engl J Med 289:1224, 1973.
130. Vayda E and Mindell WR: Variations in operative rates: what do they mean? Surg Clin North Am 62:627, 1982.
131. Vayda E and Rutkow IM: A decade of surgery in Canada, England and Wales and the United States, Arch Surg 117:846, 1982.
132. Verda DJ and Platt WR: The effectiveness of the tissue committee at the Missouri Baptist Hospital, Bull Am Coll Surg 45:124, 1968.
133. Walker Am and Jick H: Temporal and regional variation in hysterectomy rates in the United States, 1970-1975, Am J Epidemiol 110:41, 1979.
134. Warner KE and Hutton R: Cost-benefit and cost-effectiveness analysis in health care, Med Care 18:1069, 1980.
135. Weinert HV and Brill R: Effectiveness of a hospital tissue committee in raising surgical standards, JAMA 150:992, 1952.
136. Wennberg J and Gittelsohn AM: Small area variations in health care delivery, Science 182:1102, 1973.
137. Wennberg J and Gittelsohn AM: Health care delivery in Maine: patterns of use of common surgical procedures, J Maine Med Assoc 66:123, 1975.
138. Wennberg JE et al: Changes in tonsillectomy rates associated with feedback and review, Pediatrics 59:821, 1977.
139. Wetherill HG: A plea for higher hospital efficiency and standardization, Surg Gynecol Obstet 20:705, 1915.
140. Williams G: Unjustified surgery, Harper's Magazine, Feb, 1954.
141. Williams LP: How to avoid unnecessary surgery, Los Angeles, 1971, Nash Publications.
142. Wilson SE and Longmire WP: Does method of payment affect surgical care? J Surg Res 24:457, 1978.
143. Zuidema GD: The study on surgical services for the United States (SOSSUS) and its impact on American surgery, Surg Clin North Am 62:603, 1982.

WARD O. GRIFFEN, JR.

Ward O. Griffen, Jr., born in New Orleans, received his AB degree from Princeton University (1949) and his MD degree from Cornell University Medical College (1953). He took an internship in internal medicine at Bellevue Hospital, Cornell Division (1953-1954). His surgical postgraduate education was at the University of Minnesota (1954-1963) where he received a PhD (1963). From 1962 to 1967, Dr. Griffen was a Markle Scholar in Academic Medicine. He was an assistant professor of surgery at the University of Minnesota (1963-1965), associate professor of surgery and physiology and biophysics at the University of Kentucky (1965-1967), and professor and chairman of surgery and professor of physiology and biophysics at the University of Kentucky (1967-1984). He is currently the Executive Director of the American Board of Surgery and a professor of surgery at the Temple University School of Medicine.

21

Surgical Education and Certification Requirements

WARD O. GRIFFEN, JR.

HISTORICAL BACKGROUND

The education and certification of a specialist in surgery is a unique endeavor. Medicine is a service organization and must serve society in a manner that the society perceives to be appropriate and effective. If medicine is perceived as not properly fulfilling that role, the public and its representatives will seek to change the profession to meet its needs. Thus the education of an individual to the level of a certified specialist will not be complete unless it includes not only the acquisition of adequate scientific knowledge but also a cultivated awareness of societal needs.

Typically, medical students are college graduates who have obtained their degrees in a variety of subjects, mostly scientific but sometimes, and more often in recent years, in less scientific fields. They usually have met the stipulated medical school requirements embracing some study in areas such as mathematics, chemistry, physics, English, and perhaps a foreign language. Although medical education is truly graduate education, it differs enormously from most other graduate education programs. Doctoral programs in basic science, in engineering, and even in the arts are usually a continuum of college education, often conducted in the same college departments. Medical schools, although usually under a university umbrella, are often separate entities both administratively and academically, and their accreditation is obtained through the Liaison Committee for Medical Education (LCME), an agency entirely separate from college and university accrediting bodies. However, medical schools, in which the student spends 4 years, still have education as their primary goal. Successful completion of the 4 years results in a doctor of medicine degree. At the turn of the century and even into the early years of the twentieth century, the MD degree itself or the degree and an additional year of postgraduate study, previously called an internship, represented the completion of medical education. However, during the early years of this century, the seeds for the fully developed medical education system as we know it today were being sown. Even before the Flexner Report,[6] which led to establishing a solid scientific educational base for medical schools, William S. Halsted, influenced by the German apprentice-style system of educating surgeons, organized the first surgical residency program on this continent.

Thus the stage was set for postgraduate surgical education to occur in association with medical schools even though it was often conducted in large public or private hospitals. These composite institutions are now called medical centers. Certainly one of their important responsibilities, if not their primary responsibility, relates more to service than to education. This then is one aspect of postgraduate medical education differentiating it from the educational milieu where the doctor of philosophy degree is pursued. Moreover, residency programs are accredited by yet another body, the Accreditation Council for Graduate Medical Education (ACGME), which is distinct and separate from the LCME. The forerunner of the ACGME was the Advisory Committee that had been established by the American Medical Association in the 1920s. It subsequently changed its name to the Liaison Council for Graduate Medical Education (LCGME) and only recently to its current aforementioned name. This organization over the years established the system of residency review committees (RRC) whose function is to develop the special requirements for training programs in a given specialty. The ACGME establishes the general requirements that delineate training program requirements and responsibilities that are common to all programs and RRCs. The residency review committee for a specialty then develops the special requirements for residencies in that specialty.

In order to complete the understanding of the role of the accrediting and evaluation agencies, it is necessary to relate that the American College of Surgeons was founded in 1913. Because it was concerned with the practice of surgery that was conducted predominantly in hospitals, it followed that the College would concern itself with the quality of hospital care. Hence the College was instrumental in establishing the Joint Commission on Accreditation of Hospitals (JCAH) whose primary activity is to assure the proper function of hospitals as health care facilities. To carry out its charge, the JCAH must inspect hospitals periodically with regard to their administrative organizations, the medical staff, the nursing staff, the ancillary personnel, and related matters. The inspection is usually accomplished by a survey team sent to the hospital. The matter of JCAH accreditation is relevant to postgraduate surgical education: unless a hospital holds such accreditation, no residency within that hospital will receive accreditation by the ACGME.

Finally, in order to complete the background of surgical postgraduate education, it is necessary to describe the development of the specialty boards, and the umbrella organization to which all of the specialty boards belong, the American Board of Medical Specialties (ABMS). Historically, as special areas within medicine emerged and were defined requiring additional training, a mechanism was needed whereby individuals with the appropriate additional training could be suitably identified and recognized. Certifying organizations, termed boards, were organized to this end, conducting examinations and awarding certificates to indicate possession of cognitive knowledge and special skills in a given area that were requisite for establishing oneself as a qualified specialist in that field. A physician certified by a given board is referred to as board certified or as a diplomate of that board. The American Board of Ophthalmology, incorporated in 1917, was the first of these certifying bodies, followed in 1924 by the American Board of Otolaryngology, the American Board of Urology in 1933, and the American Board of Orthopaedic Surgery in 1934.

In 1935 the distinguished Canadian surgeon, Sir Edward W. Archibald, then president of the American Surgical Association, was the first to enunciate the need for a certifying body for general surgery.[4] Shortly thereafter, Dr. Evarts Graham, convinced of the need for such a certification mechanism, approached both the American College of Surgeons and the American Surgical Association for support. The American Surgical Association appointed an ad hoc committee chaired by Dr. Graham to study the situation and report back to the Association. For 2 years there were numerous meetings where many ideas were debated, but eventually a recommendation was made to establish a certifying body. When the committee had determined the structure of the board and procedures for examining applicants, the American Board of Surgery was incorporated on July 19, 1937, in Philadelphia. The first board consisted of 13 members who were sponsored as follows: three members each from the American Surgical Association, the American College of Surgeons, and the Surgical Section of the AMA and one member each from the New England Surgical Society, the Pacific Coast Surgical Association, the Southern Surgical Association, and the Western Surgical Association.

During the period when the idea of an American Board of Surgery was being developed, a conference was called in 1933 attended by representatives of the American hospital Association, the Association of American Medical Colleges, the Federation of State Medical Boards, the AMA Council on Medical Education in Hospitals, the National Board of Medical Examiners, and the four existing specialty boards. This group ultimately recommended the formation of an advisory committee composed of two delegated representatives from each specialty board then in existence or in the process of being formed as well as several other organizations. This newly formed body was known as the Advisory Board for Medical Specialties. In 1970 it was reorganized and renamed the American Board of Medical Specialties, presently comprised of 23 primary or conjoint board members. It should be mentioned, incidentally, that there are more than 100 groups whose names include "American Board of . . . ," but only the 23 that are members of the ABMS are recognized as authorized boards in the various medical specialties. No certificates are awarded by these 23 boards without examination.

CURRENT EDUCATIONAL STATUS
Undergraduate Surgical Education

Traditionally, medical education has concerned itself with imparting an understanding of normal human body structure and function, of the abnormalities that may occur, and of the ability to recognize promptly deviations from normalcy as well as an awareness of the means by which abnormalities may be rectified by intervention. The first aspect of medical education is concerned with the basic sciences that occupy the majority of the first 2 years of medical school. The second area is the discipline of pathology, perhaps to be regarded as the bridge between the basic and clinical sciences. The third aspect of medical education is the clinical realm. This portion of the undergraduate medical education is carried out exclusively in hospitals—large teaching hospitals and sometimes community hospitals—but institutions where service to patients is at least as important as the educational role, and in many instances where service predominates over education. In recent years there has been an increasing impetus for so-called primary care and thus an emphasis on the primary care specialties that are identified as family practice, internal medicine, obstetrics and gynecology, and pediatrics. Surgery tends to be viewed as no more than secondary care at best and more likely as predominantly tertiary care. Such arbitrary and artificial divisions of patient care seem false. Nothing can be more primary than cutting into the flesh of another human being to remove or repair a diseased organ. Unfortunately, the current emphasis on primary care has tended to decrease the time allotted to undergraduate surgical education, and in at least three medical schools a clinical clerkship on the surgery service is an elective rather than a required part of the curriculum.

In addition to the reduced time for the discipline of surgery to be taught in medical school, there is the additional difficulty of where, when, and how the surgical specialties enter into the curriculum. Some have argued that the surgical specialties are so highly technical and narrow that the medical student does not need to be exposed to those disciplines. Others would argue that somewhere in the curriculum a soon-to-be or a newly graduated physician, particularly one who intends to provide patient care, must be exposed to highly specialized areas if for no other reason than to know which specialist should be consulted when the patient has a particular problem. Then there is the difficulty of the elective fourth year. In many medical schools, all or most of the fourth year is an elective one. If the third-year surgical clerkship is 8 weeks and the medical student is "not interested in surgery or its disciplines," there may be no time for teaching surgical specialties. This is particularly true if the surgically uninterested student receives poor advice from his or her faculty advisor. Nevertheless, all of these trends make it imperative that the surgical clerkship be well organized and well implemented. As Lewis and Pories have stated, "Three key ingredients go into any successful clerkship: objectives, curriculum, and evaluation."[10] These may sound like terms from a school of education program. They are, and if the surgical educator is to meet the objectives of a surgical clerkship, it is important that the surgical educator learn educational methodology.

The primary goal of the surgical educator is to lead students to an understanding of surgery as a discipline.[11] Obviously the student needs to be exposed to the broad spectrum of surgical lesions, for example, thyroid nodules, breast masses, arterial aneurysms or occlusive disease, and gastrointestinal malignancies. Although this is the raw material of the surgical educational process, all lesions or abnormalities are an integral part of a living, breathing human being with feelings, fears, and desires. The surgical teaching must include not only how the surgeon thinks about a disease process, but how he or she thinks about the human aspects of the patient with the disease and the impact of that disease on the patient and others. The role of the surgical educator in teaching medical student is to demonstrate how to make the proper diagnosis of an ischemic lower extremity, to recognize the symptoms and understand their physiologic basis, to perform the simple maneuvers on physical examination, perhaps aided by relatively simple technical equipment to establish the level of obstruction, and then to direct and interpret the orderly progression of studies that might be used to determine whether an operation would be necessary. It is more important to lead the student through the proper thought processes and motor skills than it is to fill the student with the latest bypass techniques, prosthetic materials used, and similar issues. Unfortunately, far too many surgeons look upon these latter items as the essence of their instructional activities rather than teaching basic history taking and physical examination and cultivating the surgeon's thinking process.

The reduced time for teaching surgery and the need for the student to be exposed to various surgical specialties demand that the surgical clerkship be planned carefully and carried out with a schedule that will allow appropriate but not excessive emphasis on any one aspect of a particular surgical discipline. It is possible for the new third-year surgical clerk (and unfortunately, even for the easily seduced second-year student late in that year) to become enamored of a given surgical specialty. This, in combination with the assertion by some surgical specialists within the medical school that good residency positions are hard to come by, has led to what Swanson has termed "the preresidency syndrome."[15] This is a situation where a young student decides very early that he or she wishes to become an ophthalmologist, otolaryngologist, or orthopedic or neurologic surgeon. The learning of that discipline and the selection of clerkships in that discipline by the student, particularly as a fourth-year elective, is motivated largely by the questionable desire to get into position for selection in a given residency. Unfortunately, the entire process encourages the student to focus myopically on a given area within medicine, rather than obtaining a broad view of the entire field of medicine, which should be the rightful objective of a medical school education.

Lectures and conferences. All of these features of the current situation in undergraduate surgical education have been described because they are important factors in the establishment of what the surgical clerkship is in most medical schools today. Generally the two basic ingredients in the surgical clerkship are (1) lectures and conferences and (2) clinical experience. The lectures are aimed at the medical student level and generally cover general surgery as well as the surgical specialties, particularly if there has not been any other time in the 4 years of medical school when the student would have had the opportunity for acquaintance with those specialties. The value of the lectures will be limited by the availability, commitment, and enthusiasm of the teachers. Thus the timing of the lecture during the busy day of a third-year surgical clerk is terribly important and should not interfere with the clinical experience of the third-year clerks. All these considerations often leave one with the impression that there is no good time nor ideal format for the lectures. Unfortunately, professors of surgery often consider medical student teaching as a low priority item. Hence the third-year surgical clerk may or may not receive appropriate didactic teaching even when the lecture series appears well organized on paper. Perhaps some good has come out of this disappointing state of affairs in that many departments and institutions are experimenting with computer-based teaching, which has the advantage of presenting the material in a very effective mode. Moreover, the student can use the teaching packages at a time of his or her choice, which usually will lead to better assimilation of the material given. The material can also be viewed as many times as necessary for the student to learn the information thoroughly. The disadvantage, of course, is that faculty/student interaction is still further reduced.

In contrast, the conferences that are attended by faculty, residents, and students are generally directed at a level above that of the medical student. It is hoped that such conferences will illustrate the thinking process of the surgeon in dealing with a given disease entity. Rather than leaving it to chance whether a student learns something from a conference, the student can be drawn into conference participation if the moderator will take the time to ask the student about some aspect of the case with which the student should be well versed.[10] Expecting the student to comment or inquire voluntarily in the conference setting is usually not realistic.

Clinical experience. The other portion of the clerkship, that which is termed clinical experience, involves the student in all aspects of surgical care. He or she should be made to feel a member of the team and should be expected to attend all rounds on patients and to learn some basic skills in the management of patients. It is wise to have a faculty advising system so that students can identify with specific faculty members. It is also imperative that the student keep a record of the simple tasks, for example, venipuncture, arterial puncture, and insertion of urinary catheter or nasogastric tube. That record should be checked by the faculty advisor periodically to ensure that the student is in fact learning these basic skills. The student should perform and record a history and physical examination on each assigned patient. Because that is expected of the student, it is incumbent on the faculty to review and grade the student's history and physical examinations to ensure that the student is developing appropriate skills in these areas. Not to do so is demoralizing and frustrating to the student and may be even more deleterious in signaling to students that taking a history and performing a physical examination are not important in the highly technical world of surgery.

Likewise, the student's clinical experience should include attendance at the operation of the patient whom he or she examined. There is much that can be learned from the operating room experience, beginning with the means of providing for a sterile environment. The pathologic process can be observed firsthand and the means of rectifying the abnormality also seen. A good teacher in the operating room can enhance this visual or palpable feature as an educational experience by asking the student questions that emphasize the physiologic or pathologic concepts. It should be stressed to the student that the technical aspects of the operation are the least important at their level of learning. Many students, unfortunately, view these technical matters as the most important part of the operating room experience, but under today's time constraints and cost containment concerns, it is no longer feasible to allow a student even to suture an operative wound under supervision in order to gratify an interest in technique. Obviously, the design of the third-year surgical clerkship must contain some other means of allowing the student to practice manual skills. This has been accomplished in most surgical clerkships by the establishment of a motor skills laboratory.

Graduate Surgical Education

The evolution of the modern surgical residency program in the United States has been a gradual and progressive one. Unquestionably, Halsted's early residents received a superb surgical education, but the influence of a physician such as Osler and a pathologist such as Welch inevitably played a significant role in educating the neophyte surgeon. When Dr. Halsted declared his student ready for the independent performance of surgical operations, the individual was appropriately regarded as a specialist in general surgery. As the graduates of Dr. Halsted's program and others assumed ascendancy in surgery and established their own residency programs, they continued in the Halstedian mode of a guided apprenticeship format. The requirements for completion of a residency varied significantly from discipline to discipline and from institution to institution, because universities made no effort to assume responsibility for graduate surgical education. A major reason for this has been alluded to previously, namely that most graduate surgical education must, by its nature, take place in a hospital (although this may be changing with the current burgeoning of same-day or outpatient surgery). Because the hospital locale was not regarded as part of the university, not even with teaching hospitals that were associated with a university medical school, there was no entity or organization responsible for supervision of graduate surgical education. Is it any wonder that it grew like Topsy? Eventually two organizations did appear, however, that have worked in concert to establish mechanisms for the defining, accrediting, and overseeing of programs of formal graduate surgical education—the Residency Review Committee for Surgery (RRC), an arm of the Accreditation Council for Graduate Medical Education, and, for evaluating graduates of residency programs—the American Board of Surgery (ABS). It is appropriate to discuss the former in this section on graduate surgical education because the residency review committee is responsible for formulating the general and special requirements for the residency programs and also for reviewing the programs to assure their compliance with the stipulated requirements.[1]

The specific functions of the Residency Review Committee for Surgery are:
- Establish general characteristics of accredited programs
- Review content, scope, and duration of programs
- Ascertain credentials of teaching staff
- Specify resident complement of program
- Provide periodic on-site assessment surveys of programs

Before and during the residency review committee's periodic on-site visits, program directors provide documentation of the program's compliance with the requirements. Compliance means accreditation by the ACGME; lack of compliance leads to probationary approval or even withdrawal of approval.

Once the RRC and ABS came into being, graduate surgical education became more structured, resulting in the organizing of general surgery residency programs. In the 1930s the usual format of graduate surgical education was 3 years of basic instruction followed by 2 years of preceptorship under a well-recognized surgical specialist. After the establishment of the American Board of Surgery in 1937, this well-recognized surgical specialist was a board-certified general surgeon. The pattern evolved gradually into a 4-year program, structured for progressively graded responsibility and conducted at a single institution, for example, a teaching hospital or a large public hospital. With the gradual expansion of the knowledge base in general surgery, it became clear that 4 years was insufficient to instruct a young surgeon about the basic principles of surgery as well as teach him or her the technical aspects of the discipline. However, it was not until 1981 that both the RRC and the American Board of Surgery specified that a minimum of 5 years would be required for a complete and acceptable general surgery residency program. It was also clearly stated at this time that the chief or senior, residency year, in which the young surgeon takes major responsibility for patient care under supervision, was the most important year of graduate surgical education, reiterating a concept enunciated by the Board for some time.

Ingredients of a successful program. A number of ingredients make for a successful graduate surgical education program. The surgical faculty within an institution is the key element in the training environment.[13] The program director, who may or may not be the chairman of the department of surgery, or the chief of surgery at a nonuniversity teaching hospital, should be a person whose full-time commitment is exclusively to the educational environment for the resident surgeons. He or she should possess broad clinical skills, if not in the entire field of general surgery, at least in a major portion of general surgery, so that this knowledge can be passed on to faculty and residents alike. Optimally, the program director should be not only an accomplished clinician but also an investigator in the clinical and basic science arenas. He or she should possess sufficient teaching skills to conduct conferences, give formal lectures, participate in seminars, and provide for teaching at the bedside. Such an ideal program director obviously must be committed to the workload, a heavy one, and must also be committed to provide for the supervision and discipline of residents and faculty as needed. He or she must be fully informed of the requirements of the residency review committee and should be familiar enough with the requirements of the American Board of Surgery to insure that residents receive appropriate training and education to qualify them for certification.

It is impossible for a program director to provide the requisite educational environment for a number of residents without assistance. Therefore a sufficient number of faculty members must participate. The RRC for surgery suggests as a minimum at least one full-time faculty member for each chief resident in the program. It goes without saying that faculty members should be educators. Skill at surgical operations, although admirable, is not sufficient of itself to warrant a faculty position. The ability to share those skills with another individual verbally, as well as by example, and to point out the underlying principles is essential for becoming a faculty member. Ultimately, all surgical faculty should be role models for the residents.

A second ingredient for a successful residency program is the residents themselves. A surgical resident is a graduate student. Generally a graduate student learns by self-education, although he or she needs guidance and occasional didactic teaching in order to stay the course. Moreover, as the surgical graduate student progresses in the residency program, he or she is responsible for teaching medical students and the junior residents. Thus the faculty should be teaching the residents not only the principles of the discipline but also educational techniques.

The third ingredient in a successful general surgery residency program is the patient complement. Obviously, their health and well/being should be the primary concern in any residency program. Beyond this fundamental concern, it is important that there be a sufficient number of patients with a diversity of surgical diseases so that the resident can become completely familiar with the preoperative evaluation, the operative techniques, and the postoperative care in the widest possible variety of cases. It is essential that the preoperative and postoperative phases of surgical care be emphasized in the education of a surgical resident. A surgeon may be an extremely skillful technician, but if he or she possesses little diagnostic capability or the inability to recognize and treat the medical diseases that may be concurrent with the surgical disease, he or she fails as a surgeon. Likewise, if the surgeon cannot recognize postoperative complications and treat them expeditiously, the appellation "surgeon" is not deserved. Unfortunately, within some surgical residency programs and, more frequently, in a community practice of surgery, the surgeon is becoming a mere technician.

The success of a general surgery residency program also depends on the organization of the total program. To satisfy the requirements of the RRC and ABS, rotations to other specialties must be provided. It is important that these rotations take place at that residency level where optimal learning may occur. For example, if the general surgery resident should obtain operative experience in a specialty other than general surgery, it is important that he or she rotate to that specialty during the later years of the residency. It may be important for the resident to have two rotations on the specialty service, one during the first year and another during the third or fourth year. It is paramount, however, that the resident receive sufficient exposure to general surgery, and graded responsibility throughout the residency with increasing independence during later years is essential. A first-year resident must know the chain of command and must have appropriate back-up by more senior surgeons when caring for any surgical patient, particularly the critically ill patient. Despite some opinions to the contrary,[7] bedside rounds are a mainstay of surgical education. In this day of same-day surgery and shorter hospital stays, this traditional method of surgical education is being eroded. Nevertheless, it is important that the young surgeon learn by examining the postoperative patient, not just the patient's chart. As a part of that education, the senior surgeon should, usually by example, demonstrate how to converse with a patient, either preoperatively in explaining the operation and its sequelae, or postoperatively in informing the patient of the condition, be it good or bad.

Equally important is the senior surgeon's responsibility to make certain that excessive discussion of the patient's disease is not held within the patient's hearing, especially if a prognosis is grave. It is extremely important that at least once a day all members of the surgical team—faculty, residents, and students—make rounds on the surgical patients to provide appropriate care and to maximize the educational opportunity inherent in this setting.

The operating room is the faculty surgeon's classroom for the resident surgeon. It is here and only here that the faculty who teaches the more senior resident or the senior resident who teaches the more junior resident can demonstrate and highlight both the complex portions of the operation and the seemingly unimportant nuances that make for a successful procedure. In addition, faculty and residents alike can learn to interact with other personnel in the operating room as befits a professional colleague. As Organ stated,[12] "Tantrums, rude conduct, and lack of respect . . . only confirm one's insecurity. Early in their training, residents must be aware of their responsibility as leaders of the team."

A variety of conferences are usually available to a resident in a proper general surgery program. These conferences or a combination of conferences are as different as the institutions in which they are conducted. Most residency programs have some form of journal club where the residents and faculty get together each month to discuss a particular issue of a surgical journal or perhaps recent articles published about a particular surgical disease. These meetings should have definite agendas and assignments to individual residents to read and review specific articles in the literature. Specialty area conferences may also be held such as medical/surgical gastrointestinal conferences or vascular surgery conferences. A conference may deal with a specific problem, for example, surgical infection or surgical endocrine disease. Almost invariably a residency program has two specific conferences. The first is grand rounds, where a member of the department, usually a faculty person or a chief resident, presents a topic of current interest or a patient's case and then a review of the pertinent information about the disease. Grand rounds are often utilized, too, for lectures given by visiting professors to the department. Undoubtedly the most important teaching conference in any program is the weekly morbidity and mortality conference as mandated by the residency review committee.[1] It is at these conferences that the complications and deaths occurring on the surgical service are discussed and reviewed in depth to learn where errors were made and how to avoid the complication or death in the future. Here the resident surgeons must learn to take personal responsibility for the complications or deaths that occur. As Frank Spencer said, "At the mortality and morbidity conference, there is no such thing as an act of God."[14]

Finally, as with any educational program, there must be means of evaluating the progress of the resident. Most programs have now developed an advisor system whereby the residents have a designated faculty person to whom they can turn for help and advice at any time, and it is essential that such support be available. It is well recognized that the surgical residency is a time of physical and emotional stress imposed by the rigors of the residency itself. At the same time there are likely to be additional stresses, such as major events occurring in the family. In addition to sharing the resident's personal concerns, the advisor is also present to make certain that the resident is progressing in a satisfactory fashion educationally. A more structured means of evaluating the resident (and also the program itself) is the In-Training Examination of the American Board of Surgery. This is a written multiple-choice examination provided by the Board annually to each program director, who decides who will take the examination. The examination is usually conducted at the resident's own institution and monitored by the program director or another appropriate proctor. There is no set "passing score." The examination results are reported to the program director in percentiles and in relation to content areas so that it can be determined how well a resident is doing in comparison with other residents at the same level throughout the country. The program director can also scan the content percentiles to determine whether the overall performance of the residents seems to indicate inadequate knowledge in a given content area in that program.

The general surgery residency program of today should be seen as an educational endeavor devoted to producing individuals who are capable of the independent practice of general surgery. The newly graduated surgeon may then apply to the American Board of Surgery to become certified as properly qualified to practice the specialty of surgery, that is, as a specialist in general surgery. The decision to seek certification is voluntary, and the process will be discussed next.

CERTIFICATION PROCESS

The American board of Surgery is one of 23 boards holding membership in the American Board of Medical Specialties. No board awards certificates without preliminary screening of all applicants who must then successfully complete the requisite examinations. The purposes of the American Board of Surgery are promulgated as follows[2]:

1. To conduct examinations of acceptable candidates who seek certification or recertification by the Board
2. To issue certificates of qualification to all candidates meeting the Board's requirements and satisfactorily completing its prescribed examinations
3. To improve and broaden the opportunities

for the graduate education and training of surgeons

The only change in this statement of purposes since it was first enunciated in 1937 has been the addition of the words or recertification, inserted in 1986. Further, in elaborating on its purposes, the Board maintains:

> It is not concerned with the attainment of special privileges or recognition for the Diplomates in the practice of surgery. It is neither the intent nor the purpose of the Board to define the requirements for membership on the staff of hospitals or institutions involved in the practice or teaching of surgery ... The Board specifically disclaims interest in or recognition of differential emoluments that may be based upon certification or recertification.[2]

It might be mentioned that it is the third declared purpose of the Board, stated above, that sanctions its involvement with the RRC for surgery in establishing what constitutes an acceptable residency training program, in the accreditation process, and in the continuing review of such programs.

The Board also has been evolving its definition of general surgery in recent years. This most recent formulation was first approved by the Board at its June 1987 meeting.[2] It identifies eight areas of primary responsibility of the general surgeon and emphasizes a central core of knowledge of basic science underlying the practice of surgery in those areas of responsibility. In addition, the definition clearly states that a general surgeon who merits certification by the American Board of Surgery is expected to have acceptable competence in making the diagnosis and providing for preoperative, operative, and postoperative management of patients with diseases of the organ systems listed, as well as those sustaining trauma, and the critically ill patient.

Admission to the Examination Process

To be admitted to the examination process currently, the applicant must have completed satisfactorily a 5-year accredited residency program in general surgery. The applicant must be actively engaged in the practice of surgery and must hold a currently valid license to practice medicine granted by a state or other United States jurisdiction or by a Canadian province. The program director must sign a statement in which he attests that the resident is prepared for the independent practice as a specialist in surgery. In addition, the statement indicates that the program director recommends the resident for the examinations.

Qualifying Examination.

On approval of the application, the surgeon is then admitted to the qualifying examination. This written multiple-choice examination requires a full day and is administered simultaneously each fall in seven cities strategically located across the continental United States. The qualifying examination may be taken five times during a 5-year period. If the applicant is unsuccessful on five occasions, additional educational requirements must be met before the possibility of being readmitted to the qualifying examination.

Certifying Examination

On successful completion of the qualifying examination, the applicant is admitted as a candidate to the certifying examination. This oral examination is administered on six occasions annually during the Board's academic year—July 1 to June 30. Examination sites are designated regionally to minimize travel for examinees residing in the various areas. Each candidate's examination consists of three 30-minute sessions conducted by three teams of two examiners each, directed toward determining the candidate's understanding of clinical entities and the level of surgical judgment and problem-solving ability. The examining teams are composed of a director of the Board and a surgeon from the environs of the examination site who is well-known and respected and who is designated the associate examiner. Thus a candidate is examined by six examiners on the three teams who then meet on completion of the third examination session to discuss the performance of the immediately preceding candidates and to assign final grades. Although a number of boards have discontinued oral examinations, considering them to be too subjective and hence unreliable, the American Board of Surgery throughout its existence has adhered to the practice of holding oral examinations. Among other justifications, one could cite that at present there are many areas in general surgery that are controversial and for which there is no one right answer to govern appropriate management. Such a circumstance makes for excellent material for oral examinations.

Recertification

All certificates awarded by the American Board of Surgery are time-limited to 10 years. To maintain a valid certificate, a diplomate must undergo periodic reassessment. This recertification process is well established only for the parent certificate and the Certificate of Special Qualifications in Pediatric Surgery, but the requirements to be admitted to the recertification examination and the examinations themselves are similar. The diplomate must complete an application that includes a tabulation of 2 years of operative experience and documentation of some continuing medical education. A diplomate may initiate the recertification process after being certified for 7 years and may continue the process indefinitely until the written test (which is given annually) is successfully completed. The new certificate will be dated to expire 10 years after the date that appears on the previous certificate.

Questions Surrounding Certification

The question of how a valid certificate should be used or viewed is always being raised. Although the Board has expressed no interest in the recognition that a diplomate may receive on the basis of certification, it seems reasonable that because certification and recertification are obtained only by examination and that the examinations surely test for cognitive knowledge and perhaps other attributes, board certification should be used as one criterion for membership on the medical staff of a hospital. Moreover, because a candidate for certification or recertification is required to meet certain requirements before being admitted to the examinations and must then successfully complete the examinations before becoming certified, the certificate resembles a college diploma more than a license. The Board, therefore, revokes certificates only if it is determined that the admission requirements had not been met or had been falsified.

Another issue frequently raised is the future of certification. The certifying concept arose because it was recognized that surgeons on completion of a suitable postgraduate educational program should be measured by an external agency in an appropriate manner. In the early years the candidates were observed by members of the Board performing operations and providing care to surgical patients. As the number of applicants grew, on-site observation became difficult and ultimately impossible. The Board now relies on the program directors and the program faculty to document operative and patient care skills. The examinations then test for cognitive knowledge and perhaps some problem-solving abilities. This process evaluates the surgeon for appropriate knowledge and accompanying skills, which should assure the public of a competent surgeon. Competence, however, embodies other less quantitated attributes, and whether an evaluation method can be developed to test effectively for competence remains to be seen. The public desires and is becoming more insistent on a certain level of expertise in specialists, and the board certification mechanism is the best method currently available. Therefore some form of certifying, and probably on a periodic basis, will continue to be in place. The process may change, as it has in the past, but a means of certifying a certain level of knowledge and skill attainment will be retained.

SOCIOECONOMIC FEATURES OF SURGICAL EDUCATION
Undergraduate Education

Many, if not most, medical students enter medical school free of debt. However, although medical school is technically graduate school, the curriculum and hours are sufficiently demanding that the opportunity for full-time or even part-time work is usually not feasible for the medical student to meet his or her financial obligations. Some gainful employment outside of medical school may be possible during the first 2 years when the curriculum is more structured and the hours regular. But the third year, with all of its clinical duties and demands, will not permit a steady job. The fourth year has the same drawbacks as the third, although the pace may be less strenuous, and the newly acquired skills, for example, venipuncture, history-taking and physical examinations, and some clinical laboratory expertise, may allow a student at this level to work in an out-of-hours situation in a hospital.

Then there is the matter of medical school tuition. Medical school has never been an inexpensive proposition, but the recent escalation in tuition can be described as nothing less than astounding. Of interest, the better and more prestigious medical schools are likely to carry a higher tuition than the less well known schools. Moreover, state medical schools, which have always been viewed as providing a unique opportunity for residents of the state to pursue a rewarding medical career, have seen an equal escalation in tuition fees. These same schools in the rare instance when they provide a position to an out-of-state resident charge that particular individual an incredibly high fee. In comparing the fees charged by a state medical school to residents of the state with the fees of out-of-state students, the difference can be described as either extraordinary or exorbitant depending on whether you are viewing it as an economist or as a student who has to pay it (or the parent who may be helping the student to pay it). The combination of an inability to earn money while a graduate student and the hefty tuition and other expenses of medical school usually lead to the student having a substantial debt on completion of medical school.

It is necessary to look at the current trend of enrollment in medical school in order to understand still another feature of the socioeconomic forces that are impinging upon medical education. In 1987 almost 40% of the medical students in this country will be women. Many, if not most, will be well supported in their desire to become physicians. However, at least 30% of the entering female medical students will be women who have decided to pursue a medical career after other endeavors, for example, nursing, psychology, and elementary school teaching in the sciences. Often they have been in fields that are recognized as low paying, and therefore they may enter medical school either with a debt or without a visible means of continuing to support themselves while going to medical school. This phenomenon will have a palpable impact on the number of medical students entering surgical postgraduate programs. Even though only 16% of female medical students chose surgery or the surgical specialties for postgraduate study in 1986, as the entering pool of women approaches and perhaps surpasses 50%, the total number of new MDs who go into a surgical career will decrease.

The other victims of the high-tuition inability-to-work medical school atmosphere are other minorities, such as blacks and Hispanics. Often these individuals have had to "work their way through college" so that they already come to the medical school portal either in debt or close to it. They have no means of support within their family structure, and therefore their decision is either to go heavily into debt during medical school or to not pursue a medical career at all. Unfortunately, the latter is often the decision they make. These facts do not carry as great an impact on surgery and the surgical specialties, since this group represents only about 10% of students choosing surgical careers.[16]

Loans and scholarships are available to medical students from several sources. Loans are the major source of student financial aid, accounting for 76% of such support. Two programs that were enacted more than 20 years ago, the National Direct Student Loan and Health Professions Student Loan programs provided almost $42 million (21% of the more than $200 million support given to medical students in 1985 and 1986.) Other loan programs provide the remainder, with the Guaranteed Student Loan (GSL) program providing 60% of all loan funds; the Health Education Assistant Loan (HEAL) and Auxiliary Loans to Assist Students or Parietal Loans for Undergraduate Students (ALAS/PLUS) programs are the other loan funds available to medical students. Both of these programs provide loans with market-rate interest that accrues from origination of the loan but defers repayment. The other sources of medical student financial support are scholarships, which increased by 5% in 1985 and 1986 compared with 1984 and 1985, the largest increase occurring in scholarships provided by the schools themselves. Armed Forces scholarships represent the largest single source of scholarship funds but carry a military obligation in the payback.[8]

Davis has indicated that the average debt for students graduating in 1985 was about $31,000.[5] Financial burdens are becoming increasingly severe. Eighty-two percent of medical students who graduated in 1986 were in debt and for those in debt, the average was $33,499, an increase in one year of 6%. Moreover, this represents a 117.2% increase over the average debt of $15,421 for the 1980 cohort. Although the 6% increase in indebtedness is a matter of concern, the comparable figure for minority students is 14%. When this burden is added to the fact that minority students generally have greater debts on entering medical school and absent or limited family resources, the picture becomes most bleak for that group.[8]

Graduate Education (Residency)

The new physicians contemplating surgical careers already are in debt and facing 5 or more years of long hours and hard work. The mean salary for a first post-MD year (PGY 1) person is $22,006 and for a fifth post-MD year (PGY 5) is $27,322 for 1986 and 1987.[17] Despite the current controversy about the number of hours a resident shall be permitted to work, the numbers being discussed are no more than 16 hours on duty (New York) or 18 hours on duty (California) in a 24-hour period. The American Board of Medical Specialties Committee on Graduate Medical Education in a statement to the ACGME has requested that a more generic approach be taken, and that it be stated that a resident should work no more than a 90-hour week.[9] The latter approach would provide for some flexibility by recognizing the inherent irregularity of the practice of medicine: there may be times when an individual physician may be required to give 18 or more hours continuously to provide appropriate and adequate care to a patient; similarly, there will be times when the physician will be "on call" and therefore fully available, but nothing happens, and he or she has been able to sleep through most or all of the on-call situation.

Nevertheless, when the hourly wage is computed on the basis of a 90-hour week, the scale is $5.09/hour for a PGY 1 resident and $6.32/hour for a PGY 5 resident. This is not an extraordinarily high salary, particularly for a 90-hour week. Moreover, if there is truly a 90-hour week, the opportunity to earn an additional income is limited, if nonexistent. It is true that a spouse may be working and adding to the family income, but what if children have arrived and other reasons exist for only one adult member of the family working—then there is no opportunity for additional income, and debts (and interest) are deferred further. There are other financial factors that play a role in the decision made about where a resident works and how much debt the new surgeon has upon completion of the residency. For example, there are regional differences in resident salaries. Of interest, two of the cities where residents pride themselves for receiving low (that is, no) stipend, Baltimore and Boston, now have some of the highest resident salaries. Moreover, a recent *New York Times* article describes a physician who was moving after 2 years of residency from a city in the Northeast to one in the South, predominantly because housing costs were simply too high in the Northeast. The debt of residents on completing their graduate education has so many variables, including length of residency and availability (or advisability) of moonlighting, that an accurate figure is hard to identify. It is probably safe to say that most surgical residents finish with average debts higher than those of medical students.

Thus the new surgeon arrives in a new venue, deep in debt and anxious to get out from under the financial burdens. Is it little wonder that after many years of education and deprivation, the young specialist should expect appropriate recompense? It may seem extreme to the more established members of the profession, particularly in view of the meager existence some of the older members of the profession had, but it may not be so unwarranted when future expenses are envisioned, for example, malpractice premiums, equipment costs, and rent.

Costs of Practice

The physician has many practice choices. He or she may go solo; join a group—single or multispecialty; join an HMO, IPA, or other prepaid plan; become an academic surgeon; or pursue some other mode. Nevertheless, there will be costs associated with the initiation of practice that may be underwritten by a practice plan or a faculty practice plan, or they will have to be borne by the practitioner. These include the costs of the personnel and equipment to begin a practice, supply costs, malpractice and other insurance, and the costs of becoming certified.

Most residents who complete a general surgery residency will decide to seek board certification. The first step is to contact the American Board of Surgery. The surgeon will be sent a preliminary evaluation form, which will outline the training the resident has had and which must be returned before the formal application will be sent. When the application is completed and returned, a registration fee of $150 must accompany it. On acceptance of the application and supporting materials, such as license, a reply card will be sent to the surgeon. When the reply card is returned to the Board indicating an acceptance to undergo the qualifying (written) examination, a fee of $350 must be submitted. The qualifying examination is given annually in the fall. Upon successful completion of the qualifying examination, the candidate is then assigned to a certifying (oral) examination. These are conducted six times a year in strategically located areas in the continental United States and require a fee of $500. Therefore the certification process itself costs $1000. There are additional travel and lodging costs for the "privilege" of taking these examinations.

Yet the certification process is important. In a number of instances it is essential because many hospitals require board certification in order to continue as a member of the hospital staff. In some instances it is a matter of pride and recognition of the attainment of a certain expertise. Ultimately, becoming board certified will lead to greater financial rewards.[3] Thus the certification process, although costly and occurring at a time when many expenses are being experienced by the group practitioner, may prove to be the most important investment made early in a medical career. Despite the seemingly enormous initial costs, the stress of debts, and the concern about meeting payments and getting on top of things, most if not all physicians eventually achieve a comfortable and rewarding lifestyle.

References

1. Accreditation Council for Graduate Medical Education Directory of Graduate Medical Education Programs 1987-88, Chicago.
2. American Board of Surgery Booklet of Information 1987-88, Philadelphia.
3. American Medical Association News, Sept 20, 1985.
4. Archibald EW: Address of the president: higher degrees in the profession of surgery, Ann Surg 102: 481, 1935.
5. Davis CK: Financing student and resident education, Prob Genl Surg 3: 449, 1986.
6. Flexner A: Medical education in the United States and Canada, New York, 1910, Carnegie Foundation for the Advancement of Testing.
7. Hill GL et al: Teaching in clinical surgery: at the bedside or in the seminar room? J Med Educ 52: 595, 1977.
8. Jolly P, Taksei L, and Beran R: US medical school finances, JAMA 258: 1022, 1987.
9. King RB: Report of the American Board of Medical Specialties Graduate Medical Education Committee, March 17, 1987.
10. Lewis LS and Pories WJ: Medical student education: the surgical clerkship, Prob Genl Surg 3: 368, 1986.
11. Linn BS, Pratt T, and Zeppa R: The undergraduate surgical clerkship: a cutting edge which separates the clinical from the non-clinical medical specialists, Ann Surg 189: 152, 1979.
12. Organ CH Jr: The changing patterns of residency training programs, Pharos 49: 21, 1986.
13. Sheldon GF: The graduate (resident) surgical curriculum, Prob Genl Surg 3: 383, 1986.
14. Spencer FC: Personal communication.
15. Swanson AG: The "preresidency syndrome": an incipient epidemic of educational disruptions, J Med Educ 60: 201, 1985.
16. Swanson AG: Personal communication.
17. Teich JL: COTH Survey of Housestaff stipends, benefits, and funding, AAMC Publication, Washington, 1986.

BARRY M. MANUEL

Barry M. Manuel, MD, is Associate Dean and Clinical Professor of Surgery at Boston University School of Medicine. He received a BS degree (1954) and an MD degree (1958) from Boston University. He did his postgraduate training in surgery at the Boston University Hospital from 1958 to 1963.

22

The Malpractice Crisis and the Surgeon

BARRY M. MANUEL

Surgeons are aware of the extent to which professional liability affects virtually every aspect of their professional lives, from the patients they see and the tests they order to the treatments that are administered. Currently, no issue is of more concern to practicing surgeons than that of professional liability.[3-6,23]

Cost-containment mechanisms, such as diagnosis related groups, preferred provider organizations, health maintenance organizations, and gatekeepers, are affecting professional liability claims adversely because of pressure by hospitals and insurance companies to curtail the ordering of ancillary tests, reduce preoperative days, and shorten lengths of stay. The practicing physician finds himself or herself in an intolerable situation in which pressures from society require more cost-effective practice, whereas the tort system forces him to practice defensive medicine. This cost of defensive medicine is adding significantly to the already rapidly rising costs of health care.[35]

HISTORICAL PERSPECTIVE

The origins of the word malpractice date back to about 1671 when it was first used in London. It appears to have stemmed from a controversy between the seventeenth century equivalents of today's specialists and general practitioners. Evevard Maynwaring, a practitioner, wrote, "I am not daunted to oppose their male practice."[10] Although the exact meaning intended by the use of these words remains unclear, it does seem to symbolize a rebellious stance against the prevailing powerful and elitist medical contingent of the time.

A court decision several years later gave the term a legal definition of sorts. "Mala praxis is a great misdemeanor and offense at common law (whether it be for curiosity and experiment or by neglect) because it breaks the trust which the party has placed in the physician."[10]

However, the legal concepts on which the modern law of malpractice is based are much older than the evolution of the word itself. The concept evolved from English common law in the last half of the fourteenth century about 25 years after the first great plague epidemic. An accusation against a surgeon, John Swanlond, by Agnes Stratton for improper treatment of her hand was brought to trial before the Court of King's Bench. In the course of the ensuing legal argument, the principles that are still present in modern malpractice law were developed. The principles set down by Justice Cavendish in 1374 in his legal opinion is believed to be the first clear intimation that a doctor was liable in law for professional negligence.[10]

The lineage of the concept of negligence emanating from the Cavendish decision through the English decisions of the eighteenth and nineteenth centuries were assimilated into United States law. The first malpractice suit in the United States was recorded against a Connecticut physician in 1794 in Cross versus Guthrie.[15]

As early as 1885 Henry Campbell, President of the American Medical Association, devoted most of his inaugural address to the subject of malpractice. Unfavorable results from the treatment of fractures were the chief cause of such legal actions. He cited as an example a suit for $20,000 brought against a physician whose patient had been treated for a fractured patella with resultant gangrene and amputation. Although the suit was dropped, the physician suffered "loss of time, cost in fees to lawyers, and temporary injury to reputation."[9] In 1885 Campbell wrote, "We may safely say the evil of malpractice suits is but little or not at all diminished at the present day."[31] Probably as a result of these troubling issues, Campbell urged the American Medical Association even at that time to establish a Section of Medical Jurisprudence.

In January 1879, the Boston Medical and Surgical Journal published comments by Eugene Sanger who wrote regarding malpractice:

> The lawyer has plenary power to arrest or bond the surgeon for appearance at court at his own expense, damage his reputation, wound his feelings and purse, for which the surgeon has no redress unless he takes it out of the lawyer's hide.

Concerning lawmakers, Sanger wrote:

> We failed to get a bill through the last legislature to protect the science and art of surgery, mainly through the instrumentality of a low grade of lawyers, who kept out of sight their selfish and material interest in defeating it. My only reply is: Let these humane and philanthropic legislators contribute a moiety of their time and money to the suffering poor; let them run for the doctor a night, requite him for his thankless service, and, as an evidence of their sincerity and faith, become surety for the malpractice suits which they delight to encourage; let them work without retainers, relinquish their preferred claims on unsettled accounts and insolvent estates; let them step forward and cast their bread upon the waters, take the same risk that we do of prosecution for their mistakes, and the same chances of getting their pay, and their hypocritical cant will vanish into thin air.[37]

In England at this same time (1884), as a result of the conviction of a physician for felonious assault on a female patient, as well as a number of occurrences over the previous 20 years, there was growing pressure for some form of collective action by medical practitioners. In 1887 the creation of the Medical Defense Union evolved into a worldwide organization that served doctors and dentists by supporting them morally and financially in medical-legal matters, and indirectly it also benefited their patients by promoting measures to prevent mishap and malpractice.[25]

With the concept of prepaid health care in the mid-1930s came the need for review of hospital records and a meaningful analysis of the care rendered to patients. This ultimately led to investigations by review committees that disclosed inaccuracies or deficiencies in surgical and medical reporting. The Joint Commission on Accreditation of Hospitals, consisting of the American Hospital Association, the American Medical Association, the American College of Surgeons, and the American College of Physicians was formed in 1951 to 1952. Their inspections and reviews also revealed individual and hospital deficiencies, and demands were made for correction. The results of these efforts to document the need for care and appropriate treatment led to the production of records that allowed nonphysicians to inspect and judge that care and treatment. Thus by the late 1940s and early 1950s attorneys became aware that these hospital records, which before this time were privy only to physicians, might implicate physicians for substandard medical practice.[22,38] The stage was therefore set for the crisis of professional liability that gained added momentum in the 1970s and is exploding in the 1980s.

The Crisis of the 1970s

As evidenced by the previously cited historical data, the word malpractice has always had a negative connotation to physicians. But it wasn't until the early 1970s that it began to have a significant impact on clinical practice. At that time a large and unexpected increase in the frequency of claims and the severity of awards caused sudden and severe adjustments upward of professional liability rates and in many cases resulted in the termination of this product line by insurance companies.[49] Nationally, the number of commercial companies offering professional liability insurance decreased from 39 to 8. When insurance was available, frequently the premiums were prohibitive.

As a response to this crisis, more than 300 statutes were passed by the 50 states.[21,32] Some of the more common features of this legislation included:

- Establishment of a joint underwriting association that guaranteed availability
- Establishment of screening or arbitration panels to eliminate nonmeritorius claims
- Elimination of the addendum clause
- Reduction of the statute of limitation
- Limitation of physicians' liability (capping)
- Limitation of lawyers' fees
- Establishment of commissions to study medical liability problems
- Improvement of tort laws
- Development of self-insurance plan (physician mutuals) and state insurance fund
- Establishment of collateral source rule

Failures of the Remedial Tort Reform

Although these legislative initiatives provided some temporary relief at the time they were enacted, they have not afforded a permanent solution. The reasons the remedial tort reforms of the 1970s have failed to solve the professional liability problem are many.

1. The paramount reason for this lack of success is the subsequent overturning by the courts on a constitutional basis of several of the key legislative reforms, such as caps on pain and suffering, limiting of legal contingency fees and statutes of limitations.
2. Defense attorneys have expressed doubts about the effectiveness of malpractice screening panels. Indeed these panels have been found to be unconstitutional in Florida, Illinois, and Missouri and have been repealed in Nevada, North Dakota, and Rhode Island.
3. A larger number of claims are being litigated in the courtroom, and this adds to the cost of settling the disputes.
4. Lawyers have discovered the fertile field of birth defects and the enormous awards associated with them.
5. Courts are now assessing punitive damages, and physicians cannot purchase insurance against these charges.
6. Many states have changed the statute of limitations so that liability now begins at the time of discovery rather than at the time of occurrence, which, for all intents and purposes, eliminates the statute of limitations.
7. Countersuits filed by physicians seem to do well in the lower courts, but the superior courts have generally reversed the outcome of these suits, and the Supreme Court has steadfastly refused to hear appeals.
8. Increasing publicity about larger settlements is enticing patients to sue with the expectation of huge awards. Because of these large settlements, lawyers are reluctant to settle valid claims for reasonable amounts.
9. With larger and larger settlements, attorneys are getting far more sophisticated and

specialized. Some medical specialists have become lawyers and experts in plaintiff law. Others have opted to become professional plaintiffs' physicians, a group of physicians who sell their knowledge regularly to plaintiffs' attorneys.

THE PLACE FOR PROFESSIONAL LIABILITY

Professional liability does not belong in a courtroom at all for the following reasons:

1. A physician is not tried by a jury of his peers. Despite good intentions, most jurors understand very little about the practice of medicine and cannot be expected to comprehend the complex issues involved in professional liability.
2. Juries tend to be emotionally vulnerable to severely injured, handicapped, and suffering plaintiffs, which interferes with their ability to be objective.[13] Bring a poor deformed youngster before a lay jury, and their hearts go out to the child. I believe most physicians would be no different. Nonetheless, the effect has been higher and higher settlements against physicians.
3. The fine line between professional liability and maloccurrence is one that even trained experts have difficulty distinguishing.
4. Prolonged litigation causes undue hardship to the truly injured patient by delaying compensation.
5. The present system causes great injury to the physician and his family, reputation, and practice. And rarely is this famicide reversible even if he is fully exonerated by the courts.[11]
6. The costs of the present system are excessive and account for 75% of the professional liability premiums physicians pay, whereas only 25% goes to truly injured patients.
7. Physicians are being forced to practice defensive medicine, the costs of which add significantly to the total costs of health care in the United States.[20,27,28]
8. The quality of health care can be affected when physicians do not perform a procedure or conduct a test because of the fear of malpractice, even though the patient might benefit from said test or procedure. Even more disturbing is the prospect that specialists may refuse to see or accept complicated or high-risk cases, again having a negative impact on patient care.

MAGNITUDE OF THE PROBLEM

To assess the magnitude of the problem, we must look at the number of potential malpractice suits that could be filed but are not. In two separate articles in the *New England Journal of Medicine*, Nathan Couch et al. reported a study of iatrogenic illness on a surgical service of a major teaching hospital,[8] and Knight Steel et al. reported a similar study of iatrogenic illness on a medical service of another major teaching hospital.[54] They found that iatrogenic complications definitely occurred and that a small percentage of them resulted in a permanent disability or death. However, the authors were unaware of a single suit filed as a result of the complications.

The California Medical Association has conducted a well-publicized study of potentially compensable events from 20,864 case records kept by 23 representative hospitals.[42] The study found an incidence of 4.65% of potentially compensable events: 9.7% resulted in death and 3.8% in permanent disability. A statistical extrapolation of those figures to the statewide population revealed 140,000 cases of potentially compensable events. This study found that litigation was brought rarely, and purely on a chance basis. Clearly there exists a large reservoir of unlitigated maloccurrences, which further compounds the problem and emphasizes the need for a definitive solution.

Escalating Problem

The National Association of Insurance Commissioners,[33,34,40] Jury Verdict Research, Inc. of Solon, Ohio,[29,30] and most recently the General Accounting Office,[56] have each revealed that the frequency of professional liability claims has increased at a disturbing rate during the past 10 years. Jury Verdict Research, Inc. has also indicated that the average medical malpractice jury verdict has increased from $228,818 in 1975 to $1,017,716 in 1985.[30] To confirm the seriousness of the current trend, *Best's Review* in January 1987 revealed that the losses from writing professional liability insurance have increased annually since 1977 and from 1981 to 1986 have totaled $5.2 billion.[1]

RECENT EFFORTS FOR SOLUTIONS

There has been a flurry of activity during the past few years aimed at alleviating the professional liability problem. The White House, Congress, the General Accounting Office, the Department of Health and Human Services, more than 40 states, and the AMA have currently put forth legislation or suggestions to deal with this crisis. Unfortunately, the major thrust of all this activity has been in the area of remedial tort reform legislation. A blue ribbon committee of the AMA has suggested a tort reform package that includes:[50]

- Limitation of noneconomic loss
- Limit of legal contingency fees
- Collateral source rule
- Structured awards
- Elimination of punitive damages
- Defining credentials for expert witnesses
- Refining definition of statute of limitation

Because the genesis of the state legislative reforms lies with the state medical societies, it is not surprising to find that of the 41 states currently involved in tort reform legislation, the most frequent components of this legislation are as follows:[39]

- Caps on noneconomic damage
- Structured settlements
- Change in the collateral source rule
- Changes in the doctrine of joint and several liability
- Elimination of punitive damages
- Down-sliding scales for attorneys' contingency fees
- Shortening of the statute of limitations

A White House Working Group on Tort Policy was appointed by Attorney General Edwin Meese and was composed of White House personnel and representatives from 10 federal agencies.[52] Under the leadership of Deputy Attorney General Richard Willard, they have recommended the following:

- Elimination of joint and several liability
- Limitation of noneconomic damages to $100,000
- Limitation of attorney contingency fees
- Elimination of collateral source rule
- Structured awards
- Greater use of arbitration and other methods of solving disputes out of court
- Changes in the tort law that would make it more difficult for plaintiffs to win in the absence of clear fault
- Clear connection between the complaint of activity and the injury

Most recently the General Accounting Office and the Department of Health and Human Services have come out with reports dealing with professional liability.[56] The fifth and final report from the massive General Accounting Office study was released in June 1987. After 2 years of intensive study conducted at the request of Representative John Porter (Illinois) and Senator John Heinz (Pennsylvania), the government agency concluded that federal and state leadership will be required to make progress with malpractice problems. The General Accounting Office listed recommendations in four major areas:

1. Reduce the incidence of medical malpractice

2. Communicate more effectively the potential risks of medical treatment of patients
3. Improve the efficiency, predictability, and equity in the way that malpractice claims are resolved
4. Test and evaluate different ways of resolving and paying medical malpractice claims

The General Accounting Office also reported several specific state level tort reforms that hold promise of bringing more efficiency, predictability, and equity to claims resolution including:
- Shortening of statute of limitation
- Changes in the rule of joint and several liability
- Limits on lawyers' contingency fees
- Elimination of collateral source rule
- Use of periodic payments for future damages
- Caps on noneconomic damages

The Department of Health and Human Services released the results of a 1-year study on medical liability and malpractice in August 1987 that included 30 recommendations.[51] Among other suggestions, the report said states should:
1. Limit noneconomic (including punitive) damages
2. Revise their statutes of limitations for the purpose of shortening the time period in which malpractice claims can be filed
3. Eliminate the ad damnum clause
4. Institute alternative dispute resolution mechanisms, such as pretrial screening panels, to reduce the number of claims taken to trial
5. Set limits on attorneys' fees
6. Eliminate joint and several liability
7. Allow for periodic payments of damages that exceed a predetermined figure

Remedial Tort Reform and the Professional Liability Problem

The difficulty with the many recently proposed solutions is that they are amazingly similar to those that were proposed to solve the crisis of the 1970s and, as is painfully apparent, were unsuccessful. How can anyone feel that they will be any more successful now? In addition, the American Medical Association's Department of Socioeconomic Affairs has estimated that the potential savings in professional liability insurance premiums in 1986, if these components of remedial legislation were to be passed, is as follows: periodic payments, 6%; collateral source, 8%; limitation of noneconomic damages, 12%; and contingency fee limitations, 9%. Because of some overlap, the total potential savings would be 28%. These estimates have been confirmed by several state agencies and others in making their predictions of cost savings.[41] How can physicians be happy with a one-time potential savings of 28% when professional liability premiums are increasing at 40% to 50% annually? The physicians' mutual insurance companies reported an average increase in 1986 of 39%, and commercial insurers have raised their rates even higher. It is obvious that remedial legislation will not solve the crisis in professional liability even if the entire packages of reforms were passed intact.

Fault-based Administrative Alternative to the Civil Justice System

In January 1988 The American Medical Association, 31 national medical specialty societies, and the Council of Medical Specialty Societies unveiled their medical liability project—a new system of resolving medical liability disputes.[7] Specifically, it is a system in which such disputes would be adjudicated by an expert administrative agency. This agency could be either a modification of the current state licensing board or a new agency. This medical board would also have the power to take appropriate action to identify and rehabilitate or discipline physicians whose practice patterns pose a threat to patients.

The administrative system for adjudicating medical liability can be divided into three parts: (1) the prehearing and initial hearing state, (2) the final decision of the board, and (3) judicial review. The proposed system would provide a significant benefit to patients by making available to any patient who has a claim of reasonable merit an experienced attorney from the medical board's general counsel's office who will litigate the claim on behalf of the patient free of charge.

Under proposed prehearing procedures, claims reviewers from the medical board will quickly evaluate claims and dismiss those without merit. For claims with merit, the claims reviewers will submit the matter to an expert in the same field as the health care provider. The expert will review the claim and make a judgment as to whether it has merit. The claims reviewer also will help the patient evaluate the claim and any settlement offers.

If the claim is not settled, it will be assigned to one of the medical board's hearing examiners. To encourage reasonable and timely settlements, blind settlement offers by the parties will be required before a hearing. A party would be subject to sanctions if the outcome of the case is not an improvement over a settlement offer that the party has rejected. The hearing examiner also will oversee expedited discovery and ensure that the parties have valid expert evidence available to support their case. At the hearing itself, the examiner will have broad authority to conduct the proceedings, including authority to call an independent expert to provide assistance in deciding the case. The hearing examiner will be required to render a written decision within 90 days of the hearing. In that decision the hearing examiner will determine whether the health care provider is liable for the claimant's injury and, if so, will determine the size of the damage award.

The hearing examiner's decision will be subject to review by the medical board. The board will have discretion to award fees and costs incurred in an appeal if the appeal presented no substantial question. The medical board will hear these cases as an appellate body in panels of three members. The medical board will make a full independent determination whether the health care provider's conduct was inadequate and caused the claimant's injury. Appeal from the medical board's decision will be to the intermediate appellate court of the state, where the review will be limited to whether the board acted contrary to statute or the board's own rules.

In addition to acting as an adjudicator of medical liability claims, the medical board also will develop rules and substantive guidelines to complement the statutory standards. The board will have administrative authority to initiate rulemaking and to solicit public comments. A rule promulgated by the board will have the force of law and will be subject to judicial review by an appellate court to determine if it is arbitrary, capricious, or in excess of the medical board's authority.

In conjunction with its expanded authority to handle medical liability claims, the board's performance monitoring function will be strengthened. Specifically, all settlements and awards based on medical liability will be reported to the board's investigative branch. This does not mean that every or even many liability determinations will lead to disciplinary actions. What it means is that every liability determination will give rise to an initial screening of the physician's practices as reported to the medical board. The primary purpose of this endeavor, as with all performance monitoring, will be education and rehabilitation. Thus the proposal is intended to enhance the board's ability to discover physicians who are impaired, lacking appropriate medical skills, or otherwise unable to provide acceptable medical care.

In conjunction with the proposals for monitoring physician performance by the medical board, the proposal calls for enactment of three categories of changes designed to further strengthen physician credentialing. First, reporting requirements will be increased by requiring hospitals and other health care institutions to conduct periodic physician performance reviews and to report to the medical board any conclusion that a physician's performance has been substandard. Insurers will be required to report cancellations and failures to renew for reasons that are not class based. All physicians will be required to report instances of suspected incompetence, impairment, or drug or alcohol dependence to the hospital credentials committee or other credentialing entity. To facilitate physician reporting, the state will provide immunity to physicians who report suspected problems in good faith. All of these reporting requirements are designed to increase substantially the amount of information available on physician performance.

To perform the complex and sensitive functions outlined here, the existing medical boards will be restructured or a new agency will be created. Membership on the board must become full time, probably for a 5-year term. Members will be selected by the governor from a list of nominees selected by a nominating committee and approved by the legislature. The project recommends a seven-person board, of whom at least two but no more than three members are physicians.

Proper implementation of the administrative model will require substantial funding, and the use of general revenues will be necessary. In addition, the state could make an initial assessment against insurance companies that provide medical liability insurance within the state or against physicians and other health care providers.

To ensure that the administrative model of medical liability passes constitutional muster, it will be necessary to codify the liability rules to be applied by the medical board under the administrative system.

Second, this information must be maintained in a form that is accessible to those who conduct professional review activities under the proposed system. To facilitate this process, the medical board will create and maintain a clearinghouse (or utilize the one established pursuant to the Health Care Quality Improvement Act of 1986) for reports from insurers, reports from hospitals, and reports from other states. Much of the information that will be collected under this proposal overlaps with the required reporting under current federal law. The licensing board will review this information routinely every 2 years. Immediate review is required in the event of certain negative reports. The board will also have authority to conduct an on-site review of the medical practices of all physicians against whom medical liability determinations (or settlements) have been made where there are reasons to believe that the physicians' practices pose a threat to patient health. In addition, certain credentialing entities, such as hospitals, will be required to check with the clearinghouse in connection with credentialing and privilege reviews.

Finally, the project calls for the furtherance of quality assurance/risk prevention goals by requiring all physicians to complete a number of continuing medical education "credit hours" per year. A certain percentage of these hours must be directly relevant to clinical practice. In addition, all physicians will be required to participate in a risk-management program. This change is designed to ensure that physicians maintain and enhance their professional skills.

In addition to the settlements and awards that are automatically reported, performance complaints—from hospitals, physicians, the public, or employees of the medical board—will be sent to a claims reviewer at the board for investigation. As with claims of medical liability, the claims reviewer will evaluate these complaints and, if appropriate, make a recommendation to the board's general counsel's office to pursue complaints that appear meritorious. A member of the general counsel's office will then make a decision whether to initiate a disciplinary charge. Once a disciplinary charge is initiated, a member of the general counsel's office will prosecute the charge before a hearing examiner who, after an appropriate due process proceeding, will make a decision as to what, if any, action is appropriate.

The examiner's action is subject to review by the board, which is required to provide notice of any disciplinary action to credentialing entities, insurers, and other state medical boards.

In addition, the rules governing standard of care based on custom and locality would be abolished in favor of a standard that focuses on whether the challenged actions fall within a range of reasonableness, to be determined by reference to the standards of a prudent and competent practitioner in the same or similar circumstances.

A significant modification in the causation standard is also proposed. The causation standard would be modified to allow recovery if the physician's negligence was a "contributing factor" in causing the injury.

The informed consent doctrine would be codified under the current "minority" rule, which requires that the adequacy of the disclosure should be measured from the perspective of the reasonable patient.

Noneconomic damages (and punitive damages) would be capped at an amount that is tied to a percentage of the average annual wage in the state.

The rule of joint and several liability would be abolished so that defendants would be liable for damages only in proportion to their actual liability. In addition, damages exceeding $250,000 would be structured and generally would be reduced by collateral source payments.

Advantages. The major advantages for physicians proported by the authors are certainty and predictability in liability determinations and ultimately in profession liability premiums. Additional advantages would be adjudication of liability by expert reviewers with clear guidelines, caps of awards of damages, and reduction in the length of the adjudicatory process. The key benefit for patients is the right to a hearing without having to find and pay a lawyer.

Disadvantages. The disadvantages of this proposal are many. This proposal would give the medical board wide-ranging powers to define practice standards under which a claim for medical liability is established. In addition, the board would develop rules and substantive guidelines to complement the statutory standards. It would have the administrative authority to initiate rule-making and to solicit public comments. A rule promulgated by the board would have the force of law. In addition, the board would be granted enhanced powers to monitor physicians performance including, but not limited to, periodic physician performance reviews by insurers, hospitals, and other health care institutions. Reporting to the board by physicians of any suspected instances of incompetence, impairment, or drug or alcohol dependency of their colleagues would be mandatory. These enhanced powers of the board become more objectionable when one reviews the composition of the board and the method of selection. The proposal would have "a full-time seven-member board, of which at least two but no more than three members are physicians." Members will be selected by the governor and approved by the legislature. Not only does this allow for the politicizing of the board, but even more disturbing, it would allow nonphysicians to set standards and rules for the practice of medicine.

Another major objection to this proposal is that it would perpetuate the complex, expensive, inefficient, and physician-damaging necessity of establishing fault. The authors talk about efficiency, yet a claim could proceed from evaluation by claims reviewers to a medical board hearing examiner review. From there it might be heard by a three-member appellate body of the medical board. An appeal of the medical board's decision could result in a further review by the intermediate appellate court of the states. The defendant physician could find himself or herself being forced to submit to multiple separate adjudicatory hearings with all the attendant pressures, stresses, and adverse publicity for the physician and his or her family.

The result of this stress has been well documented by Dr. Sara Charles[11,12] a psychiatrist at the University of Illinois. She did a study on randomly selected physicians from the Cook County Jury Verdict Reporter during a 5-year period from 1977 to 1981.[16] Her findings detail how physically and mentally devastating the litigation process can be to a physician and to his or her family and practice. In her study, she found the following effects of being sued:

- 18.8% felt a "loss of nerve in some clinical situations."
- 14% felt less self-confident as physicians.
- 56.6% felt they and their families had suffered as a result of the suit.
- 19% felt their practices had suffered.
- 33.6% contemplated retirement as a result of the suit.

Also, two clusters of symptoms were reported by physicians:

- 39% admitted to four or five symptoms suggestive of a major depressive disorder.
- 20% acknowledged another group of symptoms including anger, change in mood, inner tension, frustration, irritability, insomnia, fatigue, and headache.
- 8% noticed the onset of physical illness; 2% had myocardial infarctions during the process.
- 8% reported aggravation of previously diagnosed illnessess.

The findings are all the more disturbing when one realizes that they occurred in physicians of whom 75% were later acquitted by the courts. "It is the process itself that is so agonizing and stressful," according to Dr. Charles.

One can only speculate on the psychologic and physical stress that will accompany a legal process that could entail multiple separate adjudicatory hearings.

EFFECT ON THE QUALITY OF HEALTH CARE

As the professional liability crisis continues unabated, what is most disturbing is its adverse effect on the quality of health care in the United States. According to two highly respected physicians, it is contributing to the deaths of thousands of patients. At a meeting of the American Cancer Society in March 1986, Dr. Vincent T. DeVita, Jr., Director of the National Cancer Institute, estimated that the number of cancer victims undergoing therapy who die as a result of less than optimal treatment—or in other words, undertreatment—may number 10,000 or more annually.[12] "Malpractice is behind it in part. Doctors are frightened to death of malpractice," said Dr. DeVita. At the same meeting, Dr. William M. Hryniuk of the Ontario Cancer Foundation stated, "Doctors tend to undertreat in this country [United States], because they fear complications will lead to a lawsuit. People are suing themselves into second-class medicine by pursuing this mentality. They are binding their physicians' hands."

A 1985 survey conducted for the American College of Obstetricians and Gynecologists revealed that 35% of the respondents had "modified" their practices to deal with the liability situation.[19] These modifications included reducing the number of deliveries performed, decreasing high-risk obstetric care, or discontinuing obstetric practice altogether. Health and Human Services Secretary, Dr. Otis R. Bowen, in announcing the findings at a press conference stated, "The net impact of all this may mean that people will have less access to necessary medical care."

The American College of Surgeons, in a survey of its membership, found that 49% of its members were no longer accepting high-risk cases in consultation, and 28% were not performing certain procedures solely because of the risk of malpractice.[47] One has to wonder, if the most highly skilled surgeons are not treating the sickest of surgical patients, who is and at what cost?

BASIC OBJECTIVES FOR A SOLUTION

To obtain a lasting solution to the professional liability crisis, several objectives must be met.

1. Any new system must be fair both to the

patient and to the physician. Under the present system, even if the courts find them innocent, physicians, their families, and their practices all suffer. A new system should be implemented in a manner that would be less destructive to them. Also, our current system compensates only a small percentage of the patients who suffer a maloccurrence, and frequently the compensation is far in excess of any real losses. A satisfactory solution, therefore, must include compensation for a greater proportion of those patients in amounts that reflect each patient's actual economic loss.

2. A new system must be timely. At present adjudicating professional liability claims can take 7 years or longer. This hardly benefits the patient or the doctor. To be meaningful, compensation should begin no later than 90 days after the occurrence.
3. The system must be efficient. Under our current system, only 25% of professional liability premiums get to the patient, with the remaining 75% for overhead, such as legal fees and insurance company overhead. Overhead should consume less than 15% of premiums.
4. The system should be affordable. Professional liability premiums are approaching levels that are simply unaffordable by practicing physicians. The cost of insuring against maloccurrences must be shared by those who are at risk.

PROPOSED SOLUTIONS

There is a solution to medicine's professional liability problem that meets all of these objectives. It requires two things. First, the issue of compensating injured patients must be separated from the issue of dealing with physicians whose practices are outside acceptable norms. Once separated, reeducation, retraining, or disciplinary actions should be adequate to handle physicians with demonstated substandard practices. Second, the public, by increasingly resorting to litigation, has indicated that compensation for all maloccurrences is desirable. Consistent with this attitude, they should therefore participate in the costs attached to this compensatory approach.

We can accomplish the goal of compensating injured patients in either of two ways. Both are fair to the patient and the physician, and both are more timely, efficient, and affordable than our current system.

Workman Compensation Model

The first alternative is a plan similar to our workman's compensation program, which has been used for many years in this country to protect the injured worker.[36,53] In terms of design, this plan could easily be state-controlled, with each state setting up a patient compensation commission. Physicians or hospitals would file claims on behalf of their patients, and, although lawyers could also represent patients before the commission, their fees would be statutorily set, eliminating the contingency fee.

The commission would award net economic loss only, and losses longer than 90 days would be structured. Pain and suffering would not be covered or recoverable. Each state would collect premiums either as a surcharge on every health and accident policy sold, a surcharge on state income tax, or from general revenues. A subcommittee of the commission, perhaps called a medical professional review board, could easily identify and review hospitals or physicians experiencing repeated claims.

To understand how the workman's compensation-type plan would work, consider the following sample case. When a patient undergoes a partial colectomy with a colocolostomy for malignant disease, there is a well-recognized risk of 3% to 4%, even among the best surgeons, that a postoperative anastomotic leak will develop. This is caused by many factors, most important, the patient's age, obesity, and the extent of the cancer, as well as the technical competence of the surgeon. The patient compensation commission would decide prospectively if it wished to cover this type of complication by first determining the number of colectomies done in the United States. To determine the actuarial cost in terms of a premium, the commission would then multiply the number of colectomies by the percentage of times that the anastomotic leak complication occurs and by the cost of this complication.

With these data, if the commission felt it necessary and affordable, the anastomotic leak complication would be covered. The exact amount of that award would be determined by the individual panel hearing the case. Awards could differ from patient to patient depending on the severity of the maloccurrence. If, however, the commission felt that this complication is related more to the patient's age, obesity, or cancer and less to the technical skill of the surgeon, they might simply conclude that a patient who undergoes removal of a portion of the colon for cancer simply has to accept this inherent risk without compensation.

Maloccurrence Insurance Model

Maloccurrence insurance (insurance for designated compensable events) is an alternative way to compensate injured patients.[24,55] This would accomplish the same objectives as the workman's compensation-type plan; it would compensate patients for all medically related injuries that are associated with a medical intervention rather than with the condition for which intervention occurs. A public insurance corporation would be created instead of a patient compensation commission. This public corporation would guarantee a high degree of independence, expertise, and stability. Under its supervision a wide cross section of medical experts would develop a finite set of compensable events. Insurance experts would then use these data and, consulting with social workers, rehabilitation counselors, and others, arrive at actuarially sound awards that are fair to the patients. The awards would include medical and other needed care, such as rehabilitation, special education, and strictly compensatory elements not covered under other programs or insurance policies.

Using the example of the patient undergoing a partial colectomy, the public insurance corporation would follow the same steps and reasoning as the patient compensation commission. The difference between the two models is that, under the maloccurrence insurance model, the size of the award would be determined by a national average, thus allowing less flexibility for individual variations based on severity of the maloccurrence. Also under this system, there would be no need for routine representation by attorneys.

Under both the workman's compensation model and the maloccurrence model, the patient could elect to decline the award and resort to the tort system to obtain relief. However, clear parameters for compensation would have been established, and it is unlikely that the courts would significantly exceed these awards. In addition, the patient who elects to pursue the tort route would be facing only a 20% chance of success because defendant physicians prevail 80% of the time in court trials. Also, the patient would face a reduction of as much as 75% of the court award for fees and expenses and might have to wait as long as 7 years for resolution of the claim. Clearly, there would be greater incentive for the patient to accept the compensatory award rather than pursue tort action. Such acceptance would prevent further tort action by the patient.

Funding. Maloccurrence insurance could exist either as a national plan, with funds collected by the federal government and administered by the public corporation, or as individual state plans administered by local boards. In either case, maintenance of professional performance would be done at the state level. Funding could be achieved in a variety of ways, as long as it included all individuals at risk—all patients. For example, the program could be funded by a surcharge on every health and accident policy sold, a tax on all employers and self-employed persons, a surcharge on state and federal income tax, or general revenues of state and federal governments. In any case, the government would have to play a major role in financing, either as a primary source or revenue for the uninsured as well as Medicare and Medicaid recipients, or as a secondary source paying only for the uninsured.

Cost Considerations

A major concern about solutions, such as those mentioned here, is cost. In other words, because more patients are receiving compensation, wouldn't the cost be greater than our present system? The answer is "no" for several reasons. First, overhead would be reduced significantly from the current 80% to less than 15%. This would leave far more money to be redirected to the patients. Second, only economic losses would be covered. Third, the enormous cost of defensive medicine would be reduced substantially.

Although it is difficult to estimate the exact costs of a compensatory system without a list of events that would be compensable, some indirect evidence can be obtained from the experience of others. Two countries currently have long-standing successful no-fault medical injury systems in place and functioning.

In 1974 New Zealand introduced the first comprehensive no-fault compensation system for personal injury caused by accidents.[8,48] It covered medical mishaps and malpractice as well as traffic accidents, home accidents, and sporting accidents. The categories covered were:
1. Medical, surgical, dental, and first-aid misadventures
2. Actual bodily harm, including pregnancy and mental or nervous shock suffered by any person because of an act of aggression of any other person
3. Incapacity resulting from an occupational disease or industrial deafness
4. The physical and mental consequences of personal injury by accident

The Accident Compensation Corporation of the government provides the money and funds, which come from general taxation, employers' contributions, and a levy on the self-employed. Compensation consists of lump sums for loss of function and continuing payments based on earnings before the accident. If the claimant is dissatisfied with the amount of compensation, he may appeal to the Accident Compensation Corporation. If still unhappy, he may appeal then to the courts. If, however, compensation is accepted, the right to go to court is lost.

On January 1, 1975, Sweden introduced its form of no-fault medical injury system.[14,17] The key to compensation under the Swedish system is an injury or illness that "has occurred as a direct consequence of examination, treatment, or any other similar procedure that does not constitute an unavoidable complication of an act justified from a medical point of view." There are some broad exclusions:
1. Infections resulting from failure to use sterile instruments or substances
2. Drug-related injuries (a separate insurance plan, Pharma Insurance, covers these cases)
3. Unavoidable results of illness or surgery (such as surgical scars)
4. Failure to diagnose

In the case of infections and failure to diagnose, negligence must be proven under the Swedish tort system for the patient to recover damages. Once negligence is proven, compensation is made through a patient insurance program. Guidelines for determining which events are compensable have been promulgated with the assistance of the medical profession.

Both systems appear to be working well.[43] The Swedish system has been in effect for longer than 12 years and has proven to be efficient, fair (not one patient has elected to opt out of the system and appeal to the courts), and cost effective (the cost is currently $1 per citizen per year).[44-46]

Another parallel may be drawn from auto insurance. In Michigan the no-fault statute provides unlimited medical coverage plus lost-wage reimbursement for as much as $72,000 for victims of auto accidents. Michigan also requires drivers to carry $20,000 of tort-liability insurance. The cost of unlimited medical coverage and $72,000 in lost wages is $63 per year, whereas the cost of $20,0000 of tort-liability insurance is $55.

New York requires $50,000 of no-fault insurance, plus coverage for medical and wage benefits, which cost a total of $46 per year. By comparison, $10,000 of tort-liability insurance, which is also required, costs on average $118. Although the auto insurance does not exactly parallel professional liability insurance, it is interesting to compare the enormous differences in cost of insuring for unlimited medical coverage and lost-wage reimbursement with tort liability.

RECENT TRENDS

Despite the preponderance of sentiment from government agencies, state legislatures, and organized medicines that still exists for the conservative approach (remedial tort reform) for solving the professional liability problem, some recent events have revealed refreshing and hopeful change in that position:

- On November 14, 1986, President Reagan signed into law legislation to create a federal no-fault compensation program for children injured in vaccine-related incidents. This law has the support of the American Academy of Pediatrics, the American Medical Association, Dissatisfied Parents Together, and the National Association of Children's Hospitals and Related Institutions.
- The state of Virginia enacted a new compensation system for severe birth-injured infants in February 1987. The Injured Infants Act drafted by the Medical Society of Virginia would create a separate system that would compensate severely injured infants through an insurance pool paid for by obstetricians, hospitals, and universities. This action followed the ruling by District Judge James H. Micheal, Jr. that Virginia's Medical Malpractice Cap enacted in 1976 was unconstitutional on the grounds that it violated the seventh amendment to the US constitution, as well as Virginia's own state constitution. The seventh amendment states that "In suits at common law, where the value in controversy shall exceed $20, the right of trial by jury shall be preserved, and no fact tried by a jury, shall be otherwise re-examined in any court of the United States, than according to the rules of the common law."
- The authors of the recently released "Health Policy Agenda for the American People" state that a "no-fault" method of handling routine professional liability disputes, such as worker's compensation, which largely bypasses the courts, deserves a trial run.[26]
- The GAO report previously discussed also states that alternative dispute resolution mechanisms should be tested, and there should be experimentation to determine their effectiveness and feasibility. The Secretary of Health and Human Services should fund a series of demonstration projects using mediation, pretrial screening panels, arbitration, and no-fault compensation programs.
- The Health and Human Services report, in addition to the recommendations noted, said that insurers and health care consumer organizations should investigate "the feasibility of patient indemnity insurance," which patients could purchase to protect themselves against adverse medical outcomes.

Clearly, decision makers in our country are beginning to recognize that after 12 years of unsuccessful tort reform legislation, we must look elsewhere for a lasting solution to the professional liability problem. It is hoped that the above recommendations will be considered.

CONCLUSION

In conclusion, professional liability is one of the most severe problems facing practicing physicians today. It is forcing doctors to practice defensive medicine, the costs of which are adding significantly to the already rising costs of health care. It is dictating the tests and procedures that physicians will perform and the cases that physicians will accept in consultation. No one can be expected to perform perfectly under all circumstances and at all times. Physicians, like other human beings, do err. The current system is unfair, untimely, and inefficient and does not benefit those to whom it was intended. Remedial legislation is not the answer. We must have a major change in our tort system that removes the entire process from the court room.

Surgeons tend to view problems very directly. When we operate on a patient with cancer, our objective is not to remove a portion of the cancer in order to palliate the patient for a few months or more. Our goal is to remove the entire malignancy in the hopes of curing the patient. This does entail some risk, but the benefits, as we all know, can be substantial.

Professional liability is a cancer that is eating away at our entire health care system. It is a particularly virulent cancer that will not render itself treatable by palliative means such as remedial tort reform. Professional liability is a cancer that requires radical surgery, because if we cannot cure this cancer, it will certainly destroy our high quality of health care.

References

1. AM Best and Company: Best's insurance management reports, Property/Casualty edition: selected issues 1976 to 1987, Oldwick, NJ.
2. American Cancer Society: Proceedings of annual meeting, Miami, Fl, March 1986.
3. American College of Surgeons: Annual report of the Board of Governors, Oct 1984.
4. American College of Surgeons: Annual report of the Board of Governors, Oct 1985.
5. American College of Surgeons: Annual report of the Board of Governors, Oct 1986.
6. American College of Surgeons: Annual report of the Board of Governors, Oct 1987.
7. American Medical Association/Specialty Society: Medical Liability Project, Chicago, Jan 13, 1988.
8. Blair AP: Accident compensation in New Zealand, ed 2, Wellington, New Zealand: Butterworth, 1983.
9. Campbell H: The past and the present: the physicians as related to tribunals of the law, JAMA 4:477, 1885.
10. Chapman C: Stratton vs. Swamlond, The Pharos, p 20.
11. Charles S and Kennedy E: Defendant—a psychologist on trial for medical malpractice: an episode in America's hidden health crisis, New York, 1985, Free Press.
12. Charles SC: Malpractice suits: their effect on doctors, patients, and families, J Med Assoc Ga 76:171, 1987.
13. Chin A and Peterson M: Deep pockets, empty pockets, Institute for Civil Justice, 1985, Rand Corporation.
14. Cohen K: The Swedish no-fault patient compensation program: provisions and preliminary findings, Insurance Law Journal, 1976.
15. Conn Med 34:182, 1970.
16. Cook County jury verdict reporter/Illinois jury verdict reporter: Calendar year summary and index to malpractice trials, Chicago, 1983.
17. Cooper JK: Sweden's no-fault patient-injury insurance, N Engl J Med 294:23, 1268, 1976.
18. Couch NP et al: The high cost of low frequency events: the anatomy and economy of surgical mishaps, N Engl J Med 304:634, 1987.
19. Department of Professional Liability Insurance and its affect: Report of a survey of ACOG's membership, American College of Obstetrics and Gynecology, Washington, 1985.
20. Duke Law J: Project: The medical malpractice threat: a study of defensive medicine, 1971.
21. Duke Law J: Comment: An analysis of state legislative responses to the medical malpractice crisis, 1975.
22. Gordon V: The origin, basis and nature of medical malpractice liability, Conn Med 35:73, 1971.
23. Harvey L and Shubat S: AMA surveys of physician and public opinion, Chicago, 1986, AMA Division of Survey Research.
24. Havighurst CC and Tancredi LR: Medical adversity insurance: a no-fault approach to medical malpractice and quality assurance, Health and Society 51:125, 1973.
25. Hawkins C: Mishap or malpractice, London, 1985, Blackwell Scientific Publications, Ltd.
26. The Health Policy Agenda for the American People, Hirt E Jill, editor, Chicago, 1987.
27. Hershey N: The defensive practice of medicine: myth or reality? Milbank Mem Fund Quart 50:69, 1972.
28. JAMA, editorial: Defensive medicine, 252:1002, 1984.
29. Jury Verdict Research, Inc: Injury valuation reports, 1981 - 1984, Reports 251, 252, 253, Solon, Ohio.
30. Jury Verdict Research, Inc: Current award trends, 1985, Solon, Ohio.
31. King L: Medicine 100 years ago. I. 257:1642, 1987. II. 257:2204, 1987.

32. A legislator's guide to the medical malpractice issue: National Conference of State Legislatures, 1976.
33. Malpractice claims: National Association of Insurance Commissioners, 1978 Dec 1978.
34. Malpractice claims: National Association of Insurance Commissioners, 1980 Sept 1980.
35. Manuel BM: A surgeon's perspective on professional liability, Bull Am Coll Surg 70:6, 1985.
36. Manuel BM: Is tort reform the answer? An alternative approach to end the malpractice Crisis, Massachusetts Medicine 2:42, 1987.
37. McCallum J: Century old complaints regarding malpractice, N Engl J Med 294:59, 1976.
38. McNeil R: Development of the malpractice problem, Clin Obstet Gynecol 20:13, 1977.
39. Medical Liability Monitor, 1975 - 1987, Winnetka, Ill.
40. Medical malpractice closed claims: National Association of Insurance Commissioners, 1975 - 1978, 1980.
41. Milliman & Robertson, Inc: Actuarial analysis of American medical association tort reform proposals, Sept 1985.
42. Mills DH, Boyden JS, and Rubsamen DS: Medical insurance feasibility study, California Medical Association and California Hospital Association, 1977.
43. Moran PT: The New Zealand experience of no-fault compensation, Med Leg J 53:222, 1985.
44. Oldertz C: The Swedish patient insurance system: 8 years of experience, Med Leg J 52:43, 1984.
45. Oldertz C: Security insurance, patient insurance, and pharmaceutical insurance in Sweden, Am J Comparative Law 34:635, 1986.
46. Oldertz C: Compensation for personal injury: The Swedish alternative in an international perspective, Unpublished personal communication, June 9, 1987.
47. Professional liability survey report: American College of Surgeons, Oct 1984.
48. Report of the Royal Commission of Inquiry: Compensation for personal injury in New Zealand, Dec 1967.
49. Report of the secretary's commission on medical malpractice, Washington, DC, 1973, Department of Health, Education and Welfare, DHEW publication.
50. Report of the special task force on professional liability and insurance and the advisory panel on professional liability, JAMA 257:810, 1987.
51. Report of the task force on medical liability and malpractice, Washington, DC, Department of Health and Human Services, Aug 1987.
52. Report of The White House Working Group on Tort Policy, 1986. Washington, DC, 1986.
53. Schneider WR: The law of Workman's Compensation, rule of procedure and computation table, ed 2, St. Louis, 1932, Thomas Law Books.
54. Steel K et al: Iatrogenic illness on a general medical service at a university hospital, N Engl J Med 304:638, 1987.
55. Tancredi LD: Designing a no-fault alternative, Law and Contemporary Problems 49:277, 281, 1986.
56. US General Accounting Office: Medical malpractice study, Washington, DC, 1987, June Reports 1 - 5.

SAL FISCINA

Sal Fiscina is the principal of Fiscina and Associates, a health law firm. He is a graduate of Harvard College (1963), the University of Rochester Medical School (1967), and the George Washington University National Law Center (1973). He is board certified in family practice. Dr. Fiscina is a past president of the American College of Legal Medicine.

23

The Surgeon in Court

SAL FISCINA

NECESSITY FOR THE EXPERT MEDICAL WITNESS

When litigation concerns medical issues, most nonphysicians have insufficient knowledge to evaluate evidence and factual testimony. Therefore the court and jury must depend on expert witness evidence. Negligence (deviation from a requisite standard of care) is established in part by expert testimony about medical science or technique.

Ordinarily a factual witness testifies at trial to matters and events about which he or she has personal knowledge. Such witnesses are sometimes referred to as "percipient witnesses" because they are competent to testify only to what they have perceived through their senses. The expert witness, however, in addition to testifying about events or observations, is permitted to draw inferences and form conclusions from acquired factual data. This allowance is granted because of the presumed skill, training, and experience of the expert. Witnesses other than experts are not permitted to render opinions or to draw inferences.

Some courts allow appointment of expert medical witnesses only with the consent of the court, recognizing an expert's property interest in his or her time and training. When an expert is asked to review evidence and apply years of training and experience, the witness is providing a necessary and valued service for the court.

Many courts, however, have either ignored or rejected the property interest concept, confirming the power of the court to compel an expert medical witness to testify in a medical malpractice case. A few courts, however, have stated that a party to a medical malpractice suit may no more compel a particular medical expert to testify than compel a particular attorney to provide representation in a case.

In a surgical malpractice case, if a plaintiff is to be able to obtain the necessary proof that a defendant surgeon was negligent, an expert witness must testify that an appropriate standard of care was not met and that the negligent care was in fact the cause of the plaintiff's injuries.

Although many courts have strongly stated that physicians have a duty to testify as have other citizens, a serious question still remains whether expert witness testimony can be compelled. Courts have generally held that, on a case-by-case basis, in the final analysis, whether a specific expert witness' testimony is necessary and relevant to the proceedings determines whether the court will order the testimony. In a case in which a well-known surgeon refused to testify against an equally distinguished surgeon, the court exercised its discretion to consider the admissibility and relevance of the surgeon's testimony in deciding whether an unwilling expert witness may be compelled to testify.

An expert witness is a person who possesses

scientific, technical, or other specialized information. Experts function in litigation by testifying to establish facts or circumstances in specialized fields of knowledge. For example, an expert may be permitted to testify about the results of tests performed or observed, about inferences that may or may not be drawn from the facts of the case, or about whether the data another expert witness has relied on in drawing opinions or inferences are generally recognized by members of the profession. Most important, a medical expert may testify about the standard of medical practice by which a defendant's professional conduct will be measured.

WEIGHT AND BASIS FOR EXPERT MEDICAL TESTIMONY

Expert medical testimony is necessary where jurors require special information to conclude that a defendant physician's conduct violated a standard of care. An expert medical witness bases his or her opinion on facts admitted by the defendant or established by the testimony of witnesses. Because the existence of facts in evidence are not within the medical expert's personal knowledge, the expert must assume them to be true as a foundation for forming an opinion. It remains the jury's role to decide whether the facts are established.

There are many rules that regulate what information reaches the jury. Irrelevant, prejudicial, and unreliable evidence is excluded. Nevertheless, some admissible evidence is less reliable than other admissable evidence; therefore the jury's responsibility is to assess the credibility of a witness, giving appropriate weight to testimonial evidence.

Most courts will not permit a medical expert to express an opinion about the ultimate conclusion concerning negligence and causation, which are to be determined by the jury. The expert medical witness may not say that the defendant was negligent or "guilty of malpractice," although he may express an opinion about how the defendant's professional conduct in the circumstances of the case was consistent (or inconsistent) with reasonable practice for a similarly situated physician.

THEORY AND PROCESS IN MEDICAL MALPRACTICE LITIGATION

Negligent medical practice consists of one or more improper acts or omissions constituting substandard practices in rendering medical services. Although professional negligence does not necessarily imply general lack of competence, it constitutes definitively more than mistake or bad therapeutic outcome.

There are a number of legal principles under which a plaintiff may bring a medical malpractice action against a physician, most notably negligence, abandonment, breach of contract, or battery. If a plaintiff establishes any one of these so called "causes of action," a monetary judgment from defendant may be awarded.

Most medical malpractice suits are based on the principles and requirements of professional negligence law. Negligence is a breach of an established duty to behave reasonably and prudently under circumstances where foreseeable harm may be caused to another by unreasonable conduct. In contrast to the legal requirements for intentional acts, such as required for a legal cause of action in battery or defamation, professional negligence is founded on several important concepts or "elements".

The first element of professional negligence is existence of a physician's duty to each patient to possess and to exercise on the patient's behalf, the knowledge, skill, and care usually exercised by reasonable and prudent physicians under similar circumstances. The prevailing state of medical knowledge and the resources available to the physician are illustrations of circumstances that may influence the standard of care required of a physician. The second element of professional negligence is a breach of the physician's duty to his patient to provide the minimum standards of care. The third element is the establishment of legal damages. If the patient has not been legally harmed, there can be no monetary recovery. Damages of several types are ordinarily compensated by money recovered in a malpractice suit. The fourth element is the establishment that the defendant physician's breach caused plaintiff's damages.

Causation, sometimes the most complex and elusive concept in a professional negligence case, consists of two branches, causation-in-fact and foreseeability. Cause-in-fact may be found when one event is the cause of a second event, if and only if a second event or result would not have occurred when and as it did, but for the preceding event. This "but for" test is met in some cases, for example, where a surgeon leaves an instrument in the abdominal cavity. Such a breach of the standard of care could be the "but for" cause of an abdominal abscess, a subsequent operation, or death of the patient, or all of these damages. In other cases, causation-in-fact may be difficult to demonstrate, as where delay in diagnosis of a disease reduces the patient's already small statistical chance of survival. The legal requirements for establishing causation vary from state to state.

Foreseeability is the second branch of the causation element. Plaintiff's damages must be reasonably foreseeable results of defendant's substandard practice, that is, they must be proximately related to defendant's conduct. Ordinarily plaintiff must prove only that injuries were the type that would have been foreseen by a reasonable physician or were likely to occur as a result of the negligence.

PROCESS IN MEDICAL MALPRACTICE LITIGATION

A medical malpractice case starts with an event or outcome in a patient's diagnosis or treatment that precipitates a claim of professional negligence. Ordinarily litigation actually commences when the patient retains an attorney and signs a retainer agreement and a statement authorizing the attorney to copy and examine the patient's medical records. The attorney will have one or more physicians review the records and perhaps examine the client to evaluate the client's condition and prognosis. Limits on investigation imposed at this stage of litigation include prohibition on contact between plaintiff's attorney and a defendant physician represented by an attorney, unless that attorney is present. Witnesses are not required to talk to an opposing attorney. Some potential factual witnesses, such as medical records custodians, may not talk to anyone without the patient's authorization.

The filing of "complaint" puts the dispute into the formal legal process. A copy of the complaint and the summons to respond is delivered to the defendant physician. The formal commencement of the lawsuit enlarges the powers of both parties of the dispute to conduct inquiries through pretrial discovery procedures. This process includes written interrogatories, oral depositions, demands to produce records, and occasionally physical or mental examination of the plaintiff. At depositions, witnesses answer questions under oath and are subject to perjury for false swearing. Attorneys have subpoena power to compel disclosure of witnesses and documents.

The rules of civil procedure that govern medical malpractice action are designed to permit pretrial discovery without intervention of the judge. The policy of courts favors full disclosure. Ordinarily parties may obtain discovery of any relevant, nonprivileged matter if the information sought appears reasonably calculated to lead to the discovery of evidence that would be admissible at trial. A privileged matter is one given special protection from disclosure. Allowing discovery of relevant evidence is much broader than the former practice of allowing discovery only of admissible evidence.

The complaint that commenced the lawsuit was a "pleading." Exchanges of pleadings are a legal procedural process to force the parties to focus on issues in dispute that will be presented and resolved at trial. The defense attorney files an answer on the defendant physician's behalf, which denies some or all of the plaintiff's allegations and sometimes asserts defenses. The complaint and answer may be freely amended if the course of discovery leads the parties to revised positions during the pretrial state. Only the issues presented in the pretrial conference will be allowed to be presented at trial. The conference is a formal meeting of opposing attorneys with a judge. It marks the end of the pretrial discovery stage of litigation.

There usually comes a point in preparation for trial when the opposing sides know substantially the contentions in case; when the content of the witness' testimony is no longer unknown; and when the documentary evidence is fully shared. Although the trial may still contain surprises, by now the characters, scenes, and dialogue of the "play" that is to be re-created are understood. What remains to be seen is what force the production of the play will command for the judge or jury.

A jury is selected on the basis of "voir dire," a series of questions intended to detect undesirable jurors. The trial begins with the attorney for plaintiff making an opening statement to the jury, outlining the plaintiff's claims and theories, and indicating what the witnesses and documents will show. The defendant's attorney may then give an opening statement or may elect to make it after the plaintiff has finished presenting the plaintiff's case-in-chief. The presentation of evidence starts the plaintiff's case-in-chief, consisting of witnesses who testify to facts or events that are intended to establish that the defendant physician was negligent and that such negligence caused compensable harm to the plaintiff. Plaintiff's witnesses will also attempt to demonstrate how much money might be appropriate to compensate the plaintiff for past, present, and future expenses and for intangible harm, such as pain and mental anguish.

Cross-examination of witnesses is intended to persuade the jury that the witness is not credible or is mistaken. After the plaintiff has presented all the evidence in the case-in-chief, the physician's attorney will offer witnesses, presenting credible defense witnesses who will deny or contradict the testimony of plaintiff's witnesses. A defense medical expert may testify that the physician, for example, followed the usual and customary practice of physicians under similar circumstances. The witness may also assert that the plaintiff did not suffer any impairment or dysfunction as a consequence of the defendant physician's treatment. The defendant can deny one or more elements of plaintiff's case without admitting the others. For example, he may deny that he was negligent or may say that even if he had been negligent, such negligence did not cause the plaintiff's injury. Even if not logically compatible with denial, the defense may present one or more instances of affirmative defense, for example, evidence that the plaintiff was contributorily negligent. Thus even if defendant was negligent, the plaintiff's damages may be caused by his own conduct because the physician's instructions were disregarded. Therefore the plaintiff's act was a cause-in-fact of the damages.

The evidence-presenting phase of the trial is closed when both sides rest. During closing arguments, each side attempts to recapitulate and persuade, recounting evidence and urging the credibility of one or another witness. Ordinarily each attorney will suggest what the jury may reasonably infer from the evidence.

TESTIMONY ON THE STANDARDS OF MEDICAL PRACTICE

A physician's duty to patients requires adherence to a reasonable standard of care. Breach of the duty involves a violation of the standard of care. The standard of care applied by a court may determine the outcome of a case. In surgery, for example, one of several standards of care may be applied by a court, namely, what the majority of surgeons would do; what a reasonable, prudent surgeon would do in applying sound and accepted medical practices; what a reasonable, prudent surgeon would do, having due regard for the welfare of the patient; or what a majority or a respectable minority of surgeons would do.

Each of these standards is a yardstick against which a surgeon's professional acts and omissions may be measured. Their effect in a professional negligence suit may change as knowledge about various medical concepts change. Some procedures have gradually become not only acceptable practice but, in some cases, may be the only acceptable practice. Tests of the standard of care include the words "under same or similar circumstances." The clinical facts and circumstances of a particular case are important qualifying factors and conditions in setting standards. Included among those circumstances is the nature of the physician's practice. A surgeon is held to the same standard as other similarly practicing surgeons. Occasionally the same standard may apply to members of different surgical specialties, such as (1) neurosurgeons and orthopedists, who both may perform diskectomies or (2) plastic surgeons and otolaryngologists who both may perform maxillofacial reconstruction. In many jurisdictions, a surgeon may be permitted to testify about the standard of care for any type of surgical practice if he asserts familiarity (not necessarily experience) with the particular surgical condition or procedure. Thus a general surgeon may be permitted to testify to the standard of care for a cardiovascular surgeon, although the amount of weight such testimony will be given by the jury is another matter.

Historically, the circumstances influencing the standard of care also included the "school" of the defendant. Thus an osteopathic surgeon might not be allowed to testify on the standard of care for an allopathic surgeon. That distinction has been diluted, caused in part by the apparent reluctance of some allopaths to testify against a professional of the same school.

The standard of care has also been influenced and limited by the locality in which the physician provided service. This limitation, however, has been expanded recently because in many jurisdictions it is now presumed that the average physician in an isolated area has had adequate training and through the use of technologic advances has the opportunity to stay as professionally current as metropolitan colleagues. Thus a surgeon in an isolated locality may be held to a national standard for specialty practices. Publications of the various specialty societies may then become accepted by some courts as documenting national standards of care for certain specialties.

There are many matters about which a physician may properly be questioned by professional colleagues but that are ordinarily inadmissible at trial. For example, a testifying surgeon may be asked whether he is aware of the standard of care for treatment of a particular disease. If the surgeon responds in the affirmative, he will then be asked to define the standard. If the witness is then asked what is done in his own practice, what he personally teaches residents or what he has written about the subject, these answers may not be admissible into evidence. The rationale is that an expert witness' personal practice and custom are irrelevant to the issue of establishing the requisite standard of care. On cross-examination, however, the opposing attorney may properly ask those questions to attack the witnesses' opinions on the standard of care.

Because of the presumed reluctance of physicians to testify that a colleague had erred, some courts have applied the doctrine of res ipsa loquitur when an adverse result is not found in the absence of negligence, and when the instrumentalities involved in the procedure are under the defendant surgeon's sole control, the defendant surgeon has the burden to prove that the services he rendered were not substandard. The burden of proof at the commencement of litigation is imposed on the plaintiff, who must prove each and all the elements of professional negligence. The doctrine of res ipsa loquitur has its greatest application to intraoperative injury, where the unconscious anesthetized patient cannot possibly contribute to the injury or to even know what transpired that may have caused the injury. When a court applies this doctrine, plaintiff's expert medical witness need not testify that certain acts or omissions of the defendant surgeon deviated from the required standard of care. The witness need only testify that such an adverse outcome rarely, if ever, results from the procedure in question if the standard of care is followed. Then the defendant surgeon must demonstrate or establish how and why the injury occurred while proving that conduct was within the standard of care.

PROOF OF CAUSATION OF PLAINTIFF'S DAMAGES

The plaintiff must prove that defendant physician's negligent conduct caused plaintiff's injuries. Under clear and obvious circumstances, courts may take judicial notice that causation has been established, and no proof of causation is required. Otherwise, causation must be established by plaintiff's expert witness testifying that the defendant surgeon's negligent conduct caused plaintiff's injury. The causation issue is a question of fact that the jury must decide in a malpractice case. Nevertheless, it is a complex legal issue susceptible to faulty scientific reasoning. Simplistic arguments, such as when an event precedes another event, the prior event must have caused the other, may be attractive to juries faced with complex medical data and contradictory expert testimony. In cases where a defendant surgeon's conduct has been exceedingly poor (as when a surgeon operates while under the influence of a chemical substance), the jury would only become inflamed if the surgeon's attorney argued that the surgeon's conduct did not actually cause plaintiff's injuries.

Causation issues are often central in cancer malpractice cases, especially those involving breast cancer, where life expectancy may not be necessarily related to a delay in diagnosis. Thus negligent delay in diagnosis may not be causally related to a patient's death from cancer. If the type of cancer in question is ordinarily curable with early detection, however, a significant delay in diagnosis may be held to be a foreseeable cause of a patient's death. Warnings regarding signs of cancer have persuaded the public that some forms of cancer are curable or controllable with early diagnosis and appropriate therapy. Ordinarily plaintiff will introduce evidence on causation purporting to establish that the cancer was at an early stage when the patient consulted the surgeon and that prompt diagnosis would probably have led to a cure. The defendant will present countervailing evidence that, even if diagnosis of cancer had been made when the plaintiff alleged was proper, the course of the disease was not alterable.

Issues of causation must be proven by expert medical testimony. Although preexisting conditions and injuries do not excuse the negligent, a defendant physician can sometimes disprove plaintiff's causation contention by establishing that the patient would have suffered the same injury or experienced the same outcome, regardless of defendant's improper conduct. In addition, the defendant may be able to prove that plaintiff's injury was substantially the result of an independent cause or intervening factor.

THE NATURE AND ROLE OF DAMAGES

The issue of damages is central to every medical malpractice claim. Compensatory damages encompass two components. Special damages include past and future medically related costs needed as a result of negligence and past and future loss of earnings or of earning capacity. General damages include pain and suffering, mental anguish, for example, from scarring and deformity, loss of consortium (sexual relations, family relationships, and love), and hedonic damages, which is loss of enjoyment of life. Exemplary, or punitive, is a separate form of damages.

Ordinarily, compensatory damages are available to injured plaintiffs in most professional negligence cases. When the question of negligent conduct has been determined in plaintiff's favor, the measure of damages awarded is determined by a consideration of the nature of the injuries sustained.

Exemplary damages are rarely awarded in medical malpractice actions, in part because the threat of compensatory damages are thought to be sufficient deterrents to antisocial professional behavior. Exemplary damages, however, are sometimes awarded for shocking or outrageous professional conduct, for improper acts or omissions that deviate so widely from the applicable standard of care that such conduct is indicative of a willful or reckless disregard for the patient's welfare. Exemplary damages are awarded to punish the defendant and to discourage similar conduct. When plaintiff has proven such gross negligence to the court, exemplary damages may be awarded as a multiple of the compensatory damages.

Many medical malpractice suits involve multiple physicians, because the plaintiff's attorney often does not know exactly whose negligence may have caused the plaintiff's injury. More than one physician may have cared for the patient and had a duty to protect the patient from the harm that materialized. In situations where the negligence of more than one defendant combined to produce a single inseparable injury, all defendants may be jointly liable for plaintiff's damages. The application of this doctrine of "joint and several liability," allows the plaintiff to collect part of the judgment from each defendant or to collect the entire sum from any one of the joint defendants. Each defendant who pays more than his share of the judgment, as determined by jury determinations of proportionate liability, may seek contribution from any other defendant who has paid less than a proper share.

Plaintiff may also sue more than one defendant to facilitate the discovery process. A surgeon named as a defendant can be required to answer a written interrogatory or to appear for a deposition. A hospital may be joined as a defendant in the case to facilitate subpoena access to the hospital's policies, procedures, and files, which may be useful to prove standards of care and may pinpoint prior knowledge of hazardous conditions.

Defendant's insurance carrier will sometimes bring other physicians into a malpractice suit as third-party defendants to add another carrier to the suit, in an effort to reduce the amount they will have to pay if plaintiff prevails.

CALLING THE EXPERT WITNESS

An attorney who calls an expert medical witness to testify must first qualify the witness as an expert. The process of qualifying an expert is addressed to the judge so that the court may declare that the witness is an expert. Qualifying questions are then asked to show that the expert witness has credentials with which to analyze a specialized or technical matter and to persuade the jury that the expert's opinion is worth accepting. When the court has declared a witness as an expert, he is then entitled to present testimony. In assessing the opinion of an expert witness, the jury weighs the credentials of opposing witnesses against each other and also considers the general impression that each expert witness makes while testifying.

A plaintiff in a malpractice suit can establish a case by the testimony of the defendant physician who may be examined regarding the standard of skill and care ordinarily exercised by similarly situated physicians under like circumstances. He may also be questioned with respect to how his professional conduct compared with the standard.

Under certain circumstances, a plaintiff in a malpractice case may make use of the expert knowledge, training, and experience of the defendant physician in establishing evidence of the standard of care. The plaintiff may subpoena the defendant as an expert witness. In most jurisdictions, one party may be permitted to call the opposing party as an adverse witness and to examine him under the procedural rules applicable for cross-examination. The rationale is that any witness who may cast light upon a fact in issue should be heard, subject to observations concerning knowledge or truthfulness.

Some courts have concluded that the importance of enabling the plaintiff to discover both the factual and opinion testimony of the defendant physician is accentuated because of the plaintiff's difficulty inherent in securing expert witnesses. The plaintiff's only recourse in many cases may be to question the defendant physician as an expert to establish the malpractice claim. Although defendants maintain that it is not fair to allow the plaintiff to force the defendant to become a plaintiff's expert, ordinarily no one is allowed to withhold material and relevant information that is needed in a judicial proceeding, because the withholding of relevant testimony obstructs the administration of justice. The duty of a witness to testify is owed to society, not to the individual parties. If the testimony will provide facts that will aid the court in arriving at a just decision, there is a duty to testify.

The trend that is followed by more and more courts is to permit a plaintiff in a malpractice case to question the defendant physician as though under cross-examination and to elicit from him or her an expert opinion based either on facts within personal knowledge or on a properly presented hypothetic question. To the extent that a plaintiff is able to obtain satisfactory answers from the defendant, the defendant's testimony obviates the need for plaintiff to obtain additional medical expert testimony.

USE OF DEPOSITION TESTIMONY

Oral depositions involve taking sworn testimony out of court to discover facts and opinions that may be presented at trial and facts that may lead to the discovery of other evidence. In addition, depositions allow attorneys to gather material for impeachment of adverse witnesses and to commemorate helpful testimony in a form that can be read at trial if a witness is unavailable to provide live testimony.

There are some important differences in testifying at a deposition and at trial. An expert medical witness deposed for the first time might be surprised by the apparent informality of the participants. Without a break in the questioning, lawyers stand up to stretch, or refill their coffee cups, or come and go during a session, and some seem to be observers rather than participants. A deposition started one day may be continued to the next or to a date several months later. Parties to the suit may be present or absent. Depositions may be taken at the expert medical witness' office, at a hospital conference room, or at a lawyer's office. A court reporter is always present to make verbatim stenographic or machine notes for later transcription to a typewritten record. The reporter administers the same oath to the witness as the witness would take in court, and he or she records every question and answer and every objection, as well as discussions and statements by attorneys regarding certain matters, unless it is agreed that the commentary be "off the record."

An attorney may ask questions at a deposition that could not be asked at trial. For example, questions that call for hearsay are acceptable during a deposition but would be subject to objection at trial. If a deposition containing inadmissible evidence is used at trial, the judge will order that such questions and their responses not be read to the jury. Attorneys at depositions, however, may not inquire into privileged matters, such as conversations between clients and their attorneys, because no judge is present at depositions to rule on attorneys' objections. Procedural rules allow attorneys to reserve most of their objections at time of the depositions and to make them before trial or even at trial. Some states require that certain technical objections to inquiries are stated on the record at time of the deposition, so the questioning attorney is given the opportunity to rephrase or restate the question in a manner less objectionable or more acceptable to the challenging attorney.

Oral depositions are often the most effective form of discovery used by attorneys. The information supplied in response to written discovery techniques, such as interrogations, however, passes through the hands of the supplying attorney, who can lawfully rephrase and perhaps defuse potentially damaging information. In an oral deposition, however, the witness may not alone be able to conceal or mollify information and attitudes that may hurt the case before a jury. If the witness is unavailable at trial, the deposition can be read to the jury, in place of live testimony. Some states allow an attorney to read a deposition or parts of it to a jury instead of calling a witness to the stand even when the witness is available. When a witness has not been prepared for deposition and has made numerous unfortunate statements on the record, an attorney for one party or the other may wish to use the transcript in this manner for impeachment and other purposes.

Deposition testimony can be used for impeachment in the cross-examination of a witness. If a witness has given a certain answer on deposition and testifies otherwise at trial, an attorney can point out the discrepancy in a manner calculated to question the witness' credibility. Where a witness has amended answers after reading this transcript, he may have to explain in court the changes and why they were made.

Most courts now permit an attorney to videotape depositions in a medical malpractice case, although videotaping is not usually a substitute for a court reporter present to make a stenographic or machine record. Videotaped depositions may be powerful trial tools because once a physician's deposition has been recorded, the attorneys can be confident that if the physician cannot personally appear at trial, the jury can see the testimony in the next best way. Moreover, many people today may be more receptive to a videoimage than to a witness in person. In addition, a "jury-friendly" video witness can employ colorful charts and models that can be introduced into evidence at trial and can then be taken to the jury room to continue "testifying" during jury deliberation.

USE OF AUTHORITATIVE LITERATURE

Medical malpractice cases, especially surgical malpractice cases, are often highly technical. Thus the standard or authoritative literature relevant to the surgical issues provides the most fertile source for questions to a defendant on the issues of standard of care, causation, and damages. The main objective of plaintiff's attorney in cross-examining a defendant's expert is to obtain agreement on as many of the fundamental issues as possible.

Because a medical witness' professional education and training consist of reading, reviewing, and in many instances, writing surgical literature, this relatively objective body of information can provide the basis for obtaining admissions from the defendant's experts. Agreement from the witness on basic propositions concerning, for example, surgical conduct and performance must be established. Unless authoritative statements in the literature are adopted and agreed to by the witness, however, such statements in the literature may remain inadmissible hearsay. Thus the plaintiff's attorney will try to establish both that the literature is standard or authoritative and that the witness agrees that the body of information is relied on by competent practitioners. Even if the witness will not agree that the literature is standard or authoritative, the plaintiff's attorney will often then seek to obtain agreement on the content of the literature.

EXAMINATION OF THE WITNESS (DIRECT AND CROSS)

Direct examination except for preliminary matters is confined to direct questions. For the medical expert witness, the process consists of identifying the witness and describing his role in the case; qualifying the witness' expertise; and eliciting evidence of the patient's treatment (if the expert actually examined the patient, it would also include the history obtained from the patient, the tests performed by the witness on the patient, and the results of those tests). Finally, based on the medical record or on a hypothetical question comprising reasonable assumed facts, the witness will present his opinion about diagnosis, causation, prognosis, and other issues. The central concept in direct examination is that the witness and not the attorney must provide the testimony. Accordingly, the examination should be conducted to allow the witness rather than the attorney to present the desired testimony. A witness will not impress the jury with the credibility of his testimony if he merely concurs in a series of statements enunciated by the attorney.

The attorney who calls a witness to the stand becomes the proponent of that witness. This attorney's examination of that witness is referred to as direct examination. An attorney other than the proponent is called the opponent of that witness. Cross-examination is examination by an opponent attorney. When a plaintiff's attorney calls the defendant physician to the stand, plaintiff attorney is technically the proponent of the physician defendant. Under such circumstances, the defense attorney technically becomes the opponent of his own client, the physician defendant. Obviously the defense attorney's cross-examination of his client would be "friendly." In the usual case, however, the aim of cross-examination is to persuade the jury that a witness is not credible. A major objective of a cross-examiner is to discredit the witness. Thus the attorney's basic approach is to secure the information needed to support questions to the jury explicitly or implicitly concerning the credibility of witnesses.

During the course of cross-examination, an expert witness should remain as objective as possible. His role in court should be that of an impartial expert trying to help court and jury ascertain and understand the medical and scientific information. The credibility of a witness is affected by the witness' bias and by presenting testimony. The witness should always endeavor to stay on sound medical and scientific ground. If a witness is persuaded to extend his expertise and experience, he will be demonstrably uncomfortable with testimony on these matters. An astute cross-examiner will detect this discomfort and cross-examine the witness on the point where he may succeed in destroying the witness' entire credibility.

By keeping within his professional expertise and by admitting his limitations, the witness also will avoid appearing like a vain know-it-all. If the witness allows the attorney to pose questions outside his field of expertise, the witness should respond that he does not feel qualified to render an opinion because of limited expertise in that area. This should protect the witness from further examination on the subject. If, on the other hand, the expert witness puffs up qualifications or elaborates on the extent of the review made of the case, such exaggeration is likely to be exposed and to cause the witness acute embarassment and loss of credibility.

In preparing to render an opinion or present testimony, the witness should review all available information about the case including, in particular, the leading literature that recognized authorities have written on the points that the witness is planning to offer as expert testimony. The viewpoints of others may help formulate the witness' own opinion, and a witness must expect to be cross-examined about the literature. The witness should insist on preparation for his testimony with the attorney who plans to offer his or her testimony. In addition, the attorney should advise the witness on what to expect on cross-examination.

Conservative courts tend to forbid cross-examination that uses professional literature unless the witness recognizes the source as an authority and also testifies having relied on it in formulating an opinion. Most courts allow an expert witness to be cross-examined on professional literature that the witness admits is considered an authority. Accordingly, the witness should be conservative in recognition of literature as authoritative and admit as "authorities" only those texts that are truly outstanding reliable standards in the field. If a witness is convinced that so-called authorities are wrong, he may disagree with them as long as sound reasons for disagreement are given.

The witness should also realize that contrary opinion of authorities will not necessarily discredit testimony. Some courts allow an expert witness to be cross-examined on professional literature that the court, after hearing evidence from other experts on the subject, determines will be the recognized authority on the point in question. A medical expert witness should always review anything he or she has personally written in the field, because there is a risk that this direct testimony will be seriously impeached on cross-examination by the expert's own writings that may express viewpoints appearing to be contrary or in conflict with his or her direct testimony. In the pretrial stage, during deposition a witness is often asked to name the literature on which he or she relied in forming an opinion, or any of his or her contributions to literature. The attorney will check those references and impeach the witness at trial if they differ from the witness' stated conclusions or opinion.

EFFECTIVENESS OF A PHYSICIAN AS AN EXPERT AND AS A WITNESS

In rendering an opinion in a medical malpractice case, the medical expert witness must understand and take into account the legal distinction between medical "possibility" and "probability." Although anything is "possible," in law nothing is "probable" unless it is more likely than not (or its chances of being so are greater than 50%). Various jurisdictions have different rules regarding this distinction. Some forbid the witness from rendering an opinion based on medical possibility, concluding that such an opinion would invade the province of the jury. In these jurisdictions, the witness is restrained to confine testimony to medical probabilities. Most courts, however, require that expert testimony be confined within the realm of "reasonable medical certainty." The attorney should inform the expert of local court rules so that the legal difference between mere "possibilities," and "probabilities" is anticipated.

The attorney who plans to call the witness should anticipate and prepare the witness for certain questions that the opposing attorney may be expected to ask. For example, the attorney may ask if the witness has talked to anybody about the case. If the witness answers "no," the jury will suspect that something is not right because a well-prepared attorney will always talk to a witness. If the witness answers "yes," the attorney will imply that the witness was told what to say. Experts should be instructed to say frankly that they talked to whomever they have, including the attorney or even the defendant physician, to ascertain the facts of the case.

An attorney may also ask the witness if he or she is getting paid to testify in the case, implying that the witness is paid to say what the payer wants. The witness should respond that he or she is not being paid to testify but is receiving compensation for time and expenses. There is no stigma attached to an expert being paid a reasonable professional rate for time expended in preparation and presentation of testimony. Reasonable rates are best calculated on the basis of the usual and customary charges made on a time basis for the professional services by physicians of similar stature, specialty, and experience. An agreement on hourly rates should be made with the attorney in advance so that questions concerning the nature or reasonableness of those charges will not elicit awkward, inconsistent, or unexpected responses.

Expert witnesses should be sure they do not testify in fields that cannot reflect the maximum benefit of their expertise. The threshold requirement to testify as an expert in most states is simply to be a licensed physician practitioner. Thus, in a technical sense, a physician would then possess legally sufficient qualifications to answer questions in other specialty areas. When it has been demonstrated that the medical expert witness has a proper medical degree and a medical license, the traditional rule has been that questions on all medical subjects are proper and the witness is qualified to give expert testimony. Nevertheless, the persuasiveness of a medical expert witness may depend on the clearly appropriate and imminent specialist testifying in his or her own field of training and experience.

Suggested Readings

1. Baum AZ: How F. Lee Bailey would cross-examine you, Med Econ, Sept 11, 1972.
2. Bell EF: How to be an expert witness, J Legal Medicine, Oct 1976.
3. Bergen RP: Medical books as evidence, JAMA 217:527, 1971.
4. Bradford RT: Medical specialists in legal medicine, J Legal Medicine, Jan/Feb 1974.
5. Bucy PC: The medical expert in malpractice suits, JAMA 232:1352, 1975.
6. Evidence and the medical witness. In Wecht CH, editor: Legal Medicine Annual, 1973.
7. Gardner RC: Malpractice and the medical expert, Case and Comment, March/April, 1986.
8. Ginsberg WH: Your courtroom attitude can break your malpractice case, Physician's Management, Aug 1984.
9. Glass LS: The physician as expert witness, Alaska Med, 27, 1985.
10. Hirsh HL: Physician as a witness: rights, duties and obligations, J Legal Medicine, Feb 1975.
11. Hirsh HL: Physician's duty to testify: right to medicolegal fees, Case and Comments, March/April 1976.
12. Holder AR: Physician's duty to testify, JAMA 219:1541, 1972.
13. Horsely JE: Testifying? Direct examination should be a breeze, Med Econ, Nov 8, 1971.
14. Horsely, JE: Testifying in court: how to figure a witness fee, Med Econ, Sep 13, 1971.
15. Horsely JE: Testifying in court: the advanced course, You can't go wrong with the right preparation Med Econ, July 5, 1971.
16. Horsely JE: Testifying: will the way you come on turn them off? Med Econ, Oct 11, 1971.
17. Horsely JE: Testifying: how to act toward judge and jury, Med Econ, Feb 28, 1972.
18. Horsely JE: Testifying: how to handle a tough cross-examiner, Med Econ, March 27, 1972.
19. Jackson TP: Presenting expert testimony, Trial Law Notes 11:21, 1975.
20. Kumin CM: The expert witness in medical litigation, Ann Intern Med 100:139, 1984.
21. Medical testimony without bias, JAMA 196:193, 1966.
22. Morris C: How not to lose a malpractice case before trial, Med Econ, March 5, 1973.
23. Payment of fees for services of medical witnesses, JAMA 201:309, 1967.
24. Rosen WD: Please take the witness stand, Mr. Medical Book, Case and Comment Jan/Feb 1979.
25. Russell F: Keeping your cool under cross-examination, Med Econ, Feb 20, 1978.
26. Sagall EL: Anatomy of a malpractice suit, Resident and Staff Physician, April 1974.
27. Sanbar S and Pataki LI: The expert witness in medical liability cases, Oklahoma Bar Association, Summer 1978.
28. Stratton WT: The physician as an expert witness, Kans Med, June 1986.
29. Usher A: The expert witness, Med Sci Law 25:111, 1985.
30. Wecht CH: What the medical expert can expect from the trial lawyer, J Legal Medicine, Jan/Feb 1974.

PART FIVE

Summary

24. RECOMMENDATIONS: A PERSONAL PERSPECTIVE
    Ira M. Rutkow

24

Recommendations: a Personal Perspective

IRA M. RUTKOW

Any attempt to summarize a work of this magnitude would be an exercise in frustration. The field is so encompassing and the many topics of more than passing interest, that I do not believe the writing of an abridged version of the current status of surgical health services research would prove successful. For these reasons I shall invoke editor's license and provide a personal perspective on the present socioeconomic situation that confronts the surgical community.

The transformation of United States' health care from a "cottage industry" to a mammoth government-industrial-medicine complex is undeniable. To the surgical profession, the central question must be how it views itself relative to this change and where it fits into the rapidly changing system. The growing prominence of large institutions, such as government, major employers, and insurers, and their consequent influence over both surgeon and patient pose perplexities previously not considered.

For surgeons to become more active in the conduct of health services research will be an important first step in this self-evaluation process. Although there will always be a need for surgeons who participate in basic biomedical research, there exists a similar want for surgeons who can conduct original investigations into the socioeconomics of the health care delivery system.

Unfortunately, at present, there are few surgeons with additional training in fields such as biostatistics, business administration, economics, epidemiology, government, health services administration, public health, policy formation, and sociology. Without a critical mass of surgeons who have this interdisciplinary approach to surgical health care, the crucial and often difficult process of making proper policy decisions will be completed in a less than optimal fashion. It is no longer sufficient to have obtained an "interest" in these fields by merely practicing surgery over an extended period of time. Any surgeon who wishes to positively affect the health care delivery system of the future will need additional education in the social sciences. The future leaders of United States' surgery must be more than just excellent clinicians who also investigate the basic sciences. They will be asked to make critical public policy decisions, and without proper education and experience, such ill-informed decisions could prove potentially damaging.

The study and analysis of health care delivery systems have become well-established academic disciplines. For various reasons, this is not yet accepted within the academic surgical community. Many surgeons feel distinctly uncomfortable discussing surgical socioeconomics. They know little about the subject and are not familiar with the literature or various research techniques. I recall in November 1974, when interviewing for surgical training programs, that a then junior faculty member (at a prestigious Eastern medical institution) told me there could never be a place in surgery for someone who had my combined interests of surgery and socioeconomics. Fortunately, that type of thinking has begun to change. Surgeons will be asked to actively participate in organizational decisions concerning, for example, resource allocation, capital budgets, manpower planning, financing of surgical care, and legal and ethical issues. To be effective in this evolving system, they must have extensive education and formal training in the management sciences.

Egdahl, in a 1970 address before the Society of University Surgeons, summarized the situation:

> We in surgery must do everything possible to legitimize and to encourage activities in the health care field by our bright young men (and women) so that their effective involvement in the multitude of challenging health care problems will provide surgery with adequate leadership from within during the all important future decades. . . It is imperative that all departments of surgery in major teaching medical centers establish formalized groups which have as their principal function the responsibility for studying and carrying out research on the organization and delivery of surgical care. . . . We must provide a forum for discussing research in the health care aspects of surgery at our national meetings or leadership will be seized from us.

Egdahl's prescient pleas fell on deaf ears. It is hoped that the leadership of surgery in this country will finally begin to understand his message and correct the current inbalance in research priorities. Surgical chairmen must not only encourage their residents to enter the basic science laboratory but also direct them into formal education in areas such as business administration and economics. If this failure continues the death knell of United States' surgery will begin to ring ever more loudly.

Surgeons must once more reevaluate themselves with a SOSSUS-like study. It has been almost 20 years since the last major report, and it is imperative that, for example, practice characteristics, demographics, and remuneration levels are better understood. National databases must be established to allow the analysis of numbers of operations that are performed and to study who is completing them and where. Without such basic background data, much of surgical health care delivery research will prove ineffective.

The surgical profession has an absolute responsiblity to be forthright with information about surgical care. Appropriate studies of the effectiveness of surgical treatment should be carried out for selected conditions, particularly those where uncertainty leads to professional disagreement. Surgeons must foster the dissemination of reliable scientifically based data to the lay public. If surgeons do not do this, the federal government or some similar large institution, such as the insurance industry, will make certain that it occurs. If this means that every individual surgeon's operative morbidities and mortalities must be publically presented, (including, of course, proper explanation of comorbidities and case mix, for example) then so be it. Nothing works like honesty and humility in health care. It is assumed that surgeons can provide more meaningful explanations of these results than a third-party payer can.

The surgical community must become comfortable with and accept the inevitable fact that changes will take place in the health care delivery system. Power is shifting, and the once dominant role of the surgeon has declined. Surgeons are no longer the heroes they were of yesteryear, and the many dramatic alterations in our surgical health care will have to be acknowledged with a sanguine outlook. To do otherwise fosters a feeling of continued resentment toward the United States' public and its desire to change the face of surgery in this country. Nothing highlights this problem more than the changed status of the surgeon/patient relationship. What was once a relationship based on trust has been replaced with a legal and economic contract.

Discussions concerning the resource-based relative value scale are just beginning. It is undeniable that this new measure will have an enormous impact on the financial future of surgeons. What is certain is that inequities exist in the current way in which surgeons and nonsurgeons are reimbursed. These differences must be reconciled in a more equitable fashion. There is little justification (financial, economic, or otherwise) for some of the current reimbursement levels for particular surgical operations. The enormous fees that are generated for cataract extraction, joint replacement, arthroscopy, vascular grafts, endoscopy, and other procedures need to be reduced. The sole purpose of surgical health care should not be to produce a subclass of physicians who have enormous wealth disproportionate to their contributions to society.

Surgeons must clarify their new-found role. They will have to realize that the practice of surgery can be conducted in a businesslike manner. This does not mean that the humanitarian aspects of medicine must be forgotten. The commitment to act on behalf of a sick patient and to be compassionate should always be preserved.

Surgical health care delivered in a highly competitive environment will undoubtedly continue to thrive. Surgeons will be in the best position to make certain this happens if they demonstrate that they remain committed to certain standard values and responsibilities.

Surgical health care is a right, not a privilege. What remains to be answered is to what dollar amount that right extends? Should every citizen of this country be guaranteed an inguinal herniorrhaphy, a porto-systemic shunt for esophageal varices, or a heart transplant?

Surgeons must provide effective leadership in determining the economic constraints that need to be imposed if expenditures are to be controlled and services made available to the poor and the uninsured. The highest priority that we, the most affluent society on this planet, can ensure is that the surgical interests of the economically and socially disadvantaged and those who have limited access to health care will be assured. Surgeons can not consider themselves among the heirs of Hippocrates if they are interested solely in patients who can pay for their care.

All of these many concerns will be properly addressed only when surgeons grasp the importance of the study of socioeconomics and its impact on overall surgical health care delivery. It is a sad truism, but another journal article on the surgical treatment of pancreatic cancer is not going to cure our inability to secure basic medical and surgical care for the poor of this nation. Neither will it help surgeons understand their role in a rapidly changing economic environment. Among the important future issues that United States' surgeons will face is not how to perform a better pancreaticoduodenectomy. Instead, they will be asked to decide the financial ramifications of performing such an operation when it is known that the patient's life expectancy is less than a year.

The challenges have been placed before the fraternity of surgeons. Whether the surgical community will seize the opportunity to study and more clearly define its own socioeconomic future will become apparent only over the course of time.

Author Index

A

Abernathy, C.M., 64
Abrams, H.B., 273
Abulencia, P.B., 49
Acheson, E.D., 91
Adamache, K., 197
Adlington, P., 255
Ahlbom, A., 255
Aiken, L.H., 63
Alexander, J., 197, 198
Alexander, M.A.J., 48
Alford, B.R., 63
Alfthan, O., 254
Alpert, J.J., 103
Alsup, P., 213
Ament, R.P., 141
Ancona-Berk, V.A., 48
Anderson, G.D., 105
Anderson, G.M., 273
Annas, G.S., 348
Ansell, J.S., 63
Archibald, E.W., 367
Arkes, H.R., 330
Arno, P., 152
Arnold, D.J., 348
Ash, A.S., 141
Ashbaugh, D.G., 225
Ashcraft, M.L.S., 275
Ashworth, A., 141
Astor, L., 214
Avorn, J., 123

B

Bach, E., 103
Backafen, J., 141
Bahnson, H.T., 63
Bailor, J.C., III, 252
Baldwin, A.D., 103, 348
Baldwin, M.F., 48
Ball, J.R., 297
Ballinger, W.F., 13
Barber-Mueller, C., 64
Barer, M.L., 273
Bar-Hillel, M., 330

Barnes, B.A., 13, 90, 91, 103, 105, 123, 252, 253, 254, 274, 330, 348
Barnett, H.J., 252
Baron, J., 330
Barr, A., 330
Barr, J.K., 179
Barry, M.J., 90
Bartlett, M.K., 48
Bauerfeind, 253
Baum, A.Z., 398
Bays, C., 197
Bean, E., 295
Bechtoldt, A.A., 50
Beck, R.G., 349
Beckner, E., 199
Begg, C.B., 253
Bell, E.F., 398
Bellin, S.S., 103
Bennett, B.M., 275
Beran, R., 367
Berenson, L., 214, 350
Berenson, R., 151, 179
Bergen, R.P., 398
Berk, A.A., 48
Berki, S., 180
Berlin, J.A., 253
Bernth-Peterson, P., 103
Berry, M.G., 253
Berry, R.E., 225
Berwick, D.M., 330
Bhaskar, R., 253
Bice, S.E., 49
Birnhaum, H., 295
Bishop, C., 197
Black, R., 253
Blackard, C.E., 254
Blackstone, E.A., 63
Blair, A.P., 383
Blanchard, R.J.W., 103, 225
Bloom, B.S., 13, 63, 123, 295
Bloor, M., 90
Bloor, M.J., 90, 91, 103
Bluestone, M.S., 180
Blum, A.L., 253
Blumberg, M.S., 151, 273, 295

Blumenthal, D., 197, 198
Blumstein, J., 197, 199
Boggs, H.G., 179
Bombardier, C., 103, 123, 348
Bonchek, L.I., 253
Bosk, C.L., 348
Bovbjerg, R.R., 151
Bowen, O.R., 225
Bourman, J.G., 348
Boyden, J.S., 384
Bradbury, R.C., 141
Bradford, R.T., 398
Bradham, D., 198
Brested, J.H., 225
Brewster, A.C., 141
Brian, A.J., 214
Brill, R., 351
Brody, J.E., 348
Brook, R.H., 103, 213, 226, 253, 273, 305
Brook, S.J., 253
Brown, B.W., 103, 348
Buchanan, B., 330
Buchanan-Davidson, D.J., 49
Buckingham, W.B., 226
Bucy, P.C., 398
Bulman, C.H., 253
Bumle, D., 179
Bunis, D., 295
Bunker, J.P., 13, 91, 103, 163, 226, 252, 253, 254, 255, 274, 330, 348, 350
Burke, J.F., 253
Burkett, G., 331
Burney, I., 151
Burns, L.A., 48
Butler, J.A., 295
Byar, D.P., 253, 254

C

Cafferata, G.L., 151
Cageorge, S.M., 274
Calore, K.A., 141
Campbell, H., 383
Campbell, P.M., 273

Campion, E.W., 295
Cannon, W.B., 48
Caper, P., 91, 124, 273, 275, 305
Cardillo, B., 255
Carey, L., 348
Carey, M.J., 105
Carper, W., 197
Carter, L.E., 151
Caswell, R., 197
Cayten, C.G., 226
Cebula, D.P., 330
Cello, I.P., 123
Chacko, G.K., 151
Chalmers, I., 253
Chalmers, T.C., 48, 253, 255, 256, 295
Chapman, C., 383
Charles, S.C., 383
Charlson, M.E., 273
Chassin, M.R., 103, 253, 295
Chernow, B., 295
Chin, A., 383
Christianson, J., 197
Civetta, J.M., 295
Clark, R., 197
Clarke, J.R., 213, 330
Clarke, J.T., 181
Clarkson, K., 197
Cleary, P., 198
Cleeman, J.I., 351
Cleveland, R.J., 63
Cleverly, W., 197
Cobb, L.A., 253
Codman, E.A., 226, 348
Coelen, C., 197
Coffey, R., 141
Cohen, K., 383
Cohen, M.M., 273
Colditz, G.A., 255
Collins, S.D., 13
Colton, T., 63
Conklin, J.E., 123, 141
Conn, H., 253
Conrad, D., 296
Cooper, B.S., 103, 226, 349
Cooper, G.S., 91
Cooper, J.K., 383
Cornfield, J., 253
Corry, B.A., 181
Couch, N.P., 295, 383
Coyne, P.S., 348
Crane, M., 13, 179, 213
Cravalho, E.G., 296

Craver, J.M., 64
Creedon, J.J., 349
Cretin, S., 273
Crile, G., 348
Crockett, J.E., 254
Cromwell, J., 91, 103, 197, 348
Cullen, D.J., 141, 295
Culliton, B.J., 213
Culp, W.J., 91, 105, 275
Cuniff, C.L., 213

D

Daniels, M., 295
Daniels, N., 179
Danzinger, R.G., 274
Danzon, P., 197
Davis, C.K., 367
Davis, H., 273
Davis, J.E., 49
Davis, K., 151
Dawes, R.M., 330
Dawson, N.V., 330
de Dombal, F.T., 91, 213
De Jong, R.H., 63
De Sy, W.A., 253
Delaney, J.P., 253
DelGuercio, L.R.M., 123
Demkovich, L., 180
Demlo, L.K., 273
Denenberg, H.S., 348
Densen, P.M., 103, 295, 348
deRouville, W.H., 348
Derson, R.A., 305
Derzon, R., 198
Detmer, D.E., 49, 50, 63, 64, 103, 226, 330, 348
Detsky, A.S., 295
Devitt, J.E., 226
Dickersin, K., 253
Dickinson, R.L., 348
Diehl, L.F., 253
Diggs, W.W., 295
Dimond, E.G., 254
Dobson, A., 152, 274
Dorsey, J.L., 180
Dorwart, R., 198
Dove, H.G., 296
Downey, W., 275
Downs, A.R., 225
Doyle, J.C., 226
Doyle, J.V., 348
Dranove, D., 295
Draper, E.A., 124, 296

Drucker, W.R., 295
Dudley, H.A., 254
Duff, R.S., 348
Duncan, P.G., 273
Dunham, M.H., 213
Dutton, B.L., 151
Duzan, K.R., 349
Dyck, F.J., 348
Dyckman, Z.Y., 151

E

Earnhart, S.W., 49
Eastaugh, S., 330, 349
Eddy, D., 163
Edhag, O., 254
Egbert, L.D., 349
Egdahl, R.H., 151, 226, 273, 349
Ehrlich, J., 226, 351
Eimerl, T., 104, 349
Einhorn, M., 295
Eisenberg, J.M., 180, 273, 295
Elliot, R.V., 349
Elliott, R.L., 64
Ellwood, P., 180
Elstein, A.S., 330
Emerson, R., 349
Emmons, D.W., 151
Engrav, L.H., 254
Enthoven, A., 13, 163, 274, 295, 305, 348, 350
Epstein, A.M., 275
Ermann, D., 197, 198
Ernest, C.B., 14, 63, 64
Etheredge, L.M., 151, 152
Evans, M., 255
Evans, R.G., 273
Ewy, D., 349

F

Fairbairn, A.S., 91
Fairbanks, D.N., 254
Farber, B.F., 349
Feder, J., 197, 198
Feigenbaum, E., 330
Feinleib, M., 273
Feinstein, A.R., 254
Feldstein, P.J., 226
Felts, J.A., 274
Fetter, R.B., 273, 295
Ficarra, B.J., 349
Fiellau-Nikolajsen, M., 254
Field, M.J., 49

Fielding, S.L., 180
Fields, W.S., 254
Fincham, J.E., 180
Fine, J., 349
Fineberg, H.V., 330
Fink, A., 151
Fink, R., 180
Finkel, M., 13, 213, 214, 226, 330, 350
Finkler, S.A., 295
Fitzgerald, J.F., 123
Fitzpatrick, G., 91
Fletcher, R.H., 254
Fletcher, S.W., 254
Flexner, A., 367
Flood, A.B., 103, 295, 349
Folse, R., 63
Ford, J.L., 50
Forthofer, R.N., 296
Fowler, F.J., 91, 275
Fowles, J., 163
Fraley, E.E., 63
Fraundorf, K., 197
Frech, H., 197
Freeborn, D.K., 180
Freeland, M., 197
Freeland, M.S., 163
Freeman, J.L., 91, 105, 275
Freiman, J.A., 254
Freiman, M.P., 63
Freireich, E.J., 254
Friedlob, A.S., 213
Friedman, J.W., 104
Frisch, C., 330
Fruen, M.A., 49
Fryback, D.G., 330
Fuchs, V.R., 103, 295, 349

G

Gabel, J., 197, 198
Gage, L., 198
Garber, A.M., 295
Garceau, A.J., 254
Garcia, A.G., 296
Gardner, R.A., 330
Gardner, R.C., 398
Garg, M.L., 295
Garnick, D.W., 163
Gavett, J.W., 295
Gartside, F., 64
Garvey, J.M., 49
Gassner, K., 330

Gaumer, G., 198
Gaus, C.R., 103, 226, 349
Gavett, J.W., 296
Geffen, N., 213
Gehan, E.A., 254
Geiger, H.J., 103
Gentry, D.W., 295
Gertman, P.M., 213, 226, 349
Gil, A.V., 103
Gilbert, J.P., 91, 254, 274
Gillick, M.R., 296
Ginsberg, W.H., 398
Ginsburg, P., 180, 198
Ginzberg, E., 123, 305
Gipson, C.D., 103
Gittelsohn, A., 91, 105, 214, 226, 305, 330, 331, 349, 350, 351
Glass, L.S., 398
Glasser, J.H., 296
Glenn, J.F., 63
Glover, J.A., 91, 103
Gold, M., 179
Goldfarb, E., 181
Goldfarb, M., 141
Goldring, S., 254
Goldstone, J., 226
Goligher, J.C., 213
Gonnella, J.S., 141
Gonzalez, M.L., 151
Goodman, L.J., 179
Goodspeed, S.W., 49
Goodwin, C.W., 254
Gordon, N.M., 151
Gordon, V., 383
Gornick, M., 103, 151
Gorry, G.A., 330
Gottlober, P., 163
Graboys, T.B., 213
Grafe, W.R., 213
Graham, N.G., 213
Gray, B., 197, 198, 199
Gray, D.T., 254
Green, S.B., 254
Greenland, S., 254
Greenlick, M.R., 180
Greifinger, T.B., 180
Griffith, J.R., 273
Griner, P.F., 296
Groves, E.W.H., 349
Gruer, R., 226
Grundy, D.J., 214
Gutman, F.H., 65

H

Haapiainen, R., 254
Hackborth, G.M., 180
Hadley, J., 151, 152, 197, 198
Haggard, W.D., 349
Halahan, J.F., 152
Harel, E.C., 273
Harrell, W.R., 254
Harris, J.E., 151
Harvey, L., 383
Hastings, J.E.F., 103
Hatcher, C.R., 64
Hauck, W.W., 63, 123
Haug, J.N., 13, 214
Havighurst, C.C., 383
Hawes, C., 198
Hawkins, B., 254
Hawkins, C., 383
Hay, J.W., 152
Heagarty, M.C., 103
Heinrich, J.J., 63
Held, P., 198
Hellinger, F.J., 349
Henderson, J.A., 49
Hendricksson, P., 254
Henley, P.G., 349
Henteleff, P.D., 91, 104, 274, 350
Herndon, D.N., 254
Herod, F., 255
Herron, D., 296
Hershey, J.C., 330
Hershey, N., 383
Hey Groves, E.W., 226
Hibbert, J., 254
Hill, A.B., 254
Hill, G.L., 367
Hillman, A.L., 179, 198, 296
Hinkley, D., 163
Hirsh, H.L., 398
Hirshman, C., 103, 226, 349
Hogarth, R.M., 330
Holahan, J.F., 151
Holder, A.R., 349, 398
Homer, C., 198
Hook, E.W., III, 296
Horn, R.A., 123, 141
Horn, S.D., 123, 141, 296
Hornbrook, M., 141, 180, 273
Horne, J.M., 349
Horsely, J.E., 398
Horton, C.A., 296
Horwitz, R.I., 273
Hsiao, W., 151

Hughes, E.F., 104
Hughes, E.F.X., 13, 63, 64, 103
Hughes, R.G., 349
Hunt, S.S., 163, 274, 349, 350
Hunt, V.B., 213
Hutton, R., 351
Hynds-Karnell, L., 13, 64

I

Iezzoni, L., 141
Iglehart, J.K., 13, 180, 296
Ironside, M.R., 226
Irwin, C.E., 350
Isershein, A.W., 179

J

Jackson, B., 49
Jackson, T.P., 398
Jacobs, C.M., 141
James, F.E., 296
Jannssen, T.J., 163
Jencks, S.F., 123, 152, 274
Jennings, M.C., 49
Jensen, J., 49, 226
Jensen, M.C., 296
Jick, H., 351
Joffe, J., 213
Johnson, D., 180
Johnson, J.M., 179
Johnson, R.E., 180
Jolly, P., 367
Jones, J., 349
Jones, K.R., 296
Jones, P.K., 124
Jordan, W.P., Jr., 254
Juba, D., 152

K

Kagay, M., 179
Kahl, L., 350
Kahn, K.A., 349
Kahn, L., 104, 180
Kahneman, D., 330, 331
Kaiser, D.L., 349
Kalaja, E., 254
Kanak, J., 197
Kane, R.L., 64
Karnell, L.H., 64
Kassan, M., 123
Kassirer, J.P., 274
Katz, H.M., 198, 305
Kay, T., 123
Kaye, R., 349

Keller, W.E., 152
Kelly, J.V., 349
Kennedy, E., 383
Kennedy, R.H., 349
King, L., 383
King, R.B., 367
Kircher, M., 179
Kirchner, M., 180, 213
Kisch, A.I., 104
Kittle, C.F., 254
Kleinfield, N.R., 305
Kline, J., 152
Klingman, D., 274
Klotz, A.P., 255
Knafl, K., 331
Knaus, W.A., 123, 296
Knoles, G.H., 163
Kobrinski, E.J., 296
Koepsell, T.D., 349
Koetting, M., 198
Kohrman, C.H., 180
Koran, L.M., 213
Kosterlitz, J., 180
Koutsilieris, M., 254
Kralewski, J., 179
Krasmiak, C.L., 124
Krentz, S.E., 49
Krischer, J.R., 296
Kumin, C.M., 398
Kurtz, L.M., 349
Kushman, J., 198
Kutner, F.R., 350

L

La Porte, V., 198
Labrie, F., 255
Lagoe, R.J., 49, 64
Lairson, D.R., 296
Lance, R., 214
Lang, S.M., 13, 64
Langfitt, T., 254
Langwell, K.M., 152
Larson, S., 226
Lave, J., 198
Lave, J.R., 141
Lave, L., 198
Lave, L.B., 141
Laws, H.L., 64
Lazaro, F.J., 214
Lazenby, H., 124, 153
Ledley, R.S., 331
Lembcke, P.A., 91, 194, 349

Leopold, D.A., 64
Letourneau, C.U., 349
Levey, G.S., 13
Levin, K.J., 50
Levine, N.S., 256
Levinson, D.F., 180
Levit, E.J., 64
Levit, K., 124, 153
Lewin, L.S., 198, 305
Lewis, C.E., 13, 91, 104, 305, 349
Lewis, L.S., 367
Lewit, E.M., 13, 63, 64
Lichtenstein, R., 180
Lichtenstein, S., 331
Lichtner, S., 91, 104
Lind, S., 296
Lindenmuth, W.W., 253
Linn, B.S., 367
Liptzin, B., 296
Litschert, R., 197
Logan, R.F.L., 104, 349
LoGerfo, J.P., 104, 226, 349
Lohr, K.N., 213, 226, 253, 273
Lomas, J., 273
Longmire, W.P., 105, 351
Loop, F.D., 64
Lorenz, M.C., 296
Lorenzo, F.V., 13, 63
Louis, D.Z., 141
Louis, T.A., 253
Louisell, D.W., 349
Lubitz, J., 13, 152, 296
Lubos, M.E., 255
Luce, R.D., 331
Luft, H., 180
Luft, H.S., 13, 152, 163, 274, 348, 349, 350
Luke, R.D., 296
Lung, J.A., 225
Lusted, L.B., 331
Luxemberg, M.N., 65
Lyttle, D., 274

M

Mackie, A., 104, 350, 351
Maerki, S.C., 274, 350
Mahler, D., 255
Majure, J.A., 64
Mankiewicz, D.A., 49
Manuel, B., 151
Manuel, B.M., 384
Marcus, A.C., 104, 180
Marcus, G.L., 153
Marder, W.D., 63, 181

Margolis, I.B., 123
Margulies, R., 198, 305
Marks, S.D., 49, 104
Marmor, T., 198
Marshak, G., 255
Martin, D., 197
Martin, S.G., 214
Marubini, E., 255
Mason, H.R., 64
Mason, L.B., 296
Matteson, A.L., 296
Maw, A.R., 255
Mawson, S.R., 255
McCall, N., 104, 296, 351
McCallum, J., 384
McCarthy, E.G., 13, 213, 214, 226, 330, 331, 350
McCurdy, J.A., Jr., 255
McDermott, W.V., 163
McElrath, D., 180
McGuire, W.J., 331
McIntosh, H.D., 214
McKee, W.J.E., 255
McKinlay, J., 197
McLean, E.R., 273
McMenamin, P., 151, 153
McMillan, A., 152
McNeil, B.J., 296
McNeil, R., 384
McNutt, D.R., 13
McPeek, B., 254, 274
McPhee, S.J., 163
McPherson, K., 91, 104, 124, 275, 350
McSherry, C.K., 226
Mechanic, D., 180
Meinert, C.L., 255
Melton, L.J., 350
Merill, J.L., 297
Merrick, N.J., 255
Miao, L.L., 255
Micciolo, R., 255
Miettinen, O.S., 255
Miller, D., 213
Miller, G.A., 331
Miller, J.I., 64
Miller, J.N., 255
Miller, L.D., 64
Miller, N.F., 350
Milliren, J.W., 49
Mills, D.H., 384
Mindell, W.R., 105, 214, 255, 351
Misek, G., 13, 64

Mitchell, J.B., 91, 103, 152, 348, 349
Mitchell, R.T., 49
Mitchell, W.E., Jr., 226
Montgomery, E., 198
Moore, F.D., 13, 64, 123, 214, 295, 297, 305
Moran, P.T., 384
Morehead, M.A., 226, 349, 351
Morgan, J.C., 123
Morgenstern, O., 331
Morison, M., 105
Morris, C., 398
Morrisey, M., 197, 198
Morrow, J.S., 296
Morton, J.H., 350
Moskowitz, M.A., 141
Mossey, J.M., 274
Mosteller, F., 13, 91, 252, 253, 254, 255, 274, 330, 348, 350
Mott, P.D., 180
Moxley, J.H., 49
Mueller, C.B., 214
Muller, C., 49
Mullner, R., 197, 198, 199
Mullooly, J.F., 180
Mullooly, J.P., 180
Munoz, E., 123, 296
Murphy, M.L., 255
Musacchio, R., 198
Myers, R.S., 350

N

Nathanson, S., 49
Neriah, Z.B., 255
Neuhauser, D., 199, 274
Neutra, R., 91, 254
Newhouse, J.P., 152
Newton, M., 152
Nickerson, R.J., 64
Nicol, J.P., 274
Nielsen, W., 198
Nilsen, S.T., 104
Nisbett, R.E., 331
Nobrega, F.T., 104
Norris, C.K., 163
Nuckton, C., 198

O

Oldertz, C., 384
Omenn, G.S., 296
O'Neil, J.A., 64
Organ, C.H., Jr., 367

Orthner, H.G., 63
O'Sullivan, J., 152
Owens, A., 152, 179
Owens, W.D., 274

P

Palfrey, J.S., 295
Pantell, R.H., 350
Paradise, J.L., 255
Paranjpe, A., 198
Pareto, V., 296
Paringer, L., 152
Paris, M., 214, 350
Parks, D.H., 254
Parmar, H., 255
Pasternak, D.P., 180
Pataki, L.I., 398
Patricelli, R.E., 274
Patterson, J.F., 50
Pattison, R.V., 198, 305
Pauker, S.G., 274
Pauly, M., 198
Pauly, M.V., 63, 152, 350
Pearse, W.H., 64
Pearson, R.J.C., 104
Peck, P., 180
Pemberton, A., 350
Perkoff, G.T., 104, 350
Perlman, M., 197
Perott, G.S., 104, 350
Perrin, J., 105, 199, 275, 351
Perry, D.J., 253
Perry, G.T., 255
Perry, H.B., 63, 64
Peterson, M., 383
Peterson, M.L., 180
Peterson, O.L., 13, 63, 64, 295
Pfeutze, K.D., 350
Pflanz, M., 91, 104
Phillips, C., 198
Phillips, R.B., 64
Phillips, R.R., 180
Piantadosi, S., 253
Pietsch, J.B., 255
Pine, P., 152, 274
Pineault, R., 50, 180
Platt, W.R., 351
Plum, F., 255
Poggio, E.C., 214
Popein, J., 253
Porell, F., 198
Pories, W.J., 367
Potsic, W.P., 255

Poullier, J.P., 104
Powell, W., 198
Pratt, L.W., 305
Pratt, T., 367
Prihoda, R., 296
Proter, L.W., 180

R

Raffel, M., 198
Raiffa, H., 331
Ralphs, D.N., 214
Ramsey, E., 274
Rand, E., 63
Rannikko, S., 253
Ransohoff, D.F., 91
Ravitch, M.M., 226
Rassman, W.R., 296
Raymond, C.A., 50
Reagan, M.D., 180, 296
Redmond, E.L., 64
Reece, R.L., 180
Reed, W.A., 50
Reinhardt, U.E., 14, 152, 274
Reitman, D., 255
Relman, A.S., 179, 198, 255, 305
Renlund, D.G., 163
Renn, S., 198
Resnick, R.H., 255
Reuter, J., 152
Rhodes, R.S., 124
Rhu, H.S., 50
Richards, D.H., 91
Richardson, F.M., 350
Riffer, J., 49
Rins, W.H., 50
Rippey, R.M., 331
Roberts, H.E., 296
Roberts, P., 181
Robertson, L., 103
Robinette, T., 198
Robins, R.B., 349
Robinson, J.C., 163, 350
Roeder, P.C., 49
Roemer, M.I., 64, 104
Roos, L.L., 91, 104, 274, 275, 350
Roos, N.P., 91, 104, 274, 350
Rosati, R.A., 255
Rosen, W.D., 398
Rosenbaum, S., 295
Rosenberg, M.J., 331
Rosenfeld, L.S., 350
Rosoff, A.J., 295

Rossiter, L., 197, 199
Rossiter, L.F., 153
Rothman, I.L., 349
Roydhouse, N., 255
Rubin, J., 198
Rubsamen, D.S., 384
Ruchlin, H., 198
Ruchlin, H.S., 13, 213, 214, 226, 330
Rufener, B.L., 50
Ruffin, J.M., 255
Rundle, R., 296
Rush, B.F., 214
Rushefsky, M., 198
Russell, F., 398
Russell, L.B., 296
Rust, J.A., 50
Rutkow, I.M., 14, 64, 104, 105, 124, 214, 296, 331, 350, 351
Rynnel-Dagöö, B., 255

S

Sabshin, M., 64
Sacks, H.S., 163, 255, 256
Sagall, E.L., 398
Sako, K., 214
Salisbury, R.E., 256
Salsberg, E., 214, 350
Sammons, J.H., 350
Samphier, M.L., 90, 91, 103
Sanbar, S., 398
Sandberg, S.I., 91
Sauter, V.L., 104
Savino, J.A., 123
Savitz, S., 181
Saward, E., 297
Schaberg, D.R., 296
Schacht, P.J., 350
Schacter, M., 214
Schaffarzick, R.W., 163
Scheff, T.J., 331
Schendler, C., 197
Schieber, G., 151
Schieber, G.J., 104
Schiratzki, H., 255
Schlenker, R., 198
Schlesinger, E., 198
Schlesinger, M., 198, 199
Schlike, C.P., 351
Schlossberg, S.M., 214
Schneck, L.H., 50
Schneider, K.C., 296
Schneider, W.R., 384
Schoonhoven, C.B., 351

Schroeder, J.L., 181
Schroeder, S.A., 274, 295, 296
Schumacher, D.N., 296, 297
Schwartz, J., 296
Schwartz, W.B., 64, 124, 152, 274
Schweiker, R., 141
Scitovsky, A.A., 104, 274, 351
Scott, H.D., 104, 351
Scott, W.R., 103, 349
Shapiro, N., 305
Shapiro, S., 64, 295
Sharkey, P.D., 123, 141, 296
Sharp, S.M., 274
Sharpe, H.R., 351
Shaughnessy, P., 198
Shaw, D.A., 256
Shaw, G., 179
Sheldon, G.F., 367
Shepard, D.S., 91
Sherman, G.J., 275
Shor, S., 256
Shortell, S., 197, 198, 199
Shortliffe, E., 330
Showstack, J.A., 152, 274, 275, 296, 351
Shubat, S., 383
Shulman, L.S., 330
Shwartz, M., 351
Siegel, A., 50
Sieverts, S., 214
Sikes, E.D., Jr., 50
Silverman, J.F., 295
Silverman, L.P., 141
Simes, R.J., 256
Simon, H.A., 331
Simon, J., 274
Simpson, A., 104
Siu, A.L., 50, 179
Sloan, F.A., 105, 152, 199, 275, 305, 351
Slovic, P., 330, 331
Smiddy, F.G., 214
Smith, D., 199
Smith, H., Jr., 256
Smith, H.L., 180, 181
Smith, M.E., 275
Smithey, R., 198
Smits, H.L., 124, 141
Snyder, R., 295
Snyder, R.K., 163
Sorensen, A., 297
Sorensen, B., 256
Spencer, F.C., 367

Spitzer, M., 305
Spitznagel, E.L., Jr., 274
Spodick, D.H., 256
Sprafka, S.A., 330
Stafford, N., 256
Starfield, B.H., 14, 104, 214, 350
Starr, P., 179, 199, 297
Stason, W., 151
Steel, K., 384
Stein, J., 181
Steinburg, M.K., 179
Steinwachs, D.M., 64
Steinwald, B., 152, 199
Stephens, S.K., 351
Stephenson, G.W., 350, 351
Stephenson, S.V., 50
Stern, A.R., 295
Stern, R.S., 275
Stevens, R., 199
Steward, D., 297
Stewart, A., 152
Still, P., 254
Stimmel, B., 14
Stone, J.P., 180
Stone, M.H., 274
Stratton, W.T., 398
Strauch, G.O., 226
Stroman, D.F., 351
Studnickl, J., 297
Suffredini, A., 331
Sugioka, K., 49
Sulvetta, M., 152
Sundt, T.M., Jr., 256
Swanson, A.G., 367
Swartwout, J.E., 179

T

Tabatabai, C., 226
Taksei, L., 367
Tancredi, L.D., 384
Tancredi, L.R., 383
Tang, J., 50
Tarlov, A.R., 64, 181
Taylor, H., 179
Taylor, J., 50
Taylor, J.W., 256
Teich, J.L., 367
Thibault, G.E., 297
Thomas, J.W., 275
Thompson, J.D., 297
Thompson, P., 256
Tilney, N.L., 295
Tolis, G., 256

Trauner, J., 179
Trussell, R.E., 226, 351
Trute, B., 275
Tucker, J., 214
Turnbull, A.D., 297
Tuttle, W.C., 180
Tversky, A., 330, 331
Tyson, T.J., 103, 214, 226, 348
Tyson, W.T., 297

U

Ullman, S., 199
Usher, A., 398

V

Valagussa, P., 255
Valvona, J., 105, 199, 275, 351
Van Der Gaag, J., 197
van der Linden, W., 256
Varco, R.L., 253
Vayda, E., 91, 105, 214, 255, 351
Venters, G.A., 90, 91, 103
Verda, D.J., 351
Viril, L.C., 255
Vladeck, B., 199
von Neumann, J., 331
Voytovich, A.E., 331
Vraciu, R., 199
Vracu, R.A., 305

W

Wagner, D.F., 296
Wagner, D.P., 124
Wagner, J., 152
Wai, H.S., 296
Wajda, A., 274, 275
Waldo, D.R., 124, 153
Walker, A., 351
Wallach, S., 198
Wallsten, T.S., 331
Wangensteen, S.L., 256
Warner, K.E., 351
Waterfall, W.K., 213
Watkins, E., 63
Watkins, R.N., 64, 105
Watson, R.E., 124, 141
Watts, C., 64
Waxman, H.A., 297
Way, L.W., 226
Webber, B.L., 330
Webster, J.R., 181
Wecht, C.H., 398
Weiner, J.P., 64

Weinert, H.V., 351
Weinstein, M.C., 256, 330, 331
Welch, W., 199
Wennberg, J., 91, 105, 124, 226, 256, 275, 305, 330, 331, 349, 351
Wenzel, R.P., 349
Wertheimer, A.I., 180
West, H., 153
West, R., 275
West, R.R., 105
Westman, J., 50
Wetchler, B.V., 50
Wetherill, H.G., 351
White, W.D., 295
Widemar, L., 256
Widmer, G.W., 214, 226, 331, 350
Wilensky, G.R., 153
William, J.S., 350
Williams, D.C., 14, 65
Williams, G., 351
Williams, H., 349
Williams, L.P., 351
Wilson, S.E., 105, 351
Winkenwerder, W., 297
Wise, L., 123, 349
Wohl, S., 199
Wolcott, M.W., 50
Wolinsky, F.D., 181
Wong, H.D., 50
Worthen, D.M., 65
Worthman, L.G., 273
Wright, P., 256

Y

Yoshida, K., 105
Yoshida, Y., 105
Young, D., 199
Young, W.W., 124, 141

Z

Zeppa, R., 367
Zervas, N., 254
Zikria, B.A., 256
Zimmerman, J., 275
Zook, C.J., 297
Zubkoff, M., 91
Zubokk, M., 105
Zuidema, G.D., 13, 65, 104, 214, 331, 350, 351

Subject Index

A

AAAHC; *see* Accreditation Association for Ambulatory Health Care (AAAHC)

Accreditation Association for Ambulatory Health Care (AAAHC), findings of, on outpatient surgery complications, 39

Accreditation Council for Graduate Medical Education (ACGME), 354, 358

Acute Physiologic and Chronic Health Evaluation (APACHE) in refinement of DRGs, 118-119

Adenoidectomy
 outpatient, complications of, 40
 per capita rate of, 95
 rate of, in fee-for-service vs. prepaid health plans, 99, 100

Advanced Cardiac Life Support (ACLS) as example of protocol and algorithm, 328

Advanced Trauma Life Support (ATLS) as example of protocol and algorithm, 328

Advisory Board for Medical Specialties, 355

Algorithms as decision-making tool, 328

Alternacare, 32

Alternative delivery systems (ADS), health care contracting and, 156

Ambiplex patients, 277, 278; *see also* Patients, high-cost
 characteristics of, 283-284

Ambiplex patients—cont'd
 clinical service utilization by, 287t
 contributors to high cost of, 285-286
 decision rights of, 291
 discharge planning for, 293-294
 do not resuscitate order and, 293
 establishing patient agents for, 290
 genesis of, 288-289
 impact of, on educational practices, 291-292
 management of, 290-294
 medical information system needs for, 294
 moral and ethical considerations with, 293
 Pareto's law and, 285
 patient management plan for, 293
 percentage of, in hospital population, 288
 recognition of, 290
 reducing hospitalization needs of, 290
 study of, 282-288
  methods of, 284-285
  results of, 285-288
 summary data for, compared with other patients, 286t
 use of hospital resources by, 287t

Ambulatory surgery, 31-50
 classification of, 35-37
 complications of, 39-41
 costs and financing of, 42-47
 defined, 35
 factors determining future of, 48
 financial savings with, 43
 health insurance and, 46-47
 history and growth of, 31
 Medicare coverage of, 39, 43, 44-45
 most common procedures in, 39
 patient preparation for, 38
 patient selection for, 37-39

Ambulatory surgery—cont'd
 as percent of total surgery, 33t
 percentage of increase in, 31-32
 preexisting conditions and, 41
 pricing decisions about, 47
 procedure classification and, 45-46
 procedure lists for, 172
 prospective pricing system for, 45
 public attitudes toward, 34
 quality control of, 41-42
 short procedure units in, 46
 third-party payment and, 43
 utilization of, 31-35

Ambulatory Surgical Facility, 38

American Board of Medical Specialties, 354, 361

American Board of Medical Specialties Committee on Graduate Medical Education, 365

American Board of Ophthalmology, 354

American Board of Orthopaedic Surgery, 354

American Board of Otolaryngology, 354

American Board of Surgery, 358
 certification process of, 361-363
 incorporation of, 355

American Board of Urology, 354

American Child Health Association, study of, on patient demand for tonsillectomy, 72-73

American College of Surgeons (ACS), 355
 founding of, 354
 on free-standing surgical centers, 32
 report of, on need for hospital standardization, 217
 response of
  to SOSSUS findings, 53
  to studies on surgeon manpower, 8-10

Page numbers in *italics* indicate illustrations.
Page numbers followed by t indicate tables.

413

American College of Surgeons (ACS)—cont'd
  study of, on surgeon workload, 58
American Hospital Association, 309, 355
American Medical Association (AMA), study of
  on characteristics of medical practice, 59-62
  on physician characteristics and distribution, 58-59
  on surgeon workload, 58
American Medical Association Council on Medical Education in Hospitals, 355
American Medical International, 32
American Society of Anesthesiologists' Physical Status Classification (ASAPS), 271
American Surgical Association, 354
Amputation, lower limb, number performed, 20t
Anesthesia for outpatient surgery, 41
Ankle arthroplasty, number performed, 20t
Aortic valve, replacement of, number performed, 26t
Appendectomy
  false-positive cases of, 81
  numbers performed, 16t
  per capita rate of, 96
  retrospective chart reviews of, 341
  systematic component of variation for, 78, 81
Arthroplasty of foot or toe, number performed, 21t
Arthroscopy, number performed, 20t
Artificial intelligence, 315-316
Association of American Medical Colleges, 355
Auxiliary Loans to Assist Students program, 365

B

Back injuries, practice style and treatment of, 77, 77
Bailey Square Surgical Center, 38
Bane Committee Report, 7

Bayne-Jones Report of 1958, 7
Bias, 316-318
  availability, 316
  ego, 318
  regret or value-induced, 317
  surgeons and, 318-320
Bile ducts, excision of, numbers performed, 17t
Blue Cross
  ambulatory surgery coverage and, 46-47
  establishment of, 184
  mandatory surgical second opinion programs of, 205
Blue Shield, establishment of, 184
Boston Inter-Hospital Liver Group, 236
  portacaval shunt study of, 233
Breast, biopsy or local incision of, numbers performed, 16t
Budget Reconciliation Act of 1988, 309, 310
Bunion, excision of, number performed, 20t
Burns, early surgical excision vs. conservative debridement for
  nonrandomized comparisons of, 249t
  randomized control trials of, 247-249, 248t

C

California Law AB-3480, 155-156
Canada, rates of surgical operations in, 93
Cancer
  hysterectomy for prevention of, 82
  metastasis of, intraobserver disagreement about, 203
Cardiac catheter ablation, coverage of, 160
Cardiac surgery, regionalization of, 162
Cardiothoracic surgery, DRGs for, description and relative weights of, 125
Carotid endarterectomy
  Boston-New Haven comparisons of, 84
  numbers performed, 16t
  per capita rate of, 96
  randomized control trials of, 238

Case management of high-cost cases, 170
CASS; see Coronary Artery Surgery Study (CASS)
Cataract extraction
  incidence of, 5
  Medicare reimbursement for, 310
  outpatient, 39
    cost factors in, 46
Catheterization, heart, coverage of investigational procedures with, 160
Center for Ambulatory Surgery, 38
Centers for Disease Control (CDC), 157
Certification of surgeon, 361-363
Cervix, conization of, repair of, 19t
Cesarean section, numbers performed, 18t
Charlson Index, 269
Chest radiographs, recommendations for frequency of, 38
Cholecystectomy
  life expectancy and, 81-82
  numbers performed, 16t
  per capita rate of, 96
  systematic component of variation for, 78
  treatment of asymptomatic gallstones with, controversy over, 81
Cholelithiasis, Computerized Severity Index criteria for, 136, 137t
Circumcision, number performed, 22t
Cirrhosis, shunt surgery for, survival of treated and control groups in, 230
Civil justice system, fault-based administrative alternative to, 374-378
Clinical Efficacy Assessment Program (CEAP), 157
Clinical judgment, defined, 315
Code of Hammurabi, 217
Colostomy, numbers performed, 17t
Commission for Physician Payment Reform, 310
Commission on Professional and Hospital Activities (CPHA), 262
Committee on Cost of Medical Care of the American Medical Association, 7

Subject Index

Communication, high-cost patient and, 288
Computer programming, artificial intelligence as discipline of, 315-316
Computerized Severity Index: ICD-9-CM Severity Modification, Adult Criteria, 136
Computerized Severity Index (CSI), 135-139
  computation process of, 136
  criteria of, for cholelithiasis, 136, 137t
  patient discharge summary applications of, 138
  quality of care applications of, 138
  severity-adjusted DRGs and, 138-139
  surgical examples of, 139-140
  utilization review applications of, 138
Consolidated Omnibus Budget Reconciliation Act (COBRA), Medicare reimbursement and, 147
Consultations, ambiplex patient use of, 286-287
Consumer-Choice Health Plan, 155
Consumer choice pricing, health care quality and, 300-301
Consumer movement, unnecessary surgery and, 335-336
Coronary artery bypass graft (CABG)
  Boston-New Haven comparisons of, 84
  case fatality rates after, *235*
  controversy over prolongation of life after, 236
  mortality rates for, in high-volume vs. low-volume hospitals, 161
  number performed, 26t
  regionalization of, 162
Coronary artery disease, three-year survival curves of surgical and medical treatment of, *231*
Coronary Artery Surgery Study (CASS), randomization in, 237
Cost and Quality of Health Care: Unnecessary Surgery, 336
Cost/benefit analysis, unnecessary surgery and, 345-346
Cost effectiveness, ProPAC's role in encouraging, 112

CPR approach to physician reimbursement, 143
  flaws in, 143-144
Craniectomy, number of, by year, 28t
Cranioplasty, number of, by year, 28t
Craniotomy
  number of, by year, 28t
  without trauma, cost factors of its DRG, 118
CSI; *see* Computerized Severity Index (CSI)
Current Procedural Terminology (CPT-4), abuses of, in charging for medical services, 149-150
Cystocele, repair of, numbers performed, 18t

D

Databases
  administrative, 260
  case mix adjustment and, 270-272
  in clinical decision analysis, 267-268
  clinical decision analysis and, 266
  enrollment files and, 270-271
  hospital-based vs. population-based, 268
  ideal, characteristics of, 259-260
  limitations of, 260-261
  population-based, 264
  quality of care and, 272-273
  record linkage and, 269
  research designs for, 261-266
  software and, 269-270
  surgery research and, 259-275
  in volume-outcome relationship analysis, 267
Debridement of wound, burn, or infection, numbers performed, 16t
Decision making, clinical, 94-103, 315-331
  about prophylactic surgery, 323, *324*
  consistency in, 325-326
  databases in analysis of, 267-268
  feedback in, 329-330
  implications of, 328-330
  improving methods of, 326-328
  as logical deduction, 315-316
  ProPAC's role in, 113
  reliability and reproducibility of, 202-204

Decision making, clinical—cont'd
  as tradeoffs, 321-325
Decision rules, defined, 316
Decision trees, 321, *322*
Department of Health and Human Services, 149
Diagnosis, physician agreement about, 202-204
Diagnosis related groups (DRGs)
  adjustment of, for severity of illness, 118-119, 133-141
  ambulatory surgery coverage and, 45
  beneficiary concerns in, ProPAC recommendations about, 114-115
  and clinical variables of admission, 120-121
  components of, 110-111
  disadvantages of, for Medicare patients, 120
  effect of
    on surgeons and hospitals, 117-118
    on surgical care, 119-121
  establishment of, 133
  and future of surgical practice, 122
  health care quality and, 301, 308
  impact of, and prospective payment assessment commission, 109-131
  implications of, for surgical practice, 307-308
  improvements in, 113-114
  medical record coding and abstracting and, 114
  payments for, ProPAC recommendations for (1988), 114
  physician-related referral behavior and, 121
  role of, in determining future health care policy, 115
  severity-adjusted, Computerized Severity Index and, 138-139
  surgical
    description and relative weights of, by specialty, 125-131
    refining, 118-119
  unprofitability of surgical procedures under, 117-118, 121-122
  updating prospective payment system payments in, 113
  variability of charges for, 117

Diagnosis related groups (DRGs)—cont'd
  weight index of, 110
Diagnostic and Therapeutic Technology Assessment (DATTA), 157
Dilation and curettage (D & C), numbers performed, 18t
Disc, intervertebral, excision or destruction of, number performed, 20t
Disease Staging System, 134
Drug formularies, mandatory, 170
Drugs, evaluation of, before outpatient surgery, 41
Duodenal ulcer, gastric freezing of
  randomized control trials of, 249-251, 250t
  vs. sham cooling, nonrandomized comparison of, 251t

E
Education
  medical
    graduate, financing of, 308-309
    increasing specialization in, 55-56
    specialist training in, 309
  surgical
    certification requirements and, 353-367
    clinical experience in, 357-358
    costs of, 364-366
    financial aid for, 365
    graduate, 358-361
    historical background of, 353-355
    socioeconomic features of, 364-367
    undergraduate, 355-358
Edwin Smith papyrus, 31, 217
Encounter, defined, 280
Endarterectomy, carotid; see Carotid endarterectomy
Endophthalmitis as complication of outpatient surgery, 40
Enthoven concept of consumer choice pricing, 300-301
Equicor, 169
Esophageal varices, shunt surgery for, survival of treated and control groups in, 230
Ethics, ambiplex patient and, 293
Evaluative clinical sciences, role of, in evaluating practice style, 84-86
Ewing Report, 7

Expected utilities, 323
Extracranial/intracranial bypass operation, randomized control trials of, 236-237

F
Fallopian tubes
  destruction or occlusion of, numbers performed, 18t
  repair of, 19t
FASA; see Freestanding Ambulatory Surgical Association (FASA)
Federal legislation, impact of
  on physician reimbursement, 309-311
  on surgical practice, 307-311
Federation of State Medical Boards, 355
Femoropopliteal bypass, inadequacy of DRG provisions for, 117
Flexner Report, 353
Food and Drug Administration (FDA), 157
Fractures
  practice style and treatment of, 76-77
  reduction and fixation of, number performed, 20t
Framing, risk aversion and, 318
Freestanding Ambulatory Surgical Association (FASA), findings of, on outpatient surgery complications, 39

G
Gambler's fallacy, 317
Gastric freezing of duodenal ulcer
  randomized control trials of, 249-251, 250t
  vs. sham cooling, nonrandomized comparison of, 251t
Gastrostomy, temporary, numbers performed, 17t
Graduate Medical Education National Advisory Committee (GMENAC)
  findings and recommendations of, about surgeon numbers and distribution, 9
  findings of, on surgeon surplus, 55
  manpower recommendations of, 308

Grafts, saphenous vein, vs. synthetic vascular prostheses, randomized control trial of, 238-239
Great Society, practice of medicine affected by, 51
Group Health Cooperative of Puget Sound, 171
Guaranteed Student Loan program, 365
Gynecologic surgery, DRGs for, description and relative weights of, 127-128

H
Hammurabi, code of, 217
HCFA; see Health Care Financing Association (HCFA)
Head and neck surgery, DRGs for, description and relative weights of, 129
Health Professions Student Loan program, 365
Health care
  access to, and form of ownership, 188-190
  consumer choice pricing of, 300-301
  cost containment of, 186-187
  costs of, 280; see also Patients, high cost
    and form of ownership, 188
    as percentage of GNP, 155
    physicians' role in, 277-278
  databases for; see Databases
  expenditures for, as percentage of gross domestic product, 94t
  fiscal competition in, 300-303
  for-profit, practice of surgery and, 183-199
  impact of medical audit on, 222-224
  impact of surgical second opinion programs on, 208-212
  increased costs of, 155
  inflation and, 143
  institutionalization of, 184-185
  managed; see also Health maintenance organizations (HMOs)
    growth of, 166-169
    impact of, on surgeons, 165-181
  Medicare and Health Professions Educational Assistance legislation and, 51
  new professions in, 304-305
  per capita cost of, 155

Health care—cont'd
  practice style and; *see* Practice style
  price-based competition among providers of, 186-187
  profit-making aspects of, 300
  Prospective Payment Assessment Commission's role in maintaining access to, 111-112
  public subsidies to, 185-186
  quality of; *see* Quality; Quality assurance
  recommendations about, 401-404
  regionalization of, patient access and, 162-163
  standardization of, as threat to health care quality, 303-304
  surgical; *see also* Surgery; Surgical procedures
    decline in quality of, and DRG system, 120
    economic impact of regionalization of, 161-162
    effects of DRGs on, 119-121
    regionalized, 155-163
Health care delivery systems
  changes in, in 1980s, 55-62
  physician performance and, 99-101
  ProPAC's role in encouraging productivity and cost-effectiveness in, 112
  surgical, expenditures of, 116t, 116-117
Health Care Financing Association (HCFA), 114
  ambulatory procedure coverage and, 44
  ambulatory procedure coverage defined by, 39
  Common Procedure Coding System of, 45
  study of, on surgical second opinion programs, 205
Health care policy, role of diagnosis related groups in determining fiscal aspects of, 115
Health care providers
  for-profit
    clinical decision making by, 190-195
    health care quality and, 301
    influence of, on physician practices, 192-195

Health care providers—cont'd
  nonprofit and for-profit
    access to care and, 188-190
    administrative constraints of, 194-195
    changing roles of, 187-188
    comparative studies of, 188-190
    health care costs and, 188
    history of, 183-188
    rate of surgery and, 221
    physicians' influence on, 191-192
    and screening for patient ability to pay, 189-190
Health Education Assistant Loan (HEAL) program, 365
Health insurance; *see also* Medicare
  ambulatory surgery and, 46-47
  health care quality and, 301-302
Health maintenance organizations (HMOs)
  advertising and selling of, health care quality and, 302
  capitation method of physician payment in, 173
  characteristics of, 166-167
  compensation under, 172-174
  cost containment in, 173
  cost control techniques used by, 170
  distribution of, 168
  enrollment in, 176
    by model type, 169t
  establishment and growth of, 165-166
  fee-for-service reimbursement in, 173-174
  for-profit vs. nonprofit, numbers of, 168
  growth of, 167, 167t
  hospital use in, vs. hospital use by Medicaid patients, 100
  level of compensation in, 175-177
  model types of, 167, 168t, 173
  national firm management of, 169, 170t
  physician financial incentives in, 174-175, 192-193
  physician satisfaction in, 177-178
  rate of discretionary surgery in, 171
  rate of surgery and, 221, 344
  salary method of physician payment in, 173
  services offered by, 166

Health maintenance organizations (HMOs)—cont'd
  utilization management in, 169-172
Health plans, fee-for-service vs. prepaid, and surgical procedure rate, 99-100
Health Policy Agenda for the American People, 382
Health Professional Educational Assistance Act of 1976 (PL 94-484), 8-9
Health Professions Educational Assistance Act of 1963 (PL 88-129), 7, 51
HealthAmerica Corporation, 169
HealthCare USA, 169
Heart transplants, surgical regionalization and, 159, 162
Hemorrhage, gastrointestinal, as indication for hospital admission, small area variation in, 83
Hemorrhoids, excision of, numbers performed, 16t
Hernia
  inguinal; *see* Inguinal hernia
  umbilical, repair of, numbers performed, 17t
Hernia equivalents, 53-54
Herniorrhaphy, inguinal; *see* Inguinal herniorrhaphy
Heuristics, 316-318
  anchor-and-adjust, 317
  availability, 316
  representative, 316
Hip arthroplasty, number performed, 20t
Hip replacement surgery, number performed, 20t
Horn Severity of Illness Index in refinement of DRGs, 118-119
Hospital admissions, unnecessary, 34
Hospital Corporation of America, 169
Hospital tissue committees, 338-339
Hospital utilization; *see* Utilization
Hospitals
  accreditation of, unnecessary surgery and, 335
  causes for admission to, small area variations in, 83-84
  decision making in, about surgical procedures, 97
  for-profit, health care quality and, 301

Hospitals—cont'd
  impact of diagnosis related groups on, 117-118
  length of stay in; see Length of stay
  proprietary, 184, 185; see also Health care providers, for-profit
  utilization measures of, 280
Hypoglycemic agents, oral, controversy over effects of, 236
Hysterectomy
  Boston-New Haven comparisons of, 84
  complications of, 82
  hospital tissue committee studies of, 339
  hospital utilization studies of, 340
  as indication for hospital admission, small variation in, 83
  numbers performed, 18*t*
  peer review studies of, 340
  prophylactic, life expectancy and, 82
  small area variation for, 82
  systematic component of variation for, 78, 82
  unnecessary, 220-221

I

Illness, severity of; see Severity of illness
Independent practice association (IPA), 98
  defined, 167
  growth of, 167, 168*t*
Infections, incidence of, in hospital vs. outpatient facilities, 39-40
Inguinal hernia, repair of, systematic component of variation for, 78
Inguinal herniorrhaphy
  incidence of, 5
  numbers performed, 16*t*
  per capita rate of, 95, 96
  small area variation in use of, 80-81
Injured Infants Act, 382
Institute of Medicine (IOM), recommendations of, for technology assessment, 157
Intelligence, artificial, 315-316
Intensive care units (ICUs), 280
International Classification of Disease, 122, 133, 260
  Computerized Severity Index and, 136

International Classification of Disease—cont'd
  diagnosis and procedure coding of, 3-4
  limitations of, 261
Intestine, excision of, numbers performed, 16*t*

J

JCAHCO; see Joint Commission for Accreditation of Health Care Organizations (JCAHCO)
Joint Commission for Accreditation of Health Care Organizations (JCAHCO), ambulatory surgery facility accreditation and, 41-42
Joint Commission on Accreditation of Hospitals (JCAH), 354
  role of, in hospital care standards, 217-218

K

Kaiser Foundation Health Plan, 168
Knee arthroplasty, number performed, 20*t*
Knee injuries, practice style and treatment of, 77, 77

L

Laboratory tests, overuse of, 277-278
Laparoscopy, diagnostic, numbers performed, 18*t*
Laparotomy, exploratory
  hospital tissue committee studies of, 339
  numbers performed, 17*t*
Large bowel procedures, severity of illness level and, 140*t*
Legislation, federal; see Federal legislation
Length of stay
  for ambiplex patients, 287-288
  cost containment and, 278
  decreased, 219
  defined, 280
Liaison Committee for Medical Education (LCME), 353
Lorenz curve, 278-279, 279
Lumpectomy, costs of, compared with those for mastectomy, 121-122
Lung
  lesions of, excision or destruction of, number performed, 26*t*

Lung—cont'd
  lobectomy of, number performed, 26*t*

M

Maine Medical Assessment Program, 84, 85
Malpractice litigation, 369-384
  authoritative literature in, 395
  cost considerations in, 381-382
  deposition testimony in, 394-395
  efforts for solutions to, 373-378
  examination of witness in, 395-397
  expert medical witness and, 387-388
  expert witness in, 393-394
  fault-based administrative alternative to civil justice system and, 374-378
  health care quality and, 378
  historical perspective on, 369-372
  incidence of claims of, 373
  legal concepts underlying, 369-370
  legislation affecting, 371-372, 382
  maloccurrence insurance model for, 380-381
  nature and role of damages in, 392-393
  1970s crisis over, 371
  physician as expert and witness in, 397-398
  and proof of causation of plaintiff's damages, 392
  proposed solutions to, 379-382
  psychologic effects of, on physicians, 377-378
  and testimony on standards of medical practice, 390-392
  theory and process in, 388-390
  workman's compensation model for, 379-380
Mastectomy
  costs of, compared with those for mastectomy, 121-122
  numbers performed, 16*t*
Maxicare Health Plans, Inc., 169
McPherson-Clifford statistic, 77
Medi-Cal, health care contracting and, 156
Medicaid
  establishment of, 185
  health care regulation and, 186

Medicaid—cont'd
  hospital use by patient with, vs. hospital use in health maintenance organizations, 100
  surgical second opinion programs and, 208
    costs savings from, 210
Medical audit, 220-224
  impact of, on patient care, 222-224
  purpose of, 220
Medical Care International, 32
Medical Illness Severity Grouping System (MedisGroups), 223
Medical information system, ambiplex patient and, 294
Medical Malpractice, 337
Medical opinion; *see also* Practice style
  significance of, in diagnosis and treatment, 68
Medical Policy Committee of Blue Shield of California, technology assessment role of, 158
Medical practice
  characteristics of, American Medical Association study of, 59-62
  testimony on standards of, 390-392
Medical technology
  assessment of; *see* Technology assessment
  health care coverage determination for, 159
  selective coverage of, 159-160
Medical testimony, expert, 388
Medical treatment, practice style and; *see* Practice style
Medicare
  abuses of, 144
  ambulatory surgery coverage by, 39, 43, 44-45
  average length of hospital stay for patients on, *111*
  cataract extraction reimbursement by, 310
  cost of, to beneficiary, 144
  databases of, 260
  disadvantages of patients on, with DRG system, 120
  establishment of, 185
  health care regulation and, 186
  impact of surgical volume-outcome relationship on, 161-162

Medicare—cont'd
  implications of, for surgical practice, 307-311
  method of payment modifications of, 109
  number of hospital admissions, 1967-1985, *112*
  part A, alterations in, 143
  part B
    increased expenditures for, 143-144
    increased use of, 156
  physician participation in, 147-148
  physician reimbursement by, 143
    Consolidated Omnibus Budget Reconciliation Act and, 147
Medicare economic index (MEI), 148
Medicine; *see* Health care
MEDISGROUPS, severity of illness quantification and, 135
Methodist Medical Center, 33
Mitral valve, replacement of, number performed, 26*t*
Mortality rates, relationship of, to volume of surgical procedures, 161
Mortality statistics, publication of, health care quality implications of, 302-303
Mt. Sinai Medical Center, 33
Mountin-Pennel-Berger forecast, 7
Mouth, excision and plastic repair of, number performed, 24*t*
Myocardial infarction as indication for hospital admission, small area variation in, 83
Myringotomy, number performed, 24*t*

N

Nasal septum, resection of, number performed, 24*t*
National Board of Medical Examiners, 355
National Center for Health Services Research and Health Care Technology, 157
National Center for Health Statistics (NCHS), operative rate data of, 3-6
National Direct Student Loan program, 365
National Institutes of Health (NIH), 157

Nephrectomy, number performed, 22*t*
Nephrotomy, number performed, 22*t*
Neurosurgery
  DRGs for, description and relative weights of, 128
  10 most frequent operations in, 28*t*
New England Surgical Society, 355
Nonrandomized comparisons (NRCs), 229-230
  cross-sectional survey of, 239, 240*t*
NRCs; *see* Nonrandomized comparisons (NRCs)
Nursing homes, nonprofit and for-profit, comparative costs of, 188

O

Office of Health Technology Assessment (OHTA), 157
Office of Technology Assessment (OTA), 156
Omnibus Budget Reconciliation Act, free-standing ambulatory surgical centers and, 43-44
Oophorectomy
  repair of, numbers performed, 18*t*
  unnecessary, 220
Ophthalmologic surgery, DRGs for, description and relative weights of, 128
Orchiectomy
  number performed, 22*t*
  versus hormonal therapy
    nonrandomized comparisons of, 245*t*
    randomized control trials of, 243, 244*t*, 245
Orthopedic surgeon, charges of, compared with podiatrist's, 57
Orthopedic surgery, DRGs for, description and relative weights of, 128-129
Ostectomy, partial, number performed, 21*t*
Otolaryngology, surgical, DRGs for, description and relative weights of, 129
Outpatient surgery, impact of, on surgical specialities, 4-6

P

Pacemakers, surgical procedures involving, number performed, 26*t*

Pareto's law, high-cost patients and, 278, 279, *279*, 285
Parietal Loans for Undergraduate Students program, 365
Patient care units (PCUs), 280
Patient management categories (PMC)
  in assessment of disease progression, 118-119
  severity of illness and, 134
Patients
  age of, and surgical risk, 38
  high-cost, 277-297; *see also* Ambiplex patient
    admissions and encounters for, *281*
    background on, 278-280
    criteria for selecting seven groups of, 284
    defined, 280
    Pareto's law and, 278-280, 285
    utilization of general hospital resources by, 282*t*
  preparation of, for ambulatory surgery, 38
  surgical risk for, by age, 38
Peak Health Care, Inc., 169
Peer review
  of ambulatory surgical procedures, 44
  unnecessary surgery and, 340
Pennsylvania Health Care Cost Containment Council, 270
Peripheral vascular surgery, DRGs for, description and relative weights of, 130
Physical Status Classification of American Society of Anesthesiologists, 271
Physician assistants, surgical, 56-57
Physician Characteristics and Distribution in the United States (PCD), data of, on physicians performing surgery, 4
Physician Payment Review Commission (PPRC), 144-150
  future concerns of, 149-150
  goals of, 145
  initial suggestions of, 145-149
  roles of, 145
  short-term recommendations of, 150
Physician reimbursement

Physician reimbursement—cont'd
  CPR approach to; *see* CPR approach to physician reimbursement
  form of
    and rate of surgery, 221, 343-344
    geographic considerations in, 146-147
    health care organization's influence on, 192-194
    in health maintenance organizations, 172-174
    under HMOs, 172-174, 176-177
    impact of federal legislation on, 309-311
  Medicare economic index and, 148-149
  Physician Payment Review Commission suggestions for, 145-150
  physician's time as component of, 146
  rate of, inherent reasonableness rule and, 147
  relative value scale and, 145
Physicians
  biases of, 318
  board-certified, 224
    increasing numbers of, 56
  characteristics and distribution of, American Medical Association study of, 58-59
  costs of practice of, 366
  credentials of, 224-225
  delineation of privileges of, 224-225
  determining cost of time of, 146
  female, age distribution of, 59
  financial incentives for
    in health care facilities, 192-193
    in HMOs, 174-175
  incompetence or malfeasance of, 224-225
  influence of, on health care organizations, 191-192
  male, age distribution of, 59
  per 100,000 population, 59*t*
  performance of
    influence of family and individual attitudes on, 98
    influence of health care delivery systems on, 99-101
    influence of patient educational level on, 98-99

Physicians—cont'd
  performance of—cont'd
    influence of patient socioeconomic status on, 98
    medical audits and, 223
    socioeconomic influences on, 98-101
  ratio of, to population, 8
  reimbursement of; *see* Physician reimbursement
  role of, in health care costs, 277-278
  sanctions against, as a result of PRO reviews, 220
  satisfaction of, with HMOs, 177-178
  studies of need and supply of, 7
  surplus of, 156
  trends threatening professional status of, 299-300
  unions for, 178
  in U.S., by gender, nationality, and year, 59*t*
Physicians Who Care, 178
PL 88-129; *see* Health Professions Educational Assistance Act of 1963
PL 94-484; *see* Health Professional Educational Assistance Act of 1976
Plain Concise Practical Remarks on the Treatment of Wounds and Fractures, 333
Plastic surgery
  DRGs for, description and relative weights of, 130
  on nose, number performed, 24*t*
Pleura, scarification of, number performed, 26*t*
PMC; *see* Patient management categories (PMC)
Podiatrists, charges of, compared with orthopedic surgeon's, 57
Portacaval shunt,
  costs of, compared with those of sclerotherapy, 122
  randomized control trials of, 232-233
PPOs; *see* Preferred provider organizations (PPOs)
PPS; *see* Prospective Payment System (PPS)

Subject Index 421

Practice style
    changes in, and changes in tonsillectomy rates, 70-72, *71*
    databases in analysis of, 266-267
    hospital utilization and, 76-78
    and rates of hospitalization for orthopedic conditions, 76-78
    and relative importance of physical examination and patient history, 73-74
    and role of evaluative clinical sciences, 84-90
    small area analysis of, 67-92
    tonsillectomy and, 68-75
Preferred provider organizations (PPOs), 98, 166
    cost containment and, 222
    fee-for-service payment in, 173-174
President's Commission on Health Needs of the Nation, 7
Primary care, increased delivery of, by specialists, 56
Primary care physician gatekeepers, 170
Probability, assignment of, 322
Process audits, 222
Professional review organizations (PROs), 219-220
Professional services review organizations (PSROs) in utilization review process, 219-220
Professional uncertainty hypothesis, 101-102
    as null hypothesis, 87-90
    and pattern variation of common operations, 80-83
Prospective Payment Assessment Commission (ProPAC)
    establishment of, 110
    role, responsibilities, and processes of, 111-115
Prospective Payment System (PPS)
    implications of, for characterizing financially at-risk populations, 118
    incentive for cost reductions under, 109-110
    legislation mandating, 109
    updating of, ProPAC recommendations about, 113, 114
Prostate, hypertrophy of, prophylactic prostatectomy and, 82-83

Prostatectomy
    number performed, 22*t*
    prophylactic use of, 82-83
        clinical sciences evaluation of, 85
    recurrent, cumulative probability for, by type of procedure, *90*
    systematic component of variation for, 78, 82
Prostheses, synthetic vascular, vs. saphenous vein grafts, randomized control trial of, 238-239
Protocols
    as decision-making tool, 328
    value of, 330
Pseudodoxia Epidemica, 203
PSRO; *see* Professional services review organizaitons (PSROs)

Q
Quality
    commercial constraints on, 299-305
    diagnosis related groups and, 308
    health care standardization and, 303-304
Quality assurance
    departmental leadership and, 225
    historical perspective on, 217-218
Quality control of ambulatory surgery, 41-42

R
Randomized control trials (RCTs)
    background on, 230-231
    biased selection of patients in, 232-233
    controversies over, 232-238
    cross-sectional survey of, 238-243, 240*t*-241*t*
    defined, 229
    learning curve problem in, 234
    negative, 235-236
    and patient reassignment after randomizing, 233-234
    recent controversies over, 236-238
    results of, compared with those of nonrandomized comparisons, 252
    surgeon experience as factor in, 234-235
RCTs; *see* Randomized control trials (RCTs)
Reasoning, errors in, 316-317

Relative value scale (RVS), physician reimbursement and, 145
Research, large databases and, 259-275
Residency Review Committee for Surgery, functions of, 358
Residency review committees (RRC), 354
Residents
    cardiothoracic, number of, by year, 27*t*
    neurologic, number of, 29*t*
    number of, by year, 17*t*
    obstetric-gynecologic, number performed, 19*t*
    orthopedic, number of, 21*t*
    otolaryngologic, number of, 25*t*
    surgical, salaries of, 365-366
    urologic, number of, 23*t*

S
Salpingo-oophorectomy, numbers performed, 18*t*
Sample size, small, variability of, 317
SAS macroprocessor and language, 272
Sclerotherapy, costs of, compared with those of portacaval shunt, 122
SCV; *see* Systematic component of variation (SCV)
Seattle Model Cities Health Care Program, appropriateness of surgical procedures performed in, 101
Severity of illness
    adjustment of DRGs for, 134-140
    computation of, with Computerized Severity Index, 136
    quantifying, 134-135
Severity of Illness Index, dimensions of, 135
Share Development Corporation, 169
Short procedure units (SPUs), 46
Sinusotomy, nasal, number performed, 24*t*
Skin graft, numbers performed, 16*t*
Small area analysis (SAA)
    database requirements for, 263-264
    of surgical practice, 67-92
    tonsillectomy and, 68-75
Small area variation, 343
    factors in, 96-97

Subject Index

Small area variation—cont'd
  inappropriate use and, 96-97
  patient demand as cause of, 72-73
  professional uncertainty and, 80-84
  role of clinical sciences in evaluation of, 84-90
SMI; *see* Supplemental medical insurance (SMI)
Social class, patient, as factor in randomized controlled trials, 233
Social Security Amendments of 1983 (PL 98-21), 307-308
  provisions of, 109
Socioeconomics
  as academic discipline, 12
  as factor in use of health care facilities, 76
  unnecessary surgery and, 346
Software, database, 269-270
SOSSUS; *see* Study on Surgical Services for the United States (SOSSUS)
Southern Surgical Association, 355
Specialty boards
  development of, 354
  surgical; *see* Surgical specialty boards
Spinal canal, exploration and decompression of, number of, by year, 28*t*
Spinal fusion, number performed, 21*t*
Storeworkers Health and Welfare Fund, 201
Stroke as indication for hospital admission, small area variation in, 83
Study on Surgical Services for the United States (SOSSUS), 51-55
  data collection in, 52
  data findings in, 52-53
    on surgeon surplus, 7-8, 9
  responses to, 53
  studies corroborating, 53-54
Supplemental medical insurance (SMI), 145
Surgeons
  age distribution of, by specialty, 61*t*
  board certification status of, by specialty, 61*t*
  cardiothoracic, number of, by year, 27*t*
  certification process of, 361-363

Surgeons—cont'd
  costs of practice of, 366
  effect of for-profit ownership on, 195-197
  geographic distribution of, 53
  GMENAC findings about numbers and distribution of, 9
  impact of diagnosis related groups on, 117-118
  impact of managed health care systems on, 165-181
  malpractice crisis and, 369-384
  neurologic, number of, 29*t*
  number of operations performed by, yearly, 53
  numbers of
    by surgical speciality (1965 to 1986), 60*t*
    by year, 17*t*
  obstetric-gynecologic, number performed, 19*t*
  orthopedic, number of, 21*t*
  otolaryngologic, number of, 25*t*
  payment preferences of, 56
  per capita rate of, by country, 95
  ratio of, to population, 347
  reimbursement of; *see also* Physician reimbursement
    under HMOs, 172-174
  response of, to surgical second opinion programs, 202
  SOSSUS findings on numbers of, 7-8
  SOSSUS findings on workload of, 52-54
  statistics on, 4
  surplus of, 156
    effects of, 10-12
    solutions to, 12-13
  urologic, number of, 23*t*
  workload of, 7-8, 61
    American College of Surgeons study of, 58
    American Medical Association study of, 58
  workweek of, 52
Surgery
  ambulatory; *see* Ambulatory surgery
  cardiothoracic, 10 most frequent operations in, 26*t*
  complications of, economic implications of, 116

Surgery—cont'd
  comprehensive studies of, 58-62
  Computerized Severity Index and, 139-140
  decisions about, reliability and reproducibility of, 202-204
  education in; *see* Education, surgical
  for-profit health care facilities and, 183-199
  future of, DRGs and, 122
  general
    defined, 362
    DRGs for, description and relative weights of, 125-126
    20 most frequent operations performed, 16*t*
  implications of federal legislation for, 307-311
  investigations of practice of, 51-55
  levels of, defined, 36
  obstetric-gynecologic, 15 most frequent operations, 18*t*
  orolaryngologic, 10 most frequence operations in, 24*t*
  orthopedic, 15 most frequent operations in, 20*t*
  otolaryngologic, outpatient, 57
  outpatient; *see* Ambulatory surgery
  payment arrangements for, 56
  pediatric, outpatient, 39
  physician-induced demand for, 93
  prophylactic, decision making about, 323, *324*
  qualifications of practitioners performing, 54
  rates of
    assessing, 343-345
    payment schemes and, 343-344
    population at risk factor in, 343
  research on; *see* Research
  risks of, by patient age, 38
  second opinions on; *see* Surgical second opinion programs
  small area analysis (SAA) of, 67-92
  socioeconomic changes relative to, 3
  unnecessary, 53, 328-329, 333-351
    consumer movement and, 335-336
    controversy over, 220-222
    cost/benefit analysis and, 345-346
    defined, 336-338
    geographic variation in, 342-343

Surgery—cont'd
unnecessary—cont'd
historical perspective on, 333-336
hospital accreditation and, 335
hospital studies of, 334-335
hospital tissue committees in monitoring of, 338-339
hospital utilization studies of, 339-340
peer review studies of, 340
public policy and, 336
recommendations about, 346-348
retrospective chart reviews of, 340-342
socioeconomic factors in, 346
and surgical second opinion programs, 344-345
urban/rural comparisons of, 54
urologic, 10 most frequent procedures in, 22t
utilization of; *see* Utilization
Surgery centers
ambulatory
accreditation of, 41
Medicare coverage and, 308
Omnibus Budget Reconciliation Act and, 43-44
free-standing, 5, 172
accreditation of, 41
corporate-owned, 32
growth projections for, 32, 32t
by type of ownership, 33t
Surgical and Allied Malpractice, 337
Surgical Care Affiliates, 32
Surgical judgment, defined, 315
Surgical physician assistants, 56-57
Surgical procedures
cardiothoracic, number of, by year, 27t
costs of different types of, for same disease, compared, 121-122
decision making about, 94-103
at individual surgeon level, 98
at professional organizational level, 97
at society-community level, 97
elective
in HMOs, 171
increased rates of, 201
evaluation of, 229-256
excess number of, 3

Surgical procedures—cont'd
experimental status of, 234
historically controlled comparisons of, 231
investigational, reimbursement for, 159-160
manpower studies of, 6-10
monitoring, 338-346
neurologic, number of, 29t
numbers of, 10
by year, 17t
obstetric-gynecologic, number performed, 19t
operative rate data on, 3-6
orthopedic, number of, 21t
otolaryngologic, number of, 25t
outpatient vs. inpatient, 4-5
per surgeon, yearly, 7
ProPAC's role in facilitating innovation in, 112
randomized control trials of, 230-231
controversies over, 232-238
rates of
care implications of, 95-97
determining, 93-105
differences of, among countries, 93-94
in fee-for-service vs. prepaid health care plans, 99
reliability of data on, 6
second opinions about; *see* Surgical second opinion programs
small area variation in, factors in, 96-97
in third world nations, 97
urologic, number of, 23t
volume of
and mortality rate, 347
relationship of, to outcome, 161-162
and surgical outcome, 262
Surgical second opinion programs, 172, 201-214
effects of, on health care costs, 212
history of, 201-204
impact of, on patient care, 208-212
mandatory, 205-207
prevalence of, 207-208
requirements of, 172
surgeon error and, 319
surgeons' response to, 202

Surgical second opinion programs—cont'd
types of, 204-207
unnecessary surgery rate and, 344-345
value of, 320-321
voluntary, 204-205
participation in, 211
Surgical signature phenomenon, 84
constancy of, over time, *88*
small area variation in, for specific procedures, *87*
Surgical specialties
studies of, 57
surgical procedures performed by, 4-5
training in, 309
Surgical specialty boards, annual certificates issued by, 62t
Sympathectomy, number of, by year, 28t
Systematic component of variation (SCV), 77

T

Technology assessment, 156-159
criteria for, 157-158
process of, 157-159
Technology Evaluation and Coverage Department of Blue Cross/Blue Shield, 157
Tonsillectomy
American Child Health Association study of patient demand for, 72-73
changes in rates of, and changes in practice style, 70-72, *71*
hospital tissue committee studies of, 339
intraobserver disagreement about need for, 203
medical care outcomes and, 69
number performed, 24t
outpatient, complications of, 40
per capita rate of, 96
practice style and, 68-75
rate of, 95
in fee-for-service vs. prepaid health plans, 99, 100
retrospective chart reviews of, 341
systematic component of variation for, 78-79
versus nonsurgical treatment

Tonsillectomy—cont'd
  versus nonsurgical treatment—cont'd
    nonrandomized comparisons of, 247t
    randomized control trials of, 245-247, 246t
Tort reform
  failures of, 371-372
  General Accounting Office proposals for, 374
  professional liability problem and, 374
Transplants, organ, regionalization of, 163
Trauma, economic costs of, 116-117
Treatment
  medical; see Medical treatment
  sources of variation in results of, 329
Turbinectomy, number performed, 24t

U

UHDDS discharge data, 119
Ulcerative colitis, intraobserver disagreement about, 203
Umbilical hernia, repair of, numbers performed, 17t
Union of American Physicians and Dentists, 178
Unions, physician, 178
United Mine Workers, 201
United States, rates of surgical operations in, 93
Ureterotomy, number performed, 22t
Urethral strictures, release of, number performed, 22t
Urologic surgery, DRGs for, description and relative weights of, 131
U.S. Public Health Service, technology assessment branches of, 156-157
Uterus, dilation and curettage of, numbers performed, 18t
Utilities, 322, 323
Utilization
  factors involved in, 76
  for orthopedic injuries, practice style and, 76-78
  practice style and, 76-78
Utilization—cont'd
  studies of, unnecessary surgery and, 339-340
Utilization management in HMOs, 169-172
Utilization review
  cost effectiveness of, 219
  historical perspective on, 217-218
  value of, 218-220

V

Vaginal vault, obliteration of, repair of, 19t
Validity, illusion of, 317
Vascular procedures, major reconstructive, severity of illness level and, 140t
Vermont Medical Society, 72
Virginia Medical Malpractice Cap, 382

W

Wangensteen, Owen, 51
Weight index of diagnosis related groups, 110
Western Surgical Association, 355
Witnesses, expert, 387-388, 393-394

NO LONGER THE PROPERTY
OF THE
UNIVERSITY OF R.I. LIBRARY